Handbook of Item Response Theory Modeling

Item response theory (IRT) has moved beyond the confines of educational measurement into assessment domains such as personality, psychopathology, and patient-reported outcomes. Classic and emerging IRT methods and applications that are revolutionizing psychological measurement, particularly for health assessments used to demonstrate treatment effectiveness, are reviewed in this new volume. World renowned contributors present the latest research and methodologies about these models along with their applications and related challenges. Examples using real data, some from NIH-PROMIS®, show how to apply these models in actual research situations. Chapters review fundamental issues of IRT, modern estimation methods, testing assumptions, evaluating fit, item banking, scoring in multidimensional models, and advanced IRT methods. New multidimensional models are provided along with suggestions for deciding among the family of IRT models available. Each chapter provides an introduction, describes state-of-the-art research methods, demonstrates an application, and provides a summary. This book addresses the most critical IRT conceptual and statistical issues confronting researchers and advanced students in psychology, education, and medicine today. Although the chapters highlight health outcomes data, the issues addressed are relevant to any content domain.

This book addresses:

- IRT models applied to noneducational data, especially patient-reported outcomes;
- Differences between cognitive and noncognitive constructs and the challenges these bring to modeling;
- The application of multidimensional IRT models designed to capture typical performance data;
- Cutting-edge methods for deriving a single latent dimension from multidimensional data;
- A new model designed for the measurement of constructs that are defined on one end of a continuum such as substance abuse;
- Scoring individuals under different multidimensional IRT models and item banking for patient-reported health outcomes; and
- How to evaluate measurement invariance, diagnose problems with response categories, and assess growth and change.

Intended for researchers, advanced students, and practitioners in psychology, education, and medicine interested in applying IRT methods, this book also serves as a text in advanced graduate courses on IRT or measurement. Familiarity with factor analysis, latent variables, IRT, and basic measurement theory is assumed.

Steven P. Reise is a full professor in quantitative psychology at UCLA.

Dennis A. Revicki is Senior Vice President of health outcomes research at Evidera and an adjunct professor at the University of North Carolina, University of Florida, and Georgetown University.

Multivariate Applications Series

Sponsored by the Society of Multivariate Experimental Psychology, the goal of this series is to apply statistical methods to significant social or behavioral issues, in such a way so as to be accessible to a nontechnical-oriented readership (e.g., non-methodological researchers, teachers, students, government personnel, practitioners, and other professionals). Applications from a variety of disciplines such as psychology, public health, sociology, education, and business are welcome. Books can be single- or multiple-authored or edited volumes that (1) demonstrate the application of a variety of multivariate methods to a single, major area of research; (2) describe a multivariate procedure or framework that could be applied to a number of research areas; or (3) present a variety of perspectives on a topic of interest to applied multivariate researchers.

Anyone wishing to submit a book proposal should send the following: (1) author/title; (2) timeline including completion date; (3) brief overview of the book's focus, including table of contents and, ideally, a sample chapter (or chapters); (4) a brief description of competing publications; and (5) targeted audiences.

For more information, please contact the series editor, Lisa Harlow, at Department of Psychology, University of Rhode Island, 10 Chafee Road, Suite 8, Kingston, RI 02881-0808; phone (401) 874-4242; fax (401) 874-5562; or e-mail LHarlow@uri.edu.

What If There Were No Significance Tests? coedited by Lisa L. Harlow, Stanley A. Mulaik, and James H. Steiger (1997)

Structural Equation Modeling with LISREL, PRELIS, and SIMPLIS: Basic Concepts, Applications, and Programming, written by Barbara M. Byrne (1998)

Multivariate Applications in Substance Use Research: New Methods for New Questions, coedited by Jennifer S. Rose, Laurie Chassin, Clark C. Presson, and Steven J. Sherman (2000)

Item Response Theory for Psychologists, coauthored by Susan E. Embretson and Steven P. Reise (2000)

Structural Equation Modeling with AMOS: Basic Concepts, Applications, and Programming, written by Barbara M. Byrne (2001)

Conducting Meta-Analysis Using SAS, written by Winfred Arthur, Jr., Winston Bennett, Jr., and Allen I. Huffcutt (2001)

Modeling Intraindividual Variability with Repeated Measures Data: Methods and Applications, coedited by D.S. Moskowitz and Scott L. Hershberger (2002)

Multilevel Modeling: Methodological Advances, Issues, and Applications, coedited by Steven P. Reise and Naihua Duan (2003)

The Essence of Multivariate Thinking: Basic Themes and Methods, written by Lisa Harlow (2005)

Contemporary Psychometrics: A Festschrift for Roderick P. McDonald, coedited by Albert Maydeu-Olivares and John J. McArdle (2005)
Structural Equation Modeling with EQS: Basic Concepts, Applications, and Programming, Second Edition, written by Barbara M. Byrne (2006)
A Paul Meehl Reader: Essays on the Practice of Scientific Psychology, coedited by Niels G. Waller, Leslie J. Yonce, William M. Grove, David Faust, and Mark F. Lenzenweger (2006)
Introduction to Statistical Mediation Analysis, written by David P. MacKinnon (2008)
Applied Data Analytic Techniques for Turning Points Research, edited by Patricia Cohen (2008)
Cognitive Assessment: An Introduction to the Rule Space Method, written by Kikumi K. Tatsuoka (2009)
Structural Equation Modeling with AMOS: Basic Concepts, Applications, and Programming, Second Edition written by Barbara M. Byrne (2010)
Handbook of Ethics in Quantitative Methodology, coedited by Abigail T. Panter and Sonya K. Sterba (2011)
Longitudinal Data Analysis: A Practical Guide for Researchers in Aging, Health, and Social Sciences, coedited by Jason T. Newsom, Richard N. Jones, and Scott M. Hofer (2011)
Structural Equation Modeling with MPlus: Basic Concepts, Applications, and Programming written by Barbara M. Byrne (2012)
Understanding the New Statistics: Effect Sizes, Confidence Intervals, and Meta-Analysis written by Geoff Cumming (2012)
Frontiers of Test Validity Theory: Measurement, Causation and Meaning written by Keith A. Markus and Denny Borsboom (2013)
Longitudinal Analysis: Modeling Within-Person Fluctuation and Change written by Lesa Hoffman (2015)
Handbook of Item Response Theory Modeling: Applications to Typical Performance Assessment coedited by Steven P. Reise and Dennis A. Revicki (2015)

Handbook of Item Response Theory Modeling

Applications to Typical Performance Assessment

Edited by
Steven P. Reise and Dennis A. Revicki

Routledge
Taylor & Francis Group
NEW YORK AND LONDON

First published 2015
by Routledge
711 Third Avenue, New York, NY 10017

and by Routledge
27 Church Road, Hove, East Sussex BN3 2FA

Routledge is an imprint of the Taylor & Francis Group, an informa business.

Library of Congress Cataloging-in-Publication Data
Handbook of item response theory modeling : applications to typical performance assessment / edited by Steven P. Reise and Dennis A. Revicki.
pages cm
Includes bibliographical references and index.
ISBN 978-1-84872-972-8 (hardback : alk. paper) — ISBN 978-1-138-78785-8 (pbk. : alk. paper) — ISBN 978-1-315-73601-3 (ebook : alk. paper) 1. Item response theory. I. Reise, Steven Paul. II. Revicki, Dennis A.
BF39.2.I84H36 2015
150.28'7—dc23
2014026950

ISBN: 978-1-84872-972-8 (hbk)
ISBN: 978-1-138-78785-8 (pbk)
ISBN: 978-1-315-73601-3 (ebk)

Typeset in Sabon
by Apex CoVantage, LLC

MIX
Paper from responsible sources
FSC® C014174

Printed and bound in the United States of America by Sheridan Books, Inc. (a Sheridan Group Company).

This book is dedicated to Roger Millsap, Ph.D., who sadly passed away in May 2014, about a month prior to this volume being in production. Roger was the world's leading expert on the topic of invariance and differential item functioning for both factor analytic and item response theory models. His research and service accomplishments are laudatory, but more importantly, Roger was highly respected in his field, for he was well known as a great person and friend, a true research collaborator, and a tremendous scholar—a rare combination, indeed. We will miss him.

Contents

About the Editors

Steven P. Reise received his Ph.D. from the Department of Psychology at the University of Minnesota in 1990. He is presently a full professor in quantitative psychology at UCLA. Dr. Reise has coauthored a popular textbook on item response theory (Embretson & Reise, 2000) and he is a fellow in the American Psychological Association Division 5 and the Society for Personality Assessment. In 1998 Dr. Reise was awarded the Raymond B. Cattell Award for outstanding early career contributions to multivariate experimental psychology, awarded by the Society of Multivariate Experimental Psychology. His research focuses on the application of item response theory (IRT) and structural equation models (SEM) to personality, psychopathology, and health outcomes measures.

Dennis A. Revicki received his Ph.D. from the University of North Carolina in 1981. He is currently a senior vice president of health outcomes research at Evidera. Dr. Revicki holds adjunct professor appointments at the University of North Carolina, University of Florida, and Georgetown University. His research primarily focuses on the development and psychometric evaluation of patient-reported outcome measures, and the application and statistical analysis of patient-reported outcome measures in clinical trials and other studies. His current methodological interests are in the application of item response theory and structural equation models in understanding the performance of patient-reported outcome measures, and in the application of latent growth curve models in evaluating the outcomes from clinical trials.

About the Editors

Contributors

Andrew J. Bodine, Ph.D., Department of Psychology, The Ohio State University

Wes E. Bonifay, C.Phil., Department of Psychology, University of California, Los Angeles

Anna Brown, Ph.D., Lecturer in Psychological Methods and Statistics, School of Psychology, University of Kent

Li Cai, Ph.D., Codirector, CRESST, Associate Professor, Education, University of California, Los Angeles

Shyh-Huei Chen, Ph.D., Medical Center Blvd., Public Health Sciences, Wake Forest School of Medicine

Wen-Hung Chen, Ph.D., Director, Psychometrics, RTI Health Solutions, Research Triangle Park, NC

Karon F. Cook, Ph.D., Department of Medical Social Sciences, Northwestern University Feinberg School of Medicine

Tim J. Croudace, Ph.D., Professor of Psychometric Epidemiology, Mental Health and Addiction Research Group (MHARG), HYMS and Department of Health Sciences, University of York

Paul De Boeck, Ph.D., Department of Psychology, The Ohio State University

Maria Orlando Edelen, Ph.D., Senior Behavioral/Social Scientist, RAND Corporation

Michael C. Edwards, Ph.D., Department of Psychology, The Ohio State University

Howard T. Everson, Professor, Educational Psychology, Director, Center for Advanced Study in Education, Graduate School and University Center, City University of New York

Pere J. Ferrando, Ph.D., Department of Psychology, Universitat Rovira i Virgili

Matthew Finkelman, Tufts University School of Dental Medicine

Heather Gunn, M.S., Department of Psychology, Arizona State University

Earl S. Hishinuma, Ph.D., Professor and Associate Chair of Research, Department of Psychiatry, University of Hawaii at Manoa

Carrie R. Houts, Ph.D., Vector Psychometric Group, LLC

Edward H. Ip, Ph.D., Medical Center Blvd., Public Health Sciences, Wake Forest School of Medicine

Joseph F. Lucke, Ph.D., Senior Statistician, Research Institute on Addictions, University at Buffalo, State University of New York

Alberto Maydeu-Olivares, Ph.D., Faculty of Psychology, University of Barcelona

John J. McArdle, Ph.D., University of Southern California, Department of Psychology

Rob R. Meijer, Ph.D., University of Groningen, Faculty of Behavioral and Social Sciences, Psychometrics and Statistics

Roger E. Millsap, Ph.D., Department of Psychology, Arizona State University

Tyler M. Moore, Ph.D., Neuropsychiatry Program, Department of Psychiatry, University of Pennsylvania

Michael Nering, Ph.D., Measured Progress, Dover, NH

Remo Ostini, Ph.D., School of Population Health, The University of Queensland

Kevin T. Petway, Ph.D., Educational Testing Service, Princeton, NJ

Kathleen S.J. Preston, Ph.D., Assistant Professor, Department of Psychology, California State University, Fullerton

Steven P. Reise, Ph.D., Department of Psychology, University of California, Los Angeles

Dennis A. Revicki, Ph.D., Senior Vice President, Health Outcomes Research, Evidera

Brian D. Stucky, Ph.D., Associate Behavioral/Social Scientist, RAND Corporation

Jorge N. Tendeiro, Ph.D., University of Groningen, Faculty of Behavioral and Social Sciences, Psychometrics and Statistics

David Thissen, Ph.D., L.L. Thurstone Psychometric Laboratory, University of North Carolina

Carole Tucker, Ph.D., Associate Professor, Department of Physical Therapy, Temple University

Rob B.K. Wanders, Ph.D., University of Groningen, Faculty of Medical Sciences, Academic Centre of Psychiatry

Jonathan P. Weeks, Ph.D., Associate Research Scientist, Educational Testing Service, Princeton, NJ

Mark Wilson, Ph.D., Graduate School of Education, University of California, Berkeley

R.J. Wirth, Ph.D., Vector Psychometric Group, LLC

Carol M. Woods, Ph.D., Associate Professor of Quantitative Psychology, Interim Director, Quantitative Psychology Program, Associate Director and Research Scientist, Center for Research Methods and Data Analysis, University of Kansas

Alex Zautra, Ph.D., Foundation Professor, Department of Psychology, Arizona State University

Preface

Over the past 30 years, item response theory (IRT) measurement models and related methods, such as differential item functioning, scale linking, and computerized adaptive testing, have been studied extensively and applied in achievement, aptitude, and ability measurement research. Only within the past decade or so, however, has IRT moved beyond the confines of educational assessment into the typical performance domains such as personality, psychopathology, and, the subject of the present text, health and patient-reported outcomes. In the domain of patient-reported outcomes measurement, for example, several large-scale NIH-funded projects—such as the Quality of Life in Neurological Disorder (NeuroQol; www.neuroqol.org/Pages/default.aspxToolbox) and Patient Reported Outcomes Measurement Information Systems (PROMIS®; www.nihpromis.org)—make extensive use of IRT methodology.

This application of IRT methods from education to noneducational assessment raises two important and related questions. First, to what extent are standard IRT methods easily exportable outside the domains of achievement, aptitude, and ability measurement? Second, what unique challenges to measurement does typical performance data, in particular item response data collected by patient-report outcomes researchers, present for IRT modeling? To begin to answer these questions, we compiled this edited volume on cutting-edge IRT models and methods as applied to noneducational data, in particular, patient-reported health outcomes data. The overarching goals of this book are to provide: (a) an outlet for leading scholars to share their latest research on IRT models and related methodologies, and (b) a reference for researchers who are considering using IRT models in their own work and, thus, need to be aware of appropriate applications, challenges, and unresolved issues.

We contacted leading psychometric researchers with the goal of attempting to cover a broad range of methodological topics in IRT. Each author was asked *not* to write an overly didactic "IRT novice-friendly" introductory guide to a specific topic, but rather to cover "cutting-edge" contemporaneous methods within a specific domain. As such, to the extent that a specific topic required highly technical presentation, authors were told to include whatever equations and derivations they believed necessary.

To fully appreciate this collection, some basic familiarity with measurement theory, in general, and IRT modeling, in particular, is required. The technical level, thus, generally is aimed at researchers who have some prior exposure to IRT and need summaries of the latest advances and critiques on foundational topics such as multidimensionality, assessment of fit, and handling non-normality, as well as applied topics such as differential item functioning and multidimensional linking. Importantly, although the substantive application illustrated in each of the chapters is predominantly health outcomes data, this text is by no means limited to such work; in fact, the issues addressed in the various chapters are relevant to any application of IRT models in any content domain.

We were fortunate to receive 21 chapters that summarize these various advanced psychometric methods, which can be used effectively to evaluate and address many of the unique challenges of applying IRT methods to health outcomes data. This book is divided into three major parts: (a) Fundamental Issues in IRT, (b) Classic and Emerging IRT Modeling Approaches, and (c) Using IRT Models in Applied Problems.

Part I, Fundamental Issues in IRT, includes chapters that raise critical differences between educational and noneducational constructs and data and the unique challenges the latter might present for IRT modeling (Chapter 1). The remaining chapters in this part cover core, fundamental topics that apply in any application of IRT modeling, such as: (a) the assessment of unidimensionality versus multidimensionality; (b) modern methods of IRT parameter estimation; (c) methods of estimating item parameters when the latent distribution is non-normal; (d) evaluating psychometric properties of a measure using nonparametric models and methods; (e) the evaluation of model fit; and (f) the evaluation of person fit.

In Part II, Classic and Emerging IRT Modeling Approaches, both new/emerging IRT models and classic IRT models are detailed. This part includes several chapters on the application of multidimensional IRT models designed to better capture the sometimes complex latent structure of typical performance data. Specifically, Part II includes chapters: (a) presenting the family of alternative multidimensional IRT models, (b) describing how multidimensional IRT models can be used to create unidimensional scales, (c) illustrating new "two-tier" IRT models appropriate for hierarchical item response data, and (d) new cutting-edge methods of deriving a single latent dimension from multidimensional data. Also included in this part are two very new modeling approaches: (a) explanatory IRT models that attempt to model item features and (b) IRT models specifically designed for the measurement of unipolar constructs, that is, constructs that are only defined on one end of a continuum (e.g., substance abuse). The last chapter is on how to decide among the large family of traditional polytomous IRT models.

Finally, in Part III, Using IRT Models in Applied Problems, are chapters on the major applications of IRT models. These include: (a) scoring individuals under different alternative multidimensional IRT models; (b) item banking for patient-reported health outcomes; (c) using IRT to evaluate measurement invariance; (d) using a nominal response model to diagnose problems with response categories; (e) linking scales to be on a common metric when the data are multidimensional; and (f) using IRT in developmental studies where the assessment of growth and change is critical. A summary chapter at the end reviews the book as a whole and considers future research directions for IRT application in health outcomes measurement.

We enjoyed reviewing these chapters and appreciate the authors' contributions immensely. We believe that researchers, graduate students, and instrument developers, for example, will find something new and helpful in these presentations and, thus, be better equipped to address the many and varied challenges in evaluating health outcome data.

Steven P. Reise
Dennis A. Revicki

Acknowledgments

The authors would like to acknowledge and thank Mark Haviland from Loma Linda University, as well as UCLA quantitative graduate students Wes Bonifay, Anthony Rodriguez, and Maxwell Mansolf for reviewing our chapters. We would also like to thank the reviewers who provided helpful insight: Lisa Harlow, University of Rhode Island, Leah Walker McGuire, University of Minnesota, Twin Cities, Carol Woods, University of Kansas, and two anonymous reviewers. Thanks also to Debra Riegert, who provided critical support and insightful advice as this volume progressed.

Part I

Fundamental Issues in Item Response Theory

1 Introduction

Age-Old Problems and Modern Solutions

Steven P. Reise and Dennis A. Revicki

The statistical foundation of item response theory (IRT) is often traced back to the seminal work of Lord, Novick, and Birnbaum (1968). The subsequent development, research, and application of IRT models and related methods link directly to the need of large-scale testing companies, such as the Educational Testing Service, to solve statistical as well as practical problems in educational assessment (i.e., the measurement of aptitude, achievement, and ability constructs). Daunting problems in this include the challenge of administering different test items to demographically diverse individuals across multiple years, while maintaining scores that are comparable on the same scale. This test score comparability problem traditionally has been addressed with "test-score equating" methods, but now more routinely, IRT-based "linking" strategies are used (see Chapter 19).

The application of IRT models and methods in educational assessment is now commonplace (e.g., see most any recent issue of the *Journal of Educational Measurement*), especially for large-scale testing firms that employ on their research staff dozens of world-class psychometricians, content experts, and item writers. The application of IRT models, and related statistical methods in the fields of personality, psychopathology, patient-reported outcomes (PRO), and health-related quality-of-life (HRQOL) measurement, in contrast, has only recently begun to proliferate in research journals. In these noneducational or "typical performance" domains, the application of IRT has gained popularity for much the same reasons as in large-scale educational assessment; that is, to solve practical and technical problems in measurement.

The National Institutes of Health (NIH) Patient Reported Outcome Measurement Information System (PROMIS®), for example, has developed multiple item banks for measuring various physical, mental, and social health domains (Cella et al., 2007; Cella et al., 2010). Similarly, the Quality of Life in Neurological Disorders (www.neuroqol.org) and NIH Toolbox (www.nihtoolbox.org) have also employed IRT methods of scale development and item analysis. One of the chief motivations underlying the application of IRT methods in these projects was to solve a long-standing and well-recognized problem in health outcomes research; namely, that for any important construct, there are typically half a dozen or so competing measures of unknown quality and questionable validity. This chaotic measurement situation, with dozens of researchers studying the same phenomena using different measurement tools, fails to promote good research and inhibits the cumulative aggregation of research results.

Large-scale IRT application projects, such as PROMIS®, have raised awareness not only of the technical and practical challenges of applying IRT models to psychological or PRO data, in general, but also has uncovered the many and varied special problems and concerns that arise in applying IRT outside of educational assessment (see also Reise & Waller, 2009). We will highlight several of these critical challenges later in this chapter to set a context for the present volume. Before doing so, however, we note that thus far, standard IRT models and methods have been imported into noneducational measurement contexts, and essentially without modification. In other words, there has been little in the way of "new models" or "new statistical methods" uniquely appropriate for PRO or any other type of noneducational data (but see Chapter 13).

This equalitarian—the same IRT models and methods should be used for all constructs, educational or PRO—was perhaps critical in early stages of IRT exploration and application in new domains. Inevitably, we believe, further progress will require new IRT-based psychometric approaches particularly tailored to meet measurement challenges in noneducational assessment. We will expand on this in the final chapter. For now, prior to previewing the chapters in this edited volume, in the following section, we briefly discuss some critical differences between educational and noneducational constructs, data, and assessment contexts, as these relate to the application of IRT models. We argue that although there are fundamental technical issues in applying IRT to any domain (e.g., dimensionality issues, assessing model to data fit), unique challenges arise when applying IRT to noneducational data due to the nature of the constructs (e.g., limited conceptual breadth, questionable applicability across the entire population), and item response data (e.g., non-normal latent trait distribution issues).

Educational Versus Noneducational Measurement

It is well recognized that psychological constructs, both cognitive and noncognitive, can be conceptualized as being hierarchically arranged, from very general to middle level, conceptually narrow to specific behaviors (Clark & Watson, 1995).[1] Since Loevinger (1957), it has also been well recognized (although not necessarily realized in practice by scale developers) that the position of a construct in this hierarchy has profound implications for all aspects of scale development, psychometric analyses, and ultimately validation of test score inferences.

Almost by definition, measures of broad bandwidth constructs (intelligence, verbal ability, negative affectivity, general distress, overall life satisfaction, or QOL) must have heterogeneous item content to capture the diversity of trait manifestations.[2] In turn, item intercorrelations, item-test correlations, and factor-loadings/IRT slopes are expected to be modest in magnitude, with low communality. Moreover, resulting factor structures may (must?) be multidimensional to some degree, perhaps with a strong general factor and several so-called group or specific factors corresponding to more content-homogeneous domains (see Chapter 2).

On the other hand, just the opposite psychometric properties would be expected for measures of conceptually narrow constructs (mathematics self-efficacy, primary narcissism, fatigue, pain interference, germ phobia). That is, in this latter context, the content diversity of trait manifestation is very limited (by definition of the construct), and as a consequence, item content is homogeneous with the conceptual distance between the item content and the

1 Interestingly, these authors attribute the apparently inexhaustible proliferation of individual difference constructs and measures to this hierarchical structure, which can be cleaved in an infinite number of ways.

2 We are assuming here that for the construct of interest, there is a latent variable underlying, or causing, variation in item response. Such a measurement model has been termed an "effects" indicator model by Bollen and Lennox (1991). If the construct of interest were better represented by a "cause" indicator measurement model, then IRT models, which assume an underlying latent trait, are questionable. Moreover, in a cause indicator model, item content diversity would be required to form a census of indicators (see Bollen & Lennox, 1991 for further discussion).

latent trait being slim. In turn, this can result in very high item intercorrelations, item-test correlations, and factor-loadings/IRT slopes. In factor analyses, essential unidimensionality would be the expectation, as would high item communalities. Finally, in contrast to broadband measures, where local independence violations are typically caused by clusters of content-similar items, in narrowband measures, local independence violations are typically caused by having the same item content repeated over and over with slight variation (e.g., "I *have problems concentrating,*" "I *find it hard to concentrate,*" "I *lose my concentration while driving,*" "*It is sometimes hard for me to concentrate at work*").

In our judgment, applications of IRT in educational measurement have tended toward the more broadband constructs, such as verbal and quantitative aptitude, or comprehensive licensure testing contexts (which also involve competencies across a heterogeneous skill domain). In contrast, we argue that with few exceptions, applications of IRT in noneducational measurement have primarily been with constructs that are relatively conceptually narrow. As a consequence, IRT applications in noneducational measurement contexts present some unique challenges, and the results of such applications can be markedly different from a typical IRT application in education.

For illustration, Embretson and Reise (in preparation) report on an analysis of the PROMIS® anger item set (see Pilkonis et al., 2010), a set of 29 items rated on a 1 to 5 response scale. Anger is arguably conceptually narrow because there simply are not that many ways of being angry (especially when rated within the past seven days); that is, the potential pool of item content is very limited, unlike a construct, say, such as spelling or reading comprehension where the pool of items is virtually inexhaustible. Accordingly, alpha was 0.96, and an eigenvalue ratio of around 15 to 1, suggesting unidimensionality, or at least a strong common factor. Fitting a unidimensional confirmatory factor analysis resulted in an "acceptable" fit by conventional standards. However, univariate and multivariate Lagrange tests indicated 407 and 157 correlated residuals needed to be estimated (set free), respectively. This unambiguous evidence against the data meeting the unidimensionality/local independence assumption was not due to the anger data being in any real sense of the term "multidimensional," with substantively interpretable distinct factors, but rather as having many sizeable correlated residuals (violations of local independence), likely caused by highly similar item content.

In sum, item responses to conceptually narrow measures such as anger are clearly highly influenced by a single common dimension (what else could items like "I *stayed angry for hours*" be measuring?), but are not, statistically speaking, truly unidimensional/locally independent, as commonly applied unidimensional IRT models assume. Importantly, item slope parameters (and, thus, test information) may be artificially high because of these unmodeled local independence violations. On the other hand, responses to measures such as anger cannot be readily fit to multidimensional models such as a correlated-factors, second-order, testlet, two-tier, or bifactor measure, because items do not cluster neatly into content domains. One either has to decide that the measure is sufficiently unidimensional such that the item parameters are estimated accurately, or start deleting items displaying local dependencies, with the realization that attempting to eliminate all local independence violations may result in a three-to-five-item bank.

As illustrated earlier, differences between educational and noneducational constructs, in particular their level of conceptual breadth, can be consequential for IRT analyses, in particular dimensionality assessment. However, it is by no means the only consequential difference. We argue that for many educational constructs where IRT models are applied, it is reasonable to assume a continuous, normally distributed latent variable in the population of relevant examinees. Often, this population is readily defined (e.g., all public school 8th graders in California), and data are collected on almost the entire population (sans absentees).

Moreover, for the test developer, it is relatively straightforward to generate multiple items that extend across the trait continuum from "easy" items requiring low-level skills to "hard" items requiring greater knowledge or skills (i.e., have item location parameters that span the latent trait range).[3] As a consequence, test information will be spread out across the latent trait range, and meaningful interpretations of latent trait scores can be made at either end of the latent trait continuum from low to high ability levels.

In the measurement of health outcomes or psychopathology, we argue that the measurement situation and the item response data often differ greatly from that discussed earlier. For example, often for constructs, such as pain interference, pain behavior, fatigue, or depression, scores are not normally distributed in the nonclinical, general population. For example, the distribution of PROMIS® pain behavior and pain interference scores in the general population are highly skewed. Based on completed IRT analyses on pain behavior items, including a sample of individuals with varying levels of chronic pain, the results supported two distributions, one of no pain and pain, and then if pain, a more normal distribution of pain behavior scores (Revicki et al., 2009). Analysts often assume a normal distribution for the latent trait during the estimation of item parameters and model fit (see Chapter 4). Violating the assumption of normal distributions for the latent trait may bias the estimates of IRT slope and threshold parameters, although the extent of this bias attributable to various levels of non-normality needs further research. Extreme cases of highly skewed and non-normal distributions may require alternative IRT modeling approaches. In the case of the PROMIS® pain behavior item bank, a hybrid nominal-partial credit IRT analysis provided very good model fit to these data (Revicki et al., 2009).

Related to this non-normal latent trait is a similar problem with a slightly different origin. Consider again the anger example described previously. The low end is not mild cynicism, negativity, irritability, being "upset" or "frustrated," but more likely the complete absence of anger reactions (within the past seven days). The construct of anger might be what Lucke (see Chapter 13) refers to as a unipolar trait—definable only on one end of the scale—and Reise and Waller have been referring to as a quasi-trait since at least 1990 (but see also Reise & Waller, 2009). The concept of a unipolar or quasi-trait is even better illustrated by constructs such as depression, sex addiction, belching/flatulence symptoms, and tobacco use. For these types of constructs, low scores are not necessarily below average on the trait, or low on the trait, but rather the trait is simply not applicable to them.

There are three obvious consequences of applying IRT models to unipolar health outcome or psychopathology traits. First, if the measure is given to a "healthy" sample, there will be many zero item scores, and total scores will be highly skewed. It is not at all clear whether even item parameter estimation strategies that can account for non-normal latent trait distributions (see Chapter 4) can salvage viable item parameters in this circumstance. Second, if the full range of the latent variable is not meaningful, then it should be difficult if not impossible to write items with location parameters that span the range of the latent variable. Instead, one would expect that they would be highly skewed. Indeed, this is exactly what is found for anger (see Pilkonis et al., 2010), where none of the first threshold parameter estimates, based on the graded response model, is below negative one and almost half of the parameters are positive.

Reise and Waller (2009) argued that application of a polytomous IRT model to noneducational measures has seldom, if ever, resulted in item location parameters spread across

3 We are by no means implying that creating a test or item bank that spans the complete ability range is an easy task. We merely are pointing out that a range of ability from low to high is more readily definable in educational assessment.

the latent trait range (see also Embretson & Reise, 2000 for a similar argument regarding a popular self-esteem scale). In fact, studies routinely report the opposite—that locations are clustered tightly at one end of the scale and that test information is highly peaked. At the very least, such findings have clear implications for the development of banks of items that provide items with differential precision across the trait range (see Chapter 16) and for the viability of computerized adaptive testing (see Reise & Henson, 2000 for further commentary). However, with those cautions raised, research has demonstrated that for the PROMIS® depression and fatigue item banks, multiple items are needed for precise assessment across the trait continuum and that CAT scores outperform static short forms (Choi et al., 2010; Lai et al., 2011).

A third consequence of applying IRT to unipolar traits, especially for clinically related patient outcomes (e.g., pain behaviors, depression), is that it is often unclear who the norming population should be. Decisions about the population for identifying the latent trait scale can affect the scale and item parameters. For example, if a clinical population is selected for item calibration and setting the scale for a depression item bank, the metric of the latent trait can be identified based on a sample of patients with depressive disorders. Selecting a clinical sample would result in an extended range of scores for the clinical depressed sample, and compression of the depression latent trait scores in the general, nonclinical population. If a general population sample is selected for item calibration and setting the metric, the opposite would occur, that is, there would be a greater spread of scores in the general population with compression of scores for the depressed clinical population. There is no right or wrong way to set the metric for the latent trait; however, decisions about the calibration population have implications for the scale metric.

Finally, and related to this issue of unipolar traits, there are a number of cases where health outcome measures are configured as presence-severity items (Liu & Verkuilen, 2013). These measures first ask the respondent to indicate whether an event or symptom is present, and if affirmative ask for a rating of severity, frequency, bother, distress or effect. For these kinds of latent constructs and item configuration, alternative models may need to be considered for the IRT analyses, such as the nominal response model (Liu & Verkuilen, 2013; Chapter 18), or new IRT models such as Lucke's unipolar models (see Chapter 13) may be required.

Brief Preview of Chapters

This summary of the unique challenges of applying IRT to noneducational data provides a context for the present volume, given that many of the examples in the various chapters illustrate IRT methods using health outcome data. To further contextualize the following chapters, we provide a very brief description of the motivation and some of the central themes of each.

Part I: *Fundamental Issues in Item Response Theory*

This part includes a set of seven chapters that tackle foundational issues relevant to the application of IRT models in any substantive domain, educational and noneducational. Because unidimensional IRT models are, by far, the most commonly applied, in Chapter 2 Steven Reise, Karon Cook, and Tyler Moore review the definition of (uni) dimensionality—as something belonging to data and not a construct—and describe how the concept of unidimensionality has been traditionally assessed using a variety of statistical indices. One unique feature of their chapter is the argument that psychological data are never strictly unidimensional, and, thus, the critical question in applied research is determining whether the multidimensionality inherent in the data is sufficient to bias item parameter estimates. In turn, they suggest a "comparison modeling" approach where the parameters from a bifactor model are evaluated relative to those estimated under a unidimensional model. This chapter sets the foundation and provides complementary material for Chapters 9 and 11, in which alternative approaches to scaling individuals on a single dimension in the presence of multidimensional data are detailed.

After establishing that the data are appropriate for application of an IRT model, perhaps the most fundamental topic in all of IRT is item parameter estimation. In Chapter 3, Li Cai and David Thissen provide a comprehensive review and discussion of modern full-information (based on the complete item response matrix) approaches to unidimensional item parameter estimation, including explanation of the Metropolis-Hastings sampler and Robbins-Monroe method. Although parameter estimation approaches in unidimensional IRT models have been around for a long time, these traditional methods are not entirely adequate to handle the computational challenges presented by new types of multidimensional IRT models, such as the bifactor or two-tier models (see Chapters 8 to 12). The methods presented in Chapter 3 have straightforward extensions to polytomous item responses and multidimensional models.

Traditional marginal maximum likelihood approaches to IRT item parameter estimation typically assume a normal prior distribution (implemented through quadrature points and weights) for the latent trait, and then item parameters are estimated assuming this distribution is reasonable. It has long been a concern that this normality assumption may not be appropriate in many noneducational measurement contexts, especially PRO measurement. Accordingly, in Chapter 4, Carol Woods describes the problems in item parameter estimation when the latent trait is non-normal and then reviews statistical methods for estimating the latent trait distribution simultaneously with the item parameters in the context of unidimensional item response theory models. It is also shown that item parameters and estimated latent trait scores are more accurate when the shape of the latent trait distribution is estimated, rather than assumed normal.

Chapter 5, authored by Rob Meijer, Jorge Tendeiro, and Rob Wanders, could have been placed as Chapter 3 because it deals with the use of nonparametric IRT methods (NIRT) to explore whether item response data are consistent with the assumptions underlying the fitting of a parametric IRT model. Nevertheless, we decided to group Chapters 5, 6, and 7 because they all are relevant to the topic of model fit, albeit approached from different vantage points. Specifically, Chapter 5 provides insight into a number of commonly used NIRT methods and demonstrates how these methods can be used to describe and explore the psychometric quality of PRO measures. The authors also emphasize consideration of the degree to which specific IRT models are "robust" to violations of assumptions and provide practical advice for applied researchers.

Chapter 6, by Alberto Maydeu-Olivares, introduces cutting-edge methods for evaluating overall IRT model fit based on analyses of the contingency table. As is well known, for any sizeable length test, the complete item response contingency table will be sparse because of many item response patterns not being observed. In turn, this has made it nearly impossible to use the discrepancy between the observed response patterns and those predicted from the estimated model to judge fit. Maydeu-Olivares reviews traditional methods for assessing the overall model fit and describes new limited information on overall goodness of fit statistics and methods for assessing approximate fit and piecewise assessment of fit. Complementing Chapter 6, Pere Ferrando, who has published extensively on the topic of person fit in noneducational settings, presents a comprehensive review of statistical methods for evaluating how consistent an individual's item response pattern is with an estimated IRT model in Chapter 7. He summarizes the importance of evaluating person fit, details the main methods for assessing person fit, and describes methods for diagnosing the causes and implications of poor person fit.

Part II: *Classic and Emerging IRT Modeling Approaches*

In this part, a number of different, cutting-edge methods for IRT modeling are summarized. Chapters 8 through 11 all deal with the emerging umbrella topic of multidimensional IRT, but in very different ways. Michael Edwards, R.J. Wirth, Carrie Houts, and Andrew Bodine, in Chapter 8, explore the concepts underlying dimensionality and present some of the challenges researchers face when trying to choose between different models. These conceptual issues are illustrated with both simulated and real data examples before turning to a broader discussion of how the issue of dimensionality may affect PROs. In Chapter 9, Brian Stucky and Maria Edelen summarize the structure of traditional multidimensional models with an emphasis on the bifactor and more recent generalizations such as the two-tier models (Chapter 10). They then describe complications that arise in interpreting multidimensional IRT item parameters and propose a method for creating unidimensional scales from multidimensional item response data using the results from a bifactor model.

Although briefly described in the preceding chapters, in Chapter 10, a two-tiered item factor analysis (or IRT) model is outlined in more detail by Wes Bonifay. A two-tier model is an IRT model with more than one general factor (which may be correlated) and multiple primary factors nested within each general factor. As such, the two-tier model is a parent model that subsumes the correlated factors, bifactor, and testlet response IRT models. Data analyses are used to demonstrate the psychometric advantages of the two-tier item factor analysis model.

The final chapter on multidimensional IRT, Chapter 11, is authored by Edward Ip and Shyh-Huei Chen. They do not propose a new multidimensional IRT model, per se, but rather a method of scaling individuals on a single dimension in the presence of multidimensionality. Specifically, this chapter details projective IRT models, which are a class of statistical methods for collapsing a multidimensional latent space down into a unidimensional latent space that reflects the common dimension assessed by all the items. Ip and Chen provide both Monte Carlo simulation results and several real-data applications to illustrate the method. They also provide a comparison of the projection methodology with the results from a bifactor model.

Chapters 12 and 13 each present "new" approaches to IRT modeling that do not fit easily into old rubrics such as "multidimensional IRT." First, explanatory IRT (EIRT) modeling is a relatively new but emerging approach to IRT modeling that heretofore has captured the interests of many educational researchers. In Chapter 12, Paul De Boeck and Mark Wilson describe how EIRT is based on finding explanatory covariates for items (i.e., variation in locations) and persons (i.e., variation in trait standing), and how in contrast to traditional IRT models, the latent variable is not viewed as causal. The authors provide a demonstration of the model in the domain of self-reported aggression and describe how the approach may be useful in PRO measurement more generally.

As noted in the first part of this chapter, it is often the case in noneducational measurement that constructs are not fully bipolar (i.e., scores are only interpretable on one end of the scale). In Chapter 13, using a gambling addiction scale as an example, Joseph Lucke introduces a new class of unipolar item response models. A distinguishing feature of these types of models is that, unlike traditional IRT models where the mean of the latent trait is defined as zero, in unipolar models, zero is the lowest possible latent trait score (corresponding to individuals with "no symptoms" or "no meaningful trait level"). Lucke also presents relevant derivatives and information functions, and discusses the fact that models can yield similar item response curves, but very different information functions.

Finally, in noneducational measurement, especially PRO measurement, polytomous item response formats are the norm, and dichotomous response formats the exception. Consequently, polytomous IRT models are more commonly used. However, there are many proposed polytomous IRT models, which begs the question, which are best for PRO data, or does it really matter? In Chapter 14, Remo Ostini, Matthew Finkelman, and Michael Nering discuss issues associated with selecting polytomous IRT models for various applications. They summarize the more commonly applied polytomous IRT models, including some of their more salient differences. The chapter also considers strategies for selecting among different polytomous IRT models and reports on some research that describes how the strategy may play out in practice.

Part III: *Using IRT Models in Applied Problems*

As we noted at the beginning of this chapter, IRT psychometric methods allow researchers to solve both statistical and practical testing problems that are otherwise either not possible or extremely challenging using traditional classical test theory–based approaches. This last part is devoted to chapters that describe how IRT models can be successfully employed in research and practice. One of the primary uses of IRT models is to estimate an individual's position on a common latent dimension or dimensions. Although methods for accomplishing this task with standard unidimensional models are fairly well known, few researchers understand estimating latent trait scores in multidimensional models. To address this, Anna Brown and Tim Croudace summarize problems and solutions for scoring individuals based on multidimensional IRT models in Chapter 15. Models described include the correlated factors, second-order, and bifactor models.

A further distinguishing feature of IRT models is that the theory promotes the development of item banks—sets of items all measuring a single construct with known IRT item parameters. The PROMIS® project, cited previously, has developed many such item banks for PRO constructs. The creation of item banks stands in marked contrast to the historical practice of researchers creating their own preferred measures. In Chapter 16, Dennis Revicki, Wen-Hung Chen, and Carole Tucker provide an overview and summary of methods for developing and evaluating item banks for patient-reported health outcomes. They cover concept identification, qualitative research, item bank development, the basics of the psychometric evaluation of an item bank and resultant measures, and review issues for future consideration in item bank development. Concepts and methods are illustrated with examples from the NIH-sponsored PROMIS® project.

Another often touted advantage of IRT models is that they provide an elegant framework for defining and assessing differential item functioning (DIF)—when the relation between the latent trait and the item responses is not equivalent across examinee populations. Accordingly, in Chapter 17, Roger Millsap, Heather Gunn, Howard Everson, and Alex Zautra summarize methods for evaluating DIF (sometimes referred to as measurement invariance research, or as item or test bias research although DIF does not necessarily imply bias). These authors review definitions of measurement invariance and how violations of invariance are distinguished from simple group mean and variance differences in scores. They then demonstrate how contemporary IRT methods are applied to empirically evaluating measurement invariance.

Yet another claimed advantage of IRT modeling is that it provides a superior method for studying the psychometric properties of items and item category functioning. To illustrate the latter, Kathleen Preston and Steven Reise (Chapter 18) discuss and summarize methods for evaluating and diagnosing problems with items using the under-used nominal response model (NRM). The NRM can be viewed as a parent model for the generalized partial credit, partial credit, and rating scale models. Preston and Reise illustrate several useful applications of the nominal response model including exploring whether category boundary discrimination parameters vary within an item, whether an item has too many response options, and whether response options are well ordered. The chapter combines Monte Carlo simulations and real data examples.

As noted previously, if individual examinees respond to different sets of test items that measure the same construct, the metrics for the two item sets must be "linked" such that scores are comparable. There is an extensive literature on linking methods for unidimensional IRT models in the educational measurement literature. In Chapter 19, Jonathan Weeks provides a foundation for understanding issues that should be considered when performing either unidimensional or multidimensional test linking. With the emergence of applications of multidimensional IRT models, this latter topic is of critical importance looking forward.

One final potential advantage of IRT lies in the domain of studying change, growth, or development. In Chapter 20, John McArdle, Kevin Petway, and Earl Hishinuma summarize the issues involved in the application of IRT methods for handling growth and changes in scale scores. A real data example of theory testing is provided based on longitudinal data collected from high school students measured in 9th, 10th, 11th, and 12th grades on the *Center for Epidemiological Studies—Depression Scale* drawn from the *Hawaiian High School Health Survey* project. To conclude this volume, in Chapter 21, Steven Reise and Dennis Revicki provide a summary of new IRT problems and future directions for IRT applications in health outcomes assessment.

References

Bollen, K., & Lennox, R. (1991). Conventional wisdom on measurement: A structural equation perspective. *Psychological Bulletin*, *110*, 305–314.

Cella, D., Riley, W., Stone, A., Rothrock, N., Reeve, B., Yount, S., et al. (2010). The Patient-Reported Outcomes Measurement Information System (PROMIS) developed and tested its first wave of adult self-reported health outcome item banks: 2005–2008. *Journal of Clinical Epidemiology*, *63*, 1179–1194.

Cella, D., Yount, S., Rothrock, N., Gershon, R., Cook, K., Reeve, B., et al. (2007). The patient-reported outcomes measurement information system (PROMIS): Progress of an NIH roadmap cooperative group during its first two years. *Medical Care*, *45*, S3–S11.

Choi, S. W., Reise, S. P., Pilkonis, P. A., Hays, R. D., & Cella, D. (2010). Efficiency of static and computer adaptive short forms compared to full length measures of depressive symptoms. *Quality of Life Research*, *19*, 125–136.

Clark, L. A., & Watson, D. (1995). Constructing validity: Basic issues in objective scale development. *Psychological Assessment*, *7*, 309–319.

Embretson, S. E., & Reise, S. P. (2000). *Item response theory for psychologists*. Mahwah, NJ: Erlbaum.

Embretson, S. E., & Reise, S. P. (in preparation). *Item response theory* (a volume in the Multivariate Applications Series). New York: Routledge/Taylor & Francis Group.

Lai, J., Cella, D., Choi, S., Junghaenel, D. U., Christodoulou, C., Gershon, R., et al. (2011). How item banks and their application can influence measurement practice in rehabilitation medicine: A PROMIS fatigue item bank example. *Archives of Physical Medicine and Rehabilitation*, *92*(10 Suppl), S20–S27.

Liu, Y., & Verkuilen, J. (2013). Item response modeling of present-severity items: Application to measurement of patient-reported outcomes. *Applied Psychological Measurement*, *37*, 58–75.

Loevinger, J. (1957). Objective tests as instruments of psychological theory: Monograph Supplement 9. *Psychological Reports*, *3*, 635–694.

Lord, F. M., Novick, M. R., & Birnbaum, A. (1968). *Statistical theories of mental test scores*. Reading, MA: Addison-Wesley.

Pilkonis, P. A., Choi, S. W., Reise, S. P., Stover, A. M., Riley, T., & Cella, D. (2010). Item banks for measuring emotional distress from the patient-reported outcomes measurement information system (PROMIS): Depression, anxiety, and anger. *Assessment*, *18*, 263–283.

Reise, S. P., & Henson, J. M. (2000). Computerization and adaptive administration of the NEO PI-R. *Assessment*, *7*, 347–364.

Reise, S. P., & Waller, N. G. (2009). Item response theory and clinical measurement. *Annual Review of Clinical Psychology*, *5*, 27–48.

Revicki, D. A., Chen, W. H., Harnam, N., Cook, K. F., Amtmann, D., Callahan, L. F., Jensen, M. P., & Keefe, F. J. (2009). Development and psychometric analysis of the PROMIS pain behavior item bank. *Pain*, *146*, 158–169.

2 Evaluating the Impact of Multidimensionality on Unidimensional Item Response Theory Model Parameters

Steven P. Reise, Karon F. Cook, and Tyler M. Moore

Introduction

Commonly applied item response theory (IRT) measurement models stipulate a *single* continuous latent variable (typically labeled "θ") to represent individual differences on a psychological construct. For example, Equation 2.1 is the item response curve for the commonly applied two-parameter logistic model (2PL) for dichotomous item responses, where α_i is an item slope, β_i is an item location, θ is a continuous latent variable, and 1.7 is a scaling factor that makes the value of the item slope parameter in logistic models comparable to a normal-ogive model. This scaling is important for researchers who wish to link IRT parameters with factor analytic results.

$$P_i(x = 1 \mid \theta) = [1 + \exp(-1.7\alpha_i(\theta - \beta_i))]^{-1} \tag{2.1}$$

Accurate estimation of IRT item parameters and subsequent applications depend critically on the degree to which item response data meet the unidimensionality assumption. Such applications include interpreting item and scale information functions, estimating individuals' trait levels, implementing computerized adaptive testing (CAT), performing cross-group investigations of differential item functioning (DIF), and conducting scale linking. However, it is almost universally agreed that item response data rarely are strictly unidimensional. Thus researchers who are considering applications of IRT models must decide whether their data are "unidimensional enough" for these models.

Herein, we argue that the critical issue in an IRT application is not whether the data are "unidimensional enough," but rather the degree to which multidimensionality impacts or distorts estimation of item parameters (see also Reise, Scheines, Widaman, & Haviland, 2013). We evaluate this criterion based on the equivalence of IRT and item-level factor analysis (Takane & de Leeuw, 1987) and propose the application of exploratory bifactor analyses (Jennrich & Bentler, 2011; Schmid & Leiman, 1957) and targeted factor rotations (Browne, 2001) to directly model and assess the impact of multidimensionality on IRT item parameter estimates. Our approach is similar in spirit, using Ip's (Chapter 11) approach to collapsing multidimensionality to more accurately identify the common latent variable underlying a set of scale items.

Although our ultimate focus is the application of IRT models, our discussion will frequently make use of factor analytic terminology. Our rationale for using factor analytic terminology is that it is accessible to a wider audience. A second reason is that parameters of item-level factor analytic models are conceptually parallel to the parameters of IRT models (e.g., Knol & Berger, 1991, pp. 460–461). Specifically, many authors such as McLeod, Swygert, and Thissen (2001, p. 199) report equations that link the multidimensional bifactor IRT model concepts of item slope and location with the item-level factor analytic (ILFA; Wirth & Edwards, 2007) concepts of loading and intercept, respectively. Moreover, the gap between ILFA and IRT is closing rapidly because of the fact that modern programs such as EQSIRT (Wu & Bentler, 2011) and IRTPRO (Cai, Thissen, & de Toit, 2011) routinely display output in both metrics.

IRT and Unidimensionality

Equation 2.1 is a unidimensional model because it contains a single parameter to represent individual differences and explain inter-item covariance. Before applying this model, it is critical to determine if the model is consistent with item response data. McDonald stated that "a set of *n* tests or of *n* binary items is unidimensional if and only if the tests or the items fit a common factor model, generally non-linear, with one common factor" (McDonald, 1981, p. 100). Hattie's conceptualization is consistent with McDonald's: "Unidimensionality is defined as the existence of one latent trait underlying the data" (Hattie, 1985, p. 139). These definitions imply that a set of item responses is unidimensional if and only if the item response matrix is locally independent after removing a single common latent factor. The weaker version of local independence holds if the partial correlations among items are zero after extracting the factor scores from the common factor, or equivalently, item residual correlations are zero after extracting a single factor.

A unidimensional factor analytic (or IRT) model is shown in Figure 2.1 as Model A. This is by far the most commonly applied or "default" IRT model. In Model A, each item has a single common cause—the latent factor—and an error variance (that includes item-specific variance and random error). This is the ideal data structure for application of IRT models such as the one defined by Equation 2.1. Assuming sufficient sample size and estimation of the correct IRT model, it can be shown that, when item response data are unidimensional:

a) IRT item parameter estimates reflect the relation between item response propensities and the common target trait (i.e., parameter estimates are not distorted by multidimensionality);
b) individuals can be scaled on a common target dimension using any subset of items regardless of content (i.e., there is no need to worry about "content representation" of the items (see Bollen & Lennox, 1991); and
c) IRT applications such as CAT and DIF assessment are valid extensions of the item and person parameter invariance property (e.g., researchers do not need to be concerned about multidimensionality as a source of DIF).

These claims are justified because, when the data are unidimensional (i.e., locally independent after extracting a single factor), the following holds.

$$L(X = x_1, x_2 \ldots x_I \mid \theta) = \Pi_1^I P_i(\theta)^{x_i} Q_i(\theta)^{1-x_i} \tag{2.2}$$

Equation 2.2 states that the likelihood of an observed dichotomous item response pattern X is the serial product of the conditional (on θ) probability of endorsing (P) when $x_i = 1$, and the probability of not endorsing an item (Q) when $x_i = 0$. In Equation 2.2 the P and $Q = 1 - P$ values are taken directly from an estimated item response curve (e.g., Equation 2.1). This likelihood is a mathematical statement of the unidimensionality assumption, and forms the mathematical basis for estimating item parameters and subsequent applications of IRT such as scoring and linking sets of items onto a common metric. Thus, its accuracy is critically important.

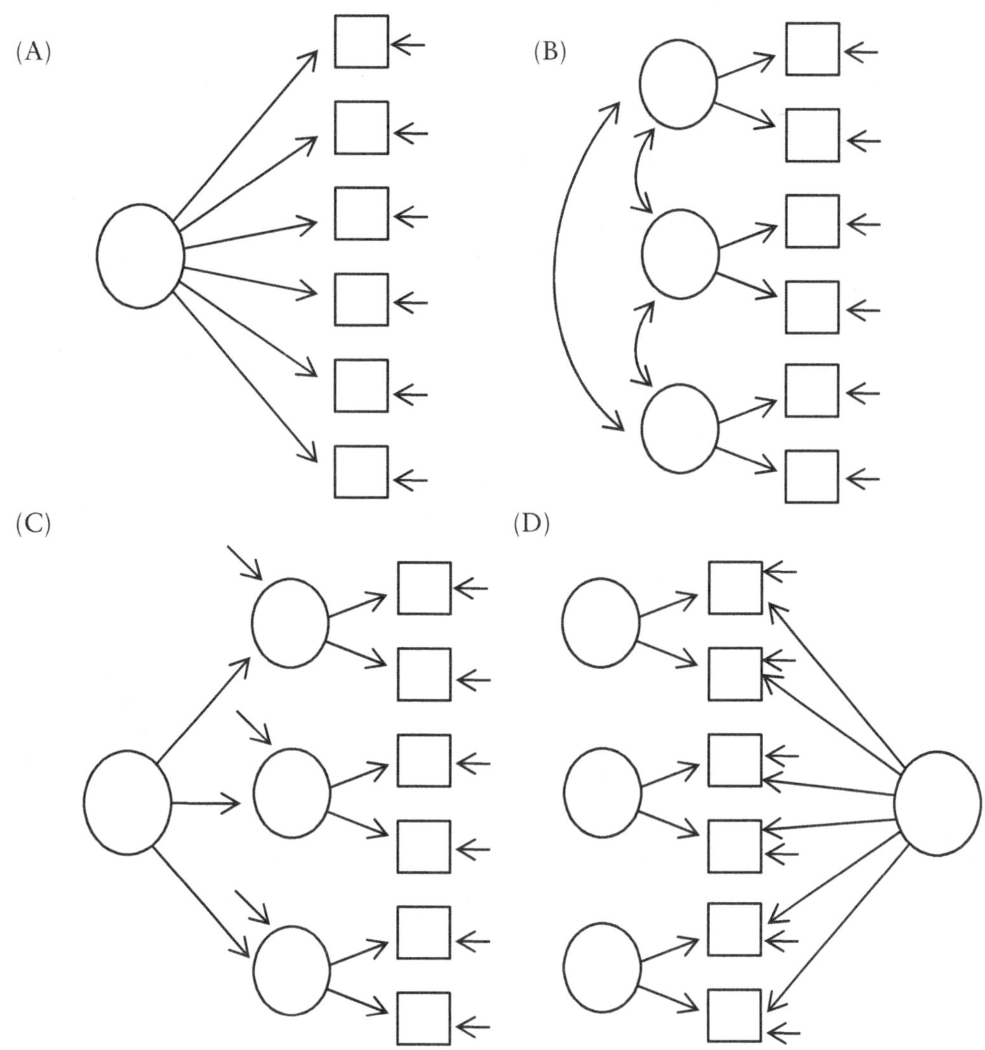

Figure 2.1 Alternative models: A—unidimensional model, B—correlated traits model, C—second-order factor model, D—bifactor model

If multidimensional data are forced into Equation 2.1, item parameter estimates may be distorted in unpredictable ways (see Steinberg & Thissen, 1996, for examples of local dependence violations), and validity coefficients are attenuated (Reise et al., 2013). If item parameters are distorted, any application based on Equation 2.2 must be questioned. For this reason, Model A is the structure researchers hope applies to their data, but this model may not be realistic or even substantively desirable (Humphreys, 1970). McDonald characterizes the prevailing view on the possibility of data strictly fitting a unidimensional model: "Such a case will not occur in application of theory" (McDonald, 1981, p. 102). Given this fact, researchers have invested much effort in: a) studying the degree to which IRT parameter estimates are robust (i.e., nearly correct) to different degrees of unidimensionality violation, and b) developing statistical guidelines for judging whether the data are reasonably close to Model A (e.g., a "strong" general trait), as reviewed next.

Unidimensional Enough for IRT

Robustness Studies

There is a substantial empirical literature based on Monte Carlo simulations exploring the robustness of IRT models to multidimensionality violations (Ackerman, 1989; Batley & Boss, 1993; De Ayala, 1994; DeMars, 2006; Drasgow & Parsons, 1983; Folk & Green, 1989; Reckase, 1979; Way, Ansley, & Forsyth, 1988). A number of factors make this literature challenging to neatly summarize. For example, robustness studies vary in: a) software program used to estimate item parameters, b) the specific IRT model evaluated, c) the criteria used to judge item or person parameter recovery, d) the type of dimensionality violation simulated, e) simulation conditions (e.g., average item slope, scale length), f) the degree to which researchers recognize that item parameters in some IRT models are not independently estimated, and g) whether estimated parameters are (mistakenly) linked back to the metric of true generating parameters.

Despite these variations in study design, a general conclusion of the robustness literature is that, if multidimensionality is due to multiple latent dimensions that are moderately correlated, or, if there is a strong general factor, IRT models are relatively robust. In this context, robust means that the item parameters are reasonably well recovered and latent trait estimates reflect individual differences on the target latent trait dimension. For example, studies that generate multidimensional data using a correlated traits approach (Model B in Figure 2.1) tend to find that item and person parameters are recovered reasonably well when the dimensions are equally correlated, the number of items per dimension is roughly the same, and the factors correlate greater than $r = 0.40$ (Kirisci, Hsu, & Yu, 2001, p. 159).

An important demonstration of robustness is the work of Drasgow and Parsons, who used the Schmid-Leiman transformation (Schmid & Leiman, 1957) of a correlated traits factor model as their basis for data simulation. This allowed them to simulate data sets with a bifactor structure (Model D in Figure 2.1) that varied in the strength of the (one) general and (five) group factors simultaneously. The item pools generated in this way were then "used to determine the degree of prepotency that is required . . . in order to recover the general latent trait and *not* be drawn to the latent trait underlying a cluster of items" (Drasgow & Parsons, 1983, p. 190).

Their first finding was that, judging by a root-mean squared deviation (RMSD) statistic, estimated item parameters reflected the general factor even in cases where the strength of the general factor was moderate (see also Reckase, 1979).[1] Only in the case of no general factor (uncorrelated traits) were item parameters poorly estimated based on the RMSD criterion. Second, they computed the correlation between the factor scores on the general factor, and the latent trait estimates based on fitting a unidimensional IRT model. These values showed that as the strength of the general factor decreases, the correlation between true and estimated latent trait scores decreases as well, and for a weak general dimension (i.e., low levels of factor intercorrelation), the trait estimates are drawn to the group factor with the highest loadings.

Considered as a whole, Monte Carlo simulations support the notion that IRT is potentially applicable to multidimensional data if the multidimensionality is due either to highly correlated latent traits, or if there is a "strong" general trait and relatively weaker group (nuisance) factors. Almost unanimously, however, the research cited earlier warns that

1 Reise and colleagues (2013) also found that parameters are recovered accurately even when the general factor is very weak, as long as the multidimensionality is properly accounted for. Such findings argue against the view that IRT is only applicable when there is a "strong" general factor.

fitting IRT models to multidimensional data is potentially problematic under certain conditions and that item parameter estimates can be seriously distorted. For example, Way, Ansley, and Forsyth conclude "it appears that using IRT in achievement test settings, or in any setting where the response data are likely multidimensional, must be done with extreme caution" (Way, Ansley, & Forsyth, 1988, p. 251).

To this we add two additional cautions in concluding, based on robustness studies, that IRT models can be applied safely to multidimensional data. First, some Monte Carlo results are not as compelling as they first appear. For example, in Drasgow and Parsons (1983) a high correlation was found between true latent trait scores on the general factor and estimated latent trait scores from a fitted unidimensional model. However, this is not convincing robustness evidence. Given a reasonably long scale, it would be unsurprising to find high correlations between true and estimated latent trait scores even when item parameters are poorly estimated. For example, in a different context, DeMar's (2006) robustness study found that latent trait estimates always correlated 0.99 regardless of whether the correct or incorrect model was used to scale individuals. She states, "If the focus is on estimated θ's and not on item parameters, any of the models will perform satisfactorily" (DeMar, 2006, p. 165).

Second, there are ambiguities in interpreting results of Monte Carlo studies, especially when multidimensional data are generated under a correlated traits model (Model B in Figure 2.1). Using the correlated traits model, it is impossible to specify what is the correct target latent trait dimension or what are the correct item parameters and individuals' scores on the target trait (see Ansley & Forsyth, 1985 for discussion). In those studies, the true item parameters (e.g., slope) often are defined as the average of the true generating item discriminations on each of the multiple dimensions, and true person parameters are defined as the average of the true generating trait levels on each of the correlated dimensions. In contrast, we note that in simulations using a bifactor model to generate data (Drasgow & Parsons, 1983; Reise et al., 2013), true item and person parameters on a target common dimension are easy to specify directly.

In sum, robustness research is of obvious and critical importance. Nevertheless, we have reservations about its overall usefulness in terms of understanding the effects of multidimensionality on particular item parameter estimates and subsequent IRT applications. Monte Carlo studies rely heavily on summaries of bias statistics, root-mean-square coefficients, and correlations between true and estimated parameters. These often are evaluated using analysis of variance (ANOVA) to gauge which independent variable (e.g., test length, average true discrimination) had the greater effect on a given dependent variable (e.g., root-mean-square). Such analyses do not directly reveal the specific impact of multidimensionality on specific item parameter estimates under specific test conditions.

Indexing "Unidimensional Enough"

Drawing from the robustness literature, IRT texts (e.g., Embretson & Reise, 2000) have suggested that the critical issue in determining the viability of an IRT application is the degree to which the data display a "strong" common dimension. The presence of a strong common dimension has been operationalized as the presence of highly correlated multiple dimensions in Model B or a strong general factor relative to group factors in Model D (see Figure 2.1). In this section we consider indices of these criteria that attempt to inform whether a particular data set is "unidimensional enough" for IRT. These indices commonly are used as "publishability statistics" in that they serve as empirical justifications to proceed with an IRT application.

Eigenvalues

Researchers have been mining eigenvalues (e.g., scree plots) for dimensionality information since long before the advent of IRT. Thus it is not surprising that eigenvalues have been used in an IRT context to judge the degree of multidimensionality. In particular, researchers have looked for a high ratio of first to second eigenvalues (e.g., 3 to 1) derived from the original correlation matrix. Hambleton and Swaminathan (1985) attribute to Reckase (1979) the criterion of a high ratio of first to second eigenvalues to define what constitutes a dominant first factor. Ackerman proposed the same notion, stating, "Evidence of multidimensionality can be seen by forming a ratio of the first to the second eigenvalue" (Ackerman, 1989, p. 119).

The comparison of relative size of eigenvalues is a logical approach to confirming whether there is a strong common factor. However, there are similar approaches that are equally, if not more, attractive. First, once a factor pattern matrix has been estimated, it can be converted back into a reproduced correlation matrix in which ones on the diagonal are replaced with communalities. Then, if eigenvalue decomposition is performed on this reproduced matrix, the ratio of the first eigenvalue to the sum of the eigenvalues indicates how much common variance is explained by the first factor (see Ten Berge & Socan, 2004). Second, given that a bifactor solution has been estimated, a researcher may compute an index such as coefficient omega ω_h (Zinbarg, Revelle, Yovel, & Li, 2005), which is the sum of the general factor loadings squared, divided by the total variance. This index can be interpreted as the degree of general factor saturation.

The ratio of first to second eigenvalues is model independent, whereas the latter two indices depend on a specified and estimated multidimensional model. Regardless, a key problem with eigenvalue-based indices of "unidimensional enough" is that they only indirectly inform about the vitiating effects of multidimensionality. As McDonald notes, "it is important to recognize that there is no direct relationship between the proportion of variance due to the first common factor and the presence or absence of additional common factors" (McDonald, 1981, p. 112). That is, even highly multidimensional item response matrices may have a high first to second eigenvalue ratio. Now with that said, if the eigenvalue ratio is unusually high, say 30 to 1, then no further consideration to dimensionality needs to be given. By the same token, the chief concern would be with too narrow a construct caused by repeated item content, and concerns about dimensionality secondary.

Fit in SEM

Statistical approaches for judging overall model fit, conducting model comparisons, and evaluating the practical adequacy of specific models have worked exceptionally well in structural equations modeling (SEM) contexts. Moreover, McDonald and Mok (1995) demonstrated the possibility of using SEM-based indices to inform the exploration of dimensionality in an IRT context. Given this, some researchers have advocated that IRT models be estimated using SEM software, and that fit indices and associated rules of thumb be used to judge dimensionality and model fit, and to compare alternative models. Some have even provided SEM-based benchmarks for judging good fit in IRT (Reeve et al., 2007).

Unfortunately, fit indices developed in SEM are of limited value in judging the viability of an IRT application. First, commonly used model-fit indices in SEM (e.g., CFI) are not designed to specifically test unidimensionality (Reise et al., 2013). Second, even when adjustments to fit indices are made for item-level ordinal data and non-normality, it is easy to demonstrate that: a) a unidimensional model that looks good under standard SEM indices can still yield item parameter estimates distorted by multidimensionality (e.g., a single correlated residual), and b) even when a unidimensional model looks poor based on SEM indices, and/or a multidimensional solution yields improved statistical fit, application of IRT may still be viable. Related to this latter point, it is well known that SEM-based indices are sensitive to trivial model violations (e.g., small correlated errors). One way to think about SEM indices in confirmatory factor analytic settings is that they reflect departures from simple structure. In a sense, they are "messiness" indices potentially useful for indicating that further data exploration is needed and more paths may need to be specified; but they are not very useful for making decisions about whether to proceed with an IRT analysis. Accordingly, we do not believe there are any SEM-based rules of thumb that can productively serve as permission slips for conducting or rejecting a particular IRT application.

Residual Analysis

A more promising approach to exploring "unidimensional enough" is inspection of the residuals after fitting a unidimensional (or multidimensional) model (see Ackerman, Gierl, & Walker, 2003; Hattie, 1985). McDonald, in reference to fitting nonlinear item factor models, stated, "If the residuals are small the fit of the hypothesis can still be judged to be satisfactory" (McDonald, 1982, p. 385). In a similar context, he stated, "the magnitudes of the residual covariances yield a non-statistical but reasonable basis for judging the extent of the misfit of the model to the data" (McDonald, 1981, p. 102). Hattie (1985) also suggests that researchers explore whether the sum of (absolute values of) residuals is small when one factor is extracted and not much smaller when two factors are extracted.

Like SEM indices, however, there is no residual value cutoff that indicates problems caused by unmodeled multidimensionality. Certainly a residual of 0.50 would be a serious concern, but the meanings of residual values of 0.20, 0.10, and 0.05 are not clear in the IRT context. Given a specific residual value, it is not possible to say how or if a particular item parameter is distorted or biased. More importantly, residuals may be small even in models where item parameters are estimated incorrectly. For example, not all local dependency problems caused by a content redundant item pair (i.e., items that share a secondary latent trait; see Steinberg & Thissen, 1996) will result in large residual values. A redundant item pair may distort parameter estimates (e.g., factor loadings go toward 1.0 or item discrimination estimates go toward infinity), even though the residual value is quite small.

Multidimensional IRT Models

When multidimensional data are forced into a unidimensional framework, Equation 2.2 must be wrong to some degree. As an alternative to searching for indices that signal conditions in which the data are "unidimensional enough" to produce reasonably accurate IRT item parameters, several scholars have advocated the potential utility of fitting multidimensional models (MIRT; Ackerman, Gierl, & Walker, 2003; Reckase & McKinley, 1991). Researchers have also suggested evaluating the unidimensionality assumption by explicit comparison of unidimensional models with multidimensional alternatives (e.g., Bartolucci, 2007; Christensen et al., 2002; Ip, 2010; Reise, Morizot, & Hays, 2007). In what follows, we argue for the utility of a particular type of comparison model, namely an unrestricted bifactor structure (Gibbons & Hedeker, 1992). In order to understand our preference, we need to review two alternative views on multidimensionality, or equivalently, two alternative views on the nature of the common target latent trait in IRT models.

In psychology, many traits are viewed as multifaceted. For example, Chen, West, and Sousa state, "Researchers interested in assessing a construct often hypothesize that several highly related domains comprise the general construct of interest" (Chen, West, & Sousa,

2006, p. 189). Hull, Lehn, and Tedlie argue, "Some of the most highly researched personality constructs in our field . . . are composed of multiple specific subcomponents" (Hull, Lehn, & Tedlie, 1991, p. 922). For measures of these types of constructs, the substantively broad construct definition almost ensures that resulting item response data are multidimensional.

If item response data are typically multidimensional by design, and thus Model A (Figure 2.1) is either unrealistic or even substantively undesirable, then what is the target latent variable of interest in IRT modeling? That is, how can researchers reconcile the notion that the construct is multifaceted and the data are multidimensional but the measurement model (Equation 2.1) allows only a single common individual difference variable to influence item responses? To address this, as Kirisci, Hsu, and Yu (2001, p. 147) recognized, researchers have taken two distinct approaches to conceptualizing the target latent variable in IRT. These frameworks also represent two ways of conceptualizing multidimensionality.

The first perspective is the correlated traits approach, and it is by far the most frequently applied model for generating data in Monte Carlo robustness studies. Under the correlated traits approach, measures are multidimensional because several correlated common factors influence item responses. A correlated traits model is shown as Model B in Figure 2.1. Under this framework, the target latent trait in IRT is what is in common among more basic primary traits or subdomains. However, to formally represent the common trait, a structure needs to be placed on the correlations among the primary dimensions in Model B. This produces Model C in Figure 2.1—a "second-order" model. In other words, the use of Model B implies that the latent trait is conceptualized as a higher-order cause of primary dimensions.

A second perspective identifiable in the literature is that the target latent variable is what is in common among the *items* (i.e., the common latent trait approach). Under this view, data are unidimensional enough for IRT to the degree that items load highly on a single common dimension and have small or zero loadings on secondary "nuisance" dimensions. The bifactor model (Holzinger & Swineford, 1937; Schmid & Leiman, 1957) shown as Model D in Figure 2.1 properly represents the common trait view. In this model, it is assumed that one common factor underlies the variance of all the scale items. In addition, a set of orthogonal group factors are specified that account for additional variation, typically assumed to arise because of item parcels with similar content.

Both the correlated traits approach (MIRT; Model B) and the common trait approach (BIRT; Model D) are reasonable conceptual models for understanding the role of multidimensionality in IRT, and both can be used productively. But for understanding the effect of multidimensionality on unidimensional IRT item parameter estimates, our preference is for the latter. A chief conceptual reason for this preference is that we believe that the BIRT model is more consistent with the hierarchical view of "traits" held by many personality and psychopathology theorists and scale developers (see Brunner, Nagy & Wilhelm, 2012; Clark & Watson, 1995). A practical reason for our preference is that if the general dimension in a bifactor model is assumed to correctly reflect the common latent dimension a researcher is interested in, it is straightforward to use the bifactor model as a comparison model as we describe next.

RESEARCH METHODS

Evaluating the Impact of Multidimensionality: A Comparison Modeling Approach

In what follows, we suggest an approach to evaluating the impact of multidimensionality for measures being considered for IRT analysis. We label this approach the "comparison modeling" method. In the comparison modeling approach a researcher first estimates a unidimensional model. Herein, this is referred to as the "restricted" model. Then a researcher estimates an "unrestricted" bifactor model that better represents the multidimensional (i.e., bifactor) data structure. Finally, item slope parameter estimates on the restricted model are compared to item slope parameter estimates on the general factor in the unrestricted model. It is assumed that the unrestricted model is a more accurate representation of the relationship between the items and the common trait being measured by the scale. Thus, the comparison of these two sets of parameter estimates provides a direct index of the degree to which item slope parameters are distorted because of forcing multidimensional data into a unidimensional model.

The value of the comparison modeling approach depends critically on the identification of a bifactor structure that is plausible, and arguably more correct than the restricted unidimensional model. This suggests the questions: 1) How do we derive an appropriate comparison model, and 2) What are the conditions under which the comparison model is likely to be accurate? In the following sections, we address these issues as we describe a two-stage procedure for identifying an appropriate comparison model: 1) exploratory bifactor analysis using a Schmid-Leiman orthogonalization (SL; Schmid & Leiman, 1957),[2] followed by 2) targeted factor rotations to a bifactor structure (Browne, 2001).

Although the following text focuses exclusively on these two methods, it is important to keep in mind that the goal is simply to find a plausible comparison model. The SL and target rotation methods are not the only tools that can inform the specification of a comparison bifactor structure (see footnote 2). Indeed, prior to implementing the direct modeling approach, we highly recommend researchers familiarize themselves with the theory underlying scale construction (i.e., what aspects of the construct are the scale developers trying to assess?) and perform extensive preliminary analyses of item psychometrics, item content cluster structure, and other forms of dimensionality analyses such as those evaluated by van Abswoude, van der Ark, and Sijtsma (2004).

Exploratory Bifactor Analysis

One obvious tool for identifying multidimensional structures is item-level exploratory factor analysis (ILFA; Wirth & Edwards, 2007) such as factor analysis of tetrachoric correlation matrices (Knol & Berger, 1991). One reason ILFA is effective for studying IRT models is that ILFA and the two-parameter normal-ogive are equivalent models (Ackerman, 2005; Knott & Bartholomew, 1999; McDonald, 1982, 2000; McDonald & Mok, 1995; McLeod, Swygert, & Thissen, 2001). As a consequence, studying the effects of model violations (e.g., multidimensionality) in one model is equivalent to studying the same phenomena in the other.

Let the latent dimensions be $p = 1 \ldots P$ and, assuming that the latent factors are uncorrelated (e.g., a bifactor model), the translations between ILFA loadings (λ) and IRT slopes (normal-ogive metric) are:

$$\lambda_{ip} = \frac{\alpha_{ip}}{\sqrt{1+\sum_{p=1}^{P}\alpha_{ip}^2}} \qquad \alpha_{ip} = \frac{\lambda_{ip}}{\sqrt{1-\sum_{p=1}^{P}\lambda_{ip}^2}}. \tag{2.3}$$

These equations allow us to study data structures using well-known factor analytic methods and then easily translate the results back into IRT terms. For example, programs for

2 Alternatively, a Jennrich and Bentler (2011) bifactor rotation can be used in place of the Schmid-Leiman. However, because this approach is so new, herein we stick with the more familiar Schmid-Leiman.

estimating multidimensional models such as IRTPRO (Cai, Thissen, & DuToit, 2011), TESTFACT (Bock et al., 2002), and NOHARM (Fraser, 1988; Fraser & McDonald, 1988) routinely provide results in both IRT and ILFA parameters.

These equations provide the grounds for using factor analytic methods to study IRT models. Familiar exploratory factor analytic rotation methods are designed to identify simple structure solutions, but in the direct modeling approach the goal is to identify a comparison model with a bifactor structure where items are free to load on a general and a set of group factors. In short, researchers will not be able to identify an exploratory bifactor structure using standard factor rotation methods such as oblimin or promax. One method that can obtain a bifactor solution is the SL procedure cited earlier. In this study, to obtain SL bifactor solutions, we used the SCHMID routine included in the PSYCH package (Revelle, 2013) of the *R* software program (*R* Development Core Team, 2013).

The SCHMID procedure works as follows. Given a tetrachoric correlation matrix, SCHMID: a) extracts (e.g., minres) a specified number of primary factors, b) performs an oblique factor rotation (e.g., oblimin), c) extracts a higher-order factor from the primary factor correlation matrix, and d) performs a SL orthogonalization to obtain the loadings for each item on the general and group factors. Specifically, assuming that an item loads on only one primary factor, an item's loading on the general factor is simply its loading on the primary factor multiplied by the loading of the primary factor on the general factor. An item's loading on a group factor is simply its loading on the primary factor multiplied by the square root of the disturbance (i.e., the variance of the primary factor that is not explained by the general factor).

The SL is clearly a complex transformation of an oblique factor rotation, and to the extent that the items have simple loading patterns (i.e., no cross-loadings) on the oblique factors, the items will tend to load on one and only one group factor in the SL. To the extent that the items lack a simple structure in an oblique rotation, the loadings in the SL become more complicated to predict as will be demonstrated shortly. Finally, to the extent that the primary factors are correlated, loadings on the general dimension in the SL will tend to be high.

The SL procedure: a) requires that a measure contain at least two (if it is assumed that the primary factors are equally related with the general) but preferably three factors (so that the primary factor correlation matrix can, in turn, be factor analyzed), b) can be affected by the particular choice of extraction and oblique rotation method, and, importantly, c) contains proportionality constraints (see Yung, Thissen, & McLeod, 1999). The proportionality constraints emerge because the group and general loadings in the SL are functions of common elements (i.e., the loading of the primary on the general and the square root of unexplained primary factor variance). Because of these proportionality constraints, we refer to the SL as a "semi-restricted" model.

Our goal of identifying a comparison model would be easy if the SL were capable of recovering a true population loading pattern under a wide variety of conditions. However, because of the proportionality constraints, the factor loadings produced from the SL are biased estimates of their corresponding population values. To demonstrate this, in Table 2.1 we show three contrived examples. In the left-hand set of columns under the "IC: Proportional" label is displayed a true population loading bifactor pattern with all items with equal loadings within factors and group and general factor loadings proportional. In the corresponding bottom portion of Table 2.1 is the result of an SL using minres extraction and oblimin rotation after converting this loading matrix to a correlation matrix. Clearly the SL results perfectly recover the true population loadings in this case.

In the second set of columns in the top half of Table 2.1 we created a small amount of loading variation within the group factors. For example, for group factor one, items 2,

Table 2.1 The Schmid-Leiman Orthogonalization Under Three Conditions

Item	*True Population Structure*											
	IC: Proportional				*IC: Not Proportional*				*IC Basis*			
	Gen	*G1*	*G2*	*G3*	*Gen*	*G1*	*G2*	*G3*	*Gen*	*G1*	*G2*	*G3*
1	.50	.60			.50	.70			.50	.60	.50	
2	.50	.60			.50	.60			.50	.60		
3	.50	.60			.50	.60			.50	.60		
4	.50	.60			.50	.60			.50	.60		
5	.50	.60			.50	.50			.50	.60		
6	.50		.50		.50		.60		.50		.50	.50
7	.50		.50		.50		.50		.50		.50	
8	.50		.50		.50		.50		.50		.50	
9	.50		.50		.50		.50		.50		.50	
10	.50		.50		.50		.40		.50		.50	
11	.50			.40	.50			.50	.50	.50		.40
12	.50			.40	.50			.40	.50			.40
13	.50			.40	.50			.40	.50			.40
14	.50			.40	.50			.40	.50			.40
15	.50			.40	.50			.30	.50			.40
Item	*Schmid-Leiman*											
	Gen	*G1*	*G2*	*G3*	*Gen*	*G1*	*G2*	*G3*	*Gen*	*G1*	*G2*	*G3*
1	.50	.60	.00	.00	.52	.69	.02	.02	.65	.49	.36	.11
2	.50	.60	.00	.00	.50	.60	.00	.00	.49	.61	.01	.02
3	.50	.60	.00	.00	.50	.60	.00	.00	.49	.61	.01	.02
4	.50	.60	.00	.00	.50	.60	.00	.00	.49	.61	.01	.02
5	.50	.60	.00	.00	.48	.52	.02	.03	.49	.61	.01	.02
6	.50	.00	.50	.00	.52	.02	.58	.02	.61	.05	.40	.38
7	.50	.00	.50	.00	.50	.00	.50	.01	.50	.01	.50	.03
8	.50	.00	.50	.00	.50	.00	.50	.01	.50	.01	.50	.03
9	.50	.00	.50	.00	.50	.00	.50	.01	.50	.01	.50	.03
10	.50	.00	.50	.00	.47	.02	.43	.03	.50	.01	.50	.03
11	.50	.00	.00	.40	.52	.02	.02	.47	.56	.45	.05	.33
12	.50	.00	.00	.40	.49	.00	.01	.41	.42	.05	.04	.48
13	.50	.00	.00	.40	.49	.00	.01	.41	.42	.05	.04	.48
14	.50	.00	.00	.40	.49	.00	.01	.41	.42	.05	.04	.48
15	.50	.00	.00	.40	.46	.03	.03	.34	.42	.05	.04	.48

Note: IC indicates independent clusters.

3, and 4 have loadings of 0.60, but item 1 has a loading of 0.70 and item 5 has a loading of 0.50. A similar increase in the loading for the first item and decrease in the loading for the fifth item procedure were used for group factors two and three. In the bottom portion of Table 2.1 are the corresponding SL results. There are two key lessons displayed. First, even with items loading on one and only one group factor (i.e., simple structure in the oblique), if there is variation of loadings within group factors, the factor loadings in the SL do not perfectly recover true population values. Second, depending on the relative size of the group loading, in the SL the general loadings may be overestimated, which results in an underestimation of the group loadings (items 1, 6, and 11). Conversely, loadings on the general factor may be underestimated and overestimated on the group factors (items 5, 10, and 15).

In the third set of columns in Table 2.1, we have added large cross-loadings to items 1, 6, and 11. The SL results shown in the corresponding bottom half of Table 2.1 are informative. Specifically, the effect of a large cross-loading is to, of course, raise an item's communality. In turn, these items have relatively large loadings in the oblimin solution that results in the SL overestimating the loadings on the general factor. In a sense, the general factor is "pulled" toward these items. As a consequence of overestimating the general factor loading, the SL underestimates the loadings on the group factors for these items. In short, the presence of large (> 0.30) cross-loadings: 1) interferes with the ability to identify a simple structure oblique rotation, and 2) results in some items having relatively large loadings on the oblique factors. The end result is that the SL results can systematically underestimate or overestimate the population loadings.

One way to summarize these results is to say, to the extent that the data have a simple structure in an oblique rotation, and loadings do not vary much within factors, the SL is a good estimator of the population loadings. To the extent that the items have large cross-loadings in an oblique rotation, the SL provides biased estimates. We would argue that for well-developed and frequently studied scales, the exploratory and confirmatory factor analytic literature suggests that the structure of psychological measures tends to fall closer to the simple structure model than the many large cross-loadings model.

Regardless of one's view on this issue, the problems with the SL may appear daunting in terms of developing a comparison model. Note that while the exact loadings in the SL may not be precise estimates of their corresponding population values, it can be shown that under a wide range of conditions, the pattern of trivial and nontrivial loadings in an SL is essentially correct. For example, Reise, Moore, and Maydeu-Olivares (2011) demonstrated that when the items have no large cross-loadings, under a wide range of true population general and group factor loading conditions, the SL can suggest a correct target matrix well over 95 percent of the time in sample sizes of 500, and nearly 100 percent of the time when sample size is 1,000 or more.

Given such results, we propose that as a first step in developing a comparison model, exploratory SL analyses be conducted on a matrix of tetrachoric correlations. The purpose of these analyses is not to identify a final comparison model, but rather to: 1) determine the number of item content clusters (i.e., group factors), 2) judge the size of the loadings on general and group factors, 3) identify items with loadings on more than one group factor (i.e., cross-loadings), and finally, 4) identify scale items that do not have meaningful loadings (< 0.30) on the general factor. These latter items should be dropped. Finally, and most importantly, we propose that the SL analysis is a useful tool for defining a target pattern (Browne, 2001) matrix. In turn, we argue that under a range of reasonable conditions, targeted rotation methods yield an appropriate comparison model.

Targeted Factor Rotations

Exploratory factor rotations to a target structure are not new (e.g., Tucker, 1940), but the rotation of a factor pattern to a partially specified target matrix (Browne, 1972, 2001) is only recently gaining attention due to the availability of software packages to implement targeted and other types of nonstandard rotation methods (e.g., *MPLUS*; Muthén & Muthén, 2012; comprehensive exploratory factor analysis, *CEFA*; Browne, Cudeck, Tateneni, & Mels, 2008). In this study, we use the freeware *CEFA* program exclusively. This program allows the user to specify a target pattern matrix where each element in the target factor pattern is treated as either specified (0) or unspecified (?). The resulting matrix "reflects partial knowledge as to what the factor pattern should be" (Browne, 2001, p. 124) and forms the basis for a rotation that minimizes the sum of squared differences between the specified elements of the target and the rotated factor pattern. It is important to recognize that a specified element of a target pattern matrix is not the same as a fixed element in structural equation modeling. In a fixed element, the estimate must equal the specified value, while in a target matrix the exploratory rotation need not match the specified value.

The use of targeted bifactor rotations to derive a comparison model suggests two important questions. The first is, given the limitations of the SL described earlier, how should the SL results be used to form an initial target? In our judgment, it is important to find any nontrivial cross-loading if it exists in the population. Thus, to guard against SL loadings being biased low, we use a very low criterion. Specifically, if in the SL a loading is greater than or equal to 0.15, then the corresponding element of the target matrix is unspecified (?) and if it is less than 0.15 it is specified (0). This criterion is admittedly subjective, but is partially based on knowledge of SL orthogonalization, experience with real data, and Monte Carlo investigation (see Reise, Moore, & Maydeu-Olivares, 2011).

The second question is given a target pattern, how well can the targeted rotation to a bifactor structure recover the true loadings? The answer to this is complicated. There is ample research (de Winter, Dodou, & Wieringa, 2009) suggesting that, at least in the case of continuous variables, factor structures can be well recovered even in very small samples if the data are well structured (i.e., high loadings, all items have simple loadings). On the other hand, the recovery of bifactor loadings in the context of targeted rotations is understudied. Although the Reise, Moore, and Maydeu-Olivares (2011) study suggests reasonable accuracy with sample sizes greater than 500 if the data are well structured and if the target matrix is correct, work remains to: a) consider alternative ILFA estimation strategies, and b) study the effects of mispecifying the target.

Comparison Modeling Demonstrations

In the following, we demonstrate the utility of the direct modeling approach and its limitations through examples. The conceptual framework underlying the following demonstrations derives from McDonald's notion of independent cluster structure (*IC*; McDonald, 1999, 2000). McDonald states, "If all the variables in a common-factor model are simple (i.e., none is complex), the model is said to have *independent clusters* (*IC*) *structure*. If each trait has sufficient simple indicators to yield identifiability, it has an *independent-clusters basis*" (McDonald, 2000, p. 102). In this latter, weaker case, items with complex loadings are allowable, but only if each orthogonal factor is defined by three items that are factorially simple, or each correlated factor has two items that are factorially simple.

In what follows, we demonstrate the fitting of targeted rotations to multidimensional data in order to evaluate the effect of unidimensionality violations. This is not a Monte Carlo study in that we make no attempt to exhaustively evaluate the impact of sets of independent variables as they may impact the accuracy of targeted rotations (see Reise, Moore, & Maydeu-Olivares, 2011). Rather, we select specific conditions that illustrate key principles. In the analyses to follow, we specify a true population factor loading matrix and then we convert that matrix into a true population tetrachoric matrix using the relation

$$\Sigma = \Lambda\Phi\Lambda' + \Psi \tag{2.4}$$

where Σ is the implied correlation matrix for the "hypothetical" latent propensities (i.e., it is an implied tetrachoric matrix), Λ is an $i \times p$ matrix of factor loadings, Φ is a $p \times p$ matrix of factor correlations, and Ψ is a $p \times p$ diagonal matrix of residual variances. In all analyses, we specify a structure with 15 items and ILFA threshold (or IRT intercept) parameters fixed to zero for all items. These parameters are irrelevant to the present approach, which focuses exclusively on the comparison of item loadings (or IRT slopes) under different models.

Independent Cluster Structures

We begin by describing the accuracy of targeted rotations when the data have perfect IC structure. In the first four columns in the top portion of Table 2.2 are population factor loadings for a bifactor structure where the items have general factor loadings of 0.70 (a very strong general trait), and the items all have group factor loadings of 0.40. When this loading pattern is transformed into a correlation matrix, the ratio of first to second eigenvalues is 7.33, clearly essentially unidimensional. In the next column, under the label Uni, are the factor loadings when these multidimensional data are forced into a unidimensional factor model. Observe that because the group factor loadings are equal across items, the effect of forcing this multidimensional structure into a unidimensional framework is to raise all loadings equally, making the items look better as measures of a common trait than they truly are.

The next set of columns displays the SL extraction (minres followed by oblimin rotation) specifying three group factors (zeros are not shown). Notice that the loadings recover the true matrix exactly. This occurs because the items are perfect IC and have the same loadings within general and group factors. If we were to allow variation of loadings within the factors, the SL loading estimates would not replicate the true population model exactly. Given that the SL results perfectly capture the true population matrix, it is not surprising that when the SL results are used as a basis for an initial target matrix, the targeted rotation produced from CEFA recovers the true model with perfect accuracy.

In the bottom portion of Table 2.2, we began with a true population structure where the items have small loadings on the general factor (0.30) and larger loadings on the group factors. In addition, the loadings across the group factors vary from 0.60 (items 1 to 5) to 0.40 (items 11 to 15). In the next column under the Uni heading we see that forcing a unidimensional solution onto these data seriously distorts the loadings. Specifically the factor is pulled toward the items with the highest communalities (i.e., items 1 to 5). Nevertheless, the SL recovers the population pattern perfectly and the resulting targeted rotation is perfect as well. Given that the eigenvalue ratio in Demonstration B is 1.6, the results suggest that a targeted rotation identifies the true relation between items and the common latent trait even if there is only a weak latent dimension. One implication of this result is that scaling individuals on a common dimension using IRT (or factor) models is feasible even if the common trait is weak as long as the multidimensionality is modeled (see also Ip, 2010).

Table 2.2 Demonstrations A & B: Performance of the SL and Targeted Rotation

Item	*Demonstration A: Strong General, Balanced Groups*												
	True Loadings				*Uni*	*Schmid-Leiman*				*Targeted Rotation*			
	General	*G1*	*G2*	*G3*		*General*	*G1*	*G2*	*G3*	*General*	*G1*	*G2*	*G3*
1	.70	.40			.73	.70	.40			.70	.40		
2	.70	.40			.73	.70	.40			.70	.40		
3	.70	.40			.73	.70	.40			.70	.40		
4	.70	.40			.73	.70	.40			.70	.40		
5	.70	.40			.73	.70	.40			.70	.40		
6	.70		.40		.73	.70		.40		.70		.40	
7	.70		.40		.73	.70		.40		.70		.40	
8	.70		.40		.73	.70		.40		.70		.40	
9	.70		.40		.73	.70		.40		.70		.40	
10	.70		.40		.73	.70		.40		.70		.40	
11	.70			.40	.73	.70			.40	.70			.40
12	.70			.40	.73	.70			.40	.70			.40
13	.70			.40	.73	.70			.40	.70			.40
14	.70			.40	.73	.70			.40	.70			.40
15	.70			.40	.73	.70			.40	.70			.40
Item	*Demonstration B: Weak General, Unbalanced Groups*												
	True Loadings				*Uni*	*Schmid-Leiman*				*Targeted Rotation*			
	General	*G1*	*G2*	*G3*		*General*	*G1*	*G2*	*G3*	*General*	*G1*	*G2*	*G3*
1	.30	.60			.62	.30	.60			.30	.60		
2	.30	.60			.62	.30	.60			.30	.60		
3	.30	.60			.62	.30	.60			.30	.60		
4	.30	.60			.62	.30	.60			.30	.60		
5	.30	.60			.62	.30	.60			.30	.60		
6	.30		.50		.27	.30		.50		.30		.50	
7	.30		.50		.28	.30		.50		.30		.50	
8	.30		.50		.27	.30		.50		.30		.50	
9	.30		.50		.28	.30		.50		.30		.50	
10	.30		.50		.28	.30		.50		.30		.50	
11	.30			.40	.23	.30			.40	.30			.40
12	.30			.40	.23	.30			.40	.30			.40
13	.30			.40	.23	.30			.40	.30			.40
14	.30			.40	.23	.30			.40	.30			.40
15	.30			.40	.23	.30			.40	.30			.40

Note: The unidimensional (Uni) model of Demonstration A had a ratio of first to second eigenvalue of 7.33, CFI of 0.93, and RMSEA of 0.09. The unidimensional model of Demonstration B had a ratio of first to second eigenvalues of 1.59, CFI of 0.87, and RMSEA of 0.05.

Independent Cluster Basis

The first set of demonstrations illustrated that when the population tetrachoric correlation matrix is known, the SL followed by a targeted rotation works when the data have a perfect IC structure. The reason is that in the perfect IC case, the SL will nearly always identify the correct pattern of loadings and thus a correct initial target matrix can be specified (see Reise, Moore, & Maydeu-Olivares, 2011). We now consider what occurs when data have an IC basis, that is, at least three items with simple loadings per group factor, but one or more items have cross-loadings. According to McDonald (1999, 2000), if data have an IC basis, the factors are identified and interpretable; the items with simple loadings are "pure" indicators of the dimension while the items with cross-loadings represent "blends" of multiple factors.

In the following, we demonstrate that while the presence of cross-loadings is not necessarily a challenge for targeted rotations, it can affect a researcher's ability to identify a correct target pattern. In the top portion of Table 2.3 is a population factor pattern with all items loading 0.50 on the general factor and 0.50 on a group factor. In addition, we have added one large (0.50) cross-loading for item 1. Consider first the unidimensional factor solution. Because item 1 has the largest communality, the factor loading for item 1 in the unidimensional solution is most inflated relative to its true value. The effect is not limited to this single item, but rather affects all the general factor loadings. Consider that items 6 through 10 have loadings around 0.61 (highly inflated) in the unidimensional solution and items 11 through 15 have loadings around 0.52 (slightly inflated).

Next consider the results in the SL solution. As in the unidimensional solution, the general factor loading for item 1 is again inflated in the SL. Also notice that for item 1, the loadings on the group factors are now underestimated for group factors one and two, and overestimated for group factor three. In addition, for items 2 through 15, all the loadings are more or less wrong compared to their true population values. Nevertheless, although every parameter estimate in the SL solution is wrong, using a criterion of 0.15 for specification, observe in the last set of columns in the top of Table 2.2 that the targeted rotation recovers the true population values exactly. This example illustrates a very important principle, namely, if you correctly specify the initial target matrix, targeted rotations can yield useful comparison models even in the presence of cross-loadings.

In Demonstration D we added more cross-loadings to this structure but have maintained an independent cluster basis. Specifically, items 1 and 2 have 0.40 loadings on group factor two, items 7 and 8 have 0.50 cross-loadings on group factor three, and items 12 and 13 have cross-loadings on group factor one. In the unidimensional solution, items 1, 2, 7, 8, 12, and 13 have relatively inflated loadings and the size of the inflation parallels the size of the cross-loading (or in this case the size of the item's communality). This illustrates that the item's communality in a multidimensional solution has a profound impact on the degree to which the item slope in a unidimensional solution is distorted. The SL loadings are clearly wrong, but because all the relevant SL loadings are above a 0.15 cutoff and all true zero loadings are below, the initial target pattern matrix is correct. In turn, the targeted rotation recovers the true loadings correctly.

Demonstrations C and D illustrate what occurs when the initial target pattern is correctly specified. However, there are conditions under which a data set can have an independent cluster basis, but the size and configuration of cross-loadings can make it nearly impossible for an SL to suggest a reasonable initial target pattern. In Table 2.4 are two sets of true pattern matrices (demonstrations E and F) where there are no cross-loadings on group factor one, four items with cross-loadings on group factor two, and two items with cross-loadings on group factor three. The only difference

Table 2.3 Demonstrations C & D: Performance of the SL and Targeted Rotation

Item	*Demonstration C: Independent Cluster Basis, One Cross-Loading*												
	True Loadings				*Uni*	*Schmid-Leiman*				*Targeted Rotation*			
	Gen	*G1*	*G2*	*G3*		*Gen*	*G1*	*G2*	*G3*	*Gen*	*G1*	*G2*	*G3*
1	.50	.50	.50		.74	.65	.36	.35	.09	.50	.50	.50	
2	.50	.50			.56	.51	.49	.02	.04	.50	.50		
3	.50	.50			.56	.51	.49	.02	.04	.50	.50		
4	.50	.50			.56	.50	.49	.02	.04	.50	.50		
5	.50	.50			.56	.51	.49	.01	.04	.50	.50		
6	.50		.50		.61	.52	.01	.48	.03	.50		.50	
7	.50		.50		.61	.51	.01	.48	.03	.50		.50	
8	.50		.50		.62	.52	.01	.48	.03	.50		.50	
9	.50		.50		.61	.52	.01	.48	.03	.50		.50	
10	.50		.50		.61	.52	.01	.48	.03	.50		.50	
11	.50			.50	.52	.44	.01	.01	.55	.50			.50
12	.50			.50	.53	.45	.01	.01	.55	.50			.50
13	.50			.50	.53	.45	.01	.01	.55	.50			.50
14	.50			.50	.53	.45	.01	.01	.55	.50			.50
15	.50			.50	.52	.45	.01	.01	.55	.50			.50
Item	*Demonstration D: Independent Cluster Basis, Six Unbalanced Cross-Loadings*												
	True Loadings				*Uni*	*Schmid-Leiman*				*Targeted Rotation*			
	Gen	*G1*	*G2*	*G3*		*Gen*	*G1*	*G2*	*G3*	*Gen*	*G1*	*G2*	*G3*
1	.50	.50	.40		.68	.56	.51	.28	.03	.50	.50	.40	
2	.50	.50	.40		.68	.56	.51	.28	.03	.50	.50	.40	
3	.50	.50			.53	.43	.55	.05	.09	.50	.50		
4	.50	.50			.53	.43	.56	.05	.09	.50	.50		
5	.50	.50			.53	.43	.55	.05	.08	.50	.50		
6	.50		.50		.57	.48	.11	.49	.02	.50		.50	
7	.50		.50	.50	.77	.65	.06	.43	.35	.50		.50	.50
8	.50		.50	.50	.77	.65	.06	.44	.35	.50		.50	.50
9	.50		.50		.57	.47	.11	.49	.02	.50		.50	
10	.50		.50		.57	.48	.11	.49	.02	.50		.50	
11	.50			.50	.58	.48	.01	.03	.50	.50			.50
12	.50	.30		.50	.68	.56	.22	.05	.48	.50	.30		.50
13	.50	.30		.50	.68	.56	.22	.05	.48	.50	.30		.50
14	.50			.50	.59	.48	.01	.03	.50	.50			.50
15	.50			.50	.59	.49	.01	.03	.50	.50			.50

Note: The unidimensional (Uni) model of Demonstration C had a ratio of first to second eigenvalue of 3.08, CFI of 0.82, and RMSEA of 0.10. The unidimensional model of Demonstration D had a ratio of first to second eigenvalues of 3.74, CFI of 0.81, and RMSEA of 0.12.

between the true pattern matrices in the top and bottom portions of Table 2.4 is the size of the cross-loading, namely, 0.50 versus 0.30.

In both demonstrations, the size of the factor loading in the unidimensional solution is inflated, especially for items 7, 8, 12, and 13. Items 1 and 2 also have inflated loadings but not to the same degree as the other items. To understand this, it must be recognized that because of the pattern of cross-loadings (i.e., none on group factor one, four on group factor two and two on group factor three), the unidimensional solution is being pulled toward what is in common among group factors two and three.

Inspection of the SL loading patterns for demonstrations E and F is informative. In demonstration E where the cross-loadings are 0.50 (as large as the group and general factor loadings), the SL loadings are clearly not good estimators of their population values. More importantly, using a 0.15 cutoff, the resulting target pattern matrix is wrong in several ways. In turn, although the target rotation recovers the general factor loadings perfectly, the group factor loadings are in error. On the other hand, when this same pattern of cross-loadings is lowered to a value of 0.30 (demonstration F), the SL results in an accurate target and the targeted rotation recovers the population solution perfectly. The critical lesson to be learned here is that if cross-loadings are numerous and sizable, great caution should be used in applying target rotations. On the other hand, it is hard to foresee a situation where real data have such a structure and a researcher would still be interested in applying any IRT model.

Application

The demonstrations featured earlier in this chapter illustrated some key points of direct modeling but relied entirely on ILFA methods. However, the main focus of comparison modeling is on evaluating the effects of multidimensionality on IRT item parameter slope estimates. It is these parameters that are critically affected by multidimensionality violations. Thus for a final demonstration, we will conduct a real data analysis to illustrate how comparison modeling can be used in considering the application of unidimensional IRT models. A secondary goal of this real data analysis is to illustrate that although ILFA and IRT parameters are simple transforms (Equation 2.3), in multidimensional models equivalent IRT and ILFA models can appear very different in terms of data structure.

The data used for illustration is a correlation matrix taken directly from Mohlman and Zinbarg (2000, p. 446). The correlation matrix was derived from item responses to a 16-item scale called the Anxiety Sensitivity Index (ASI; Peterson & Reiss, 1992). In the article, the authors used confirmatory factor analysis to demonstrate that this scale is consistent with a bifactor structure with items loading on a general (anxiety sensitivity) and three group factors (social, physical, and mental incapacitation).

This scale is ideal for our purposes because, as the authors note, much debate exists in the literature as to whether this measure is unidimensional or consists of multiple correlated sub-domains. Relatedly, researchers debate whether the measure can produce meaningful subscale scores. In our view, such debates are a very common situation in psychology, namely, a scale that produces item response matrices that are consistent with both unidimensional and multidimensional models and researchers debating whether to score the scale as a whole or as subscales.

Using the reported correlation matrix, in the first column of the top portion of Table 2.5 are the factor loadings from a unidimensional solution (minres extraction). Clearly, all the items have reasonable loadings on a single factor and the first to second eigenvalue ratio of 7.2/1.4 suggests a single "strong" common factor. In the corresponding bottom portion are the IRT loadings. In the unidimensional case, factor loadings and IRT slopes are

Table 2.4 Demonstrations E & F: Performance of the SL and Targeted Rotation

Item	*Demonstration E: Second Group Factor Dominated by Cross-Loadings*												
	True Loadings				*Uni*	*Schmid-Leiman*				*Targeted Rotation*			
	Gen	*G1*	*G2*	*G3*		*Gen*	*G1*	*G2*	*G3*	*Gen*	*G1*	*G2*	*G3*
1	.50	.50	.50		.69	.72	.33	.18	.29	.50	.50	.35	.35
2	.50	.50	.50		.69	.72	.32	.18	.29	.50	.50	.35	.35
3	.50	.50			.42	.58	.38	.06	.11	.50	.50		
4	.50	.50			.42	.58	.38	.06	.11	.50	.50		
5	.50	.50			.42	.59	.38	.06	.11	.50	.50		
6	.50		.50		.62	.46	.08	.38	.30	.50		.35	.35
7	.50		.50	.50	.83	.51	.01	.69	.03	.50		.71	
8	.50		.50	.50	.83	.51	.01	.69	.03	.50		.71	
9	.50		.50		.63	.46	.08	.38	.30	.50		.35	.35
10	.50		.50		.62	.46	.08	.38	.30	.50		.35	.35
11	.50			.50	.55	.37	.05	.46	.37	.50		.35	-.35
12	.50		.50	.50	.84	.51	.01	.70	.03	.50		.71	
13	.50		.50	.50	.83	.51	.00	.69	.03	.50		.70	
14	.50			.50	.56	.37	.05	.46	.38	.50		.35	-.35
15	.50			.50	.56	.37	.05	.46	.37	.50		.35	-.35
Item	*Demonstration F: Second Group Factor Dominated by Weak Cross-Loadings*												
	True Loadings				*Uni*	*Schmid-Leiman*				*Targeted Rotation*			
	Gen	*G1*	*G2*	*G3*		*Gen*	*G1*	*G2*	*G3*	*Gen*	*G1*	*G2*	*G3*
1	.50	.50	.30		.63	.54	.51	.16	.04	.50	.50	.30	
2	.50	.50	.30		.63	.54	.51	.16	.04	.50	.50	.30	
3	.50	.50			.49	.41	.58	.05	.05	.50	.50		
4	.50	.50			.49	.41	.57	.05	.05	.50	.50		
5	.50	.50			.49	.41	.58	.05	.05	.50	.50		
6	.50		.50		.62	.56	.07	.42	.02	.50		.50	
7	.50		.50	.30	.72	.64	.01	.36	.21	.50		.50	.30
8	.50		.50	.30	.72	.64	.01	.36	.21	.50		.50	.30
9	.50		.50		.62	.56	.07	.41	.01	.50		.50	
10	.50		.50		.61	.56	.07	.41	.01	.50		.50	
11	.50			.50	.56	.47	.05	.03	.52	.50			.50
12	.50		.30	.50	.70	.61	.01	.18	.43	.50		.30	.50
13	.50		.30	.50	.70	.60	.01	.18	.43	.50		.30	.50
14	.50			.50	.56	.47	.05	.03	.52	.50			.50
15	.50			.50	.56	.47	.05	.03	.53	.50			.50

Note: The unidimensional model of Demonstration E had a ratio of first to second eigenvalue of 3.74, CFI of 0.85, and RMSEA of 0.11. The unidimensional model of Demonstration F had a ratio of first to second eigenvalues of 3.46, CFI of 0.88, and RMSEA of 0.09.

simply nonlinear transforms (Equation 2.3) and the interpretation is completely symmetric: items with relatively large loadings on a single factor have high slopes and vice versa.

In the next set of columns are the SL (minres extraction, oblimin rotation) factor loadings (top) and corresponding IRT slope parameters (bottom). Inspection of SL loadings reveals that all items load highly on the general factor. In addition 12 of the 16 items appear to have simple loading patterns on the group factors. The exceptions are items 3, 8, 12, and 14. These cross-loading items illustrate a challenge to the comparison modeling approach. Specifically, although the loadings are above a 0.15 cutoff, several of these items appear not to load well on any group factor and sometimes a loading just barely misses the cutoff (item 3 group factor one). These types of patterns certainly call for judgment in specifying a target. Of course, there is nothing wrong with trying alternative targets and inspecting how that impacts the results.

Sticking with our 0.15 criterion for specifying a target, the target rotation is shown in the last set of columns in Table 2.5. Notice first that some cells that were unspecified (?) in the target had near zero loadings in the targeted rotation (e.g., item 8). This illustrates a kind of self-correcting nature of targeted rotations and is an advantage over confirmatory procedures. Second, notice that the IRT and ILFA results are not symmetrical. For example, the bottom of Table 2.5 shows that in an unrestricted IRT bifactor model, items 1 and 2 have equal slopes on the general factor. However, they have different general factor loadings in the ILFA bifactor model. This is not a math error. Close inspection of Equation 2.3 reveals that in converting from ILFA to IRT, the communality of the item must be considered. Thus, in a multidimensional factor solution, a researcher must be cognizant that the IRT slopes may not convey the same message as the factor loadings, even when the models are completely equivalent.

This non-symmetry of interpretation of parameters in multidimensional models does not imply that the effects are incomparable across the two models. Indeed, it is easy to confirm that data generated under the target factor rotation in the top portion of Table 2.5 will produce estimated IRT parameters similar to the corresponding IRT values in the bottom portion of Table 2.5 and vice versa. Moreover, programs for estimating multidimensional models such as EQSIRT (Wu & Bentler, 2011), IRTPRO (Cai, Thissen, & du Toit, 2011), TESTFACT (Bock et al., 2002), and NOHARM (Fraser, 1988; Fraser & McDonald, 1988) routinely provide results in both IRT and ILFA metrics using the exact transforms in this study. Nevertheless, because of this non-symmetry of interpretation, we recommend that final model comparisons be made solely on the IRT parameters. This is sensible given the fact that it is the IRT model that is actually being considered for application.

The final step of direct modeling is to address the key question, are the item slopes in the unidimensional model distorted by multidimensionality or not? A comparison of the slopes from the restricted unidimensional model with the slopes from the general factor of the unrestricted bifactor model suggests in this case the answer is no. Despite the multidimensionality, a unidimensional IRT model could be fit to this data without distorting the parameters to a significant degree. The one exception may be item 9, which has a slope of 0.97 in the unidimensional model but a slope of 1.48 on the general in the bifactor. Finally, an inspection of the slopes on the group factors suggests that a researcher would be hard pressed to gain reliable information from subscales (group factors) that is independent of the general factor. In short, breaking this scale down and scoring subscales is not recommended (see Reise, Bonifay, & Haviland, 2013, for further discussion).

Discussion

Commonly applied IRT models are unidimensional; that is, item responses are assumed locally independent (Equation 2.2) after controlling for one common factor. However,

Table 2.5 Example Data Analysis

Item	*Item–Level Factor Analysis*								
	Uni	*Schmid–Leiman*				*Target Rotation*			
	λ	λ_g	λ_1	λ_2	λ_3	λ_g	λ_1	λ_2	λ_3
1	.55	.51	.00	.02	**.47**	.56	.02	.00	**.43**
2	.59	.51	.03	**.58**	.01	.49	.04	**.61**	.02
3	.71	.64	.14	**.17**	**.24**	.71	.04	.10	.05
4	.61	.56	**.24**	.04	.20	.65	.10	–.13	–.03
5	.40	.38	.00	.03	**.37**	.37	.05	.01	**.62**
6	.75	.71	**.42**	.04	.08	.71	**.42**	–.04	.08
7	.53	.48	.06	.06	**.31**	.53	.00	.02	**.21**
8	.71	.64	**.18**	.14	**.20**	.73	.06	.04	–.02
9	.70	.66	**.44**	.06	.09	.57	**.71**	.14	.05
10	.73	.70	**.47**	.02	.02	.72	**.39**	–.06	–.10
11	.64	.59	**.29**	.08	.06	.61	**.23**	.05	–.04
12	.68	.60	.05	**.26**	**.24**	.66	–.02	**.21**	.10
13	.64	.56	.05	**.37**	.12	.59	.01	**.33**	.02
14	.72	.64	.11	**.16**	**.29**	.76	–.08	.06	.01
15	.58	.51	.02	**.58**	.08	.47	.09	**.63**	.01
16	.73	.64	.03	**.46**	.13	.69	–.05	**.42**	–.03
Item	*Item Response Theory*								
	α	α_g	α_1	α_2	α_3	α_g	α_1	α_2	α_3
1	0.66	0.71	0.01	0.03	0.65	0.79	–0.03	0.00	0.61
2	0.73	0.81	0.05	0.91	0.01	0.79	0.06	0.98	0.03
3	1.02	0.91	0.20	0.24	0.34	1.02	0.06	0.14	0.07
4	0.77	0.73	0.32	0.05	0.26	0.88	0.13	–0.18	–0.04
5	0.44	0.44	0.00	0.03	0.44	0.54	0.07	0.01	0.90
6	1.14	1.29	0.76	0.06	0.15	1.27	0.75	–0.07	0.14
7	0.63	0.59	0.07	0.07	0.38	0.65	0.00	0.02	0.26
8	1.02	0.91	0.26	0.2	0.29	1.07	0.09	0.06	–0.03
9	0.97	1.10	0.73	0.1	0.14	1.48	1.84	0.36	0.13
10	1.07	1.29	0.87	0.04	0.03	1.28	0.69	–0.11	–0.18
11	0.83	0.78	0.38	0.11	0.07	0.81	0.30	0.07	–0.05
12	0.92	0.84	0.08	0.37	0.34	0.92	–0.03	0.29	0.14
13	0.82	0.76	0.06	0.5	0.16	0.80	0.01	0.45	0.03
14	1.03	0.93	0.16	0.24	0.43	1.18	–0.12	0.09	0.02
15	0.71	0.80	0.02	0.91	0.12	0.77	0.15	1.03	0.02
16	1.06	1.07	0.05	0.77	0.22	1.18	–0.09	0.72	–0.05

many psychological constructs have substantive breadth and thus their measures have heterogeneous item content that results in multidimensional item response data. The standard paradigm in IRT applications, building on Monte Carlo simulation research, is to use a combination of SEM fit indices, residual values, and eigenvalue ratios to judge whether data are unidimensional enough for IRT. Once a data set is deemed acceptable under these criteria, IRT applications proceed under the assumption that the item parameters are correct.

A notable concern with this standard approach is that the researcher cannot be confident that the common target latent trait is identified correctly or that the estimated item parameters properly reflect the relation between item responses and the common latent trait. Thus, we propose a complementary "comparison modeling" approach that allows researchers to estimate the degree to which multidimensionality interferes with the ability to obtain good item parameter estimates under unidimensional IRT models. Our approach is consistent with the evaluation of essential unidimensionality (Stout, 1990) that assumes: a) the existence of a common trait running among the items, and b) multidimensionality arises through sampling items from diverse content domains. However, the testing of essential unidimensionality focuses on distortion of trait level estimates, not item parameters.

In our view, a useful approach to judging whether a measure is appropriately modeled by unidimensional IRT is to compare item slope parameter estimates when multidimensionality is modeled (unrestricted model) versus not (unidimensional restricted model). The suggestion that fitting multidimensional models provides added value over traditional analysis is not new. Ackerman (1989, 1992, 2005) demonstrated the utility of multidimensional IRT in multiple contexts including DIF assessment and judging an instrument's measurement fidelity. Moreover, as cited earlier, several researchers have suggested evaluating the unidimensionality assumption by explicit comparison of unidimensional models with multidimensional alternatives (e.g., Bartolucci, 2007; Christensen et al., 2002; Reise, Morizot, & Hays, 2007).

Most interesting and relevant to our work is Ip's recent study that shows that "a multidimensional item response theory model is empirically indistinguishable from a locally dependent unidimensional model of which the single dimension represents the actual construct of interest" (Ip, 2010, p. 1). Ip's work suggests that multidimensionality in the item response data need not require the application of multidimensional IRT models. Our direct modeling approach is very similar to Ip's with the exception that we require local dependencies to be modeled by a bifactor structure while his locally dependent unidimensional models do not necessarily require such an identified formal structure.

Specifically, the comparison modeling approach involves the following steps: 1) Fit a unidimensional item-level factor model and convert the factor loadings to IRT slope parameters. This is labeled the "restricted" model; 2) Use a Schmid-Leiman (Schmid & Leiman, 1957) orthogonalization to find a plausible and identified bifactor structure with one general and two (but preferably three) or more identified group factors; 3) Use the factor loadings from the SL orthogonalization to suggest a target pattern matrix of specified and unspecified elements; 4) Based on the target matrix conduct a targeted pattern rotation (Browne, 2001) to a bifactor structure; 5) Convert the resulting targeted pattern rotation matrix to IRT slope parameters. This is called the "unrestricted" or "comparison" model; and 6) Compare the estimated IRT slopes from the unidimensional model (restricted) with the slopes on the general factor from the bifactor (unrestricted) solution.

These steps suggest two major questions: 1) Under what conditions does the direct modeling approach correctly identify an appropriate comparison model? and 2) How should a researcher use the results in applied work? This latter question can be rephrased as, when does multidimensionality truly matter? In the following we address these issues in turn.

Strengths and Limitations of Comparison Modeling

The overarching virtue of the comparison modeling approach is that, if the comparison model (or models) is plausible and accurate, a researcher can directly judge the impact of multidimensionality on unidimensional IRT parameters. However, there are several steps in developing the comparison model: a) estimating a tetrachoric correlation matrix, b) identifying the number of group factors, c) selecting an extraction and rotation method for implementing the SL, d) using the SL to specify a target pattern, and e) using software (e.g., *CEFA*) to perform a target rotation. Each of these steps presents its own unique set of challenges. Rather than tediously reviewing potential pitfalls of each step, we offer the following summaries.

First, the comparison modeling approach outlined here is not appropriate for identifying small model violations such as a single item pair that displays a local dependence violation. Such violations are usually obvious and easily solved by deleting an item. Second, comparison modeling will not work if the data do not have at least an IC basis (i.e., group factors identified). Finally, comparison modeling will also not be productive on measures with highly narrow item content (i.e., the scale consists of essentially the same question asked repeatedly with slightly different content). In contrast, comparison modeling works best when item content is diverse and multidimensionality is well structured, that is, caused by the inclusion of multiple items that share similar content drawn from different content domains.

In addition, our research (Reise, Moore, & Maydeu-Olivares, 2011) suggests that comparison modeling is optimal when: a) sample size is more than 500, b) the data are well structured (not many large cross-loadings), and c) items have strong loadings on the general and group factors. Although reasonable minds may disagree about the possibility of independent cluster structures (see Church & Burke, 1994; Marsh et al., 2009), our view is that such conditions exist for many psychological scales and thus comparison modeling will be of wide interest. That is, scales like the ASI analyzed in this report, where researchers debate unidimensionality versus multidimensionality, are common. For such measures, the comparison modeling approach may not only inform the application of an IRT model, but also help inform the decision to score subscales or not. In other words, by virtue of estimating slopes for items on group factors, the bifactor model provides important information regarding how discriminating an item is with respect to a content domain, independent of its contribution to the general construct.

In closing this section, it is clear that a comparison model plays a critically important role. Nevertheless, we argue that the comparison model does not necessarily have to precisely reflect the true population model (if there really is such a thing). Rather, it must be a plausible, identifiable, multidimensional alternative to the more restricted unidimensional model. Many data sets may be consistent with several alternative multidimensional models. Despite the existence of dozens of approaches to identifying the dimensionality of a data matrix, there is no magic formula that can guarantee the identification of the "correct" number of latent dimensions or group factors in our case. We agree with de Winter, Dodou, and Wieringa, who argue that the structural modeling literature suggests that "it is better to think in terms of 'most appropriate' than 'correct' number of factors" (de Winter, Dodou, & Wieringa, 2009, p. 176).

Using Comparison Modeling With Real Data: When Is Multidimensionality Ignorable?

An often repeated phrase in standard texts and review articles is that IRT models are useful to the degree to which they fit item response data. It would follow that whenever multidimensional data are forced into IRT (Model A), the estimated model parameters must be distorted in some way, and any applications based on those parameters are suspect. Multidimensionality matters the most when the parameters obtained with a unidimensional model do not truly reflect the relations among items and the common target latent dimension. When said parameters are distorted, the information functions and trait level estimates are wrong, and linking and DIF analyses are highly questionable.

In comparison modeling the degree to which unidimensional parameters are wrong is judged by comparison of estimated slope parameters from restricted and unrestricted models. We cannot offer precise guidelines or even rules of thumb for deciding when an observed difference is a meaningful difference. The reason is that the consequences of a difference depend on many factors. For example, when scaling individual differences, even large slope differences may not matter; but when conducting linking or DIF analysis, even small differences may be highly consequential. The applied importance of a parameter difference also depends on the size of the parameter. For example, because it is the highly discriminating items that do the heavy lifting in a measurement application, a difference in slope of 0.5 matters much more when the difference is between items with slopes of 1.5 and 1.0 than it does between items with slopes between 0.3 and 0.8.

The bottom line of comparison modeling is that the researcher must make one of three decisions. First, the slope parameter differences between the restricted and unrestricted models may be small and after inspecting item and scale information functions under unidimensional and bifactor models, might conclude that the unidimensional model is "good enough." The virtue of the comparison modeling approach is that after fitting the multidimensional alternative, the researcher now has strong evidence to support the claim that the unidimensional model is sufficient. For example, in the demonstration reported here on the ASI scale, we concluded that a unidimensional model is acceptable despite the obvious and interpretable multidimensionality. The fact that slopes change very little between the unidimensional and the general factor of the bifactor comparison model supports this contention strongly.

A second alternative is to conclude that in the unidimensional model the item slopes are too distorted by multidimensionality to be useful in any meaningful application. Alternatively, a researcher may simply argue that the unrestricted model "fits" better than a unidimensional model, and by virtue of modeling the multidimensionality, better reflects the relation between items and common latent trait. In either case the researcher may decide to simply use the multidimensional model as a basis for applications. However, there are good reasons why, to date, multidimensional models have not replaced unidimensional IRT models in applied contexts.

Relative to a unidimensional model: a) it is much harder to use multidimensional models as bases for applications (e.g., determining which item to administer in CAT can be greatly complicated when considering multiple dimensions simultaneously), b) the item parameters in multidimensional models are more challenging to interpret (e.g., the location parameter in MIRT compared to IRT) and, c) in order to fully understand an item's functioning, new indices, such as multidimensional discrimination, need to be calculated (Reckase & McKinley, 1991). On the other hand, Segall (2001) has shown the beneficial effects of using multidimensional models, such as a bifactor, to score individuals appropriately on the general trait. This approach is a nice compromise because it focuses on the general trait that researchers are most interested in while at the same time recognizing and making full use of the multidimensional data structure.

The third option is to conclude that the data have no interpretable structure, either unidimensional or multidimensional, and that even if a few items were deleted from the scale, the data are not analyzable under any parametric latent variable modeling framework. For example, there are many small two-item unidentified group factors (i.e., no IC basis), large cross-loadings, murky dimensionality, and so on. Such scales are more likely found among older measures not developed through factor analytic techniques or subject to the repeated scrutiny of confirmatory factor analyses. In such cases, a researcher would not want to force a latent variable measurement framework onto an inappropriate data structure.

Summary

We proposed a comparison modeling procedure for evaluating the impact of multidimensionality on the parameter estimates of unidimensional IRT models. The approach centers around the comparison of estimated slope parameters from a unidimensional model with slope parameters from an unrestricted bifactor model derived from a target rotation (Browne, 2001). Like all latent variable modeling procedures, the method arguably works best when the data are well structured (e.g., an IC loading pattern). However, we would argue that even in situations where the methodology is less effective in achieving a definitive comparison model, the process of considering multidimensional alternatives, and learning how item parameters may change under different models, is highly informative in its own right. We suggest that in any proposed unidimensional IRT application, alternative multidimensional models be reported as a complement to traditional indices such as eigenvalue ratios, fit indices, or residuals.

Author Notes: This work was supported by: the NIH Roadmap for Medical Research Grant AR052177 (PI: David Cella); and the Consortium for Neuropsychiatric Phenomics, NIH Roadmap for Medical Research Grants UL1-DE019580 (PI: Robert Bilder), and RL1DA024853 (PI: Edythe London). The content is solely the responsibility of the authors and does not necessarily represent the official views of the funding agencies.

References

Ackerman, T. A. (1989). Unidimensional IRT calibration of compensatory and noncompensatory multidimensional items. *Applied Psychological Measurement, 13*, 113–127.

Ackerman, T. A. (1992). A didactic explanation of item bias, item impact, and item validity from a multidimensional perspective. *Journal of Educational Measurement, 29*, 67–91.

Ackerman, T. A. (2005). Multidimensional item response theory modeling. In A. Maydeu-Olivares & J. J. McArdle (Eds.). *Contemporary psychometrics*. Mahwah, NJ: Erlbaum (pp. 3–26).

Ackerman, T. A., Gierl, M. J., & Walker, C. M. (2003). Using multidimensional item response theory to evaluate educational and psychological tests. *Educational Measurement: Issues and Practice, 22*, 37–53.

Ansley, T. N., & Forsyth, R. A. (1985). An examination of the characteristics of unidimensional IRT parameter estimates derived from two-dimensional data. *Applied Psychological Measurement, 9*, 37–48.

Bartolucci, F. (2007). A class of multidimensional IRT models for testing unidimensionality and clustering items. *Psychometrika, 72*, 141–157.

Batley, R. M., & Boss, M. W. (1993). The effects on parameter estimation of correlated dimensions and a distribution-restricted trait in a multidimensional item response model. *Applied Psychological Measurement, 17*, 131–141.

Bock, R. D., Gibbons, R., Schilling, S. G., Muraki, E., Wilson, D. T., & Wood, R. (2002). TESTFACT 4 [Computer Program]. Chicago, IL: Scientific Software International.

Bollen, K., & Lennox, R. (1991). Conventional wisdom on measurement: A structural equation perspective. *Psychological Bulletin, 110*(2), 305.

Browne, M. W. (1972). Orthogonal rotation to a partially specified target. *British Journal of Mathematical and Statistical Psychology, 25*, 115–120.

Browne, M.W. (2001). An overview of analytic rotation in exploratory factor analysis. *Multivariate Behavioral Research, 35*, 111–150.

Browne, M.W., Cudeck, R., Tateneni, K., & Mels, G. (2008). CEFA: Comprehensive exploratory factor analysis, Version 2.00 [Computer software and manual]. Retrieved from http://quantrm2.psy.ohio-state.edu/browne/.

Brunner, M., Nagy, G., & Wilhelm, O. (2012). A tutorial on hierarchically structured constructs. *Journal of Personality, 80*, 796–846.

Cai, L., Thissen, D., & du Toit, S. (2011). IRTPRO 2.1 for Windows. Chicago, IL: Scientific Software International.

Chen, F.F., West, S.G., & Sousa, K.H. (2006). A comparison of bifactor and second-order models of quality-of-life. *Multivariate Behavioral Research, 41*, 189–225.

Christensen, K.B., Bjorner, J.B., Kreiner, S., & Petersen, J.H. (2002). Testing unidimensionality in polytomous Rasch models. *Psychometrika, 67*, 563–574.

Church, T.A., & Burke, P.J. (1994). Exploratory and confirmatory tests of the big five and Tellegen's three and four-dimensional models. *Journal of Personality and Social Psychology, 66*, 93–114.

Clark, L.A., & Watson, D. (1995). Constructing validity: Basic issues in objective scale development. *Psychological Assessment, 7*, 309–319.

De Ayala, R.J. (1994). The influence of multidimensionality on the graded response model. *Applied Psychological Measurement, 18*, 155–170.

DeMars, C.E. (2006). Application of the bi-factor multidimensional item response theory model to testlet-based tests. *Journal of Educational Measurement, 43*, 145–168.

De Winter, J.C.F., Dodou, D., & Wieringa, P. A. (2009). Exploratory factor analysis with small sample sizes. *Multivariate Behavioral Research, 44*, 147–181.

Drasgow, F., & Parsons, C.K. (1983). Application of unidimensional item response theory models to multidimensional data. *Applied Psychological Measurement, 7*, 189–199.

Embretson, S.E., & Reise, S.P. (2000). *Item response theory for psychologists.* Mahwah, NJ: Erlbaum.

Folk, V.G., & Green, B.F. (1989). Adaptive estimation when the unidimensionality assumption of IRT is violated. *Applied Psychological Measurement, 13*, 373–389.

Fraser, C. (1988). NOHARM: Computer software and manual. Australia: Author.

Fraser, C., & McDonald, R. P. (1988). NOHARM: Least squares item factor analysis. *Multivariate Behavioral Research, 23*(2), 267–269.

Gibbons, R.D., & Hedeker, D.R. (1992). Full-information item bi-factor analysis. *Psychometrika, 57*, 3, 423–436.

Hambleton, R.K., & Swaminathan, H. (1985). *Item response theory: Principles and applications.* Boston, MA: Kluwer-Nijhoff.

Hattie, J. (1985). Methodology review: Assessing unidimensionality of tests and items. *Applied Psychological Measurement, 9*, 139–164.

Holzinger, K.J., & Swineford, R. (1937). The bifactor method. *Psychometrika, 2*, 41–54.

Hull, J.G., Lehn, D.A., & Tedlie, J.C. (1991). A general approach to testing multifaceted personality constructs. *Journal of Personality and Social Psychology, 61*, 932–945.

Humphreys, L.G. (1970). A skeptical look at the factor pure test. In C.E. Lunneborg (Ed.) *Current problems and techniques in multivariate psychology: Proceedings of a conference honoring Professor Paul Horst* (pp. 23–32). Seattle: University of Washington.

Ip, E.H. (2010). Empirically indistinguishable multidimensional IRT and locally dependent unidimensional item response models. *British Journal of Mathematical and Statistical Psychology, 63*, 395–416.

Jennrich, R.I., & Bentler, P.M. (2011). Exploratory bi-factor analysis. *Psychometrika, 76, 537–549.*

Kirisci, L., Hsu, T., & Yu, L. (2001). Robustness of item parameter estimation programs to assumptions of unidimensionality and normality. *Applied Psychological Measurement, 25*, 146–162.

Knol, D. L., & Berger, M. P. F. (1991). Empirical comparison between factor analysis and multidimensional item response models. *Multivariate Behavioral Research*, *26*, 457–477.

Knott, M., & Bartholomew, D. J. (1999). *Latent variable models and factor analysis* (No. 7). Edward Arnold.

Marsh, H. W., Muthén, B., Asparouhov, T., Ludtke, O., Robitzsch, A., Morin, A. J. S, & Trautwein, U. (2009). Exploratory structural equations modeling, integrating CFA and EFA: Application to students' evaluations of university teaching. *Structural Equation Modeling*, *16*, 439–476.

McDonald, R. P. (1981). The dimensionality of tests and items. *British Journal of Mathematical and Statistical Psychology*, *34*, 100–117.

McDonald, R. P. (1982). Linear versus non-linear models in latent trait theory. *Applied Psychological Measurement*, *6*, 379–396.

McDonald, R. P. (1999). *Test theory: A unified treatment*. Psychology Press.

McDonald, R. P. (2000). A basis for multidimensional item response theory. *Applied Psychological Measurement*, *24*(2), 99–114.

McDonald, R. P., & Mok, M. M. C. (1995). Goodness of fit in item response models. *Multivariate Behavioral Research*, *30*(1), 23–40.

McLeod, L. D., Swygert, K. A., & Thissen, D. (2001). *Factor analysis for items scored in two categories*. In D. Thissen & H. Wainer (Eds.). *Test scoring* (pp. 189–216). Mahwah, NJ: Erlbaum.

Mohlman, J., & Zinbarg, R. E. (2000). The structure and correlates of anxiety sensitivity in older adults. *Psychological Assessment*, *12*, 440–446.

Muthén, L. K., & Muthén, B. O. (2012). *Mplus: Statistical Analysis with Latent Variables (Version 4.21)* [Computer software]. Los Angeles: Author.

Peterson, R. A., & Reiss, S. (1992). *Anxiety sensitivity index manual* (2nd ed.). Worthington, OH: International Diagnostic Systems.

R Development Core Team (2013). *R: A language and environment for statistical computing. R Foundation for Statistical Computing*, Vienna, Austria. ISBN 3–900051–07–0, URL www.R-project.org.

Reckase, M. D. (1979). Unifactor latent trait models applied to multifactor tests: Results and implications. *Journal of Educational Statistics*, *4*, 207–230.

Reckase, M. D., & McKinley, R. L. (1991). The discriminating power of items that measure more than one dimension. *Applied Psychological Measurement*, *15*, 401–412.

Reeve, B. B., Hays, R. D., Bjorner, J. B., et al. (2007). Psychometric evaluation and calibration of health-related quality of life item banks: Plans for the Patient-Reported Outcomes Measurement Information System (PROMIS). *Medical Care*, *45 Suppl 1*, S22–S31.

Reise, S. P., Bonifay, W. E., & Haviland, M. G. (2013). Scoring and modeling psychological measures in the presence of multidimensionality. *Journal of Personality Assessment*, *95*, 129–140.

Reise, S. P., Moore, T. M., & Maydeu-Olivares, A. (2011). Targeted bifactor rotations and assessing the impact of model violations on the parameters of unidimensional and bifactor models. *Journal of Educational and Psychological Measurement*, *71*, 684–711.

Reise, S. P., Morizot, J., & Hays, R. D. (2007). The role of the bifactor model in resolving dimensionality issues in health outcomes measures. *Quality of Life Research*, *16*, 19–31.

Reise, S. P., Scheines, R., Widaman, K. F., & Haviland, M. G. (2013). Multidimensionality and structural coefficient bias in structural equation modeling: A bifactor perspective. *Educational and Psychological Measurement*, *73*, 5–26.

Revelle, W. (2013). Psych: Procedures for psychological, psychometric, and personality research. R package version 1.3–2. http://personality-project.org/r, http://personality-project.org/r/psych.manual.pdf.

Schmid, J., & Leiman, J. (1957). The development of hierarchical factor solutions. *Psychometrika*, *22*, 53–61.

Segall, D. O. (2001). General ability measurement: An application of multidimensional item response theory. *Psychometrika*, *66*, 79–97.

Steinberg, L., & Thissen, D. (1996). Uses of item response theory and the testlet concept in the measurement of psychopathology. *Psychological Methods*, *1*, 81–97.

Stout, W. F. (1990). A new item response theory modeling approach with applicaitons to unidimensionality assessment and ability estimation. *Psychometrika*, *55*, 293–325.

Takane, Y., & de Leeuw, J. (1987). On the relationship between item response theory and factor analysis of discretized variables. *Psychometrika*, *52*, 393–408.

Ten Berge, J.M.F., & Socan, G. (2004). The greatest lower bound to the reliability of a test and the hypothesis of unidimensionality. *Psychometrika*, *69*, 613–625.

Tucker, L. R. (1940). A rotational method based on the mean principal axis of a subgroup of tests. *Psychological Bulletin, 5*, 289–294.

Van Abswoude, A.A.H., van der Ark, A., & Sijtsma, K. (2004). A comparative study of test data dimensionality assessment procedures under nonparametric IRT models. *Applied Psychological Measurement*, *28*, 3–24.

Way, W.D., Ansley, T.N., & Forsyth, R.A. (1988). The comparative effects of compensatory and noncompensatory two-dimensional data on unidimensional IRT estimated. *Applied Psychological Measurement*, *12*, 239–252.

Wirth, R. J., & Edwards, M. C. (2007). Item factor analysis: current approaches and future directions. *Psychological methods*, *12*(1), 58.

Wu, E.J.C., & Bentler, P.M. (2011). *EQSIRT – A User-Friendly IRT Program*. Encino, CA: Multivariate Software, Inc.

Yung, Y.F., Thissen, D., & McLeod, L.D. (1999). On the relationship between the higher-order factor model and the hierarchical factor model. *Psychometrika*, *64*, 113–128.

Zinbarg, R.E., Revelle, W., Yovel, I., & Li, W. (2005). Cronbach's α, revelle's β, and McDonald's ω_h: Their relations with each other and two alternative conceptualizations of reliability. *Psychometrika*, *70*, 123–133.

3 Modern Approaches to Parameter Estimation in Item Response Theory

Li Cai and David Thissen

Introduction

Entire volumes (e.g., Baker & Kim, 2004) have been dedicated to the discussion of statistical parameter estimation techniques for item response theory (IRT) models. There has also been much recent development in the technical literature on improved methods for estimating complex IRT models (e.g., Cai, 2010a, 2010b; Edwards, 2010; Rijmen & Jeon, 2013). We offer here a map to help researchers and graduate students understand the fundamental challenges of IRT parameter estimation, and appropriately contextualize the underlying logic of some of the proposed solutions. We assume that the reader is familiar with elementary probability concepts such as prior, posterior, and likelihood, as well as the equations for describing statistical models for categorical observed data, for example, logistic regression. For methodologically inclined readers interested in studying IRT parameter estimation and in trying out some of the approaches discussed here, the combination of conceptual sections and more technical sections should be sufficient as a basis of software implementation.

We do not discuss limited-information estimation methods derived from categorical factor analysis or structural equation modeling (see, e.g., Bolt, 2005), but not because estimators based on polychoric correlation matrices and weighted least squares are not useful. They certainly may be, when conditions are appropriate (see, e.g., Wirth & Edwards, 2007), and for a long time, limited-information methods provided the only practically viable means for conducting formal model appraisal; although on that latter point, the situation has changed dramatically in the past few years (see, e.g., Maydeu-Olivares, 2013). In choosing to focus exclusively on full-information approaches that are based on either likelihood or Bayesian derivations, we believe that we provide readers with insight that tends to be obscured by the technicality that tends to accompany limited-information approaches. That is, the latent variables in IRT models are missing data, and had the latent variable scores been available, estimation for IRT models would have been a rather straightforward task. For the sake of simplicity, we contextualize our discussion with unidimensional logistic IRT models for dichotomously scored outcomes, but the missing data formulation applies generally across a far wider range of statistical modeling frameworks, IRT modeling included.

RESEARCH METHODS

Univariate Logistic Regression

Some Notation

We begin our discussion with a familiar framework, a univariate logistic regression model for dichotomous outcomes. Let there be $j = 1, \ldots, J$ independent cases. For each case, let

Y_j denote a binomial random variable with conditional success probability μ_j, that depends on x_j, the value of a fixed and observed covariate/predictor. The number of trials can be understood as a weight variable n_j attached to case j, and Y_j is the number of successes out of n_j independent Bernoulli trials each with success probability μ_j.

We assume that the log-odds of success is described by a linear model

$$\log\left(\frac{\mu_j}{1-\mu_j}\right) = \eta_j = \alpha + \beta x_j, \tag{3.1}$$

in which α and β are the regression intercept and slope parameters, respectively. From Equation (3.1), the conditional probability μ_j may be expressed using the inverse transformation, that is, a logistic cumulative distribution function (CDF):

$$\mu_j = \frac{1}{1+\exp(-\eta_j)} = \frac{1}{1+\exp\left[-(\alpha+\beta x_j)\right]}. \tag{3.2}$$

Note that Equation (3.2) resembles the two-parameter logistic IRT model with the key distinction that in IRT, the predictor is a latent variable, whereas x_j is observed.

Given a sample of data, we may write the likelihood function of the regression parameters. The goal is to find the set of parameters that would serve to maximize the likelihood (or log-likelihood) given the observed data. The parameter estimates are the maximum likelihood estimates (MLEs). The nonlinearity of the model implies that direct, analytical solutions such as those found in the case of least squares linear regression analysis are not feasible, and iterative algorithms such as Newton-Raphson or Fisher Scoring must be employed.

Maximum Likelihood Estimation for Logistic Regression

For case j, omitting constant terms, the binomial likelihood function is

$$L(\alpha,\beta \mid y_j, x_j) \propto \mu_j^{y_j}(1-\mu_j)^{n_j - y_j}, \tag{3.3}$$

where μ_j is as in Equation (3.2), and y_i is the realized/observed value of Y_j. Invoking the assumption of independence of observations across cases, for the entire sample, the likelihood function becomes a product of individual likelihood contributions:

$$L(\alpha,\beta \mid \mathbf{y},\mathbf{x}) = \prod_{j=1}^{J} L(\alpha,\beta \mid y_j, x_j) = \prod_{j=1}^{J} \mu_j^{y_j}(1-\mu_j)^{n_j - y_j}, \tag{3.4}$$

where the vector $\mathbf{y}$ collects together all the observed outcomes, and $\mathbf{x}$ contains all the predictor values. At this point it is convenient to take the natural logarithm of the likelihood function in Equation (3.4), and the log-likelihood is a sum of individual case contributions

$$l(\alpha,\beta \mid \mathbf{y},\mathbf{x}) = \log L(\alpha,\beta \mid \mathbf{y},\mathbf{x}) = \sum_{j=1}^{J} y_j \log\mu_j + (n_j - y_j)\log(1-\mu_j). \tag{3.5}$$

To maximize the log-likelihood, one would need its first-order partial derivatives (also known as the gradient vector). Using the chain rule, we have:

$$\begin{aligned} \frac{\partial l(\alpha,\beta|\mathbf{y},\mathbf{x})}{\partial\alpha} &= \sum_{j=1}^{J}\left(\frac{y_j}{\mu_j}\frac{\partial\mu_j}{\partial\eta_j}\frac{\partial\eta_j}{\partial\alpha} - \frac{(n_j-y_j)}{1-\mu_j}\frac{\partial\mu_j}{\partial\eta_j}\frac{\partial\eta_j}{\partial\alpha}\right), \\ \frac{\partial l(\alpha,\beta|\mathbf{y},\mathbf{x})}{\partial\beta} &= \sum_{j=1}^{J}\left(\frac{y_j}{\mu_j}\frac{\partial\mu_j}{\partial\eta_j}\frac{\partial\eta_j}{\partial\beta} - \frac{(n_j-y_j)}{1-\mu_j}\frac{\partial\mu_j}{\partial\eta_j}\frac{\partial\eta_j}{\partial\beta}\right). \end{aligned} \tag{3.6}$$

From Equation (3.2), one can verify a convenient fact about the logistic CDF:

$$\frac{\partial\mu_j}{\partial\eta_j} = \mu_j(1-\mu_j).$$

Furthermore, the derivatives of the linear function η_j are conveniently:

$$\frac{\partial\eta_j}{\partial\alpha} = \frac{\partial}{\partial\alpha}(\alpha+\beta x_j) = 1, \quad \frac{\partial\eta_j}{\partial\beta} = \frac{\partial}{\partial\beta}(\alpha+\beta x_j) = x_j.$$

Inserting these identities into Equation (3.6), we see that the expressions simplify considerably and the gradient vector of the log-likelihood is:

$$\mathbf{g}(\alpha,\beta|\mathbf{y},\mathbf{x}) = \begin{pmatrix} \dfrac{\partial l(\alpha,\beta|\mathbf{y},\mathbf{x})}{\partial\alpha} \\ \dfrac{\partial l(\alpha,\beta|\mathbf{y},\mathbf{x})}{\partial\beta} \end{pmatrix} = \begin{pmatrix} \sum_{j=1}^{J}(y_j - n_j\mu_j) \\ \sum_{j=1}^{J}(y_j - n_j\mu_j)x_j \end{pmatrix}. \tag{3.7}$$

Setting these derivatives to zero, the likelihood equations have remarkably direct interpretations. They amount to equating the observed counts in y to the expected counts in μ, summed over the individual contributions. We see that the likelihood equations are, however, nonlinear in α and β. Hence they cannot be solved analytically. We can use the Fisher Scoring method to solve the likelihood equations. To do so, we would need the second-order derivatives of the log-likelihood. Continuing from Equation (3.7), we see that

$$\begin{aligned} \frac{\partial^2 l(\alpha,\beta|\mathbf{y},\mathbf{x})}{\partial\alpha^2} &= \frac{\partial}{\partial\alpha}\sum_{j=1}^{J}(y_j - n_j\mu_j) = -\sum_{j=1}^{J} n_j\frac{\partial\mu_j}{\partial\eta_j}\frac{\partial\eta_j}{\partial\alpha} = -\sum_{j=1}^{J} n_j\mu_j(1-\mu_j), \\ \frac{\partial^2 l(\alpha,\beta|\mathbf{y},\mathbf{x})}{\partial\beta^2} &= \frac{\partial}{\partial\beta}\sum_{j=1}^{J}(y_j - n_j\mu_j) = -\sum_{j=1}^{J} n_j\frac{\partial\mu_j}{\partial\eta_j}\frac{\partial\eta_j}{\partial\beta}x_j = -\sum_{j=1}^{J} n_j\mu_j(1-\mu_j)x_j^2, \\ \frac{\partial^2 l(\alpha,\beta|\mathbf{y},\mathbf{x})}{\partial\alpha\partial\beta} &= \frac{\partial}{\partial\alpha}\sum_{j=1}^{J}(y_j - n_j\mu_j)x_j = -\sum_{j=1}^{J} n_j\frac{\partial\mu_j}{\partial\eta_j}\frac{\partial\eta_j}{\partial\alpha}x_j = -\sum_{j=1}^{J} n_j\mu_j(1-\mu_j)x_j. \end{aligned} \tag{3.8}$$

The information matrix, which is minus one times the matrix of second-order derivatives of the log-likelihood function (with the latter known as the Hessian matrix), is equal to

$$-\mathcal{H}\left(\alpha,\beta|y,x\right)=-\begin{pmatrix}\dfrac{\partial^2 l\left(\alpha,\beta|y,x\right)}{\partial\alpha^2} & \\ \dfrac{\partial^2 l\left(\alpha,\beta|y,x\right)}{\partial\alpha\partial\beta} & \dfrac{\partial^2 l\left(\alpha,\beta|y,x\right)}{\partial\beta^2}\end{pmatrix}. \tag{3.9}$$

If we choose as starting values some provisional estimate of intercept and slope, say, α_0 and β_0, and evaluate the gradient and information matrix at these provisional values, we would obtain $g\left(\alpha_0,\beta_0|y,x\right)$ and $-\mathcal{H}\left(\alpha_0,\beta_0|y,x\right)$. The gradient vector and inverse of the information matrix may be combined to obtain a correction factor so that improved estimates become

$$\begin{pmatrix}\alpha_1\\ \beta_1\end{pmatrix}=\begin{pmatrix}\alpha_0\\ \beta_0\end{pmatrix}+\left[-\mathcal{H}\left(\alpha_0,\beta_0|y,x\right)\right]^{-1}g\left(\alpha_0,\beta_0|y,x\right).$$

In general, from provisional estimates α_k and β_k, $k = 0, \ldots,$ Fisher Scoring uses the iterations

$$\begin{pmatrix}\alpha_{k+1}\\ \beta_{k+1}\end{pmatrix}=\begin{pmatrix}\alpha_k\\ \beta_k\end{pmatrix}+\left[-\mathcal{H}\left(\alpha_k,\beta_k\,|\,y,x\right)\right]^{-1}g\left(\alpha_k,\beta_k\,|\,y,x\right), \tag{3.10}$$

to gradually improve the provisional estimates. Under general conditions, the sequence of estimates generated by the Fisher Scoring iterations converges to the MLE as k increases without bounds. At the converged solution, the inverse of the information matrix provides an estimate of the large sample covariance matrix of the parameter estimates.

Item Response Theory Model as Multivariate Logistic Regression

Some Notation

Suppose a hypothetical assessment is made up of $i = 1, \ldots, I$ dichotomously scored items. An item score of one indicates a correct or endorsement response, and zero otherwise. Furthermore, suppose that the assumption of unidimensionality holds for this set of items. Let us use the standard notation of θ_j to denote the latent variable score for individual j. The two-parameter logistic (2PL) item response model specifies the conditional response probability curve (also known as the traceline) of a correct response or endorsement as a function of the latent variable and the item parameters:

$$T_i\left(\theta;\alpha_i,\beta_i\right)=\frac{1}{1+\exp\left[-\left(\alpha_i+\beta_i\theta\right)\right]}, \tag{3.11}$$

where α_i and β_i are the item intercept and slope parameters. The parentheses in $T_i\left(\theta;\alpha_i,\beta_i\right)$ highlight the fact that the response probabilities are conditional on θ_j, and that they also depend on the item parameters. Let Y_{ij} be a Bernoulli (0–1) random variable representing individual i's response to item j, and let y_{ij} be a realization of Y_{ij}. This suggests a formulation of the conditional probability of the event $Y_{ij} = y_{ij}$ similar to Equation (3.4),

$$P\left(Y_{ij} = y_{ij} \mid \theta; \alpha_i, \beta_i\right) = \left[T_i\left(\theta; \alpha_i, \beta_i\right)\right]^{y_{ij}} \left[1 - T_i\left(\theta; \alpha_i, \beta_i\right)\right]^{1-y_{ij}}. \tag{3.12}$$

Under the assumption of unidimensionality, the latent variable θ alone explains all the observed covariations among the items. In other words, conditionally on θ, the item response probabilities are independent for an individual, that is, the probability of response pattern $\boldsymbol{y}_j = \left(y_{1j}, \ldots, y_{Ij}\right)$ factors into a product over individual item response probabilities:

$$\begin{aligned} P\left(\boldsymbol{y}_j \mid \theta; \boldsymbol{\gamma}\right) &= \prod_{i=1}^{I} P\left(Y_{ij} = y_{ij} \mid \theta; \alpha_i, \beta_i\right) \\ &= \prod_{i=1}^{I} \left[T_i\left(\theta; \alpha_i, \beta_i\right)\right]^{y_{ij}} \left[1 - T_i\left(\theta; \alpha_i, \beta_i\right)\right]^{1-y_{ij}} \end{aligned} \tag{3.13}$$

where on the left-hand side we collect all item intercept and slope parameters into $\boldsymbol{\gamma} = (\alpha_1, \ldots, \alpha_I, \beta_1, \ldots, \beta_I)$, a $2I$-dimensional vector. The joint probability of the observed and latent variables is equal to the product of the conditional probability of the observed variables given the latent variables, times the prior probability of the latent variables:

$$P\left(\boldsymbol{y}_j, \theta; \boldsymbol{\gamma}\right) = \prod_{i=1}^{I} \left[T_i\left(\theta; \alpha_i, \beta_i\right)\right]^{y_{ij}} \left[1 - T_i\left(\theta; \alpha_i, \beta_i\right)\right]^{1-y_{ij}} h(\theta), \tag{3.14}$$

where $h(\theta)$ is prior (population) distribution of the latent variable θ. In IRT applications, it is customary to resolve the location and scale indeterminacy of the latent variable by assuming that the θ's are standard normal, so $h(\theta)$ does not contain free parameters.

From Equation (3.14), a natural derived quantity is the marginal probability of the response pattern, after integrating the joint probability over θ:

$$P\left(\boldsymbol{y}_j; \boldsymbol{\gamma}\right) = \int \prod_{i=1}^{I} \left[T_i\left(\theta; \alpha_i, \beta_i\right)\right]^{y_{ij}} \left[1 - T_i\left(\theta; \alpha_i, \beta_i\right)\right]^{1-y_{ij}} h(\theta)\, d\theta. \tag{3.15}$$

Unfortunately Equation (3.15) is already the simplest form that we can obtain, given the combination of the IRT model and normally distributed latent variable. Note that the marginal probability does not depend on the unobserved latent variable scores; it is a function solely of the observed item response pattern and the item parameters.

As in the case of logistic regression, we assume the individuals are independent, with latent variable scores sampled independently from the population distribution. Let $\mathbf{Y}$ be a matrix of all observed item responses. If we treat the item responses as fixed once observed, the marginal likelihood function for all the item parameters in $\boldsymbol{\gamma}$, based on observed item response data, can be expressed as:

$$L(\boldsymbol{\gamma} \mid \mathbf{Y}) = \prod_{j=1}^{J} \int \prod_{i=1}^{I} \left[T_i\left(\theta; \alpha_i, \beta_i\right)\right]^{y_{ij}} \left[1 - T_i\left(\theta; \alpha_i, \beta_i\right)\right]^{1-y_{ij}} h(\theta)\, d\theta. \tag{3.16}$$

Because the marginal likelihood $L(\boldsymbol{\gamma} \mid \mathbf{Y})$ does not depend on the unobserved θ values, it may be referred to as the *observed* data likelihood.

Under some circumstances, this likelihood function can be optimized directly, again using Newton Raphson or Fisher Scoring-type algorithms (see, e.g., Bock & Lieberman, 1970), but those circumstances are rather limited. In particular, Bock and Lieberman (1970) noted that this direct approach does not generalize well to the case of many items and many parameters because of computing demands. We would add that even as computers have become faster and storage cheaper, what the direct approach glosses over is a *missing data formulation* of latent variable models that is central to our understanding of IRT and of other modern statistical techniques such as random effects regression modeling, or modeling of survey nonresponse. This missing data formulation was made transparent by Dempster, Laird, and Rubin's (1977) classical paper that coined the term *Expectation-Maximization (EM) algorithm.*

Missing Data Formulation and Fisher's Identity

Implicit in the "observed data" terminology is a realization that θ contains the "missing" data. If we treat the item responses as fixed once observed, and also suppose the latent variable scores were observed, then after some algebra that follows directly from Equation (3.14), we see that the so-called complete data likelihood function of the vector of item parameters is:

$$
\begin{aligned}
L(\boldsymbol{\gamma}|\mathbf{Y},\boldsymbol{\theta}) &= \left[\prod_{j=1}^{J} h(\theta_j)\right]\left[\prod_{j=1}^{J}\prod_{i=1}^{I}[T_i(\theta_j;\alpha_i,\beta_i)]^{y_{ij}}[1-T_i(\theta_j;\alpha_i,\beta_i)]^{1-y_{ij}}\right] \\
&\propto \prod_{i=1}^{I}\prod_{j=1}^{J}\left[T_i(\theta_j;\alpha_i,\beta_i)]^{y_{ij}}[1-T_i(\theta_j;\alpha_i,\beta_i)\right]^{1-y_{ij}},
\end{aligned}
\tag{3.17}
$$

where $\boldsymbol{\theta}$ is a vector that collects together all J latent variable scores. The proportionality on the second line holds because $h(\theta_j)$ does not depend on item parameters in our model, and given θ_j, it becomes a constant. Had the latent variable scores been observed, Equation (3.17) makes it clear that the complete data likelihood function would be a constant multiple of I item-specific likelihoods, each representing a logistic regression model. Thus the IRT model can be understood as multivariate logit analysis, if one could observe the predictor variable θ.

Of course, the latent variable θ is not observed, but that does not imply the situation is hopeless. Instead, it forces us to pay close attention to the posterior distribution of the latent variable given the observed item responses:

$$
P(\theta|\mathbf{y}_j;\boldsymbol{\gamma}) = \frac{P(\mathbf{y}_j,\theta;\boldsymbol{\gamma})}{P(\mathbf{y}_j;\boldsymbol{\gamma})} = \frac{\prod_{i=1}^{I}[T_i(\theta;\alpha_i,\beta_i)]^{y_{ij}}[1-T_i(\theta;\alpha_i,\beta_i)]^{1-y_{ij}}h(\theta)}{\int\prod_{i=1}^{I}[T_i(\theta;\alpha_i,\beta_i)]^{y_{ij}}[1-T_i(\theta;\alpha_i,\beta_i)]^{1-y_{ij}}h(\theta)d\theta}. \tag{3.18}
$$

This is an analytically intractable distribution, but it follows directly from the application of the Bayes rule to Equations (3.14) and (3.15). It also has some interesting characteristics that deserve comments. First, given item parameter values and the observed item response pattern y_j, the denominator is a constant that can, in principle, be computed. This is a normalization factor that makes (3.18) a proper probability density function. Second, given item parameter values, the posterior is proportional to the joint distribution in the numerator, which is more tractable than the posterior itself. Third, with the help of the posterior distribution, one may verify that given item parameter values, the following equality holds (it is known as Fisher's Identity; Fisher, 1925) assuming mild regularity conditions:

$$
\frac{\partial \log P(\mathbf{y}_j;\boldsymbol{\gamma})}{\partial\boldsymbol{\gamma}} = \int\frac{\partial \log P(\mathbf{y}_j,\theta;\boldsymbol{\gamma})}{\partial\boldsymbol{\gamma}}P(\theta|\mathbf{y}_j;\boldsymbol{\gamma})d\theta. \tag{3.19}
$$

Fisher's Identity states that the gradient of the observed data log-likelihood *log* $L(\gamma|Y)$ is equal to the conditional expectation of the gradient of the completed data log-likelihood *log* $L(\gamma|Y, \theta)$ over the posterior distribution of the latent variables given the observed variables. This powerful insight suggests that instead of trying to maximize the observed data likelihood, which is direct but often difficult, one should consider iteratively maximizing the conditional expected complete data likelihood (i.e., the right-hand side of Equation 3.19), which can be an indirect route but more computationally tractable. This is because the complete data model is no more than a set of logistic regressions, which is a problem we already know how to solve. We will demonstrate this argument via two approaches, beginning with Bock and Aitkin's (1981) classical application of the EM algorithm, and then turning to its modern cousin, Cai's (2008) Metropolis-Hastings Robbins-Monro algorithm.

Bock-Aitkin EM Algorithm

Bock and Aitkin (1981) began with the insight that the marginal probability can be approximated to arbitrary precision by replacing the integration with a summation over a set of Q quadrature points over θ:

$$P(y_j;\gamma) \approx \bar{P}_j = \sum_{q=1}^{Q}\prod_{i=1}^{I}\left[T_i(X_q;\alpha_i,\beta_i)\right]^{y_{ij}}\left[1-T_i(X_q;\alpha_i,\beta_i)\right]^{1-y_{ij}} W_q, \tag{3.20}$$

where X_q is a quadrature point, and W_q is the corresponding weight. In the simplest case, one may take the quadrature points as a set of equally spaced real numbers over an interval that captures sufficiently the probability mass of the population distribution, for example, from –6 to +6 in increments of 0.1, and the corresponding weights as a set of normalized ordinates of the quadrature points from the population distribution $W_q = h(X_q)/\sum_{q=1}^{Q} h(X_q)$.

Another important insight of Bock and Aitkin (1981) is that the height of the posterior distribution at quadrature point X_q can be approximated to arbitrary precision as well:

$$P(X_q|y_j;\gamma) \approx \frac{\left[T_i(X_q;\alpha_i,\beta_i)\right]^{y_{ij}}\left[1-T_i(X_q;\alpha_i,\beta_i)\right]^{1-y_{ij}} W_q}{\bar{P}_j}. \tag{3.21}$$

Ignoring constants involving the prior distribution $h(\theta_j)$ from Equation (3.17), the complete data log-likelihood for the item parameters can be written as:

$$\log L(\gamma|Y,\theta) = \sum_{j=1}^{J}\sum_{i=1}^{I} y_{ij}\log T_i(\theta_j;\alpha_i,\beta_i) + \sum_{j=1}^{J}\sum_{i=1}^{I}(1-y_{ij})\log\left(1-T_i(\theta_j;\alpha_i,\beta_i)\right). \tag{3.22}$$

Following the logic inspired by the Fisher Identity, the conditional expected complete data likelihood given provisional item parameter values $\gamma^* = (\alpha_1^*,\ldots,\alpha_I^*,\beta_1^*,\ldots,\beta_I^*)$ can be approximated by quadrature, case by case, as follows:

$$\begin{aligned} Q(\gamma|\mathbf{Y};\gamma^*) \approx & \sum_{j=1}^{J}\sum_{q=1}^{Q}\sum_{i=1}^{I} y_{ij} log T_i(X_q;\alpha_i,\beta_i)P(X_q|y_j;\gamma^*) \\ & + \sum_{j=1}^{J}\sum_{q=1}^{Q}\sum_{i=1}^{I}(1-y_{ij}) log(1-T_i(X_q;\alpha_i,\beta_i))P(X_q|y_j;\gamma^*). \end{aligned} \tag{3.23}$$

The third and arguably most important insight from Bock and Aitkin (1981) is that by interchanging the order of summation, they realized that the posterior probabilities can be accumulated over individuals first:

$$\begin{aligned} Q(\gamma|\mathbf{Y};\gamma^*) &\approx \sum_{i=1}^{I}\sum_{q=1}^{Q}\log T_i(X_q;\alpha_i,\beta_i)\left(\sum_{j=1}^{J} y_{ij}P(X_q|\mathbf{y}_j;\gamma^*)\right) \\ &\quad + \sum_{i=1}^{I}\sum_{q=1}^{Q}\log\left(1-T_i(X_q;\alpha_i,\beta_i)\right)\left(\sum_{j=1}^{J}(1-y_{ij})P(X_q|\mathbf{y}_j;\gamma^*)\right) \\ &= \sum_{i=1}^{I}\sum_{q=1}^{Q} r_{iq}\log T_i(X_q;\alpha_i,\beta_i) + \sum_{i=1}^{I}\sum_{q=1}^{Q}\bar{r}_{iq}\log(1-T_i(X_q;\alpha_i,\beta_i)), \end{aligned} \tag{3.24}$$

where $r_{iq} = \sum_{j=1}^{J} y_{ij}P\left(X_q|\mathbf{y}_j;\gamma^*\right)$ is understood as the conditional expected proportion of individuals that respond positively/correctly to item i, and $\bar{r}_{iq} = \sum_{j=1}^{J}\left(1-y_{ij}\right)P\left(X_q\,|\,\mathbf{y}_j;\gamma^*\right)$ is the conditional expected proportion of individuals that respond negatively/incorrectly to item i, at quadrature point X_q. Taken together, let $n_{iq} = r_{iq} + \bar{r}_{iq} = \sum_{j=1}^{J} P\left(X_q\,|\,\mathbf{y}_j;\gamma^*\right)$ be the conditional expected proportion of individuals at quadrature point X_q, then we have:

$$Q\left(\gamma|\mathbf{Y};\gamma^*\right) \approx \sum_{i=1}^{I}\sum_{q=1}^{Q} r_{iq}\log T_i(X_q;\alpha_i,\beta_i) + (n_{iq}-r_{iq})\log\left(1-T_i(X_q;\alpha_i,\beta_i)\right). \tag{3.25}$$

Equation (3.25) highlights the fact that the conditional expected complete data log-likelihood is a set of I independent logistic regression log-likelihoods, with the quadrature points X_q serving as the predictor values, and weights given by n_{iq}, and r_{iq} serving as the positive outcome "frequency" at X_q. The inner summation over the quadrature points bears striking similarity to the log-likelihood given in Equation (3.5). The only difference is that in standard logistic regression, the weights n_j and number of successes y_j are integers, whereas in the case of Bock-Aitkin EM, n_{iq} and r_{iq} may be fractional and will change from cycle to cycle, given different item parameter values. With the Fisher Scoring algorithm developed in Section 2, optimization of $Q(\gamma|\mathbf{Y};\gamma^*)$ is straightforward, which leads to updated parameter estimates that may be used in the next cycle.

In general, Bock-Aitkin EM (or any EM algorithm) alternates between the following two steps from a set of initial parameter estimates, say $\gamma^{(0)}$, and it generates a sequence of parameter estimates $\gamma^{(0)},\ldots,\gamma^{(k)},\ldots$, where $\gamma^{(k)} = \left(\alpha_1^{(k)},\ldots,\alpha_I^{(k)},\beta_1^{(k)},\ldots,\beta_I^{(k)}\right)$, that converges under some very general conditions to the MLE of γ as the number of cycles k tends to infinity (Wu, 1983):

E-step. Given $\gamma^{(k)}$, evaluate the conditional expected complete data log-likelihood $Q\left(\gamma|\mathbf{Y};\gamma^{(k)}\right)$, which is taken to be a function of γ.

M-step. Maximize $Q\left(\gamma|\mathbf{Y};\gamma^{(k)}\right)$ to yield updated parameter estimates $\gamma^{(k+1)}$. Go back to E-step and repeat. The cycles are terminated when the estimates from adjacent cycles stabilize.

The application of the EM algorithm to IRT epitomizes the elegance of the missing data formulation in statistical computing. Finding MLEs in logistic regression analysis is a task that statisticians already know how to do. The goal of the E-step, then, is to replace the missing data with conditional expectations that depend on values of θ, represented using a set of discrete quadrature points. Once the missing data are filled in, complete data estimation can be accomplished with tools that are already available. Leveraging the conditional independence built into the IRT model, the M-step logit analyses can even be run in parallel and the overall demand on computing resources is rather low. Although the EM algorithm is only first-order (linearly) convergent, and may be slow (by optimization researchers' standard), the statistical intuition is simply too elegant to ignore. Thissen (1982) extended the unconstrained Bock-Aitkin EM to handle parameter restrictions and used it to estimate the Rasch IRT model.

Metropolis-Hastings Robbins-Monro Algorithm

Motivations of MH-RM

One issue with Bock-Aitkin EM is that while it deftly handles unidimensional IRT parameter estimation with many items, it does not generalize well to the case of multidimensional IRT. This is because the posterior expectations must be accumulated over grids of quadrature points formed by the direct product of the quadrature rule. Even with a moderate number of quadrature points, the exponentially increasing size of the grid as the number of dimensions increases presents major computational challenges. Adaptive quadrature helps somewhat by requiring fewer points than fixed quadrature rules (see, e.g., Schilling & Bock, 2005), but does not solve the problem completely. Various authors (e.g., Wirth & Edwards, 2007) referred to this as the "challenge of dimensionality." As assessments become more complex, multidimensional IRT models are increasingly in demand, but estimating the item parameters has been difficult.

Cai (2006, 2008, 2010a, 2010b) realized that a solution already resides in Fisher's Identity. It is worth repeating that equation:

$$\frac{\partial \log P(\mathbf{y}_j;\boldsymbol{\gamma})}{\partial \boldsymbol{\gamma}} = \int \frac{\partial \log P(\mathbf{y}_j,\theta;\boldsymbol{\gamma})}{\partial \boldsymbol{\gamma}} P(\theta|\mathbf{y}_j;\boldsymbol{\gamma})d\theta.$$

Cai reasoned that if one can randomly draw plausible values or imputations of θ from its posterior predictive distribution $P(\theta|\mathbf{y}_j;\gamma^*)$, with provisional item parameter estimates γ^*, the right-hand side can be approximated by Monte Carlo, that is,

$$\frac{\partial \log P(\mathbf{y}_j;\gamma)}{\partial \gamma} \approx \frac{1}{M}\sum_{m=1}^{M}\frac{\partial \log P(\mathbf{y}_j,\theta_{jm};\gamma)}{\partial \gamma}, \tag{3.26}$$

where θ_{jm} are the random draws from $P(\theta|\mathbf{y}_j;\gamma^*)$. Because the cases are independent, we also see that:

$$\begin{aligned}\frac{\partial \log L(\gamma|\mathbf{Y})}{\partial \gamma} &= \sum_{j=1}^{J}\frac{\partial \log P(\mathbf{y}_j;\gamma)}{\partial \gamma} \approx \frac{1}{M}\sum_{m=1}^{M}\sum_{j=1}^{J}\frac{\partial \log P(\mathbf{y}_j,\theta_{jm};\gamma)}{\partial \gamma}\\ &= \frac{1}{M}\sum_{m=1}^{M}\frac{\partial \log L(\gamma|\mathbf{Y},\boldsymbol{\theta}_m)}{\partial \gamma},\end{aligned} \tag{3.27}$$

where $(\mathbf{Y}, \boldsymbol{\theta}_m)$ may be taken as the *m*th complete data set, and $\boldsymbol{\theta}_m$ is the augmented missing data. We end up with the first insight that motivates the MH-RM algorithm: *The Monte Carlo average of complete data log-likelihood gradients gives the same likelihood ascent direction as the observed data log-likelihood gradient vector.*

An immediate problem with the Monte Carlo approximation is that it contains error, and unless the Monte Carlo size M becomes large, the random sampling error obscures the true direction of likelihood ascent. This is a known issue in the context of Monte Carlo EM (Booth & Hobert, 1999), where the solution is to adaptively increase the size of the Monte Carlo sampling, so that increasingly accurate approximations can be found as the estimates converge. Unfortunately, as will be explained later, while computing random draws of the $\boldsymbol{\theta}$'s has become an increasingly manageable task, with help from Markov chain Monte Carlo (MCMC; Hastings, 1970; Metropolis, Rosenbluth, Rosenbluth, Teller, & Teller, 1953), it is still a nontrivial matter for fitting of IRT models in practical settings, because of the multitude of nonlinear functions (exponential, for instance) that must be evaluated for the IRT model's likelihood functions. The amount of computing time required to draw the imputations frequently dwarfs the amount of time needed to compute the complete data derivatives by several orders of magnitude. Thus it is necessary, if only for computational efficiency, to find a method that utilizes Monte Carlo sampling effectively.

Cai (2010a) noted that instead of treating the Monte Carlo noise as a nuisance to be contained, it may in fact be employed more productively. By drawing an analogy to the engineering applications of Robbins and Monro's (1951) classical Stochastic Approximation (SA) method, the Monte Carlo noise provides the stochastic excitations that drive an underlying stochastic process. The noise is gradually filtered out with the use of an appropriately chosen sequence of gain constants, as the parameters are recursively updated.

This leads to the second insight that leads to MH-RM: *In Robbins and Monro's context, they were attempting to find roots of noise-corrupted regression functions, where the noise may be due to observational measurement error; in our context, we purposefully inject Monte Carlo noise by imputing the missing data (the latent variable scores), so that we can observe an approximate direction of likelihood ascent.* It is not necessary that the approximate ascent direction be made precise, especially in the beginning stages of the iterative scheme. In fact, it is possible to let M be identically equal to one (a single imputation per iteration) and still obtain a point-wise convergent algorithm to the MLE (see Cai, 2010a, for a proof).

Definition of the Algorithm

With the IRT model, cycle $k+1$ of the MH-RM algorithm consists of three steps:

Imputation. Given provisional parameter estimates $\gamma^{(k)}$ from the previous cycle (or initial parameter values $\gamma^{(0)}$ if this is the first cycle), random samples of the latent variables $\boldsymbol{\theta}_m^{(k+1)}$ are imputed. For each individual, the draws may come from a Metropolis-Hastings sampler that has, as its unique invariant distribution, the posterior predictive distribution $P\left(\theta_j \mid y_j; \gamma^{(k)}\right)$ of the missing data given the observed data and provisional parameter values. In other words, the complete data sets are formed as $\left(\mathbf{Y}, \theta_m^{(k+1)}\right)$.

Approximation. In the second step, based on the imputed data, the complete data log-likelihood and its derivatives are evaluated so that the ascent directions for parameters can be determined. The complete data gradient (score) function is approximated as:

$$s_{k+1} = \frac{1}{M}\sum_{m=1}^{M}\frac{\partial \log L\left(\gamma^{(k)} \mid \mathbf{Y}, \theta_m^{(k+1)}\right)}{\partial \gamma}, \tag{3.28}$$

Note that for each item, the complete data gradient vector is simply $g\left(\alpha_i^{(k)}, \beta_i^{(k)} \mid \mathbf{y}_i, \theta_m^{(k+1)}\right)$, as defined in Equation (3.7), where $\mathbf{y}_i$ is a vector that collects together all J observed responses to item i. At the same time, to improve stability and speed, we also evaluate a Monte Carlo approximation to the conditional expected complete data information matrix:

$$\mathbf{H}_{k+1} = -\frac{1}{M}\sum_{m=1}^{M}\frac{\partial^2 \log L\left(\gamma^{(k)} \mid \mathbf{Y}, \theta_m^{(k+1)}\right)}{\partial\gamma\partial\gamma'}. \tag{3.29}$$

Again, because of conditional independence given the latent variables in the IRT model, the complete data information matrix is block-diagonal, with each item's information matrix equal to $-\mathcal{H}\left(\alpha_i^{(k)}, \beta_i^{(k)} \mid \mathbf{y}_i, \theta_m^{(k+1)}\right)$, as defined in Equation (3.9).

Robbins-Monro Update. In the third step, Robbins-Monro stochastic approximation filters are applied when updating the estimates of item parameters. First, the Robbins-Monro filter is applied to obtain a recursive stochastic approximation of the conditional expectation of the complete data information matrix:

$$\Gamma_{k+1} = \Gamma_k + \epsilon_k\left(\mathbf{H}_{k+1} - \Gamma_k\right), \tag{3.30}$$

where ϵ_k is a sequence of non-negative *gain constants* such that $\epsilon_k \in (0,1], \sum_{k=0}^{\infty}\epsilon_k = \infty, \sum_{k=0}^{\infty}\epsilon_k^2 < \infty$. Next, we use the Robbins-Monro filter again when updating the parameters:

$$\gamma^{(k+1)} = \gamma^{(k)} + \epsilon_k\left(\Gamma_{k+1}\right)^{-1}\mathbf{s}_{k+1}. \tag{3.31}$$

The iterations are started from some initial parameter values $\gamma^{(0)}$ and terminated when the estimates stabilize. Cai (2008, 2010a) showed that the sequence of parameters converges with probability 1 to a local maximum of $L(\gamma \mid \mathbf{Y})$. Typically, the sequence of gain constants are taken to be $\epsilon_k = 1/(k+1)$, in which case the initial choice of Γ_0 becomes arbitrary. Cai (2010a) contains formulas for recursively approximating the parameter error covariance matrix, as well as further discussions about convergence checking.

Implementing the Metropolis-Hastings Sampler

At this point, a critical missing link is a method to draw random values of $\theta_m^{(k+1)}$ from its posterior predictive distribution. Cai (2006) proposed the use of the Metropolis-Hastings method, for several reasons. First, we see from Equation (3.18) that while the posterior predictive distribution is analytically intractable in that it does not belong to any "named" distribution family, it is proportional to the joint probability of observed item responses and latent variables:

$$P\left(\theta \mid \mathbf{y}_j; \gamma^{(k)}\right) \propto \prod_{i=1}^{I}\left[T_i\left(\theta; \alpha_i^{(k)}, \beta_i^{(k)}\right)\right]^{y_{ij}}\left[1 - T_i\left(\theta; \alpha_i^{(k)}, \beta_i^{(k)}\right)\right]^{1-y_{ij}} h(\theta). \tag{3.32}$$

The Metropolis-Hastings method is ideally suited to the task of sampling a posterior when the normalization constant is not readily available. In addition, the right-hand side of Equation (3.32) is the complete data likelihood at $\gamma^{(k)}$, which is evaluated in any event to compute the item gradients and information matrices required in the approximation step of MH-RM. Furthermore, the sampling of the θ values can be accomplished in parallel, as the individual $P(\theta_j|y_j;\gamma^{(k)})$'s are fully independent. Finally, the Monte Carlo approximation in Equation (3.28) remains unbiased even if the draws are not independent, for example from a Markov chain.

Implementing the Metropolis-Hastings method is straightforward. For each individual j, we begin with some initial value of θ_j, say, θ_j^c, and let us call it the current state of θ_j. We now draw a random increment from an independent normal sampler, with mean 0 and standard deviation equal to σ. Let this increment value be denoted δ_j. By adding the increment to the current state, we have produced a proposal for a new state of θ_j: $\theta_j^p = \theta_j^c + \delta_j$. We now evaluate the right-hand side of Equation (3.32) at both current and proposal states, and form the following likelihood ratio:

$$R(\theta_j^p, \theta_j^c) = \frac{\prod_{i=1}^{I}\left[T_i\left(\theta_j^p; \alpha_i^{(k)}, \beta_i^{(k)}\right)\right]^{y_{ij}}\left[1 - T_i\left(\theta_j^p; \alpha_i^{(k)}, \beta_i^{(k)}\right)\right]^{1-y_{ij}} h(\theta_j^p)}{\prod_{i=1}^{I}\left[T_i\left(\theta_j^c; \alpha_i^{(k)}, \beta_i^{(k)}\right)\right]^{y_{ij}}\left[1 - T_i\left(\theta_j^c; \alpha_i^{(k)}, \beta_i^{(k)}\right)\right]^{1-y_{ij}} h(\theta_j^c)}. \tag{3.33}$$

If $R(\theta_j^p,\theta_j^c)$ is larger than 1.0, meaning that the proposed move to a new state increased the likelihood relative to the current state, we accept the move and set the proposal state as the new current state. If $R(\theta_j^p,\theta_j^c)$ is smaller than 1.0, meaning that the proposed move decreased the likelihood, we accept the move with probability equal to the likelihood ratio. This can be accomplished by drawing, independently, a uniform (0,1) random number u_j, and comparing it to $R(\theta_j^p,\theta_j^c)$. If u_j is smaller than $R(\theta_j^p,\theta_j^c)$, we accept the proposed move and set the proposal state as the new current state. If u_j is larger than the likelihood ratio, we reject the proposal, and remain at the current state. Iterating this sampler will produce a Markov chain that converges to $P(\theta_j|y_j;\gamma^{(k)})$ in distribution.

As the chain evolves, dependent samples from this chain can be regarded as samples from the target distribution. To avoid excessive dependence on the initial state, one can drop the samples in the so-called burn-in phase of the chain. For the IRT model, experience suggests that this burn-in phase typically amounts to not more than 10 iterations of the Metropolis-Hastings sampler. Of course, this assumes that the chain is appropriately tuned by monitoring the rate of acceptance of the proposed moves and scaling the increment density standard deviation σ up (for decreased acceptance rate) or down (for increased acceptance rate). Roberts and Rosenthal (2001) discussed the statistical efficiency of Metropolis-Hastings samplers, and its relationship to optimal scaling. Asymptotically efficient chains can be obtained by tuning the acceptance rate to around 25 percent.

Application

We analyze a well-known data set (Social Life Feelings), analyzed by Bartholomew (1998), among others, to illustrate the Bock-Aitkin EM and MH-RM algorithms. The data set contains responses from $J = 1{,}490$ German respondents to five statements on perceptions of social life. The responses were dichotomous (endorsement vs. non-endorsement of the statements). Table 3.1 presents the $2^5 = 32$ response patterns and their associated observed response frequencies.

Let us first examine the most frequently encountered response pattern (0, 1, 1, 0, 0), wherein 208 respondents endorsed items 2 and 3 and none of the others. Following the logic of Bock-Aitkin EM, we must first choose a set of quadrature points for

Table 3.1 Social Life Feelings Data in Response Pattern by Frequency Form

Item Response Pattern					*Observed Frequency*
0	0	0	0	0	156
0	0	0	0	1	26
0	0	0	1	0	14
0	0	0	1	1	9
0	0	1	0	0	127
0	0	1	0	1	26
0	0	1	1	0	66
0	0	1	1	1	16
0	1	0	0	0	174
0	1	0	0	1	35
0	1	0	1	0	36
0	1	0	1	1	13
0	1	1	0	0	208
0	1	1	0	1	65
0	1	1	1	0	195
0	1	1	1	1	129
1	0	0	0	0	8
1	0	0	0	1	2
1	0	0	1	0	1
1	0	0	1	1	3
1	0	1	0	0	4
1	0	1	0	1	4
1	0	1	1	0	18
1	0	1	1	1	9
1	1	0	0	0	8
1	1	0	0	1	2
1	1	0	1	0	5
1	1	0	1	1	3
1	1	1	0	0	19
1	1	1	0	1	10
1	1	1	1	0	31
1	1	1	1	1	68
					Total = 1,490

approximating the E-step integrals. Here we use a set of 49 quadrature points equally spaced between –6 and +6. Next we must also choose a set of initial values for the item parameters. For the sake of variety, we let the initial values of the item intercepts be $\alpha_1 = -1.5$, $\alpha_2 = -1$, $\alpha_3 = 0$, $\alpha_4 = 1$, $\alpha_5 = 1.5$, and let all initial slopes be equal to 1.0. We are now ready to begin our first E-step.

Figure 3.1 contains a set of three plots showing the relationship between the prior distribution, the likelihood function for response pattern (0,1,1,0,0) evaluated at the initial values of the item parameters, and the implied posterior distribution—formed by multiplying the likelihood and the prior, point by point over the quadrature points, and then normalized to sum to one. The prior and the posterior distributions are shown as discrete probability point masses over the quadrature points. The ordinates of the normalized prior distribution have been multiplied by the observed sample size (1,490), and those of the posterior distribution have been multiplied by the observed frequency associated with the response pattern (208).

For each item, depending on the response (0 or 1), the posterior probabilities are accumulated as per Equation (3.24). For instance, item 1's response is zero, which means

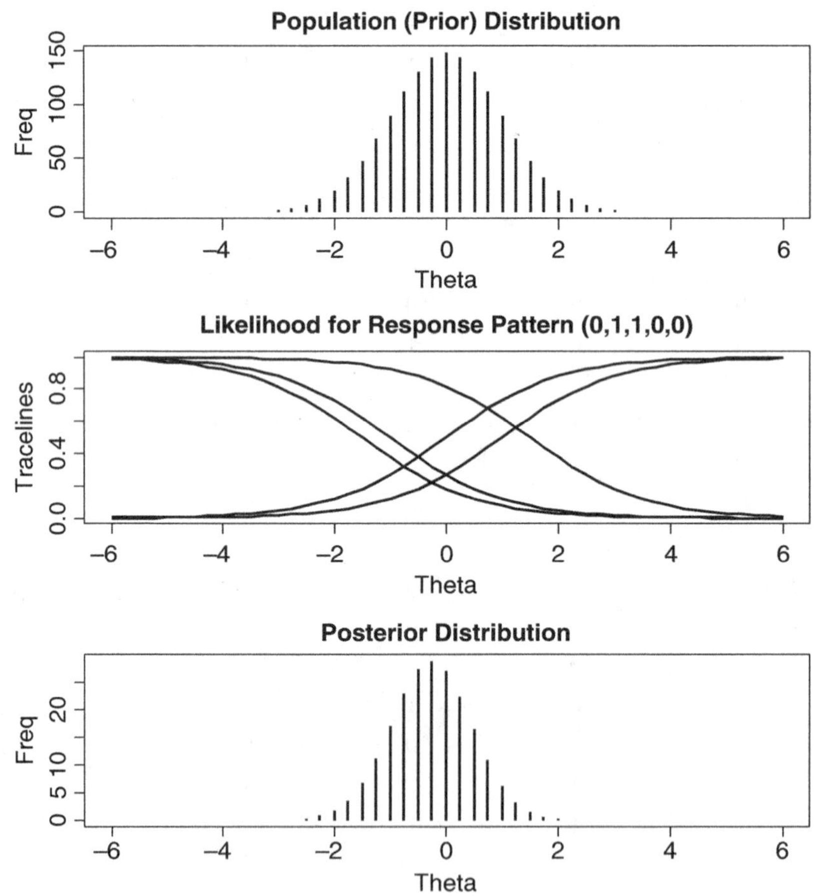

Figure 3.1 Multi-panel plot showing the relationship among the prior (population) distribution, the likelihood (products of tracelines shown) for response pattern (0,1,1,0,0), and the posterior.

that the current set of posterior probabilities must be added into the $\bar{r}_{1q}$ values over the Q quadrature points. Similarly, because item 2's response is one, for that item, the posterior probabilities are added into the r_{2q} values for all q. Regardless of the response, the posterior probabilities are added into n_{iq} for all items and quadrature points.

For each response pattern, there is a set of corresponding three-panel plots that generate the posterior probabilities over the same set of quadrature points. These posterior probabilities are accumulated into the item-specific r_{iq} and n_{iq} values, depending on the item response. At the end of the E-step, the weights n_{iq} and (artificial) response frequencies r_{iq} are submitted to the M-step for logit analyses.

Figure 3.2 presents the current and updated tracelines for item 1 after one cycle of E- and M-step. The current tracelines (dashed curves) are at their initial values of $\alpha_1 = -1.5$ and $\beta_1 = 1$. The ordinates of the solid dots are equal to r_{1q} / n_{1q}, representing the conditional expected probability of the endorsement response for item 1 at each of the quadrature points. The size of each of the solid dots is proportional to the conditional expected number of respondents at each of the corresponding quadrature points. The updated tracelines (solid curves) correspond to $\alpha_1 = -2.12$ and $\beta_1 = 1.11$. It is obvious that the updated tracelines are much closer approximations of the "data" generated by the E-step conditional expectations. Other items can be handled similarly. Thus iterating the E- and M-steps leads to a sequence of item parameter estimates that eventually converges to the MLE. At the maximum, the following item parameters are obtained: $\alpha_1 = -2.35$, $\alpha_2 = 0.80$, $\alpha_3 = 0.99$, $\alpha_4 = -0.67$, $\alpha_5 = 1.10$, $\beta_1 = 1.20$, $\beta_2 = 0.71$, $\beta_3 = 1.53$, $\beta_4 = 2.55$, $\beta_5 = 0.92$.

Let us now turn to the application of the MH-RM algorithm. The MH-RM algorithm also requires the characterization of the posterior distribution of θ, but it uses it differently than Bock-Aitkin EM: The Metropolis-Hastings sampler is used to generate dependent draws from this posterior, given provisional item parameter values and the

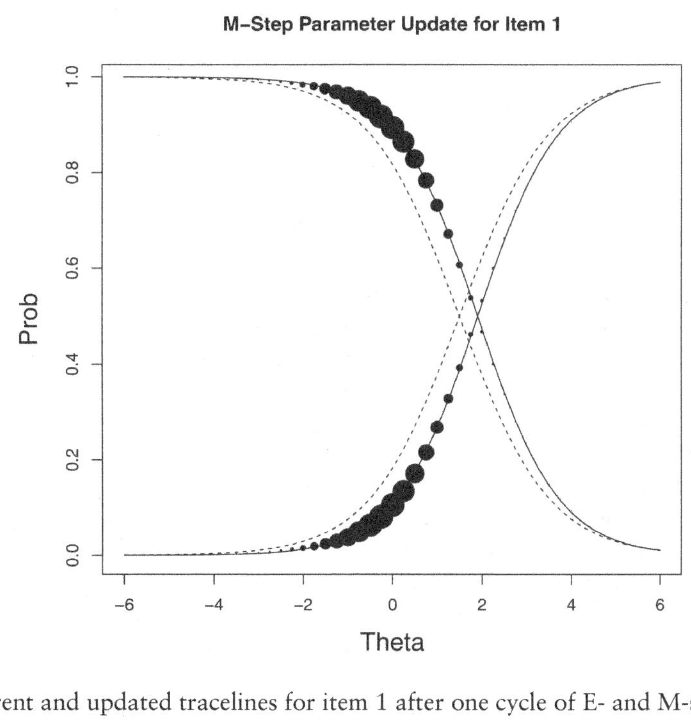

Figure 3.2 Current and updated tracelines for item 1 after one cycle of E- and M-step.

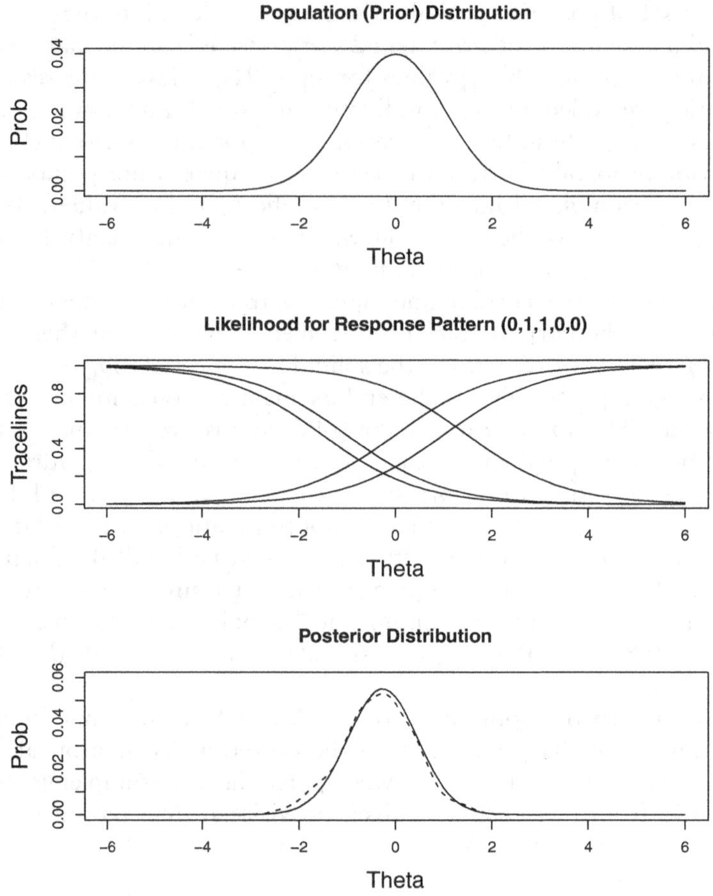

Figure 3.3 Multi-panel plot showing the relationship among the prior (population) density, the likelihood (products of tracelines shown) for response pattern (0,1,1,0,0), and the posterior density approximated in two ways. The solid posterior curve is found by numerically evaluating the normalized posterior ordinates over a range of θ values. The dashed posterior curve is found by plotting the empirically estimated density of the posterior from the random draws produced by a Metropolis-Hastings sampler for θ.

samples are used in complete data estimation with the Robbins-Monro method. Figure 3.3 plots the relationship among the prior density (standard normal), the likelihood function for response pattern (0,1,1,0,0) evaluated at the initial values of the item parameters ($\alpha_1 = -1.5, \alpha_2 = -1, \alpha_3 = 0, \alpha_4 = 1, \alpha_5 = 1.5, \beta_1 = \ldots \beta_5 = 1.0$), and the implied normalized posterior distribution. The prior and the posterior are represented as smooth solid curves.

There are 208 individuals associated with this response pattern. For each individual, we iterate the Metropolis-Hastings sampler 10 times and take the last draw as the posterior sample. We then empirically estimate a density function from the 208 posterior samples. The estimated density is shown as the dashed curve superimposed on the true implied posterior density. The two are obviously quite close, indicating the Metropolis-Hastings method can generate adequate posterior samples. For our sampler, the tuning constant (proposal dispersion σ) is equal to 2.0. The starting value of θ is equal to the standardized total score associated with response pattern (0,1,1,0,0). The total score for this response pattern is 2.0. The sample average total score over all response patterns is 2.17, and

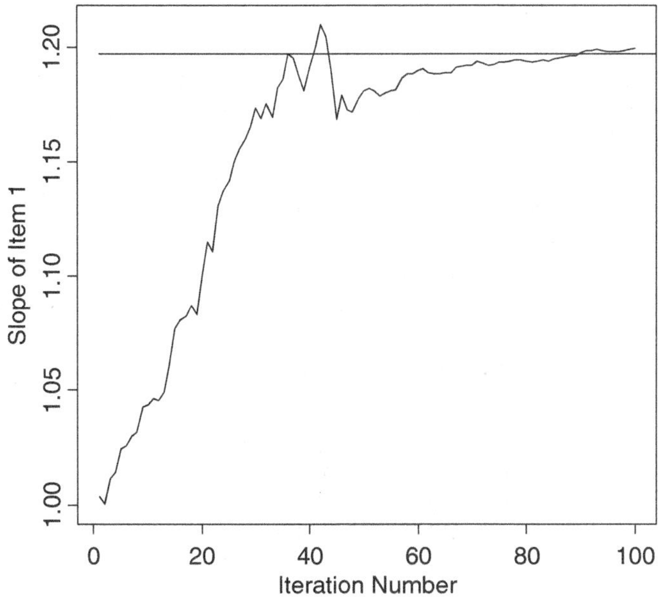

Figure 3.4 The iteration history of the slope parameter estimate for item 1 from MH-RM. The solid line is the MLE.

the sample standard deviation of the total score is 1.32, so the standardized total score is –0.13.

Together with the observed item responses, the posterior samples for all 1,490 individuals form the complete data set, with the posterior draws serving the role of predictor values. Complete data derivatives are evaluated and the item parameters are updated according to Equation (3.31) with the Robbins-Monro method. Figure 3.4 shows a sequence of parameter estimates from 100 iterations of the MH-RM algorithm for the slope parameter of item 1. The solid line is the MLE of that parameter from the Bock-Aitkin EM algorithm ($\beta_1 = 1.20$). The MH-RM estimates contain random error initially, but as the number of cycles increases, the Robbins-Monro method filters out the error to achieve convergence near the MLE.

Discussion and Conclusion

The key emphasis of our discussion of IRT and IRT parameter estimation is on a missing data formulation: The unobserved latent variable θ amounts to missing data. Had the missing data been observed, IRT parameter estimation would be standard logit analysis. Motivated by this missing data formulation, we described estimation algorithms that augment the observed data by replacing the missing data either deterministically by their posterior expected values or stochastically by multiple imputations from the posterior predictive distribution of θ. The former approach (Bock-Aitkin EM) requires numerical integration with quadrature. The latter approach (MH-RM) requires the combination of elements of Markov chain Monte Carlo (Metropolis-Hastings sampler) with stochastic approximation (Robbins-Monro method). In both approaches, it is revealed that an insight due to Fisher (1925) provided the key equation that connects the complete data and observed data models. We illustrated the estimation algorithms with an empirical data set.

This presentation has been restricted to parameter estimation for unidimensional IRT models for dichotomous responses, to keep the focus on the essential ideas. The procedures described here straightforwardly generalize to either multidimensional IRT models, or IRT models for polytomous responses, such as those used in the PROMIS® measures (Reeve et al., 2007), or both. We have alluded to the generalization to multidimensional IRT; that simply adds multidimensional quadrature grids, or vector-valued random draws, to the procedures described in the previous sections. Parameter estimation for IRT models for polytomous responses requires that the computations described in this chapter for each of the two dichotomous responses be carried out for each of the several polytomous responses, and that the values of partial derivatives be calculated for each parameter of the model. The necessary partial derivatives for most commonly used IRT models are available from a variety of sources, and are brought together in the book-length treatment of this topic by Baker and Kim (2004).

Author's Note: Li Cai is supported by grants from the Institute of Education Sciences (R305D140046 and R305B080016) and National Institute on Drug Abuse (R01DA026943 and R01DA030466). David Thissen has been supported by a PROMIS® cooperative agreement from the National Institutes of Health (NIH) Common Fund Initiative (U01AR052181). The views expressed here belong to the authors and do not reflect the views or policies of the funding agencies or grantees.

References

Baker, F.B., & Kim, S.-H. (2004). *Item response theory: Parameter estimation techniques.* New York: Dekker.

Bartholomew, D.J. (1998). Scaling unobservable constructs in social science. *Journal of the Royal Statistical Society – Series C, 47*, 1–13.

Bock, R.D., & Aitkin, M. (1981). Marginal maximum likelihood estimation of item parameters: Application of an EM algorithm. *Psychometrika, 46*, 443–459.

Bock, R.D., & Lieberman, M. (1970). Fitting a response model for *n* dichotomously scored items. *Psychometrika, 35*, 179–197.

Bolt, D. (2005). Limited and full information estimation of item response theory models. In A. Maydeu-Olivares & J.J. McArdle (Eds.). *Contemporary psychometrics* (pp. 27–71). Mahwah, NJ: Earlbaum.

Booth, J.G., & Hobert, J.P. (1999). Maximizing generalized linear mixed model likelihoods with an automated Monte Carlo EM algorithm. *Journal of the Royal Statistical Society—Series B, 61*, 265–285.

Cai, L. (2006). *Full-information item factor analysis by Markov chain Monte Carlo stochastic approximation.* Unpublished master's thesis, Department of Statistics, University of North Carolina at Chapel Hill.

Cai, L. (2008). *A Metropolis-Hastings Robbins-Monro algorithm for maximum likelihood nonlinear latent structure analysis with a comprehensive measurement model.* Unpublished doctoral dissertation, Department of Psychology, University of North Carolina at Chapel Hill.

Cai, L. (2010a). High-dimensional exploratory item factor analysis by a Metropolis-Hastings Robbins-Monro algorithm. *Psychometrika, 75*, 33–57.

Cai, L. (2010b). Metropolis-Hastings Robbins-Monro algorithm for confirmatory item factor analysis. *Journal of Educational and Behavioral Statistics, 35*, 307–355.

Dempster, A.P., Laird, N.M., & Rubin, D.B. (1977). Maximum likelihood estimation from incomplete data via the EM algorithm. *Journal of the Royal Statistical Society—Series B, 39*, 1–38.

Edwards, M.C. (2010). A Markov chain Monte Carlo approach to confirmatory item factor analysis. *Psychometrika, 75*, 474–497.

Fisher, R.A. (1925). Theory of statistical estimation. *Proceedings of the Cambridge Philosophical Society, 22*, 700–725.

Hastings, W.K. (1970). Monte Carlo simulation methods using Markov chains and their applications. *Biometrika, 57*, 97–109.

Maydeu-Olivares, A. (2013). Goodness-of-fit assessment of item response theory models. *Measurement: Interdisciplinary Research and Perspectives, 11,* 71–101.

Metropolis, N., Rosenbluth, A.W., Rosenbluth, M.N., Teller, A.H., & Teller, E. (1953). Equations of state space calculations by fast computing machines. *Journal of Chemical Physics, 21,* 1087–1092.

Reeve, B.B., Hays, R. D., Bjorner, J.B., Cook K.F., Crane, P.K., Teresi, J.A., Thissen, D., Revicki, D.A., Weiss, D.J., Hambleton, R.K., Liu, H., Gershon, R., Reise, S.P., Lai, J.S., & Cella, D (2007). Psychometric evaluation and calibration of health-related quality of life items banks: Plans for the patient-reported outcome measurement information system (PROMIS). *Medical Care, 45,* S22–31.

Rijmen, F., & Jeon, M. (2013). Fitting an item response theory model with random item effects across groups by a variational approximation method. *Annals of Operations Research, 206,* 647–662.

Robbins, H., & Monro, S. (1951). A stochastic approximation method. *Annals of Mathematical Statistics, 22,* 400–407.

Roberts, G.O., & Rosenthal, J.S. (2001). Optimal scaling for various Metropolis-Hastings algorithms. *Statistical Science, 16,* 351–367.

Schilling, S., & Bock, R.D. (2005). High-dimensional maximum marginal likelihood item factor analysis by adaptive quadrature. *Psychometrika, 70,* 533–555.

Thissen, D. (1982). Marginal maximum likelihood estimation for the one-parameter logistic model. *Psychometrika, 47,* 175–186.

Wirth, R.J., & Edwards, M.C. (2007). Item factor analysis: Current approaches and future directions. *Psychological Methods, 12,* 58–79.

Wu, C.F.J. (1983). On the convergence properties of the EM algorithm. *Annals of Statistics, 11,* 95–103.

4 Estimating the Latent Density in Unidimensional IRT to Permit Non-normality

Carol M. Woods

Introduction

A premise of item response modeling is that observed item responses are indicators of an underlying latent variable (or more than one). Often, for parameter estimation, the latent variable is presumed to be normally distributed. However, many psychological constructs like ambition or dysthymia are unlikely to be normally distributed in the general population. Non-normality could result from the sampling of one or more distinct populations such as those with or without a "disorder" (as defined by contemporary criteria). Alternatively, variables representing symptoms of pathology that are rare in the general population may be skewed because they exist in low levels for most people and in high levels for a few (with other people in between). Simulation studies about item response modeling have shown that when a non-normal latent variable is presumed normal, item parameters and scores for persons can be biased (Abdel-fattah, 1994; Boulet, 1996; Kirisci & Hsu, 1995; Stone, 1992; Woods, 2006a, 2007a, 2007b, 2008a; Woods & Lin, 2009; Woods & Thissen, 2006; Yamamoto & Muraki, 1991; Zwinderman & van den Wollenberg, 1990).

The present chapter deals with item response theory (IRT) in which there is one latent variable (θ), and item parameters are estimated using Bock and Aitkin's (1981) marginal maximum likelihood (MML) estimation implemented using an expectation maximization (EM) algorithm (Dempster, Laird, & Rubin, 1977). In this approach, θ is random, meaning the model specifies a distribution of latent trait or proficiency values for the population of people. Most commonly, a model with a logistic item response function is used along with a normal population distribution for θ.

However, models with logistic item response functions (IRFs) and normal latent densities are not flexible enough for all contexts. As mentioned earlier, many latent variables are not likely to be normally distributed. Flexibility can be introduced in either the shape of the IRF, or in the shape of the latent density, $g(\theta)$. Either one can be fixed to an alternative parametric form. For example, $g(\theta)$ can be fixed to a beta distribution, or the IRF can be fixed to the complementary log-log function. However, the most flexible strategy is to estimate either the regression relationship between the latent variable and the probability of responding (i.e., the IRF), or to estimate $g(\theta)$. A model that estimates both the IRF and $g(\theta)$ simultaneously is not identified, so one has to choose.

Equivalent fits to data may be obtained from a model with a normal $g(\theta)$ combined with nonparametrically estimated IRFs, versus a model with a nonparametrically estimated $g(\theta)$ combined with logistic IRFs. An example method for estimating the IRFs with a normal $g(\theta)$ is Ramsay's (1991) kernel smoothing approach implemented in TestGraf software. This method produces graphical depictions of IRFs without requiring iteration. However, with nonparametric IRFs, interpretable item parameters (e.g., "discrimination" and "guessing"), which are valuable for evaluating item properties, are lost. Also, the idea of an underlying response process (i.e., latent variable underlying the categorical item response) fits well theoretically with logistic (or normal ogive) IRFs, but not with nonparametric IRFs; thus, the nonparametric approach represents a fundamental change to the psychometric theory on which IRT is based (Holland, 1990; Lord & Novick, 1968, pp. 370–373; Thissen & Orlando, 2001, pp. 84–89).

Although there are some purposes for which an IRF-estimating approach may be preferred, the present chapter is focused on the strategy of permitting flexibility by estimating the shape of $g(\theta)$ while maintaining logistic IRFs. Such methods are appropriate when interpretable item parameters are desired, a latent response process is hypothesized, and one wishes to permit the latent variable to be non-normal in the population of people instead of forcing it to be normal. The methods to be described in this chapter include normal $g(\theta)$ as a special case so they can be considered, at the least, tools for testing the usual assumption about the normality of $g(\theta)$. If non-normality is evinced, improved item parameters and scores for persons using the estimated $g(\theta)$ can result.

What's Wrong With Violating Normality?

Although Bock and Aitkin (1981) speculated that the shape of $g(\theta)$ would have minimal impact on the item parameter estimates from EM MML fittings, simulation research indicates otherwise. This is not always observed, but some of the older studies are based on a single replication (e.g., Reise & Yu, 1990; Yen, 1987), and the degree to which bias is observed depends in part on the shape of $g(\theta)$. Bartholomew (1988) showed analytically that any *symmetric* $g(\theta)$ will predict essentially the same first- and second-order marginals, rendering it unlikely to influence the IRT results. Consistently, simulated densities that are non-normal but symmetric — with a platykurtic, uniform, or even bimodal shape, usually do not produce biased IRT results (De Ayala, 1995; Kirisci & Hsu, 1995; Kirisci, Hsu, & Kaohsiung, 2001; Reise & Yu, 1990; Roberts, Donoghue, & Laughlin, 2002; Stone, 1992; Woods & Lin, 2009; Woods & Thissen, 2006). It also seems that bias is not demonstrated when simulated item parameters are moderate (e.g., difficulty = –1, 0, or 1 in Seong, 1990), because bias is more pronounced for more extreme parameters, and averaging over item parameters of different magnitudes (frequently done) dilutes the amount of bias.

By contrast, when $g(\theta)$ is non-normal and nonsymmetric, EM MML estimates of item parameters are nontrivially biased when $g(\theta)$ is presumed normal and if $g(\theta)$ is skewed, the bias increases as the skewness increases (Abdel-fattah, 1994; Boulet, 1996; Kirisci & Hsu, 1995; Stone, 1992; Woods, 2006a, 2007a, 2007b, 2008a; Woods & Lin, 2009; Woods & Thissen, 2006; Yamamoto & Muraki, 1991; Zwinderman & van den Wollenberg, 1990).

IRT scores for persons are also less accurate when latent normality is assumed mistakenly (Kirisci & Hsu, 1995; Roberts, Donoghue, & Laughlin, 2002; Stone, 1992; Woods, 2006a, 2007a, 2007b, 2008b; Woods & Lin, 2009; Woods & Thissen, 2006). This finding has not been observed in all studies, but some use *maximum a posteriori* (MAP) scores whereas some use *expected a posteriori* (EAP) scores, and some are based on only few (e.g., 1 or 5) replications. Perhaps most importantly, the extent of bias usually varies over the range of the θ they estimate (Stone, 1992; Woods, 2006a, 2007a, 2007b, 2008a; Woods & Lin, 2009; Woods & Thissen, 2006), so averaging all scores together (as done in many studies) likely obscures the bias. EAPs tend to be well estimated for θ values in the part of $g(\theta)$ where there is substantial mass, so scores from the normal model will be biased for only some parts of a skewed $g(\theta)$.

Given that not all latent variables are expected to be well approximated as normal and that the bias is nontrivial when normality is assumed mistakenly for density shapes likely to be observed, it is important to have sound methods for fitting IRT models that do not assume $g(\theta)$ is normal. There are three main strategies for circumventing the assumption that $g(\theta)$ is normal (in the context of ML, conditional on logistic IRFs). One is to fit IRT models without a population distribution using joint maximum likelihood (JML; Birnbaum, 1968), and another is to use EM MML and assume an alternate parametric shape (or family of shapes) for $g(\theta)$ with distributional parameters estimated from the data. The third (preferred) is to estimate the shape of the density from the data using EM MML. The first two are reviewed primarily for didactic and historical interest. Readers primarily interested in "what is recommended now" may wish to skip ahead one section.

Early Work Relevant to IRT Without a Normal g(θ)

Before EM MML was introduced (Bock & Aitkin, 1981; Bock & Lieberman, 1970), IRT models were fitted without a population distribution using JML so the concern about the shape of $g(\theta)$ was moot. JML became obsolete because JML parameter estimates are biased and inconsistent, JML θ estimates are not finite when all, or no, items are endorsed (Baker, 1987; Embretson & Reise, 2000), and JML is theoretically mis-specified (Lord, 1986), because θ is treated as a fixed parameter rather than a random latent variable.

A better option is to use EM MML and assume an alternate parametric shape (or family of shapes) for $g(\theta)$ with distributional parameters estimated from the data. The beta distribution and mixtures of normals were proposed for this purpose (Andersen & Madsen, 1977; Engelen, 1989, chapter 4; Mislevy, 1984), both of which can assume a variety of forms. Though proposed on paper, these ideas did not evolve into widely used methodologies, probably because implementation was obscure or lacking in the context of IRT. Finite normal factor mixture models (Bauer & Curran, 2004; Lubke & Muthén, 2005; Lubke & Neal, 2008) represent an alternate formulation and are now quite popular. Nevertheless, distinct classes are not applicable to all research contexts and many latent variables are thought to be continua, varying quantitatively and not qualitatively, among persons. Thus, more flexible options are desirable.

A more flexible option due to Thissen (1991) is to assume $g(\theta)$ is one of a family of distributions developed by Johnson (1949), with the first four moments free to vary according to the data. Thissen's Johnson curve method is the most flexible of these parametric approaches, and was implemented (MULTILOG; Thissen, 1991) and applied to real data (e.g., van den Oord, 2005; van den Oord, Pickles, & Waldman, 2003). Unfortunately, the Johnson curve method tended to be unstable. It often failed to converge under exactly the conditions when it should be most necessary—for highly non-normal $g(\theta)$. A limitation of all approaches wherein a particular parametric form is assumed for $g(\theta)$ is that any a priori assumption may constitute a misspecification and is limited compared to nonparametrically estimating the density from the data.

Perhaps the ideal way to avoid assuming $g(\theta)$ is normal is to fit IRT models without making any assumptions about $g(\theta)$ (except of course that it is a proper density). In what is perhaps the earliest attempt at estimating something like $g(\theta)$, Lazarsfeld discussed the estimation of "latent structure," that included latent classes as well as latent continua (Lazarsfeld, 1950, p. 370), $\int_{-\infty}^{+\infty}\phi(x)f_i(x)f_j(x)f_k(x)\ldots = p_{ijk\ldots}$, where $\phi(x)$ is the population distribution, *f*s are IRFs for items i, j, and k, and p_{ijk} is the probability of a response pattern (he omitted "dx"). Lazarsfeld (1950) assumes the IRFs are polynomial, and derives formulas for the moments of $\phi(x)$. Unfortunately, the number of distributions with the same moments is not finite; thus, these methods do not yield a unique population distribution. Also, polynomial IRFs use different (and, in many cases, more) parameters than modern IRT models.

Finally, the issue of Rasch-family models fitted with conditional maximum likelihood (CML; Andersen, 1970; Rasch, 1960) should be addressed here as well. First, CML is only applicable to Rasch-family models. Rasch-family models force item discrimination to be equal for all items, which is often unrealistic, but renders the summed score a sufficient statistic for θ so that CML is possible (conditioning is with respect to the summed score). CML appears not to require an assumption about the shape of $g(\theta)$, so it appears initially appealing as a solution to circumventing the normality assumption about $g(\theta)$.

However, although there is no explicit $g(\theta)$ in CML (even after estimation), there is an implicit one. It turns out that a Rasch model estimated with CML is isomorphic with a certain log-linear model estimated with MML (Baker & Subkoviak, 1981; Blackwood & Bradley, 1989; Cressie & Holland, 1983; de Leeuw & Verhelst, 1986; Engelen, 1989, chapter 2; Follman, 1988; Holland, 1990; Kelderman, 1984; Mellenbergh & Vijn, 1981; Thissen & Mooney, 1989; Tjur, 1982). Some of the parameters of the log-linear MML model are moments of the implicit CML $g(\theta)$, and Cressie and Holland (1983) described moment inequalities that must be met for the implicit $g(\theta)$ to be a proper density. These moment inequalities are not always met for CML solutions, meaning that the implicit $g(\theta)$ from CML is not always a proper density. When fitting Rasch-family models to data, it is better to use EM MML (e.g., Thissen, 1982) so that $g(\theta)$ is a proper density and one can be clear about its shape.

Research Methods

Introduction to Modern Estimation of $g(\theta)$

We move now to methods for estimating $g(\theta)$ that are considered, at the time of this writing, reasonable to use. They are not without limitations, but all of them permit substantial flexibility in the shape of $g(\theta)$, are implemented in software, can be used with realistic numbers of items and people, include normal $g(\theta)$ as a special case, and have been shown in simulations to improve the accuracy of item parameters when used in lieu of assuming normality when the true density is known to be non-normal. Three methods are described here: (a) empirical histograms, (b) Ramsay curves, and (c) Davidian curves.

Because each of these methods constitutes a (different) small change to the standard EM MML approach to fitting an item response model, it is useful if readers already understand EM MML estimation in some detail. The following section describes EM MML (Bock & Aitkin, 1981; Bock & Lieberman, 1970) using a normal $g(\theta)$, and may be skipped by readers already familiar with the standard approach.

EM MML Estimation

The likelihood and estimation procedures are described here for the two-parameter logistic (2PL; Birnbaum, 1968) model but generalize to other IRFs (note, however, that some shorthand is used for responses coded 0 or 1 that would not exactly generalize for polytomous item responses). Let $\mathbf{a}$ = vector of discrimination parameters for all items, and $\mathbf{b}$ = vector of difficulty or location parameters for all items. Further, let u_{ij} represent a 0 or 1 response to item i by person j, where items are counted $i = 1$ to k and people are counted $j = 1$ to n, and let $\mathbf{u}$ refer to a response pattern.

With locally independent items, the likelihood of **u** is:

$$f(\mathbf{u} \mid \mathbf{a},\mathbf{b};\theta) = \prod_i T_i^{u_i}(1-T_i)^{1-u_i}, \tag{4.1}$$

where T_i is the 2PL IRF: $T(u_i = 1 \mid \theta) = \dfrac{1}{1+e^{[-a_i(\theta-b_i)]}}$. Each **u** has a different likelihood at each value of θ. Thus, to consider the likelihood of **u** over all possible values of θ, the integral is taken, over the latent distribution, $g(\theta)$:

$$P(\mathbf{u} \mid \mathbf{a},\mathbf{b}) = \int_{-\infty}^{+\infty}\left(\prod_i T_i^{u_i}(1-T_i)^{1-u_i}\right)g(\theta)d\theta. \tag{4.2}$$

The integration is carried out numerically with rectangular quadrature.

Next, consider all response patterns simultaneously. Because each person's pattern assigns him or her to one of 2^k mutually exclusive categories, the combination of likelihoods follows a multinomial distribution, with persons assumed independent:

$$L = \frac{n!}{\prod_{\mathrm{u}} r_{\mathrm{u}}}\prod_{\mathrm{u}}[P(\mathbf{u} \mid \mathbf{a},\mathbf{b})]^{r_{\mathrm{u}}}, \tag{4.3}$$

where r_{u} is the frequency with which each pattern occurs in the data set (i.e., the number of people who gave that pattern).

The log of the likelihood is maximized for computational convenience and the multinomial coefficient may be omitted because it does not depend on the item parameters and is an additive constant to the log likelihood:

$$\ell \propto \sum_{\mathrm{u}} r_{\mathrm{u}} \log[P(\mathbf{u} \mid \mathbf{a},\mathbf{b})]. \tag{4.4}$$

Solutions for the parameters are not known to exist in closed form, but Bock and Aitkin (1981) described an EM approach for maximizing it iteratively, alternating so-called E-steps and M-steps until convergence.

The primary goal of the E-step is to compute the number of people expected to respond "1" and "0" to each item, at each level of θ (the continuum has "levels" because it is represented using quadrature). The item parameters are treated as known (from the previous M-step or arbitrary starting values), and $g(\theta)$ is standard normal. The "number of people" is actually fractional (an expected frequency), and is calculated using posterior distributions. Derived from Bayes's theorem, the posterior distribution for response pattern **u** is the normalized product of the likelihood of the data (i.e., product of the IRFs), and $g(\theta)$:

$$S_{\mathrm{u}} = \frac{\mathrm{f}(\mathbf{u} \mid \mathbf{a},\mathbf{b};\theta)\,\mathrm{g}(\theta)}{\mathrm{P}(\mathbf{u} \mid \mathbf{a},\mathbf{b})}. \tag{4.5}$$

For the E-step, first consider the expected fraction of people at each quadrature point, irrespective of which response they gave. Each normalized posterior is multiplied by the observed frequency of people at each quadrature point: $S_{\mathrm{u}}r_{\mathrm{u}}$, rendering the total area of each posterior equal to r_{u} instead of 1. Then the expected frequency of people at each quadrature point is obtained by summing all of the rescaled posteriors:

$$N(\theta_q) = \sum_{\mathrm{u}} S_{\mathrm{u}} r_{\mathrm{u}}, \tag{4.6}$$

where θ_q is the latent variable represented using quadrature, with points $q = 1, 2, ..., Q$. Second, N is further divided into people who gave the "1" versus "0" response, which is item specific. For data coded 0 or 1, the item response may be included as a multiplier as shown below, where r_{1i}^* is the expected frequency of people who responded "1" to item i at each level of θ: $r_{1i}^*(\theta_q) = \sum_u u_{ij} S_u r_u$ and $r_{0i}^*(\theta_q) = N - r_{1i}^*$ is the expected frequency of people who responded "0" to item i at each level of θ.

In the M-step, the E-step frequencies are used to maximize a separate likelihood for each item:

$$L_i^* \propto \prod_q T_i^{r_{1i}^*} (1 - T_i)^{N - r_{1i}^*}, \tag{4.7}$$

(binomial coefficient omitted). An iterative algorithm such as the Newton-Raphson is used to solve each individual likelihood. The item-specific likelihood is maximized separately for each item before the next E-step is initiated.

Empirical Histogram (EH) Estimation of g(θ)

When introducing EM MML, Bock and Aitkin (1981) included the suggestion to estimate $g(\theta)$ as an empirical histogram (EH) instead of fixing it at normal. Mislevy (1984) elaborated on this idea, and versions of the BILOG program (e.g., Mislevy & Bock, 1990; Zimowski, Muraki, Mislevy, & Bock, 2003) have been capable of estimating $g(\theta)$ as an EH simultaneously with the item parameters for many years. The method was also implemented in Mx software (Schmitt, Mehta, Aggen, Kubarych, & Neale, 2006). BILOG and the Mx approach cited here analyze binary-coded responses. There is also a Fortran implementation due to Tzamourani that is used in several papers about binary responses (e.g., Knott & Tzamourani, 2007; Nader, Tran, & Formann, 2011; Tzamourani & Knott, 2002). Woods (2007b) produced and evaluated, in simulations, a C++ implementation for EH with ordinal responses using Samejima's (1969, 1997) graded model. Perhaps the most flexible implementation of EH available at the time of this writing is in flexMIRT software (Cai, 2012), which performs EH estimation for unidimensional models and the general dimension of a bifactor model (Gibbons & Hedeker, 1992) with any of several binary and ordinal logistic IRFs.

The EH approach is to estimate the height of $g(\theta)$ at each quadrature point instead of computing the heights based on the normal density. The standard EM MML algorithm already includes an approximation of the number of people expected at each level of θ, $N(\theta_q)$ (see Equation 4–6). The EH approach is produced when every current E-step uses the previous E-step's estimate of $g(\theta)$, the $N(\theta_q)$, instead of the normal distribution [with an arbitrary $g(\theta)$ for the very first E-step]. This influences the expected frequencies and therefore the item parameter estimates, rendering them more accurate if the true latent density is non-normal (Woods, 2007b). To decide whether a latent density is non-normal, one may examine a plot of the EH, but to reduce the ambiguity of this decision, a likelihood ratio difference significance test can be used to compare the EH and normal models (Schmitt et al., 2006).

Limitations of EH

Although it is generally better to use the EH versus normal solution if $g(\theta)$ is non-normal (Schmitt et al., 2006a; Woods, 2007b, 2008a), there are limitations. For one, the results are sensitive to the quadrature scheme (i.e., range and number of points). Woods (2007b) tested four rectangular quadrature schemes and found that estimation failure was more likely when a small number of points were spread over a wide range (e.g., 15 points between –6 and 6), and item parameters were less accurate with fewer points (spread over either a wide or small range). The recommended scheme was 81 points between –4 and 4. Nader, Tran, and Formann (2011) found that the EH approach was also sensitive to starting values for the item parameters (but there was no comparison to other methods, which may be similarly sensitive).

An alternative to user-specified rectangular quadrature is automated quadrature selection (i.e., adaptive quadrature), and this may improve the performance of EH. It certainly avoids user decision making, which can be attractive. An adaptive quadrature scheme is implemented in versions of BILOG software, including BILOG-MG 3 (Zimowski et al., 2003), and an adaptive algorithm is studied and implemented by Tzamourani and Knott (2002). Simulation evaluations of EH performance with adaptive quadrature are scant, and I am not aware that EH has been evaluated in a single study with, versus without, adaptive quadrature. Nevertheless, the EH implementation in BILOG-MG 3 (Zimowski et al., 2003) has produced highly accurate item parameter estimates for non-normal true $g(\theta)$ using the 2PL and 3PL IRFs (Woods, 2008a; Woods & Lin, 2009), and Tzamourani and Knott's approach recovered the true non-normal density well, conditional on adequate test length (2002).

Another limitation of the EH approach is that the characterization of $g(\theta)$ does not produce a smooth curve. An example plot from an EH analysis of an anxiety scale (5,913 people, 13 binary items), from Woods and Thissen (2006), is shown in Figure 4.1. The EH plot can be kernel smoothed to create a better picture (cf. Knott & Tzamourani, 2007), but this does not change the fact that all the parameters were estimated to create the EH in the first place, and is not expected to improve accuracy. When plotted in natural EH form, it is common for plots of EH solutions to be choppy, or to have sharp twists and turns. Indeed, one can conceptualize an EH as a latent class model, where each quadrature point represents a latent class (Bartolucci & Pennoni, 2007). But this is inconsistent with the definition of θ in IRT; it is supposed to be a continuum, with quadrature for numerical integration. The choppy EH does not appear to be a problem for improving the accuracy of item parameter

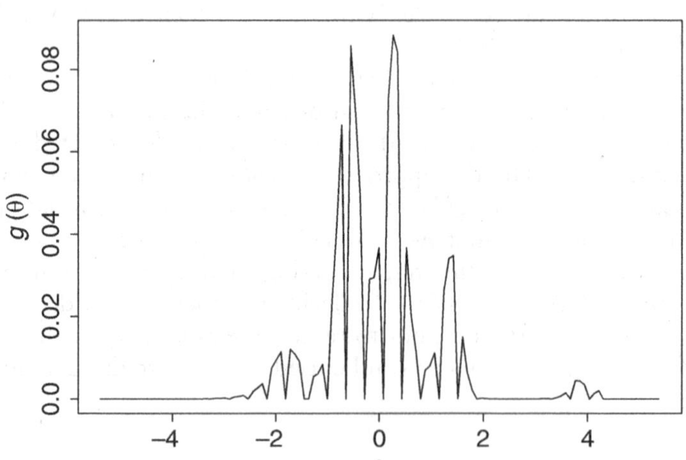

Figure 4.1 Example empirical histogram: Anxiety scale.

estimates, but scores and density recovery from EH models have been less accurate than those from Ramsay- or Davidian-curve IRT (Woods, 2008a; Woods & Lin, 2009). The disadvantage is key when the shape of $g(\theta)$ is of substantive interest: It is difficult to accept a choppy EH characterization as an accurate representation of a latent continuum.

A final limitation of the EH approach is that the number of additional parameters required is often large. The height at every quadrature point is a free parameter. The number of free parameters needed for an EH is equal to the number of quadrature points minus three constraints: The heights have to sum to 1 and the mean and variance of the histogram are 0 and 1, respectively. Thus, if the number of quadrature points is 81, the number of EH-related free parameters is 78. To compute accurate standard errors (SEs) for the item parameters, parameters for $g(\theta)$ should be considered; thus, the huge number of EH parameters leads to suboptimal efficiency for the item parameters. I am not aware of any currently available implementations of EH for which the item parameter SEs incorporate information from the $g(\theta)$ as they should.

Scale Identification When $g(\theta)$ Is Estimated

Typically in IRT, the latent scale is identified by fixing the mean and variance of θ to 0 and 1 (respectively). This is preferable to other approaches, such as fixing a discrimination parameter to 1 for one of the items, because selection of an extreme item could produce an implausible, strange shape for $g(\theta)$. When $g(\theta)$ is assumed normal, or any another distribution for which the mean and variance are its parameters or simple functions of its parameters, it is easy to fix the mean and variance. However, when $g(\theta)$ is estimated as an EH, or using other methods to be discussed here, $g(\theta)$ cannot be standardized directly, and an alternative strategy is needed. The scale identification strategy used for Ramsay curves, for Davidian curves, and for some implementations of EHs (Woods, 2007b) is an interpolation-extrapolation algorithm designed by David Thissen (Woods & Thissen, 2006). This strategy is described next.

The algorithm is to standardize the histogram of expected frequencies in the E-step, and then translate the standardized histogram back to the original quadrature points so that the quadrature points remain constant throughout the EM cycles. As mentioned earlier, the E-step involves computation of the number (fraction) of people expected at each level of θ, $N(\theta_q)$ (see Equation 4–6). This is a histogram of expected frequencies that may be standardized by subtracting the mean and dividing the standard deviation from each (weighted) quadrature point. Standardization is a linear transformation that alters neither the number of quadrature points nor the equal spacing between them. However, the particular values change, which is problematic because the quadrature must remain constant throughout EM cycles. The solution is to translate the standardized histogram back to the original quadrature using linear interpolation and extrapolation.

Let N represent an expected frequency at each quadrature point, q, and let N^* and q^* represent N and q after standardization, with subscripts indicating the point, from the smallest (0) to the largest (Q). If $q \le q_0^*$ or $q \ge q_Q^*$, extrapolation is used to calculate N. Specifically, if $q \le q_0^*$, then $N_q = \left[\left(\frac{N_0^*}{N_1^*}\right)^{\frac{q_0^* - q}{\Delta}}\right] N_0^*$ where Δ is the distance between any two q or, equivalently, between any two q^*. Conversely, if $q \ge q_Q^*$, then $N_q = \left[\left(\frac{N_Q^*}{N_{Q-1}^*}\right)^{\frac{q - q_Q^*}{\Delta}}\right] N_Q^*$.

For q between any two q^*, interpolation is used: $N_q = \left[\left(\frac{q-q^*}{\Delta}\right)\left(N^*_{q^*+1} - N^*_{q^*}\right)\right] + N^*_{q^*}$.
After standardization and translation back to the original quadrature, the histogram is renormalized, and used for the M-step.

Ramsay Curve IRT for the Estimation of g(θ)

Ramsay curve IRT (RC-IRT; Woods, 2004, 2006a; Woods & Thissen, 2006) improves upon the EH approach because the estimate of $g(\theta)$ is smooth, not particularly sensitive to the user-specified rectangular quadrature scheme, and requires at most 10 additional free parameters. Although a Ramsay curve also appears in the mathematical statistics literature as a logspline density (e.g., Kooperberg & Stone, 1991; Stone & Koo, 1986), the name "Ramsay" was assigned because of Ramsay's (2000) accessible description of the density estimation method. RC-IRT should not be confused with Ramsay's (1991) kernel density approach to the estimation of IRFs that is implemented in TestGraf software. The next section provides background related to splines because Ramsay curves are spline-based densities.

Preliminaries About Splines

Splines (named by Schoenberg, 1946) are linear combinations of polynomial functions joined together smoothly at breaks or knots. They were developed in an attempt to retain the virtues, but offset the disadvantages, of polynomial functions. Polynomial functions are smooth, provide curvature, and can be evaluated, differentiated, and integrated easily and in finitely many steps using basic arithmetic operations (de Boor, 2001, p. 1). However, they often fit data poorly because of their global dependence on local properties. If the function to be approximated is badly behaved *any*where in the interval of approximation, then a polynomial approximation is poor *every*where (de Boor, 2001, p. 17). The use of the piecewise polynomial spline, with a separate polynomial between each pair of knots, makes use of the desirable properties of polynomials, but the behavior in one section of the spline is not unduly influenced by the behavior in another. Usually, the polynomials that compose a spline are all of the same order. Following de Boor (2001), the order of a polynomial is one more than the degree.

A spline is linear in the parameters, thus analogous to the usual linear regression model, except that the "predictors" are functions. Within a set (defined by the order of the polynomials), all splines can be written as linear combinations of the predictor functions; thus, the predictor functions are called basis functions. A matrix containing values of each basis function at each value of the variable being approximated is simply "the basis," and is analogous to the predictor or design matrix in linear regression. Coefficients for a spline are estimated in the same ways as for linear regression (e.g., ordinary least squares or maximum likelihood).

A widely used class of splines are the basis-splines, usually called B-splines (de Boor, 2001 attributes them to Curry & Schoenberg, 1947). Around the same time, de Boor (1972) and Cox (1972) derived the recurrence relation expression for a B-spline, which has computational advantages over the original formulation of B-splines. The recurrence relation for a B-spline of degree 1 (order 2) or higher is (adapted from de Boor, 2001):

$$B_x^d(\theta) = \frac{\theta - \kappa_x}{h} B_x^{d-1}(\theta) + \frac{\kappa_{x+d+1} - \theta}{h} B_{x+1}^{d-1}(\theta), \quad (4.8)$$

where d is the degree, κ is a knot on θ, x is the knot at which a given B-spline starts, and h is the distance between the knots. The distance between the knots need not be uniform (a more general expression of the recurrence relation appears in, e.g., de Boor, 1978, p. 131). However, so-called cardinal B-splines (Schoenberg, 1969, 1973), with equally spaced knots, are easiest to work with and are used for Ramsay curves.

Three properties of B-splines are (de Boor, 2001; Nürnberger, 1989): (a) they are 0 everywhere except a finite interval, (b) the set of B-splines of a given order, evaluated at any θ, partitions unity, and (c) all nonzero values are positive. Also, B-splines are themselves piecewise polynomial. Thus, a spline made with a B-spline basis is a piecewise polynomial composed of piecewise polynomials, providing heuristic insight about why splines with B-spline bases are very flexible.

The recurrence relation shows that B-splines are functions of lower-order B-splines defined over the same knots. The lowest degree possible is 0. 0th-degree (order 1) B-splines are step functions composed of 0s and 1s. Consider the simple example of linear (degree 1, order 2) B-splines, fitted for θ between -5 and 5 (in one-unit increments). In this context, two B-splines can join in only one place; however, there must always be knots at the endpoints of a fitting range. Thus, a minimum of two knots is required, and they occur at -5 and 5 for this example. Note that calculation of a B-spline requires two more knots than the user specifies. This is what de Boor refers to as the "not-a-knot" condition, and is usually done because nothing is known about the two endpoint derivatives (de Boor, 2001, p. 44). For the present problem, the invisible endpoint knots, used only for the computations, are κ_0 and κ_3, whereas κ_1 and κ_2 are specified by the data analyst. For equally spaced knots, the placement of the invisible endpoint knots on θ is easily calculated: θ is depicted in one-unit increments, and the distance between -5 and 5 is 10; thus $\kappa_0 = -15$ and $\kappa_3 = 15$.

In general, the order (or degree) and the number of knots determine the number of B-spline functions:

$$m = (d + 1) + \text{number of knots} - 2. \tag{4.9}$$

Given two knots and $d = 1$, Equation (4.9) shows that there are two B-splines. One extends from κ_0 to κ_1, and the other extends from κ_1 to κ_2 (alternatively, these can be calculated so that the first extends from κ_1 to κ_2 and the second from κ_2 to κ_3). By substitution into Equation (4.8), the first B-spline function is $B_0^1(\theta) = \frac{\theta - \kappa_0}{10} B_0^0(\theta) + \frac{\kappa_2 - \theta}{10} B_1^0(\theta)$, and computations are shown in Table 4.1. Calculation of the second B-spline function is very similar: x is just incremented by one. This calculation is shown in Table 4.2.

Ramsay's (2000) Density Approximation Procedure

Linear combinations of B-splines have desirable mathematical properties. However, when a curve is estimated with a spline, it is not necessarily a probability density function. Thus, to employ splines in the estimation of a density like $g(\theta)$, constraints must be imposed so that the result integrates to one, and is everywhere non-negative. In work similar to Silverman (1982), Ramsay (2000) showed how to impose these constraints. His approach is founded on a differential equation: an equation that involves derivatives in which the unknown is a function.

Table 4.1 The First Degree-1 B-Spline Function

θ	*knots*	$\frac{\theta-\kappa_0}{10}$	$B_0^0(\theta)$	+	$\frac{\kappa_2-\theta}{10}$	$B_1^0(\theta)$	=	$B_0^1(\theta)$
−5	κ_1	1.0	0		1.0	1		1.0
−4		1.1	0		0.9	1		0.9
−3		1.2	0		0.8	1		0.8
−2		1.3	0		0.7	1		0.7
−1		1.4	0		0.6	1		0.6
0		1.5	0		0.5	1		0.5
1		1.6	0		0.4	1		0.4
2		1.7	0		0.3	1		0.3
3		1.8	0		0.2	1		0.2
4		1.9	0		0.1	1		0.1
5	κ_2	2.0	0		0.0	1		0.0

Note. θ = latent variable represented with example quadrature points here; B = a B-spline, with a superscript equal to the degree and subscripts keeping track of how many B-splines there are of that degree; κ_j = knot at point j.

Table 4.2 The Second Degree-1 B-Spline Function

θ	*knots*	$\frac{\theta-\kappa_1}{10}$	$B_1^0(\theta)$	+	$\frac{\kappa_3-\theta}{10}$	$B_2^0(\theta)$	=	$B_1^1(\theta)$
−5	κ_1	0.0	1		2.0	0		0.0
−4		0.1	1		1.9	0		0.1
−3		0.2	1		1.8	0		0.2
−2		0.3	1		1.7	0		0.3
−1		0.4	1		1.6	0		0.4
0		0.5	1		1.5	0		0.5
1		0.6	1		1.4	0		0.6
2		0.7	1		1.3	0		0.7
3		0.8	1		1.2	0		0.8
4		0.9	1		1.1	0		0.9
5	κ_2	1.0	1		1.0	0		1.0

Note: θ = latent variable represented with example quadrature points here; B = a B-spline, with a superscript equal to the degree and subscripts keeping track of how many B-splines there are of that degree; κ_j = knot at point j.

Given that a smooth function has at least one derivative, there exists a differential equation that describes the relation, **w**, between the unknown (smooth) function $g(\theta)$ and its first derivative:

$$\frac{\partial g(\theta)}{\partial \theta} = \mathbf{w}g(\theta), \tag{4.10}$$

where **w** is a spline function with a B-spline basis, **B**: **w** = **Bc**, and **c** is an m by 1 vector of coefficients, estimated from the data. Because $g(\theta)$ must be non-negative, solving Equation (4.10) for **w** is equivalent to defining **w** as the derivative of the log of $g(\theta)$: $\mathbf{w} = \frac{1}{g(\theta)}\left(\frac{\partial g(\theta)}{\partial\theta}\right) = \frac{\partial \log[g(\theta)]}{\partial\theta}$. Then, an expression for $g(\theta)$ may be obtained by integrating and exponentiating **w** and $\frac{\partial \log[g(\theta)]}{\partial\theta}$: $g(\theta) \cong \exp\int_{\theta_o}^{\theta}\mathbf{w}(\zeta)d\zeta$, where θ_o is the smallest value of θ, and ζ is a variable of integration. Finally, the norming constant ensures that $g(\theta)$ integrates to 1:

$$g(\theta) = \frac{\exp\int_{\theta_o}^{\theta}\mathbf{w}(\zeta)d\zeta}{\int_{-\infty}^{+\infty}\left[\exp\int_{\theta_o}^{\theta}\mathbf{w}(\zeta)d\zeta\right]d\theta}. \tag{4.11}$$

We call Equation (4.11) a Ramsay curve (Woods & Thissen, 2006). The advantage of re-expressing $g(\theta)$ is that **w** need not exist as a probability density function and therefore may be estimated as a spline.

Estimation of RC-IRT Models

Two changes to standard EM MML IRT produce RC-IRT. First, the current estimate of $g(\theta)$ is used in place of the normal distribution in every E-step. Second, after all of the item parameters are re-estimated as usual in the M-step, there is one more Newton-Raphson maximization to estimate Ramsay curve parameters. This uses a separate likelihood for the Ramsay curve parameters: $L_g \propto \prod_q g(\theta_q)^{N(\theta_q)}$, where $N(\theta_q)$ is the E-step estimate of the total number of (fractions of) people at each quadrature point (Equation [4.6]), and $g(\theta_q)$ is the Ramsay curve given by Equation (4.11), subscripted here to reflect its computation with quadrature points.

However, Ramsay curve parameters are sometimes difficult to estimate. For at least some problems, the fact that a skewed Ramsay curve has virtually no mass at one end will cause one or more Ramsay coefficients to become unidentified because little or no information is available in the lower region fitted by that part of the basis. When this happens, estimation of the entire set of coefficients fails.

To prevent one or more coefficients from becoming unidentified, the coefficients are Bayesian maximum a posteriori estimates, computed using a diffuse prior density. By Bayes's Theorem, the Ramsay curve posterior (*RCP*) density is the product of the Ramsay curve likelihood and an m-variate normal prior, where m is the number of coefficients (Equation [4.9]). With the normalization constant for the posterior omitted, the RCP at each quadrature point is:

$$RCP_q\left(\mathbf{c} \mid N(\theta_q)\right) \propto \left(g(\theta_q)^{N(\theta_q)}\right)\left(\frac{1}{(2\pi)^{\frac{m}{2}}|\Sigma|^{\frac{1}{2}}}\exp\left[-\frac{1}{2}(\mathbf{c}-\mu)'\Sigma^{-1}(\mathbf{c}-\mu)\right]\right), \tag{4.12}$$

where μ is the vector of means consisting of coefficients that make the resulting $g(\theta)$ normal, and Σ is a diagonal matrix with nonzero elements equal to the prior variance (SD^2; identical value for each coefficient). Conditioning is on the heights of $g(\theta_q)$ as estimated in the E-step (pseudo counts of fractions of people), and the vector of estimated coefficients maximizes the RCP.

Although some scientists argue that classic Bayesian analysis is characterized by undesirable subjectivity, it should be recognized that the prior employed for the estimation of Ramsay coefficients is minimally informative and therefore exerts small influence on the coefficient estimates in most cases. Further, the coefficients are not of direct interest in RC-IRT, and small variations in the coefficients usually have only small consequences on the shape of the resulting Ramsay curve. What little influence the prior may have on the results will be in the direction of bias toward normality of the population distribution; thus, tests for its non-normality may be a little conservative. This bias will decrease as the sample size and the number of items increase. To minimize the influence of the prior on the estimated coefficients, the largest value for the SD that permits successful estimation should be used (analysts can find this by trial and error). Prior SDs equal to 500 are often enough to provide successful estimation; however, in Woods's (2006a) simulations, the estimation success rate increased when prior SDs were 75, without any meaningful deterioration in the results (compared to SDs = 500). Additional estimation details about RC-IRT appear in Woods (2004) and Woods and Thissen (2006).

A development (Monroe & Cai, 2013) that is very new at the time of this writing is the estimation of RC-IRT models with the Metropolis-Hastings Robbins-Monro algorithm (MH-RM; Cai, 2010). The first simulation study shows item parameter and density estimates that are nearly identical for MH-RM and EM-MML (Monroe & Cai, 2013), with the advantage that the observed information matrix (thus SEs) are part of estimation with MH-RM. The MH-RM may be the most promising estimation strategy for RC-IRT to follow as it develops in the future.

How to Do RC-IRT

At the time of this writing, RC-IRT is implemented for unidimensional models only, along with any of several different logistic IRFs. The first implementation was in RCLOG (Woods, 2006b; Woods & Thissen, 2004), which is a C++ program lacking the flexibility typical of commercial software, but is free, fast, and well tested. A more accessible and user-friendly implementation of a procedure closely related to RC-IRT is implemented in EQSIRT (Wu & Bentler, 2011). Also note that there is an implementation using MH-RM estimation (Monroe & Cai, 2013). All of the details and simulation results reviewed in this chapter are specific to the RCLOG implementation. RCLOG implements the 2PL, 3PL, and graded IRFs, but many other IRFs could be used in combination with RC-IRT.

To carry out RC-IRT, the data analyst fits several candidate RC-IRT models, which vary according to the order and number of knots, to a single data set. The RC-IRT model with $g(\theta)$ equivalent to the normal distribution (2-breaks-order-2, or "2–2") is always fitted first, and subsequent models use more knots and higher order, up to user-specified maxima, usually 6 for both. Therefore, the number of Ramsay coefficients for the models varies from 2 (normal) to 10 (6 + 6 −2, see Equation [4.9]), and the data analyst must select a model to interpret among 25 possibilities.

Often, the item parameters (and EAPs) from RC-IRT models with similar-looking Ramsay curves differ minimally, and the choice among several similar models is minimally consequential. The goal of model selection is to identify a good model, not the single, perfect, or "true" model (all models are wrong to some degree). As in other model selection contexts, one balances parsimony with good fit when selecting an RC-IRT model.

Based on what is known about RC-IRT to date, the following steps are recommended for selecting an RC-IRT model to interpret. First, create a plot of all candidate models (R code for this purpose is distributed with RCLOG). Exclude models that did not converge. Look at the shape of the density estimated with the maximum number of coefficients. If this shape is replicated in other models with fewer coefficients, it is probably the target shape. Sometimes the evidence will point toward approximate normality, and then standard software and methods may be used, or the results of the order-2, 2-knots RC-IRT model may be interpreted.

For additional assistance, several statistical criteria are implemented in RCLOG, which were compared in Woods (2006a). Simulations indicated that the most useful was the Hannan-Quinn (Hannan, 1987) criterion: $HQ = -2\text{LogL} + 2m(\log(\log(n)))$, where log = natural log, m = number of spline coefficients and n = sample size. Smaller values indicate better fit, and it may be used for non-nested models (the only known nesting relationships among Ramsay curves are the normal within all the others). Therefore, analysts should seriously consider the HQ-best model for interpretation. Further, if a non-normal model is selected, it should be significantly different from normal by the Kolmogorov-Smirnov test (Kolmogorov, 1933; Smirnov, 1939) and a likelihood-ratio difference test comparing it to the normal model.

An example plot of candidate Ramsay curves for the Physical Concerns subscale of the Agoraphobic Cognitions Questionnaire (ACQ; Chambless, Caputo, Bright, & Gallagher, 1984) appears in Figure 4.2 for data (N = 1,005; 7 ordinal response items) analyzed by Woods (2006a). Plots are missing for 2 of the 25 candidate models (3-breaks-order-2, 4-breaks-order-2) because they did not converge. The consistency in the plots provides evidence against the normal model, and suggests that many non-normal models will yield similar results. The HQ-best model is the 5-knot, order-2 model with five coefficients. This model is significantly different from the normal by the KS test (d = .18, $p < .001$) and the likelihood ratio difference test ($\chi^2 = -65.60 - -45.77 = 111.37$, $df = 3$, $p < .001$). As shown in Table 4.3, parameter estimates from Samejima's (1969, 1997) graded-model IRFs produced by the HQ-best model differ noticeably from those produced by the normal model. Item parameter estimates from RC-IRT are interpreted as those from classic IRT.

Davidian Curve IRT for the Estimation of $g(\theta)$

This section describes a third method available for the estimation of $g(\theta)$ simultaneously with the item parameters using EM MML: Davidian curve IRT (DC-IRT; Woods & Lin, 2009). Like RC-IRT, DC-IRT provides a smooth representation of $g(\theta)$, and is not particularly sensitive to the user-specified rectangular quadrature scheme. However, it improves upon RC-IRT because it requires fewer tuning parameters, estimation is more stable, and model selection is easier. A "Davidian curve" is a "seminonparametric" (SNP) density function described by Gallant and Nychka (1987). Though the contributions of several individuals are acknowledged, the name "Davidian" was given because Davidian and her collaborators described the curves accessibly and developed a useful reparameterization (Davidian & Gallant, 1993; Davidian & Giltinan, 1995, chapter 7; Zhang & Davidian, 2001).

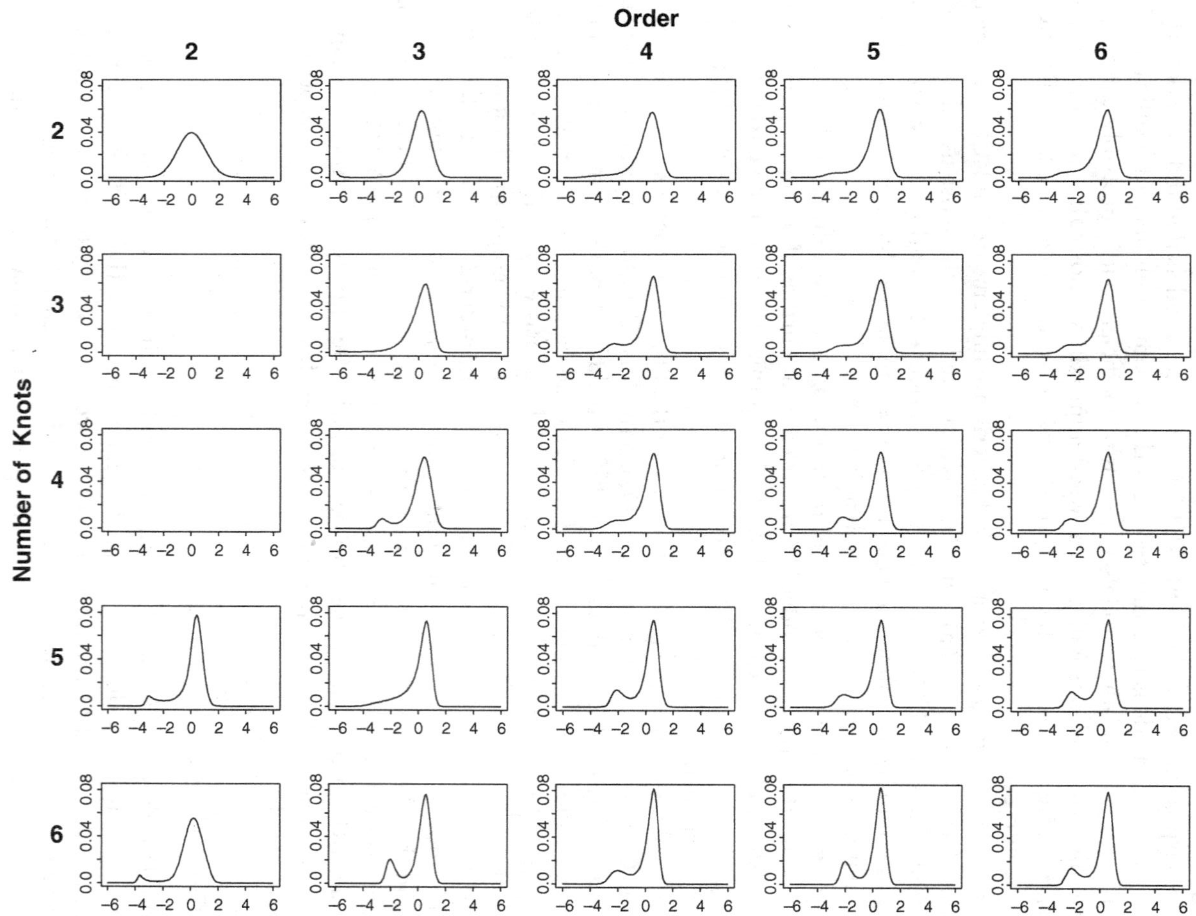

Figure 4.2 Example set of candidate Ramsay curves: Physical Concerns Scale.

Table 4.3 Item Parameter Estimates: Normal and HQ-best Models for the Physical Concerns Scale

Item	*Model*	*a*	b_1	b_2	b_3	b_4
1	normal	0.86	−1.06	1.51	2.96	4.69
	HQ-best	1.36	−0.66	1.08	1.99	3.08
2	normal	1.38	0.26	2.06	3.12	3.97
	HQ-best	2.40	0.33	1.36	1.95	2.44
3	normal	3.04	1.47	2.22	3.03	
	HQ-best	6.69	0.96	1.31	1.67	
4	normal	2.83	1.29	2.09	2.65	3.34
	HQ-best	6.37	0.88	1.24	1.49	1.80
5	normal	2.80	1.65	2.55	3.00	
	HQ-best	6.10	1.05	1.46	1.67	
6	normal	2.36	1.65	2.40		
	HQ-best	5.11	1.05	1.39		
7	normal	4.77	1.75	2.36		
	HQ-best	10.76	1.09	1.37		

Note: a = discrimination parameter estimate from Samejima's graded IRT model, b_j = the jth threshold parameter estimate from Samejima's graded IRT model.

Davidian Curves

In DC-IRT, g(θ) is represented as a unidimensional Davidian curve and estimated as described by Zhang and Davidian (2001). A Davidian curve is the product of a squared polynomial and the standard normal density function, φ:

$$h(\theta) = P_k^2(\theta)\varphi(\theta) \ . \tag{4.13}$$

P_k is a polynomial of order k: $P_k^2(\theta) = \left\{\sum_{\lambda=0}^{k} m_\lambda \theta^\lambda\right\}^2$, where λ is a non-negative integer and there are k + 1 coefficients: **m** = (m_o, m_1,...m_k), where $m_k \neq 0$. For example, if k = 1, $P_k^2(\theta) = (m_o + m_1\theta)^2$, a constraint is needed to ensure that h(θ) integrates to 1: $E\left[P_k^2(Z)\right] = 1$, where Z~N(0,1).

In matrix notation, the constraint can be re-expressed as:

$$E\left[P_k^2(Z)\right] = E\left[\left(\mathbf{m}^T\mathbf{U}\right)^2\right] = \mathbf{m}^T\left[E\left(\mathbf{U}\mathbf{U}^T\right)\right]\mathbf{m} = \mathbf{m}^T\mathbf{M}\mathbf{m} = 1\,, \tag{4.14}$$

where **M** = E(**UU**^{T}) is a symmetric positive definite, square matrix of dimension k + 1 and **U** = (1, Z, ...Z^k)^T. For k = 1, the constraint (Equation [4.14]) is: $\mathbf{m}^T\mathbf{M}\mathbf{m} = \begin{bmatrix} m_o & m_1 \end{bmatrix} \left[E\begin{Bmatrix} 1 & Z \\ Z & Z^2 \end{Bmatrix}\right]\begin{bmatrix} m_o \\ m_1 \end{bmatrix} = \begin{bmatrix} m_o & m_1 \end{bmatrix}\begin{bmatrix} 1 & 0 \\ 0 & 1 \end{bmatrix}\begin{bmatrix} m_o \\ m_1 \end{bmatrix} = 1$. Davidian curve parameters can then be estimated by constrained maximum likelihood estimation.

To improve the numerical stability of this constrained optimization, Zhang and Davidian (2001) introduced a reparameterization of the coefficients (m_o, m_1,...m_k) using a polar coordinate transformation. Because **M** is symmetric and positive definite, there exists a $k+1$ by $k+1$ positive definite matrix **B** such that $\mathbf{B}^T\mathbf{B} = \mathbf{M}$, where **B** can be obtained by singular value decomposition. If we let $\mathbf{c} = \mathbf{Bm}$, the constraint (Equation [4.14]) becomes: $\mathbf{m}^T\mathbf{B}^T\mathbf{B}\mathbf{m} = \mathbf{c}^T\mathbf{c} = 1$. Because $-\mathbf{c}$ leads to an identical density for θ, **c** must lie on a half-unit sphere in the domain of real numbers, and may be represented using a polar coordinate transformation:

$$\mathbf{c} = \begin{bmatrix} \sin(\phi_1) \\ \cos(\phi_1)\sin(\phi_2) \\ \ldots \\ \cos(\phi_1)\cos(\phi_2)\ldots\cos(\phi_{k-1})\sin(\phi_k) \\ \cos(\phi_1)\cos(\phi_2)\ldots\cos(\phi_{k-1})\cos(\phi_k) \end{bmatrix}, \text{ where } -\frac{\pi}{2} < \varphi_j \leq \frac{\pi}{2} \text{ for } j = 1, 2, \ldots k.$$

Using this reparameterization, $h(\theta)$ automatically integrates to 1. Thus, the squared polynomial becomes:

$$P_k^2(\theta) = \left\{ \left[\mathbf{B}^{-1}\mathbf{c}\right]^T \begin{bmatrix} 1 \\ \theta \\ \ldots \\ \theta^k \end{bmatrix} \right\}^2 . \tag{4.15}$$

For $k = 1$, $\mathbf{c} = \left[\sin(\varphi_1), \cos(\varphi_1)\right]^T$, which satisfies the constraint: $\mathbf{c}^T\mathbf{c} = \left[\sin(\varphi_1), \cos(\varphi_1)\right] \begin{bmatrix} \sin(\varphi_1) \\ \cos(\varphi_1) \end{bmatrix} = \sin^2(\varphi_1) + \cos^2(\varphi_1) = 1$. With the reparameterization, the number of Davidian curve parameters (ϕ_j) is equal to the tuning parameter, k.

Davidian Curve IRT (DC-IRT; Woods & Lin, 2009)

DC-IRT is a modification of classic EM MML IRT. In every E-step, the current estimate of $g(\theta)$ is used in place of the normal distribution. In every M-step, after all of the item parameters are re-estimated, there is one more Newton-Raphson maximization to estimate Davidian curve parameters. The Davidian curve likelihood is $L_g = \prod_{q=1}^{Q} g(\theta_q)^{N(\theta_q)}$, where $q = 1, 2, \ldots, Q$ counts quadrature points, $N(\theta_q)$ is the expected number (fraction) of people at each quadrature point, and $g = h$ from Equation (4.13). Further details are given in Woods and Lin (2009).

DC-IRT requires only one tuning parameter: the order of the polynomial in Equation (4.13), k. Complicated shapes including multimodality and skewness can be approximated with small values of k such as 1 or 2 (Zhang & Davidian, 2001, p. 796). However, when the mean of the density is constrained to 0, as done in DC-IRT to identify the scale of the latent variable, $k = 1$ imposes normality (Davidian & Gallant, 1993). Thus, for DC-IRT, both $k = 0$ and $k = 1$ produce the normal model. The constraint on the mean also sometimes increases the value of k required to obtain adequate fit (Davidian & Gallant, 1993). Therefore, DC-IRT uses larger values of k than are used by Davidian and her colleagues. DC-IRT is currently implemented for $k = 1, 2, \ldots, 10$.

Woods and Lin (2009) implemented DC-IRT in a C++ program that calls SAS (proc IML code from Zhang & Davidian, 2001) for the part of every M-step that estimates the Davidian curve parameters. The software fits 10 different DC-IRT models, with varying k, to the same data set, and the user selects a model to interpret. The model selection task is similar to that for RC-IRT; however, there are only 10 models to choose among instead of 25. The HQ criterion has worked well for model selection in Davidian's work (Davidian & Gallant, 1993; Zhang & Davidian, 2001), and for DC-IRT (Woods & Lin, 2009). The same advice given for model selection for RC-IRT applies to model selection with DC-IRT.

Application

Empirical Example of DC-IRT

DC-IRT will be illustrated using wave I of the Patient Reported Outcomes Measurement Information System (PROMIS®)[1] public use data, which consists of patient-reported health status outcomes about physical, mental, and social well-being. Here, responses to the Anger Questionnaire (AQ) given by a sample of 847 adults from the general population (441 male, 433 female; mean age = 50.89, SD = 18.24) were analyzed with DC-IRT. The AQ consists of 12 items with Likert-type responses ranging from 1 (extremely uncharacteristic of me) to 5 (extremely characteristic of me).

Samejima's graded model was used with Davidian curves fitted to the data with $k = 1$ through $k = 10$ using the implementation of DC-IRT from Woods and Lin (2009). The HQ-best model was non-normal with $k = 4$. The first six candidate densities ($k = 1$ through $k = 6$) are shown in Figure 4.3 with the corresponding HQ (less 23,330 to

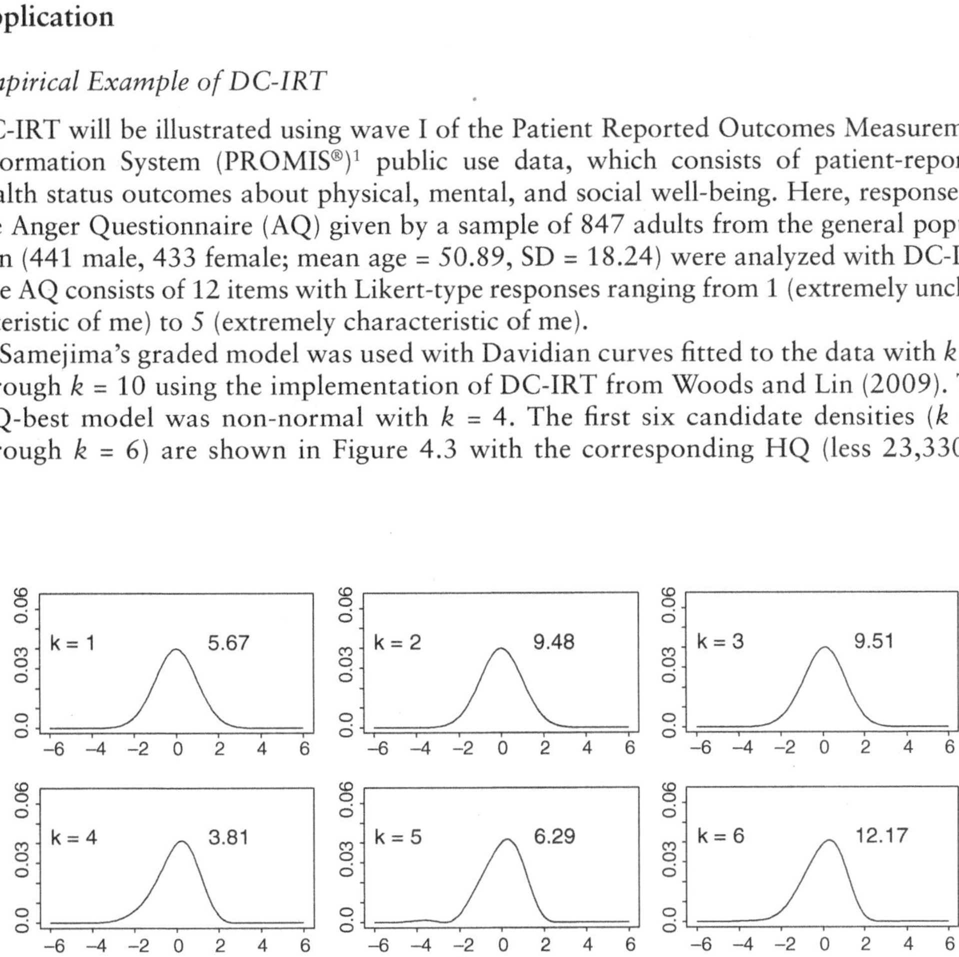

Figure 4.3 Candidate Davidian curves for PROMIS® Anger Questionnaire.

1 PROMIS® was funded with cooperative agreements from the National Institutes of Health (NIH) Common Fund Initiative (U54AR057951, U01AR052177, U54AR057943, U54AR057926, U01AR057948, U01AR052170, U01AR057954, U01AR052171, U01AR052181, U01AR057956, U01AR052158, U01AR057929, U01AR057936, U01AR052155, U01AR057971, U01AR057940, U01AR057967, U01AR052186). The contents of this chapter use data developed under PROMIS®. These contents do not necessarily represent an endorsement by the U.S. federal government or PROMIS®. See www.nihpromis.org for additional information on the PROMIS® initiative.

highlight differences among models). For this example, the HQ-best model is not dramatically non-normal, but item parameter estimates (and EAPs if desired) from the $k = 4$ DC-IRT model should be more accurate than those from the normal model. Item parameter estimates for the normal ($k = 1$) and HQ-best ($k = 4$) models are given in Table 4.4. Differences in the estimates between models are small but evident for

Table 4.4 Item Parameter Estimates: Normal and HQ-best Models for the PROMIS® Anger Questionnaire

Item	*Model*	a	b_1	b_2	b_3	b_4
1	normal	2.34	0.53	1.00	1.65	2.81
	HQ-best	2.48	0.54	0.98	1.59	2.67
2	normal	0.50	−5.98	−2.90	−0.97	3.11
	HQ-best	0.50	−5.94	−2.87	−0.96	3.09
3	normal	1.68	−0.24	0.66	1.60	2.85
	HQ-best	1.72	−0.21	0.67	1.57	2.78
4	normal	1.43	−0.41	1.14	1.96	2.88
	HQ-best	1.45	−0.39	1.14	1.94	2.84
5	normal	1.10	−1.15	−0.22	0.91	2.64
	HQ-best	1.11	−1.12	−0.20	0.91	2.60
6	normal	0.97	−1.04	0.19	1.17	3.18
	HQ-best	0.98	−1.01	0.20	1.16	3.13
7	normal	2.77	0.34	0.95	1.51	2.34
	HQ-best	2.96	0.36	0.93	1.45	2.21
8	normal	1.44	−1.47	−0.28	0.35	2.52
	HQ-best	1.44	−1.47	−0.26	0.36	2.49
9	normal	1.55	−1.04	0.11	1.32	2.96
	HQ-best	1.58	−1.01	0.12	1.30	2.89
10	normal	2.39	0.77	1.17	1.70	2.60
	HQ-best	2.57	0.76	1.13	1.63	2.46
11	normal	2.02	−0.07	0.53	1.22	2.57
	HQ-best	2.11	−0.04	0.53	1.20	2.46
12	normal	2.60	0.73	1.19	1.85	2.60
	HQ-best	2.83	0.73	1.15	1.75	2.44

Note: a = discrimination parameter estimate from Samejima's graded IRT model, b_j = the jth threshold parameter estimate from Samejima's graded IRT model.

most parameters. Item parameter estimates from DC-IRT are interpreted as those from classic IRT.

Summary

Simulation Results and Comparisons Among EH, RC-IRT, and DC-IRT

This section summarizes what is known to date from simulation research about all three methods, and concludes with distinctions among them. For methods that estimate $g(\theta)$, sample sizes needed for accurate estimation of item parameters and EAPs are about the same as for usual EM MML IRT: At least about 500 with the 2PL and graded IRFs (Woods, 2006a, 2007a; Woods & Thissen, 2006), but more like 1,000 for the 3PL (Woods, 2008a). These are rough guidelines and the requisite sample size depends on the purpose of the analysis and is influenced by study characteristics that differ in the various real-life situations in which IRT is applied.

The number of items is important because it provides information about θ needed to estimate its shape. With fewer than 10 items, EH and RC-IRT have failed to detect latent non-normality (Knott & Tzamourani, 2007; Woods, 2006, 2007a). It is reasonable to expect that item discrimination ability, the number of item response categories, and the degree to which $g(\theta)$ is non-normal would influence power to detect non-normality also. Specifically, it should be easier to detect normality when the items are more discriminating and have more response categories, and when $g(\theta)$ is more extremely skewed.

Expected a Posteriori Scores (EAPs)

For non-normal $g(\theta)$, EH, RC-IRT, and DC-IRT produce EAPs that are more accurate than those from the normal model (Woods, 2006a, 2007a, 2007b, 2008a; Woods & Lin, 2009; Woods & Thissen, 2006). However, the EAPs are estimated with different degrees of accuracy depending on the range of θ. With skew curves, the proportion of people with θ values in the long tail of the distribution is often so low that the EAPs for that range of θ are actually estimated better from the normal model (Woods, 2006a, 2007a, 2007b, 2008a; Woods & Lin, 2009; Woods & Thissen, 2006). One solution is to avoid interpreting EAPs from the tail of a skewed distribution. (The rest of the EAPs could be interpreted.) At least with the non-normal (versus mis-specified normal) approaches, one has a depiction of $g(\theta)$, and therefore knows that there is a long tail about which to make only tentative interpretations.

Specification of the IRF

There is evidence from simulations that if the IRF is mis-specified as 2PL when the data are actually generated from a 3PL IRF, this will be absorbed by the estimate of $g(\theta)$ from either EH or RC-IRT (Woods, 2008b). Thus, what appears to be non-normal $g(\theta)$ can be only IRF misspecification, or a combination of non-normal $g(\theta)$ and IRF misspecification. It is expected that this would hold for other types of IRF misspecification, such as (for example) a 1PL fit when item discrimination actually varies over items. Fortunately, the likelihood ratio difference test comparing the 2PL and 3PL IRFs from models with normal $g(\theta)$ is statistically accurate even with a non-normal true $g(\theta)$ (Woods, 2008b). Then the item parameters (and most of the EAPs) are further improved if the correct IRF is re-fitted permitting non-normal $g(\theta)$. Thus, a two-stage process of IRF selection with normal $g(\theta)$, followed by estimation of $g(\theta)$, is recommended (Woods, 2008b).

Comparisons Among Methods

Both RC-IRT and DC-IRT are preferable to EH. EH is the simplest, but the least accurate (Woods & Lin, 2009). In one study using the 3PL IRF, I concluded that EH and RC-IRT have complementary strengths, because recovery of item parameters was a little better with EH, whereas RC-IRT provided a better approximation of $g(\theta)$, and less biased EAPs (Woods, 2008a). However, this study was unusual (compared to other simulations about RC-IRT) because the only outcome measure of item parameter recovery was the maximum difference between the true and estimated IRF, and this was averaged over all item parameters. In a later comparison between RC-IRT and EH (Woods & Lin, 2009), bias was the outcome measure, and (2PL) item parameters were estimated as accurately by RC-IRT (and DC-IRT) as by EH, and were more variable from EH. Also, the density and EAPs were better estimated by RC-IRT and DC-IRT than by EH.

For the most part, SEs for item parameters that incorporate information about $g(\theta)$ are not available for the methods reviewed in this chapter. One exception is the MH-RM implementation of RC-IRT mentioned earlier (Monroe & Cai, 2013), which produces the observed information matrix (thus SEs) as part of estimation. This seems to be a more tractable strategy than the alternative idea of using the supplemented EM algorithm (Meng & Rubin, 1991) to compute SEs for EM MML item parameter estimates (Cai, 2008). I am not aware of any implementations of this supplemented EM approach for SEs with an estimated density. Bootstrap SEs have also been suggested for RC-IRT (Gu, Skorupski, Hoyle, & Kingston, 2011), but this requires much more computation after estimation is complete. SEs from the EH approach are expected to lack efficiency because of the large number of additional free parameters needed. Research on SEs for DC-IRT is needed.

An alternate use of bootstrapping is to obtain information about the variability of the density estimate, which has been used with EHs (Knott & Tzamourani, 2007). This is an interesting idea, and more interpretable and feasible than it would be to try to compute an SE for the weight at every quadrature point. I am not aware of any work on the variability of the density estimate from RC-IRT or DC-IRT.

Both RC-IRT and DC-IRT provide a smooth representation of $g(\theta)$, require few additional free parameters, and will not inspire the alternate interpretation that there are as many latent classes as there are quadrature points (as could be argued with the EH approach). RC-IRT and DC-IRT have been compared in only one study (Woods & Lin, 2009). Nevertheless, they performed almost equivalently, except that DC-IRT EAPs were more accurate. RC-IRT is the most studied approach, but unwieldy compared to DC-IRT. Overall, DC-IRT seems to be the most promising because it has two advantages over RC-IRT: it requires only one tuning parameter (this leads to simpler model selection), and it is already generalized to the multidimensional case (Zhang & Davidian, 2001).

Future Directions

This chapter focused on three methods for estimating $g(\theta)$ simultaneously with the item parameters in EM MML IRT, conditional on logistic IRFs. Although it is reasonable to use EH and RC-IRT, and software is more accessible for these methods, DC-IRT is the most promising approach for the future. Notably, there are other ways to estimate a smooth latent density that can be used in the EM MML framework, so an entirely new alternative is also possible.

For DC-IRT to become prominent, several developments would be needed. One is software that is fully stand-alone, user-friendly, and flexible. Another is SEs computed using either the supplemented EM algorithm (Cai, 2008; Meng & Rubin, 1991), or from the observed information matrix if MH-RM can be used as it has been for RC-IRT (Monroe & Cai, 2013). Then, the empirical performance of SEs and the influence of variables like density shape and assumption violations on the detection of non-normality could be further studied. It will also be important to attend to appropriate starting values for both the item parameters and density parameters in any method estimating $g(\theta)$ (Nader et al., 2011). Because Davidian curves are already generalized to multiple dimensions (Zhang & Davidian, 2001), it is reasonable to pursue multidimensional non-normal DC-IRT, which would be a valuable contribution and present a variety of methodological questions and challenges for the future.

References

Abdel-fattah, A. (1994, April). *Comparing BILOG and LOGIST estimates for normal, truncated normal, and beta ability distributions.* Paper presented at the annual meeting of the American Educational Research Association, New Orleans.

Andersen, E.B. (1970). Asymptotic properties of conditional maximum likelihood estimators. *Journal of the Royal Statistical Society, Series B, 32,* 283–301.

Andersen, E.B., & Madsen, M. (1977). Estimating the parameters of a latent population distribution. *Psychometrika, 42,* 357–374.

Baker, F.B. (1987). Methodology review: Item parameter estimation under the one-, two-, and three-parameter logistic models. *Applied Psychological Measurement, 11,* 111–141.

Baker, F.B., & Subkoviak, M.J. (1981). Analysis of test results via loglinear models. *Applied Psychological Measurement, 5,* 503–515.

Bartholomew, D. (1988). The sensitivity of latent trait analysis to choice of prior distribution. *British Journal of Mathematical and Statistical Psychology, 41,* 101–107.

Bartolucci, F., & Pennoni, F. (2007). On the approximation of the quadratric exponential distribution in a latent variable context. *Biometrika, 94,* 745–754.

Bauer, D.J., & Curran, P.J. (2004). The integration of continuous and discrete latent variable models: Potential problems and promising opportunities. *Psychological Methods, 9,* 3–29.

Birnbaum, A. (1968). Some latent trait models. In F.M. Lord & M.R. Novick (Eds.), *Statistical theories of mental test scores.* Reading, MA: Addison & Wesley.

Blackwood, L.G., & Bradley, E.L. (1989). The equivalence of two methods of parameter estimation for the Rasch model. *Psychometrika, 54,* 751–754.

Bock, R.D., & Aitkin, M. (1981). Marginal maximum likelihood estimation of item parameters. Application of the EM algorithm. *Psychometrika, 46,* 443–459.

Bock, R.D., & Lieberman, M. (1970). Fitting a response model for *n* dichotomously scored items. *Psychometrika, 35,* 179–197.

Boulet, J. R. (1996). The effect of nonnormal ability distributions on IRT parameter estimation using full-information and limited-information methods (item response theory, nonlinear factor analysis). Dissertation abstracts online, University of Ottawa (Canada).

Cai, L. (2008). SEM of another flavour: Two new applications of the supplemented EM algorithm. *British Journal of Mathematical and Statistical Psychology, 61,* 309–329.

Cai, L. (2010). High-dimensional exploratory item factor analysis by a Metropolis-Hastings Robbins-Monro algorithm. *Psychometrika, 75,* 33–57.

Cai, L. (2012). flexMIRT: Flexible multilevel item factor analysis and test scoring [Computer software]. Seattle, WA: Vector Psychometric Group, LLC.

Chambless, D.L., Caputo, G.C., Bright, P., & Gallagher, R. (1984). Assessment of "fear of fear" in agoraphobics: The Body Sensations Questionnaire and the Agoraphobic Cognitions Questionnaire. *Journal of Consulting and Clinical Psychology, 52,* 1090–1097.

Cox, M. G. (1972). The numerical evaluation of B-splines. *Journal of the Institute for Mathematics and its Applications, 10,* 134–149.

Cressie, N., & Holland, P.W. (1983). Characterizing the manifest probabilities of latent trait models. *Psychometrika, 48,* 129–141.

Curry, H. B., & Schoenberg, I. J. (1947). On spline distributions and their limits: The Polya distribution functions. *Bulletin of the American Mathematical Society, 53,* 1114.

Davidian, M., & Gallant, A.R. (1993). The nonlinear mixed effects model with a smooth random effects density. *Biometrika, 80,* 475–488.

Davidian, M., & Giltinan, D.M. (1995). *Nonlinear models of repeated measurement data.* London: Chapman & Hall.

De Ayala, R. J. (1995, April). Item parameter recovery for the nominal response model. Paper presented at the Annual Meeting of the American Educational Research Association, San Francisco.

de Boor, C. (1972). On calculating with B-splines. *Journal of Approximation Theory, 6,* 50–62.

de Boor, C. (1978). *A practical guide to splines.* New York: Springer-Verlag.

de Boor, C. (2001). *A practical guide to splines, revised edition.* New York: Springer-Verlag.

de Leeuw, J., & Verhelst, N. (1986). Maximum likelihood estimation in generalized Rasch models. *Journal of Educational Statistics, 11,* 183–196.

Dempster, A.P., Laird, N.M., & Rubin, D.B. (1977). Maximum likelihood from incomplete data via the EM algorithm. *Journal of the Royal Statistical Society, Series B, 39,* 1–38.

Embretson, S.E., & Reise, S.P. (2000). *Item response theory for psychologists.* Mahwah, NJ: Lawrence Erlbaum Associates.

Engelen, R.J.H. (1989). *Parameter estimation in the logistic item response model.* Unpublished doctoral dissertation. Universiteit Twente, Netherlands.

Follman, D. (1988). Consistent estimation in the Rasch model based on nonparametric margins. *Psychometrika, 53,* 553–562.

Gallant, A.R., & Nychka, D.W. (1987). Semi-nonparametric maximum likelihood estimation. *Econometrica, 55,* 363–390.

Gibbons, R.D., & Hedeker, D. (1992). Full-information item bifactor analysis. *Psychometrika, 57,* 423–436.

Gu, F., Skorupski, W., Hoyle, L., & Kingston, N. (2011). Standard errors and confidence intervals from bootstrapping for Ramsay-curve item response theory model item parameters. *Applied Psychological Measurement, 35,* 562–565.

Hannan, E.J. (1987). Rational transfer function approximation. *Statistical Science, 2,* 135–161.

Holland, P.W. (1990). On the sampling theory foundations of item response theory models. *Psychometrika, 55,* 577–601.

Johnson, N.L. (1949). Systems of frequency curves generated by methods of translation. *Biometrika, 36,* 149–176.

Kelderman, H. (1984). Loglinear Rasch model tests. *Psychometrika, 49,* 223–245.

Kirisci, L. & Hsu, T. C. (April, 1995). The robustness of BILOG to violations of the assumptions of unidimensionality of test items and normality of ability distribution. Paper presented at the annual meeting of the National Council on Measurement in Education, San Francisco.

Kirisci, L., Hsu, T., & Kaohsiung, L. (2001). Robustness of item parameter estimation programs to assumptions of unidimensionality and normality. *Applied Psychological Measurement, 25,* 146–162.

Knott, M., & Tzamourani, P. (2007). Bootstrapping the estimated latent distribution of the two-parameter latent trait model. *British Journal of Mathematical and Statistical Psychology, 60,* 175–191.

Kolmogorov, A. (1933). Sulla Determinazione Empirica di una Legge di Distributione. *Giornale dell'Istituto Italiano degli Attuari, 4,* 1–11.

Kooperberg, C., & Stone, C. (1991). A study of logspline density estimation. *Computational Statistics and Data Analysis, 12,* 327–347.

Lazarsfeld, P.F. (1950). The logical and mathematical foundation of latent structure analysis. In S.A. Stouffer, L. Guttman, E.A. Suchman, P.F. Lazarsfeld, S.A. Star, & J.A. Clausen (Eds.), *Measurement and prediction* (pp. 362–412). Princeton, NJ: Princeton University Press.

Lord, F.M. (1986). Maximum likelihood and Bayesian parameter estimation in item response theory. *Journal of Educational Measurement, 23,* 157–162.

Lord, F.M., & Novick, M.R. (1968). *Statistical theories of mental test scores.* Reading, MA: Addison-Wesley.

Lubke, G., & Muthén, B. (2005). Investigating population heterogeneity with factor mixture models. *Psychological Methods, 10,* 21–39.

Lubke, G., & Neale, M.C. (2008). Distinguishing between latent and continuous factors with categorical outcomes: Class invariance of parameters of factor mixture models. *Multivariate Behavioral Research, 43,* 592–620.

Mellenbergh, G.J., & Vijn, P. (1981). The Rasch model as a loglinear model. *Applied Psychological Measurement, 5,* 369–376.

Meng, X.-L., & Rubin, D.B. (1991). Using EM to obtain asymptotic variance-covariance matrices: The SEM algorithm. *Journal of the American Statistical Association, 86,* 899–909.

Mislevy, R. (1984). Estimating latent distributions. *Psychometrika, 49,* 359–381.

Mislevy, R.J., & Bock, R.D. (1990). *BILOG-3: Item analysis and test scoring with binary logistic models* [Computer software]. Mooresville, IN: Scientific Software.

Monroe, S., & Cai, L. (2013). Estimation of a Ramsay-curve item response theory model by the Metropolis-Hastings Robbins-Monro Algorithm. *Educational and Psychological Measurement,* published online first September 3, 2013.

Nader, I., Tran, U., & Formann, A. (2011). Sensitivity to initial values in full non-parametric maximum likelihood estimation of the two-parametric logistic model. *British Journal of Mathematical and Statistical Psychology, 64,* 320–336.

Nürnberger, G. (1989). *Approximation by spline functions.* New York: Springer-Verlag.

Ramsay, J.O. (1991). Kernel smoothing approaches to nonparametric item characteristic curve estimation. *Psychometrika, 56,* 611–630.

Ramsay, J.O. (2000). Differential equation models for statistical functions. *Canadian Journal of Statistics, 28,* 225–240.

Rasch, G. (1960). *Probabilistic models for some intelligence and attainment tests.* Copenhagen: Danish Institute for Educational Research.

Reise, S. P., & Yu, J. (1990). Parameter recovery in the graded response model using MULTILOG. *Journal of Educational Measurement, 27,* 133–144.

Roberts, J. S., Donoghue, J. R., & Laughlin, J. E. (2002). Characteristics of MML/EAP parameter estimates in the generalized graded unfolding model. *Applied Psychological Measurement, 26,* 192–207.

Samejima, F. (1969). Estimation of latent ability using a response pattern of graded scores. *Psychometrika Monograph,* No. 17.

Samejima, F. (1997). Graded response model. In W.J. van der Linden & R.K. Hambleton (Eds.), *Handbook of modern item response theory.* New York: Springer.

Schmitt, J.E., Mehta, P.D., Aggen, S.H., Kubarych, T.S., & Neale, M.C. (2006). Semi-nonparametric methods for detecting latent non-normality: A fusion of latent trait and ordered latent class modeling. *Multivariate Behavioral Research, 41,* 427–443.

Schoenberg, I. J. (1946). Contributions to the problem of approximation of equidistant data by analytic functions, Part A: On the problem of smoothing or graduating, a first class of analytic approximation formulas. *Quarterly of Applied Mathematics, 4,* 45–99.

Schoenberg, I. J. (1969). Cardinal interpolation and spline functions. *Journal of Approximation Theory, 2,* 167–206.

Schoenberg, I. J. (1973). Cardinal spline interpolation. *Monographs of the Conference Board of the Mathematical Sciences, 12.* SIAM: Philadelphia.

Seong, T. (1990). Sensitivity of marginal maximum likelihood estimation of item and ability parameters to the characteristics of the prior ability distributions. *Applied Psychological Measurement, 14,* 299–311.

Silverman, B.W. (1982). On the estimation of a probability density function by the maximum penalized likelihood method. *Annals of Statistics, 10,* 795–810.

Smirnov, N. (1939). Sur les Écarts de la Courbe de Distribution Empirique. *Recueil Mathématique, 6,* 3–26.

Stone, C. A. (1992). Recovery of marginal maximum likelihood estimates in the two-parameter logistic response model: An evaluation of MULTILOG. *Applied Psychological Measurement, 16,* 1–16.

Stone, C., & Koo, C. (1986). Logspline density estimation. *Contemporary Mathematics, 59,* 1–15.

Thissen, D. (1982). Marginal maximum likelihood estimation for the one-parameter logistic model. *Psychometrika, 47,* 175–186.

Thissen, D. (1991). *MULTILOG user's guide: Multiple categorical item analysis and test scoring using item response theory*: Chicago: Scientific Software, International.

Thissen, D., & Mooney, J. A. (1989). Loglinear item response models, with applications to data from social surveys. *Sociological Methodology, 19,* 299–330.

Thissen, D., & Orlando, M., (2001). Item response theory for items scored in two categories. In D. Thissen & H. Wainer (Eds.), *Test scoring* (pp. 73–137). Mahwah, NJ: Erlbaum.

Tjur, T. (1982). A connection between Rasch's item analysis model and a multiplicative Poisson model. *Scandinavian Journal of Statistics, 9,* 23–30.

Tzamourani, P., & Knott, M. (2002). Fully semiparametric estimation of the two-parameter latent trait model for binary data. In G. A. Marcoulides & I. Moustaki (Eds.), *Latent variable and latent structure models* (pp. 63–84). Mahwah, NJ: Erlbaum.

van den Oord, E. (2005). Estimating Johnson curve population distributions in MULTILOG. *Applied Psychological Measurement, 29,* 45–64.

van den Oord, E., Pickles, A., & Waldman, I. (2003). Normal variation and abnormality: An empirical study of the liability distribution underlying depression and delinquency. *Journal of Child Psychology and Psychiatry, 44,* 180–192.

Woods, C. (2004). *Item response theory with estimation of the latent population distribution using spline-based densities*. Unpublished dissertation, University of North Carolina at Chapel Hill.

Woods, C. M. (2006a). Ramsay-curve item response theory to detect and correct for nonnormal latent variables. *Psychological Methods, 11,* 253–270.

Woods, C. M. (2006b). RCLOG v.2: Software for item response theory parameter estimation with the latent population distribution represented using spline-based densities. Technical Report. Washington University in St. Louis.

Woods, C. M. (2007a). Ramsay-curve IRT for Likert-type data. *Applied Psychological Measurement, 31,* 195–212.

Woods, C. M. (2007b). Empirical histograms in IRT with ordinal data. *Educational and Psychological Measurement, 67,* 73–87.

Woods, C. M. (2008a). Ramsay-curve item response theory for the 3PL item response model. *Applied Psychological Measurement, 32,* 447–465.

Woods, C. M. (2008b). Consequences of ignoring guessing when estimating the latent density in item response theory. *Applied Psychological Measurement, 32,* 371–384.

Woods, C. M., & Lin, N. (2009). Item response theory with estimation of the latent density using Davidian curves. *Applied Psychological Measurement, 33,* 102–117.

Woods, C. M., & Thissen, D. (2004). *RCLOG v.1: Software for Item Response Theory Parameter Estimation with the Latent Population Distribution Represented Using Spline-Based Densities.* (Tech. Rep. No. 1). Chapel Hill: University of North Carolina, L.L. Thurstone Psychometric Laboratory.

Woods, C. M., & Thissen, D. (2006). Item response theory with estimation of the latent population distribution using spline-based densities. *Psychometrika, 71,* 281–301.

Wu, E. J. C., & Bentler. P. M. (2011). EQSIRT—A User-Friendly IRT Program. Encino, CA: Multivariate Software, Inc.

Yamamoto, K., & Muraki, E. (1991, April). Non-linear transformation of IRT scale to account for the effect of non-normal ability distribution on the item parameter estimation. Paper presented at the annual meeting of the American Educational Research Association, Chicago, IL.

Yen, W. M. (1987). A comparison of the efficiency and accuracy of bilog and logist. *Psychometrika, 52,* 275–291.

Zhang, D., & Davidian, M. (2001). Linear mixed models with flexible distributions of random effects for longitudinal data. *Biometrics, 57,* 795–802.

Zimowski, M., Muraki, E., Mislevy, R., & Bock, D. (2003). BILOG-MG 3. [Computer software]. Lincolnwood, IL: Scientific Software International.

Zwinderman, A. H., & van den Wollenberg, A. L. (1990). Robustness of marginal maximum likelihood estimation in the Rasch model. *Applied Psychological Measurement, 14,* 73–81.

5 The Use of Nonparametric Item Response Theory to Explore Data Quality

Rob R. Meijer, Jorge N. Tendeiro, and Rob B. K. Wanders

Introduction

The aim of this chapter is to provide insight into a number of commonly used nonparametric item response theory (NIRT) methods and to show how these methods can be used to describe and *explore* the psychometric quality of questionnaires used in patient-reported outcome measurement and, more in general, typical performance measurement (personality, mood, health-related constructs). NIRT is an extremely valuable tool for preliminary data analysis and for evaluating whether item response data are acceptable for parametric IRT modeling. This is in particular useful in the field of typical performance measurement where the construct being measured is often very different than in maximum performance measurement (education, intelligence; see Chapter 1 of this handbook). Our basic premise is that there are no "best tools" or "best models" and that the usefulness of psychometric modeling depends on the specific aims of the instrument (questionnaire, test) that is being used. Most important is, however, that it should be clear for a researcher how sensitive a specific method (for example, DETECT, or Mokken scaling) is to the assumptions that are being investigated. The NIRT literature is not always clear about this, and in this chapter we try to clarify some of these ambiguities.

NIRT may serve two aims (Sijtsma & Meijer, 2007): (1) providing a theoretical framework that may serve as a basis for IRT modeling (e.g., Hemker, Sijtsma, Molenaar, & Junker, 1997) and (2) providing methods and procedures that can be used to analyze test and questionnaire data mainly to explore data quality. In this chapter we are primarily interested in how to apply NIRT as an exploratory model to obtain information about the data structure. Software for nonparametric IRT analyses can be found in the R-packages *irtoys* (Partchev, 2013), *KernSmoothIRT* (Mazza, Punzo, & McGuire, 2012), *mokken* (van der Ark, 2007, 2012), and *PerFit* (Meijer, Niessen, & Tendeiro, 2014; Tendeiro, 2014).

There are several good introductions written on NIRT at varying levels of technical sophistication. For example, Santor and Ramsay (1998) and Meijer and Baneke (2004) provided an introduction and empirical examples of the usefulness of NIRT in the context of personality and psychopathology measurement. Sijtsma and Molenaar (2002) wrote a monograph on NIRT and Sijtsma and Meijer (2007) provided an extensive psychometric and statistical overview of the foundations of NIRT. Also Stout and colleagues (e.g., Stout, 1987; Stout, Habing, Douglas, & Kim, 1996) wrote many theoretical and empirical papers on NIRT.

In general, the advantage of NIRT approaches is that through inspecting the simple covariance structure between items and using tools like nonparametric regression (a) results are obtained that can be interpreted very easily by practitioners, (b) data are not forced into a structure they do not have, and (c) analyses can be run through user-friendly software programs. Finally, NIRT models may serve as alternatives to model data to parametric models to answer the question of "the robustness of conclusions under variations in model choice" (Molenaar, 2004).

Interesting in this respect was a study by Chernyshenko, Stark, Chan, Drasgow, and Williams (2001), who found that nonparametric maximum-likelihood formula scoring models to noncognitive dichotomous and polytomous data provided a better description of these data than the two- and three-parameter logistic model and the graded response model. Meijer and Baneke (2004) also argued that for data for which the response process is not well understood, such as noncognitive and clinical data (see Reise & Waller, 2009), NIRT may provide an interesting basis to investigate data quality. This is not to argue for an overall replacement of parametric by nonparametric models. Parametric IRT models lead to point estimates of the latent trait. Such scales can be very convenient, for example, for comparing the results from different questionnaires selected from the same item bank or for the study of change. However, we do think that NIRT approaches may serve as handy tools to describe and explore item response data. As Molenaar (2004) stated, "The question whether misfit is significant or not is in my view less relevant than the exploration, detection, and description." Exploring data quality may help researchers to uncover the structure of the data so that, when needed, appropriate confirmatory parametric models can be chosen.

Although NIRT models are based on weaker assumptions than parametric IRT models, NIRT models often do make several assumptions about the data. Sijtsma and Meijer (2007) stated that "the reason for calling one class of IRT models nonparametric and another parametric, is that the former only puts order restrictions on response functions and the latter assumes a specific parametric function, such as the logistic or the normal ogive." Thus in this sense the parametric assumptions are weakened. For example, NIRT typically assumes that there is a monotone relationship between the probability of endorsing an item and the latent variable. On the other hand programs like TESTGRAF do not specify this relationship.

In this chapter, we present and explore the usefulness of methods to investigate nonparametric assumptions in typical performance data and we apply these methods to data from an Aggression Questionnaire and a Physical Functioning scale. We present a critical evaluation of a number of often-used NIRT models and, in particular, we explore some recently proposed methods to investigate invariant item ordering (IIO). A set of items possesses the IIO property when the ordering of the items according to their mean score is the same for persons with different latent variable scores. There are three reasons why we consider this an interesting property to investigate for typical performance data: (1) many applied researchers and practitioners seem unaware of the fact that the item ordering according to the mean score in the population does not necessarily hold at the individual level, (2) the few studies that investigate IIO in clinical practice often use the wrong methods, and experience on how to interpret results has to accumulate as more applications become available, and (3) investigating IIO gives us a good idea about the general quality of the data. In particular it may provide us information about the psychometric quality of items in a particular population.

Research Methods

Both parametric and nonparametric IRT models try to explain the structure in the manifest item and test responses by assuming the existence of a latent scale (θ) on which persons and items have a position. Because an IRT model places restrictions on the data, a researcher can check whether the data fit the model. Models have been formulated for both dichotomous (e.g., true-false) and polytomous (e.g., disagree-neutral-agree) items. We start with the models for dichotomous items. For dichotomous items, most IRT models assume unidimensionality (UD assumption) and a specified form for the so-called item response function (IRF). The IRF denotes the probability that an item i is answered correctly or is endorsed in the keyed direction as a function of the latent trait θ and is denoted $P_i(\theta)$. We refer to Chapter 2 of this handbook for a discussion of unidimensionality and "essential unidimensionality." From this chapter it is clear that dimensionality depends on the population of persons. Especially in clinical and outcome measurement, this is a constant source of worry because in clinical assessment it is often unclear what the exact population is. Unidimensionality implies the assumption of *local independence* (LI assumption), which states that the responses in a test are statistically independent conditional on θ. Furthermore, it is assumed that the probability of endorsing an item is *monotonically* non-decreasing in θ (M assumption).

Nonparametric IRT models differ from parametric models in that the form of the IRFs is not parametrically defined. In parametric IRT models, like the well-known two- and three-parameter logistic models, the IRF is specified through the logistic function and through item parameters like the discrimination parameter (*a* parameter) and the item difficulty or threshold parameter (*b* parameter). In nonparametric models there are no restrictions with regard to the form of the IRFs, except that they should be non-decreasing. Furthermore, in parametric IRT often specific distributions are required for the trait scores; this is not the case in nonparametric IRT.

Because NIRT models do not parameterize the response function, there is no θ metric available as in parametric models. However, dichotomous NIRT models imply an ordinal scale in the sense that the latent variable θ is stochastically ordered by the total score X_+ (Sijtsma & Molenaar, 2002). Thus, in practice any IRT model that is based on UD, LI, and M implies the ordering of respondents on the latent variable θ by means of the ordering of respondents on the observable sum score X_+, except for error.

Mokken Models

Two models that are based on the three assumptions of UD, LI, and M are Mokken's (Mokken, 1971) monotone homogeneity model (MHM) and Mokken's double monotonicity model (DMM). These models are probably the most researched and applied nonparametric IRT models, and chapters have been devoted to these models in several psychometric handbooks (e.g., Mellenbergh, 2011; Rao & Sinharay, 2007; van der Linden & Hambleton, 1997). Furthermore, there is a stand-alone computer program MSP5.0 (Molenaar & Sijtsma, 2000) and an R program package *mokken* (van der Ark, 2007, 2012) that can be used to analyze data through these models. In this chapter, we therefore use these Mokken models as the basis to discuss nonparametric data analyses. This is not to say that we are not critical about some of the methods suggested in the literature to check the fit of these models. However, we believe that these models provide a good basis to discuss useful nonparametric data analyses for typical performance measurement, as we show later in this chapter.

As mentioned earlier, the MHM assumes UD, LI, and increasing IRFs. The DMM also assumes UD, LI, and increasing IRFs, and an additional assumption is that the IRFs do not intersect. This makes the DMM a special case of the MHM, which means that when the DMM holds the weaker MHM also holds, but the reverse is not true. The assumption of nonintersecting IRFs implies IIO. More formally, when IIO holds for a set of k items and the items are ordered in decreasing popularity (or decreasing proportion-correct score), it applies that:

$$P_1(\theta) \geq P_2(\theta) \geq \ldots \geq P_k(\theta), \text{ for all } \theta. \tag{5.1}$$

Molenaar (1997) discussed polytomous versions of Mokken's original dichotomous models, which are based on the same set of assumptions as the dichotomous models. Central in his approach is the item step response function (ISRF). Let X_i be the score on item i, with values $x_i = 0, \ldots, m$; thus for five-point rating scales, this means $x_i = 0, \ldots, 4$. The ISRF is the probability of obtaining an item score of at least x_i and is denoted $P(X_i \geq x_i \mid \theta)$ for $x_i = 1, \ldots, m$, thus ignoring $x_i = 0$ because this probability by definition equals one. Molenaar (1997) also discussed the DMM for polytomous items, which adds to the MHM the assumption that the ISRFs of different items do not intersect.

The polytomous DMM, however, does *not* imply that items can be invariantly ordered, it only implies that the ISRFs do not intersect across items. This was extensively discussed in Sijtsma, Meijer, and van der Ark (2011) and Meijer (2010), but it has been a source of confusion in a number of empirical papers. For example, Watson, Deary, and Austin (2007) claimed to investigate whether sets of the items have IIO. In that study, however, methods were used that were sensitive to checking whether sets of ISRFs do not intersect, *not* whether items have IIO.

Methods to Check Nonparametric IRT

As discussed earlier, NIRT models do not offer estimates of item parameters, neither do they allow for point estimates of θ. However, several methods have been proposed to check the assumptions of the NIRT models without using model parameters. In the following paragraphs we discuss methods for each model assumption.

Monotonicity Assumption

To investigate whether IRFs or ISRFs are non-decreasing in the latent variable, several nonparametric regression methods are available. An approach that obtained some popularity especially in applied clinical testing is TESTGRAF (Ramsay, 1991, 2000). For example, Santor, Ramsay, and Zuroff (1994) used TESTGRAF to inspect the IRFs for a depression questionnaire. Through TESTGRAF, category response functions (CRFs) can be plotted. A CRF gives the probability of endorsing each response category as a function of the trait score (here approximated by the total score). In general, good items should have CRFs with steep trace lines that exceed all other response functions in one interval of the total score. When the categories are ordered in increasing order, the total score values for which a response function is optimal should reflect the order in which the response choices of an item are presented. If this is not the case, two or more response functions may be combined to one response function. Items with flat or unsatisfactory response functions may be reformulated or may be removed from a questionnaire.

TESTGRAF uses so-called kernel smoothing to estimate IRFs/CRFs. This technique takes weighted averages at each trait score value; the weights are determined by the kernel function. The formula is given by:

$$\hat{P}_{im}(\theta_q) = \sum_{a=1}^{N} \frac{K\left[(\theta_a - \theta_q)/h\right]}{\sum_{b=1}^{N} K\left[(\theta_b - \theta_q)/h\right]} y_{ima}, \tag{5.2}$$

where i, m, index the item and the response category, respectively, and a, b, and q index persons (ranked by total score), respectively, K is the kernel function, h is a smoothing parameter, and y_{ima} is an indicator variable (1 if person a chose option m of item i; 0 otherwise). The trait score θ_q of person q is estimated as a quantile of the standard normal distribution, taking the ranking of the persons by the total sum score into account. The kernel function $K()$ is chosen so that larger weights are given to trait values in the neighborhood of θ_q; common options are the uniform, quadratic, and Gaussian functions (Ramsay, 1991). The user-specified bandwidth value h controls the trade-off between bias and sampling variation. Low values of h yield estimated functions with large variance and small bias, and high values of h yield estimated functions with small variance but large bias. Generally, the bottom line is to choose a bandwidth minimizing the mean-square error, which is the sum of the variance and the squared bias (i.e., MSE = Bias^2 + Variance).

It should be realized that smoothing can be affected by the bandwidth and that one should be careful in choosing a bandwidth, especially when there are not many observations. TESTGRAF uses the value $1.1N^{-1/5}$ as default. Note that kernel smoothing does not enforce monotonicity in θ, and as such it may be a handy tool to investigate local deviations from monotone increasing IRFs.

The *KernSmoothIRT* (Mazza et al., 2012) R package provides another possibility for performing nonparametric regression smoothing to estimate IRFs. As an alternative, both the MSP5.0 and the R package *mokken* provide a simpler method to investigate monotonicity. Here the discrete estimates of IRFs and ISRFs based on binning are constructed. That is, groups of persons who have similar total scores (or rest scores, that is the total score minus the score on the researched item) are formed for each item i, and for each group the proportion that answers item i correct is calculated. These proportions are plotted as a function of the total scores. This approach yields a limited number of plots (at most the number of items in the test). For two sample proportions it can be tested whether the item proportions are non-decreasing. This graph then forms the IRF or in the case of polytomous items the ISRF. The reason why sometimes a rest score is used instead of total score is that, theoretically, it can be shown that for polytomous item scores the total score does not need to have monotonicity in θ (Sijtsma & Meijer, 2007, p. 732).

The assumption of monotonicity can be fairly easily investigated using graphical methods, eyeball inspection, and simple statistical significance testing. In general, however, there seems to be a great reluctance by especially trained psychometricians to use graphs. We often see fit statistics and large tables full of numbers that certainly do not provide more information than graphs (see also Wainer, 2005, for a more thorough presentation of this topic). As we discuss later in this chapter, graphs are also excellent tools to inspect the assumption of invariant item ordering.

Unidimensionality Assumption

When reviewing the NIRT literature, it is not always clear how sensitive the different methods are to investigating the unidimensionality assumption. Later in this chapter, we discuss a number of techniques that are all presented under the label of unidimensionality assessment tools but that are sensitive to sometimes different characteristics of the data.

As mentioned in Sijtsma and Meijer (2007), nonparametric unidimensionality analysis is based on *conditional association* (Holland & Rosenbaum, 1986). Let $\mathbf{X}$ denote a vector of ordered item scores. Split $\mathbf{X}$ in two disjoint vectors, $\mathbf{X} = (\mathbf{Y},\mathbf{Z})$. Let f_1 and f_2 denote non-decreasing functions in the ordered item scores from **Y**, and let g be some function of the item scores in **Z**. Conditional association (CA) means that:

$$\text{Cov}[f_1(\mathbf{Y}), f_2(\mathbf{Y}) \mid g(\mathbf{Z})=z] \geq 0, \tag{5.3}$$

for all z. CA is a necessary condition for UD, LI, and M. Therefore, necessary conditions for NIRT model fit based on CA are available after proper specification of **Y**, **Z**, f_1, f_2, and g. One such condition that can be used to check unidimensionality for the MHM states that all $k(k\text{-}1)/2$ inter-item covariances within a test should be non-negative in the sample. Strictly speaking, one negative covariance indicates misfit of the MHM. However, important is that if one finds only positive signs in the data this does not mean that the MHM fits. Hence, having nonnegative inter-item covariances is a necessary, but not sufficient, condition for unidimensionality to hold.

To investigate the unidimensionality assumption in the context of the Mokken models, several methods have been proposed. A popular method, but sensitive to specific item characteristics as we discuss later in this chapter, is the automated item selection algorithm (AISP). This algorithm uses the scalability coefficient H. H is defined at the item(step)-pair level (H_{ij}) and item level (H_i). All coefficients can be expressed as ratios of (sums of) observed covariances and maximum possible covariances. For the interpretation of H, Sijtsma and Molenaar (2002, p. 60) give the following guidelines. The scale H coefficient should be above 0.3 for the items to form a scale. When $0.3 \leq H < 0.4$ the scale is considered weak, when $0.4 \leq H < 0.5$ the scale is considered medium, and when $H \geq 0.5$ the scale is considered strong. There is, however, a lack of literature with respect to the exact meaning of these benchmarks.

The AISP is based primarily on the inter-item covariances and the strengths of the relationship between items and the rest score as expressed by the item H_i coefficients. Based on such information, clusters of related items may be identified. The AISP "bottom-up" procedure starts by selecting the pair of items for which (a) H_{ij} is significantly larger than 0 and (b) H_{ij} is the largest among the coefficients for all possible item pairs. Then a third item l is selected that (c) correlates positively with the items already selected, (d) has an H_l coefficient that is larger than 0, and (e) has an H_l coefficient that is larger than a user-specified value c. The procedure continues to select items as long as items are available that satisfy conditions c, d, and e. The end result may be one or more item clusters such that each taps a different latent trait or latent trait composite. The substantive interpretation of the clusters is done on the basis of the content of the clustered items and the substantive knowledge one has about the data structure. For Mokken scale analysis the AISP plays a crucial role. Sijtsma and Molenaar defined a Mokken scale as a set of items that "a) measure a common trait . . . with b) reasonable discriminative power determined by lowerbound c" (Sijtsma & Molenaar, 2002, p. 68).

The AISP is a bottom-up selection algorithm that selects an item only once, without the possibility of taking back the assignment later on. Thus, AISP does not consider all possible item partitionings. Straat, van der Ark, and Sijtsma (2013) suggested a new selection algorithm that uses a genetic search (GA) algorithm that avoids this problem. In contrast to the AISP algorithm, this GA is probabilistic and approximates all possible subdivisions. As a result it may produce different item partitionings than the AISP procedure.

Because for a fixed distribution of θ both H and H_i are increasing functions of the slopes of logistic IRFs, this selection procedure selects items that have (together) high discrimination parameters. Thus, what is very important to understand is that *the monotonicity assumption* forms the basis of the dimensionality analysis in Mokken procedures. This may have important consequences for the selection of items in the noncognitive area.

Theoretically, selecting items on the basis of monotonicity may result in selecting items within a cluster that are locally dependent. As several authors have shown for parametric IRT models (e.g., Chen & Thissen, 1997), item discrimination parameters may be inflated when the items are locally dependent. How strong this effect is in the AISP procedure is not clear from the literature. Recently, Straat (2012, chapter 6) suggested a number of statistics to detect violations of local independence, but there is not yet much experience with these statistics.

Local Independence

Chen and Thissen (1997) showed that, for parametric IRT models, item discrimination parameters may be inflated when the items are locally dependent. To investigate what the effect of local dependence on the H_i scalability coefficient is we replicated and extended the study by Chen and Thissen (1997, p. 266) as follows. A data set with scores of 1,000 subjects on six items was generated using the 2PL model; the true *a* and *b* parameters that were used are shown in Table 5.1 (second and third columns). Two cases were considered: Local independence (LI) and local dependence (LD). The LI case consisted of using the generated data set without any further changes. In the second data set LD was simulated using the same item scores for both item 3 and item 6 (like in the Chen & Thissen, 1997 study). Item parameters *a*'s, *b*'s and scalability coefficients H_i were then estimated for each case (LI, LD) using IRTPRO (using default program options) and the R *mokken* package, respectively. Results are depicted in Table 5.1. It is clear that the estimation of the parameters of items 3 and 6 in the LD case was greatly affected by the fact that their scores are dependent (equal in this case). Moreover, the associated H_i values seem to be larger, on average, than the H_i values for items that do not contribute to the LD problem. This effect was confirmed by replicating the experiment 100 times, as shown in Table 5.2 (second column).

The study was further extended by increasing the number of items from 6 to 12. Only item scalability H_i values were computed. Table 5.3 shows the results for one data set only; Table 5.2 (third column) shows the average results of more than 100 replications. It can be seen that the effect of LD on the H_i values was somewhat reduced, implying that test length is an important factor. More specifically, the scalability of locally dependent

Table 5.1 True Item Parameters, Estimated Item Parameters, and Item Scalability Coefficients H_i Under Local Independence and Local Dependence of Items 3 and 6

	True parameters		*First case: LI*			*Second case: LD (item 3 = item 6)*		
Item	*a*	*b*	*a (SE)*	*b (SE)*	H_i *(SE)*	*a (SE)*	*b (SE)*	H_i *(SE)*
1	1.0	−1.0	1.07 (.14)	−0.88 (.11)	0.27 (.03)	0.62 (.08)	−1.42 (.18)	0.27 (.03)
2	1.0	−0.5	1.11 (.14)	−0.45 (.08)	0.25 (.02)	0.54 (.07)	−0.85 (.15)	0.24 (.03)
3	1.0	0.0	0.98 (.13)	−0.05 (.08)	0.22 (.02)	207.75 (*)	−0.11 (**)	0.44 (.02)
4	1.0	0.5	1.10 (.14)	0.53 (.09)	0.25 (.02)	0.52 (.07)	0.89 (.17)	0.24 (.03)
5	1.0	1.0	1.03 (.14)	0.98 (.12)	0.27 (.03)	0.66 (.08)	1.31 (.17)	0.27 (.03)
6	1.0	0.0	1.06 (.14)	0.02 (.07)	0.23 (.02)	207.75 (*)	−0.11 (**)	0.44 (.02)

Note: * = 51964.62. ** = 37.64. LI = local independence. LD = local dependence.

Table 5.2 Mean (SD) H_i Values Across 100 Replications for Data Sets With 6 and 12 Items

	$k = 6$	$k = 12$
LI	0.24 (.03)	0.23 (.03)
LD	0.43 (.02)	0.32 (.02)

Note: k = number of items. LI = local independence. LD = local dependence.
All H_i values in each replicated data set are used in the LI cases.
Only H_i values concerning items 3 and 6 ($k = 6$) and items 6 and 12 ($k = 12$) in each replicated data set are used in the LD cases.

Table 5.3 True Item Parameters and Item Scalability Coefficients H_i Under Local Independence and Local Dependence of Items 6 and 12

	True parameters		*First case: LI*	*Second case: LD (item 3 = item 6)*
Item	*a*	*b*	H_i *(SE)*	H_i *(SE)*
1	1.0	−1.25	0.26 (.03)	0.24 (.03)
2	1.0	−1.00	0.26 (.02)	0.26 (.02)
3	1.0	−0.75	0.24 (.02)	0.25 (.02)
4	1.0	−0.50	0.25 (.02)	0.25 (.02)
5	1.0	−0.25	0.24 (.02)	0.25 (.02)
6	1.0	0.00	0.21 (.02)	0.32 (.02)
7	1.0	0.25	0.23 (.02)	0.23 (.02)
8	1.0	0.50	0.22 (.02)	0.21 (.02)
9	1.0	0.75	0.19 (.02)	0.20 (.02)
10	1.0	1.00	0.29 (.02)	0.29 (.02)
11	1.0	1.25	0.23 (.03)	0.24 (.03)
12	1.0	0.00	0.21 (.02)	0.32 (.02)

Note: LI = local independence. LD = local dependence.

items may become less problematic if the number of items violating the LI assumptions is relatively small with respect to the total number of items. More studies are needed to clarify which proportions of locally dependent items are admissible in a data set to still allow for good scaling of individual differences.

Maximizing H *Values: Some Drawbacks*

In the literature there is a strong emphasis on selecting items with H_i values larger than some lower bound as, say, $H_i = 0.3$. Egberink and Meijer (2011) observed, however, that a researcher should also be careful when H_i values are very high. They argued that repeating items with a similar content will result in scales with high H_i values but, sometimes, scales that measure extremely narrow-band constructs. That is, strong Mokken scales may very reliably differentiate persons, but at the cost of construct validity. High H_i values may also point at items that define the construct ("*I am often depressed*" in a depression questionnaire).

Following this line of reasoning, Meijer, de Vries, and van Bruggen (2011) also argued to consider the 18 items of the BSI-18 scale (Derogatis, 1983) as one scale instead of forming subscales with each higher H_i value. Often subscales of clinical questionnaires contain items that are semantically similar, like "*I get a sort of frightened feeling as if something awful is about to happen*" and "*I get a sort of frightened feeling like butterflies in the stomach*" (both items from the Anxiety scale in the HADS questionnaire, Zigmond & Snaith, 1983), or "*I still enjoy the things I used to enjoy*" and "*I look forward with enjoyment to things*" (Depression items from the HADS). These items will result in high H_{ij} values, but a researcher may question whether it is strictly necessary to have both items in the same scale. A similar observation was reported by Reise (2009). He reported that fatigue and sleep disturbance are conceptually narrow and have a limited pool of item indicators. The Mokken scalability coefficient for the fatigue item bank equaled $H = 0.71$. As Reise (2009) remarked, there is little conceptual distance between the symptoms (items) and the construct. In this case one may conclude that it is not necessary to ask several questions, but that asking a few questions may suffice to estimate a person's standing on the latent trait scale.

Because the AISP focuses on the monotonicity assumption, several studies showed that this procedure performs worse in recovering the correct dimensionality structure than other methods (Mroch & Bolt, 2006; Smits, Timmerman, & Meijer, 2012; van Abswoude, van der Ark, & Sijtsma, 2004). In particular, those studies revealed that Mokken scale analysis does not function well in conditions in which the traits correlate (Mroch & Bolt, 2006; van Abswoude et al., 2004), or in which the items load on more than one trait (Smits et al., 2012; van Abswoude et al., 2004).

DETECT

Several alternative procedures have been proposed to assess unidimensionality in nonparametric contexts. In this chapter we restrict ourselves to DETECT because it is the most often used alternative to Mokken scale analyses and alternatives such as DIMTEST are based on assumptions that assume the knowledge of existing unidimensional subtests. DETECT uses conditional covariances between items to assess dimensionality and it is based on the early work by Stout (1987, 1990). He defined essential unidimensionality (Stout, 1987), essential independence, and weak monotonicity. Essential unidimensionality states that there is one dominant latent variable and several nuisance parameters. In this respect, it resembles common (general) factors and unique (group) factors as in factor analysis. Essential independence states that for infinitely many items the mean inter-item covariance conditional on θ equals 0. Also weak monotonicity assumes that the mean of the k IRFs is monotone on θ. This means that assumption M is dropped as a requirement for individual IRFs but that it is active for the test response function under the name of weak monotonicity. A drawback of these procedures is that the properties implied by UD, LI, and M with respect to stochastically ordering persons on θ by means of the total score are lost. Therefore, we restrict ourselves here to dimensionality analyses.

To check the dimensionality assumption, Stout and coworkers based their method on a special case of conditional association, namely that the covariance between items i and j must be nonnegative for subgroups that have the same rest score. Assuming that the items measure Q latent variables to a different degree, we may assume that θ_q is a linear combination of these variables. The performance on the Q latent variables is estimated by means of total score or rest scores that both summarize test performance but ignore multidimensionality. Zhang and Stout (1999), however, showed that the sign of $\text{cov}(X_i, X_j \mid \theta_q)$ provides useful information about the dimensionality of the data. It is positive when two items measure the same latent variable and negative when they clearly measure different latent variables. This observation forms the basis of DETECT that divides a data set of items into clusters that together approach essential independence as well as possible given all possible item clusters.

Assume that several of the latent variables measured by the items are dominant and that others are nuisance variables. Consider an arbitrary partitioning, denoted P, of the set of items into disjoint clusters; and let $d_{ij}(P) = 1$ if items *i* and *j* are in the same cluster and $d_{ij}(P) = -1$ if they are not. DETECT is then defined as:

$$d(P) = \frac{2}{k(k-1)} \sum_{i=1}^{k-1} \sum_{j=i+1}^{k} d_{ij}(P) E[cov(X_i, X_j \mid \theta)]. \tag{5.4}$$

The DETECT procedure tries to find the partitioning of the items, denoted P*, that maximizes Equation (5.4). This is the item clustering that best approximates weak LI between item sets, and it is taken as the best description of the dimensionality of the data. Thus, important here is that DETECT is sensitive to violations of LI, whereas Mokken scaling is sensitive to the monotonicity assumption. Several studies suggested rules of thumb that can be used to decide whether a data set is unidimensional or multidimensional. Stout and colleagues (1996) considered DETECT values smaller than 0.1 indicating essential unidimensionality and DETECT values larger than 1 as indicating multidimensionality. Roussos and Ozbek (2006) suggested the following rules of thumb; $DETECT < 0.2$: weak multidimensionality/approximate unidimensionality; $0.2 < DETECT < 0.4$: weak to moderate multidimensionality; $0.4 < DETECT < 1.0$ = moderate to large multidimensionality, and $DETECT > 1.0$: strong multidimensionality. Recently, however, Bonifay, Reise, Scheines, and Meijer (2014) discussed that these values are sensitive to the factor structure of the data set and the relation between general and group factors. Thus, these values should be used with care. We will return to this in the data analyses we discuss at the end of this chapter.

Invariant Item Ordering

The measurement of patient-reported outcomes through questionnaires sometimes assumes that the items used in these questionnaires represent different levels of intensity with respect to the attribute of interest. For example, when we consider two items of the Aggression Questionnaire that we analyze later, then it is assumed that an item "Sometimes I fly off the handle for no good reason" represents a much higher level of aggression than the item "I tell my friends openly when I disagree with them." On the other hand, we often encounter questionnaires that consist of items that are repetitions of similar questions and with conditional item means that cluster together, suggesting that there are no differences between the intensity of the items. The question then is whether the item ordering according to severity (or mean score) established at the *group* level can be used for persons at different *individual* trait levels, that is, whether IIO holds (Ligtvoet, van der Ark, te Marvelde, & Sijtsma, 2010; Sijtsma et al., 2011). Thus the IIO assumption holds when the ordering of the items according to their severity is the same across different values of the latent variable.

Methods to Investigate IIO

Several methods have been developed to establish IIO for dichotomously scored items (see Sijtsma & Junker, 1996, for an overview). Meijer and Egberink (2012) suggested, however, to first inspect plots of item-rest score regression before checking possible violations of IIO. Then, to further investigate IIO for dichotomous items, the rest-score method, the P-matrix method, and the coefficient H^T can be used. These methods are implemented in the R package *mokken*.

It should be emphasized that two different kinds of methods can be used together. One type of method checks whether IRFs intersect (e.g., the rest-score method and the P-matrix methods, see later in this chapter). The other method (H^T) provides information about the spread of IRFs, that is, how far the IRFs are apart. The idea is that when the IRFs are further apart, we may have more confidence in IIO.

Rest-Score Method

Under the null hypothesis of nonintersecting IRFs Equation (5.1) applies. In the rest-score method the IRFs for each pair of items are estimated and compared using the item rest-score functions. For the dichotomous case, item rest-score functions relate the rest score (summed score minus the item score) on the x-axis with the observed response proportions for each rest-score group on the y-axis. Rest scores are grouped together when there are not enough persons at each possible rest score to compute reliable item proportions. For each pair of items i and j, with item j more popular than item i in the total group, it is checked whether:

$$P\left(X_j = 1 \mid R_{(ij)} = r\right) \geq P\left(X_i = 1 \mid R_{(ij)} = r\right), \text{ for } r = 0, \ldots, k-2, \tag{5.5}$$

with $R_{(ij)}$ denoting the summary score that contains neither X_i nor X_j. Thus, when two item rest-score functions are compared, the conditioning is based on the remaining $k - 2$ items. When IIO holds, the order of the item proportions for the different rest-score groups is the same as the ordering of the item proportions for the total group. Rest-score functions for all item pairs are compared to investigate whether IIO holds for a set of k items. A violation is reported when the response proportion is reversed in a rest-score group as compared to the response proportion order for the total group. The null hypothesis of equal item proportions can be tested against the one-sided alternative that the proportion of item i is larger than the proportion of item j.

Because significant violations sometimes have low impact, Molenaar and Sijtsma (2000) discuss an effect size measure named *Crit* that consists of a weighted number of different indicators of violations for which the following guidelines have been suggested: *Crit* values smaller than 40 indicate no serious violations; *Crit* values between 40 and 80 indicate minor violations, and *Crit* values larger than 80 indicate serious violations. The numerical values are based on several practical data analyses but should be interpreted with care. For example, there are no simulation studies that endorse these values. We will use these *Crit* values to get an idea about the seriousness of model violations in our data analyses.

The P-Matrix Method

To investigate nonintersection of the IRFs, the P-matrix method uses two square symmetric k x k matrices in which the items are ordered from difficult to easy (based on the probabilities in the overall group). The cells in the first matrix, P(+ +), contain all joint proportions $P_{ij}(1,1)$ of persons "passing" both items i and j. The cells in the second matrix, P(− −), contain all joint probabilities $P_{ij}(0,0)$ of persons "failing" both items i and j. Nonintersection of the IRFs means that the rows and columns of the P(+ +) matrix are non-decreasing and of the P(− −) matrix non-increasing. A violation is reported when there is a decrease in one of the rows or columns of the P(+ +) matrix and when there is an increase in one of the rows or columns of the P(− −) matrix. Like the rest-score method, significance testing is done using the McNemar's test.

Coefficient H^T

Coefficient H^T (Sijtsma & Meijer, 1992) can be used as a measure for the accuracy of the item ordering. A low H^T value suggests that the IRFs are close together, whereas a high value of H^T suggests that the IRFs are further apart. When IIO holds for k items, it can be shown that $0 \leq H^T \leq 1$. For practical purposes, Sijtsma and Meijer (1992) suggested using $H^T \geq 0.3$ as a lower bound. It is important to emphasize that H^T is only related to all k items together, and cannot be used to assess which items cause intersections. Therefore, Sijtsma and Meijer (1992) suggested combining information from H^T with the results from other methods such as the rest-score method and the P-matrix method.

Polytomous Data: Method Manifest IIO

Ligtvoet and colleagues (2010) developed a method to investigate IIO for polytomous items, which is named method manifest IIO. Method manifest IIO (MIIO) compares the ordering of the item means for all item pairs for different rest-score groups. This is investigated by numbering and ordering the items in increasing order of difficulty (i.e., from easy to difficult) for the entire test. IIO holds when:

$$E\left(X_i \mid R_{(ij)} = r\right) \geq E\left(X_j \mid R_{(ij)} = r\right), \text{ for all } r \text{ and all } i < j, \tag{5.6}$$

and with $R_{(ij)}$ denoting, once more, the total test score excluding the scores on items i and j. Then, one-sided one-sample t-tests are conducted to test the significance of each sample violation of the IIO condition stated earlier. The null hypothesis is that the expected conditional item means are equal, and it is tested against the alternative that the expected conditional mean of item j exceeds that of item i, which is a violation of IIO. A violation is reported when there is a reverse ordering of the conditional sample means for a particular rest score. To prevent taking very small violations seriously, these reverse orderings are only reported when they exceed a minimum value, denoted *minvi*.

Reliability in Nonparametric IRT

In *parametric* IRT a latent trait variable is estimated and the variance of this estimate across (hypothetical) repeated test administrations of the same test is the variance of the trait score. When this variance is small the estimate is precise, when it is large it is not precise. Because this variance is defined for a particular person it is within-person precision. Often the reciprocal of the within-person variance of the trait estimate is used, which is the test information at the given trait estimate.

In parametric IRT, reliability is concerned with the differentiation between trait scores of different persons. When the trait score can be precisely predicted from the test score reliability is satisfactory and it is unsatisfactory when it cannot.

Because in *nonparametric* IRT there are no θ estimates, Mokken (1971) proposed a method in the context of the DMM model that is based on the same definition as classical reliability and that results in a reliability estimate. TESTGRAF gives plots for a reliability estimate conditional on the estimated score.

Fit of Item Score Patterns

Thus far, we have discussed model data fit from the perspective of the items and set of items. Once a researcher concluded that a set of items can be described by an NIRT model, it can be checked whether there are persons who do not comply to the model assumptions.

Psychologists and clinicians have become increasingly aware of the need to evaluate carefully and routinely the veracity of information obtained from testing, clinical interviews, and other methods that are based on self-report. Deliberate exaggeration, or fabrication of problems to obtain a desired external goal, may invalidate test scores. Thus, feedback provided by simple statistics about the consistency of answering behavior can be useful, especially in clinical treatment and outcome measurement settings.

In personality and clinical assessments a tradition exists to detect invalid test scores using different types of validity scales. The utility of validity scales to detect "faking bad" or exaggerating symptoms has generated quite some debate. For example, Pinsoneault (2007) found that different MMPI validity scales had enough power to be used in practice. However, other authors have questioned the usefulness of validity scales to detect "faking good" or social desirability. One of the problems of validity scales is that they may be confounded with valid personality trait variance and show a relationship with other content scales. For example, Ones, Viswesvaran, and Reiss (1996) found that social desirability measures correlate with Emotional Stability ($r = 0.37$), Conscientiousness ($r = 0.20$), and Agreeableness ($r = 0.14$) in normal (honest) assessment situations. Because of this, a high social desirability score can indicate either legitimate favorable trait elevations or dissimulation. Also, many clinical scales do not have separate validity scales.

As an alternative, some authors have suggested using consistency measures (Tellegen, 1988). Since the 1980s with the increased use of item response theory modeling, statistics have been proposed to identify item score patterns that are unlikely under an IRT model. These unlikely patterns can be identified and further inspected. Although many statistics can be used to identify invalid score patterns (see Meijer & Sijtsma, 2001 for an overview), only a few studies show their practical usefulness (e.g., Meijer, Egberink, Emons, & Sijtsma, 2008).

Despite this lack of empirical evidence, we think that although a particular questionnaire can be a good measure of a psychological construct for a group of persons, it may be a poor measure of the construct for a particular individual, and that checking the consistency of answering behavior on questionnaires may be of help in outcome measurement. Perhaps it is the lack of easy-to-use software and the lack of the presence in often-used software programs (such as Multilog or IRTPRO) that make this technique relatively unpopular. However, the recently developed R packages *irtoys*, *PerFit*, and *mirt* (Chalmers, 2012) contain parametric person-fit statistics, which may increase the use of these statistics.

Application

To illustrate the different nonparametric IRT methods described so far we used two different data sets we obtained from the PROMIS® Wave 1 data (www.nihpromis.org). First, we analyzed data from two subscales of the Aggression Questionnaire (Buss & Perry, 1992): the Verbal Aggression scale and the Anger scale. We analyzed the 12 items of the combined subscales as one scale (denoted as AQ) because this enabled us to illustrate the performance of the different nonparametric IRT methods. Items were scored on a five-point Likert scale from 0 (*extremely uncharacteristic of me*) through 4 (*extremely characteristic of me*). Second, we analyzed data from the Physical Functioning (PF) scale of the SF-36

(Ware & Sherbourne, 1992) consisting of 10 items scored from 0 through 2 (0 = *limited a lot*; 1 = *limited a little*; 2 = no, not *limited at all*).

Aggression Scale

The sample consisted of 819 persons of the normal population (M_{age} = 51.3, *SD* = 18.21); 50.7 percent were men. Sijtsma and colleagues (2011) suggested a procedure for analyzing data according to the DMM. Because the DMM implies the MHM this procedure nicely fits the aim of the present study. For dichotomous items they distinguished the following steps: (1) investigate scalability/unidimensionality through an automated item selection procedure (AISP), (2) investigate monotonicity through inspecting item rest-score regressions, (3) investigate IIO through inspecting methods like rest score and P-matrix, and finally (4) investigate the precision of the item ordering through the H^T coefficient.

For polytomous data, a similar methodology was proposed by Sijtsma and colleagues (2011), with the exception that the method manifest IIO proposed by Ligtvoet and colleagues (2010) should be used to investigate IIO. We will loosely follow this methodology. That is, our aim is to illustrate how the data can be checked with respect to the MHM and the DMM. Analyses were performed using the *R* package *mokken*.

For the methodology as proposed by Sijtsma and colleagues (2011) it is not strictly necessary to use $c = 0.3$ as a lower bound in the AISP procedure. An alternative is to check whether all inter-item covariances are positive, thus using $H_{ij} = 0$ as a lower bound.

For both data sets, we started with the AISP procedure with $c = 0$. Although this lower bound is seldom used, it provides interesting information about which items comply to the minimum requirements of the MHM. Then we checked monotonicity by inspecting the IRFs.

Second, we used a lower bound of $c = 0.30$ for the AISP, *minvi* = 0.03 to investigate monotonicity, and *minvi* = 0.03 times the number of item step response functions (m) to investigate IIO. Ligtvoet and colleagues (2010) investigated the sensitivity and specificity of method manifest IIO. They used different *minvi* values and their simulation study showed that a *minvi* of 0.03 times m is an appropriate choice for investigating IIO with polytomous items. Furthermore, we used the following rules of thumb for the H^T coefficient: $H^T < 0.3$ implies that the item ordering is too inaccurate to be useful; $0.3 \leq H^T < 0.4$ implies low accuracy of item ordering; $0.4 \leq H^T < 0.5$ implies medium accuracy; and $H^T \geq 0.5$ implies high accuracy.

Ligtvoet and colleagues (2010) suggested the following sequential data-analysis procedure for method manifest IIO. First, for each of the k items the number of significant violations (i.e., that exceed *minvi*) is determined and the item with the highest number of violations is removed. When different items have the same number of significant violations, the item with the smallest H_i coefficient may be removed, but other criteria might also be considered, for example the item content. Second, this procedure is repeated for the remaining items until none of the remaining items have significant violations, which means that IIO holds for all items. When IIO holds for the (remaining) items, the H^T coefficient for polytomous items can be computed. This coefficient is a generalization of the original H^T coefficient to polytomous data and it allows checking the accuracy of the item ordering.

Results

Descriptive Statistics

Table 5.4 shows the content of the items, the mean item scores, and the item-total score correlation. A first observation is that the distribution of the item scores is skewed to the right; that is, most persons chose options 0, 1, or 2. This is as expected because most persons in

Table 5.4 Descriptive Statistics for the Aggression Scale

Item	*Subscale*	*Item content*	*Mean*	*SD*	*Item-total correlation*
1	Anger	Some of my friends think I am a hothead	0.66	1.04	0.70
2	Verbal	I tell my friends openly when I disagree with them	2.54	1.12	0.39
3	Verbal	I can't help getting into arguments when people disagree with me	1.06	1.13	0.67
4	Anger	I am an even-tempered person (reverse scored)	1.01	1.08	0.55
5	Anger	I flare up quickly but get over it quickly	1.69	1.28	0.54
6	Verbal	When people annoy me, I may tell them what I think of them	1.51	1.28	0.56
7	Anger	I have trouble controlling my temper	0.74	1.09	0.72
8	Anger	When frustrated, I let my irritation show	1.90	1.21	0.64
9	Verbal	I often find myself disagreeing with people	1.48	1.09	0.64
10	Anger	I sometimes feel like a powder keg ready to explode	0.55	1.02	0.63
11	Verbal	My friends say that I'm somewhat argumentative	1.12	1.22	0.71
12	Anger	Sometimes I fly off the handle for no good reason	0.53	0.97	0.66

the general population will not endorse statements that indicate (very) aggressive behavior. In Figure 5.1 we depicted the conditional reliability as calculated through TESTGRAF. As can be seen, reliability was highest for scores between 5 and 15 (to be further discussed later in this chapter). To obtain a first impression about the relative first-factor strength to assess unidimensionality we determined the ratio of the first to second eigenvalues—the larger this ratio, the more appropriate the item response data are thought to be for unidimensional IRT modeling. The ratio between first and second order factors was 4.7/1.5 = 3.1 for the Aggression scale and 6.3/1.0 = 6.0 for the Physical Functioning scale, so there is a stronger general factor running through the PF data than the AQ data.

Checking Monotonicity and Scalability

We start with inspecting the mean ISRF plots to obtain a first impression about the functioning of the items across different rest-score groups (see Figure 5.2). Note that we grouped many rest scores at the higher end of the total scores because there are relatively few persons with a high rest score. This plot already teaches us some interesting things about the item quality. It tells us (1) which items are most related to the underlying latent variable, aggression (steepest functions) and (2) in what range of the rest scores the items discriminate best. From Figure 5.2 it is clear that the item rest-score functions for all items are non-decreasing, although the mean ISRF of item 2 "*I tell my friends openly when I disagree with them*" is rather flat (i.e., not discriminating well between different rest scores). The rest-score function of item 11 "*My friends say that I'm somewhat argumentative*" has one of the steepest item rest-score functions. Note that one should be careful in interpreting the steepness of the IRFs because high rest scores are pooled together, thus the x-axis is not interval scaled.

Also note that items 10 and 12 discriminate well in the high rest-score range, but do not discriminate in the low rest-score range. Another observation is that for low rest-score levels the mean scores on items 2, 5, 6, and 8 are far from zero and for high rest-score

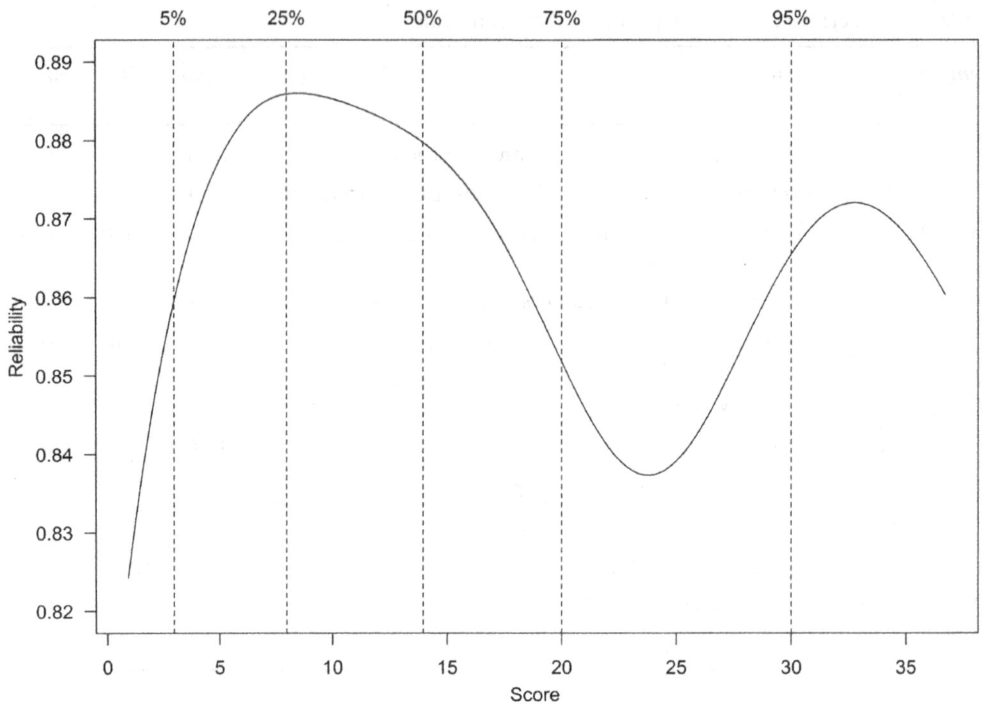

Figure 5.1 Conditional reliability for the Aggression scale scores.

levels this mean score is below three out of a maximum of four, thus indicating that the upper asymptote is far from the maximum category. This would suggest that for these data a parametric IRT model with an upper asymptote parameter lower than one is needed. These plots and similar results can also be obtained using TESTGRAF. To further explore item quality we return to the descriptive statistics in Table 5.4; these statistics confirm some of the observations obtained from inspecting the graphs in Figure 5.2. For example, item 2 does have a relatively low item-test correlation and the scores are skewed to the right.

Next, we ran the AISP using $c = 0$. Interesting is that 11 out of 12 items were selected; only item 2 was not selected because of a negative correlation with item 4. From these first analyses, it is clear that item 2 is a candidate for removal from the scale. When we ran the AISP with $c = 0.3$ as a lower bound item 6 was also removed from the scale because of an H_i value smaller than 0.3. When using the new AISP approach proposed by Straat and colleagues (2013) we found the same results; that is, both items 2 and 6 were not selected in the final scale.

Checking the monotonicity assumption for the remaining 10 items, we observed that the most problematic case concerned item 4. In Figure 5.3 we depicted the ISRFs of item 4. Note that there are five options (scores from 0 through 4) and thus four ISRFs. The figure shows that ISRF 1 is (almost) non-decreasing, but that the remaining ISRFs decrease between rest-score groups (3–4) and (5–6). ISRF 3 is also decreasing between rest-score groups 9–11 and 12–14 and ISRF 4 is also decreasing between rest-score groups 5–6 and 7–8. This results in a decreasing mean item step (bold line) and thus a violation of the MHM model.

To explain how monotonicity is checked consider Figure 5.3. There are eight rest-score groups with a varying number of persons (with a minimum of 81 persons per group in the present analysis). For each item step we now compare the proportions across the

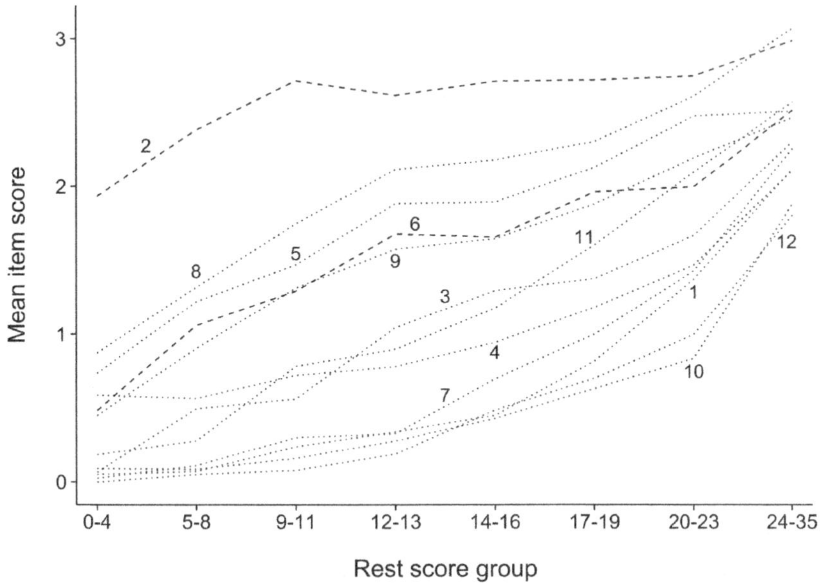

Figure 5.2 Mean ISRFs for the 12 items of the Aggression Questionnaire.

rest-score groups and a decrease larger than 0.03 is indicated as a violation against monotonicity. For example, for item step 2 there were violations for rest-score groups 1 and 3, 2 and 3, and 2 and 4.

To further explore this and to investigate how serious these violations are, in Table 5.5 we depicted some relevant statistics for all 10 selected items, but we concentrate on item 4 (in bold). In Table 5.5 we give the H_i values, the so-called number of *active pairs*, number of violations, and *Crit* values. The number of *active pairs* is the number of pairs that are taken into account when comparing the proportion-correct scores for each ISRF.

As can be seen in Table 5.5, item 4 had 15 violations out of 108 active pairs.[1] Between each two rest-score groups an observed decrease in proportion could be due to sampling variation. For example, for item step 2, the maximum violation was found when comparing the proportions of rest-score groups 3–4 and 5–6; the conditional probability $P(X_{(4)} \geq 2|R_{(4)})$ decreased 0.05. This decrease could be due to random fluctuation and not necessarily due to a large difference between both rest-score groups. This can be tested in a 2*2 table containing the number of persons in the rest-score groups 2 and 3 and the number of persons with item step < 2 and item step ≥ 2. Using a normal approximation for this hypergeometric distribution resulted in $z = 0.91$, thus we conclude that this specific violation is not significant. The same line of reasoning allows us to confirm that no significant violations exist for item steps 1 and 2. For item step 3 there were 4 violations (all significant) and for item step 4 there were 8 violations (6 significant). Thus in total there were 10 significant violations that resulted in a *Crit* value of 92. The researcher may consider removing this item from the item set.

1 There are 108 active pairs for item 4 because there are eight rest-score groups (see Figure 5.2) and there are four ISRFs per item. For each item there are thus (8*7/2)*4 = 112 possible comparisons. However, because there were zero results for the fourth rest group, the comparisons with rest-score groups 5, 6, 7, and 8 did not exist. Hence the number of active pairs for item 4 is 112 – 4 = 108.

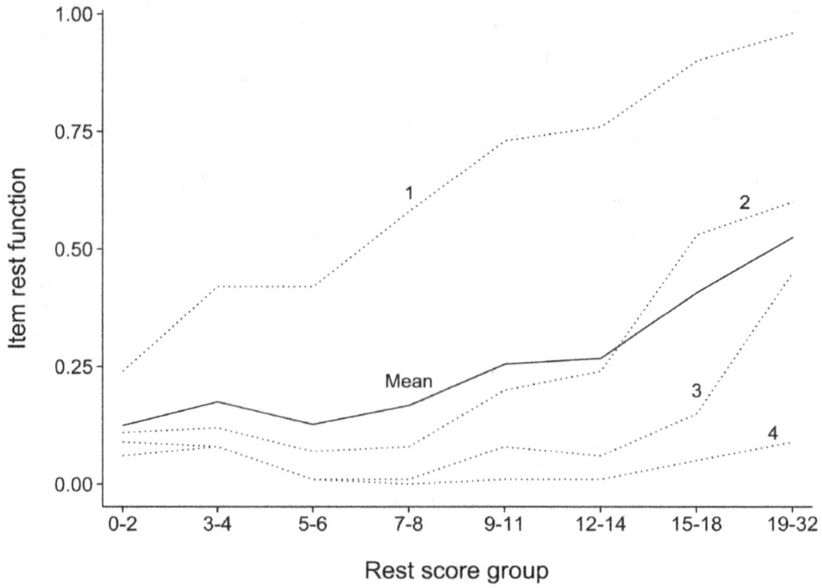

Figure 5.3 ISRFs for item 4, Aggression scale.

Table 5.5 Item H_i Values and Monotonicity Checks for 10 Items of the Aggression Questionnaire

Item	H_i	*# Ac pairs*	*# violations*	*# sign Z-test*	*crit*
1	.47	72	2	0	12
3	.41	112	1	1	33
4	**.37**	**108**	**15**	**10**	**92**
5	.32	112	3	0	21
7	.51	92	1	0	3
8	.43	105	3	0	19
9	.42	97	2	0	12
10	.47	92	0	—	—
11	.45	103	0	—	—
12	.49	64	0	—	—

Note: # Ac pairs = number of active pairs. # violations = number of violations. # sign Z-test = number of significant z tests. crit = *Crit* values.

Sijtsma and Molenaar (2002) suggested investigating multidimensionality by increasing the lower bound c values in the AISP. When this increase clearly resulted in the creation of different scales that are easy to interpret, multidimensionality may exist. If not, then the scale may be considered unidimensional. When we used $c = 0.4$ we found two scales: a first scale with items (10, 12, 7, 8, 1, 11, 9, 3) and a second scale with items (2, 6); items 4 and 5 were unscalable. With a lower bound of $c = 0.5$ there were two scales (10, 12, 7, 8, 1) and (11, 9, 3) and items 2, 4, and 6 are unscalable. There was no clear distinction between anger items and verbal aggression items. As we discussed earlier, maximizing H values leads to clusters of items that are very narrow in content. For example, item cluster (3, 9, 11) only consists of verbal disagreeing items and these items are thus very similar in content. On the basis of this analysis we conclude that there is no clear multidimensionality present in the data, and that items 2, 4, and 6 are candidates for removal from the scale.

Results Using DETECT

The DETECT procedure was used to further study the dimensionality of the data. We used the stand-alone program polyDETECT described in Zhang (2007) and obtained from the author. For the AQ items, DETECT selected three subscales: one consisting of items from the Anger subscale (items 1, 4, 7, 10, 12), another subscale consisted of Verbal Aggression items (items 2, 3, 6, 9, 11), and a cluster of two items (5, 8) formed a third subscale. The maximum DETECT value equaled 6.1, indicating multidimensionality. When we forced the data to have two dimensions, both the Anger and the Verbal Aggression subscales were identified. We will further elaborate on these results in relation to the Mokken analyses results when we discuss the results for the Physical Functioning scale.

Invariant Item Ordering

We checked for violations of IIO without items 2, 4, and 6. There was only one violation for items 10 and 12 and this violation was not significant according to MIIO, therefore these items were kept in the scale. For the subscale consisting of the remaining nine items we found $H^T = 0.38$, which following the rules of thumb tentatively proposed by Ligtvoet and colleagues (2010) indicates that the accuracy of the ordering of the items is low. This is also reflected in the plots of the mean ISRFs (see Figure 5.2). The ISRFs of items 1, 7, 10, and 12 cluster together and even cross (although not resulting in a significant different ordering of the items, as discussed earlier). Note that MIIO only investigates a reversed ordering and that item response functions may cluster together without violating the assumption of IIO. Important now is that it is clear that many mean ISRFs cluster together as is typical for many clinical scales (Meijer & Egberink, 2012).

How can we apply this information for further analyses? Based on these analyses one may choose a parametric model with a fixed *a*-parameter to describe the data. Another implication is that there is not a strong item ordering according to the *p*-values (i.e., the items' proportion-correct). Note that item 2 is not a good item because it does not differentiate between respondents with a low and high total score, although the item is responsible for a larger spread in the mean ISRFs; removing this item results in a decrease of the H^T coefficient from 0.41 to 0.31.

Physical Functioning Scale

The sample consisted of 714 persons ($M_{age} = 51.1$, $SD = 18.94$); 48.9 percent were men. An interesting conceptual difference between the AQ and the PF scale is that the AQ measures a psychological construct, whereas the PF scale measures physical activities and clearly not a psychological construct. As our results show, this has a strong influence on the psychometric quality of the scale. Because the questions of the PF scale refer to concrete activities a person can perform and because there seems to be a clear ordering of those activities from easy to difficult, the scale seems to be much more like a Guttman (1950) scale than

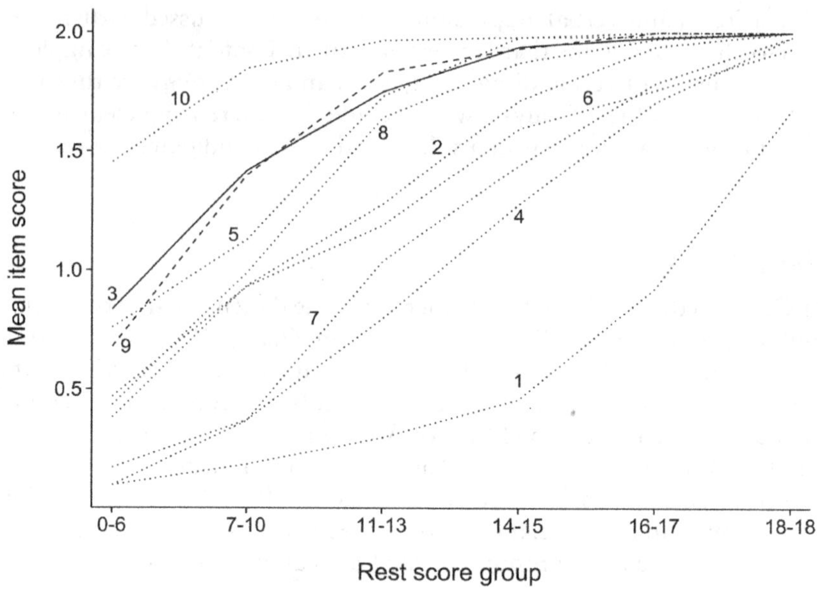

Figure 5.4 Mean ISRFs for the 10 items of the Physical Functioning scale.

the AQ. Thus, for the PF scale there is much similarity between the construct and the items that measure the construct. In contrast, for the AQ items the difference between the construct and the indicators (items) is larger than for the PF items and as a result scalability is lower. This is indeed reflected in the mean ISRF for the PF scale as compared to the AQ scale: Compared to the PF scale, the mean ISRFs of the AQ scale are less steep.

Table 5.6 gives the descriptive statistics for the 10 items of the PF scale. As expected, item-test correlations and H_i values are very high. H_i values varied between 0.69 and 0.80, resulting in an overall H value of 0.77 and thus indicating a very strong scale. As a consequence all items were selected by the AISP procedure using $c = 0.3$ (and thus also for $c = 0$). Inspecting the mean ISRFs of the PF items it is clear that most items discriminate much better across groups with different rest scores than the mean ISRFs of the Aggression scale (see Figure 5.4).

This is also reflected in the result from the IIO analyses. There were no violations against IIO with $H^T = 0.65$ indicating a high precision of the item ordering according to the rules proposed by Ligtvoet and colleagues (2010). However, one should be careful when interpreting this value. As Meijer and Egberink (2012) showed, H^T is sensitive to outliers. The mean ISRFs of items 1 and 10 are far apart from the other IRFs and these mean ISRFs are partly responsible for the high H^T value. When we removed these items, H^T dropped from 0.65 to 0.40. Thus, it is important to inspect the IRFs to get an idea about the spread of the IRFs.

Furthermore, it is clear that the IRFs of item 3 (*Lifting or carrying groceries*) and item 9 (*Walking one block*) almost coincide, indicating that these items do not reflect a different severity of physical functioning, at least in this population (note that the mean value of both items is 1.78). Given the fact that these items are so highly related ($H_{ij} = 0.69$), one may consider removing one of these items from the scale because each item does not overly contribute to the item ordering in the presence of the other. Also the mean ISRFs of items 2 and 6 are close together.

Table 5.6 Descriptive Statistics of the PF Scale

Item	*Item content*	*Mean*	*SD*	*Item-total correlation*	H_i
PF1	Vigorous activities, running, lifting	1.00	0.83	.74	.79
PF2	Moderate activities, moving table	1.60	0.63	.87	.79
PF3	Lifting or carrying groceries	1.78	0.50	.77	.74
PF4	Climbing several flights of stairs	1.38	0.78	.85	.78
PF5	Climbing one flight of stairs	1.75	0.53	.82	.78
PF6	Bending, kneeling, or stooping	1.52	0.66	.77	.69
PF7	Walking more than a mile	1.43	0.75	.88	.80
PF8	Walking several blocks	1.68	0.62	.84	.78
PF9	Walking one block	1.78	0.52	.80	.78
PF10	Bathing or dressing yourself	1.91	0.35	.55	.72

Results Using DETECT

Concerning data dimensionality, for the PF scale DETECT identified three subscales: (1,4,5), (2,3,6,10), and (7,8,9) with a maximum DETECT value of 0.89, implying some multidimensionality (Roussos & Ozbek, 2006). Note that cluster (7,8,9) consists of the "walking items" and two out of the three items from the cluster (1,4,5) are about "climbing stairs."

What should we make of these results? It is clear that the much lower DETECT value for the PF data as compared to the AQ data is the result of the stronger general factor in the PF data than the AQ data. As we mentioned earlier, there are several rules of thumb (e.g., Roussos & Ozbek, 2006) that would classify the AQ scale as multidimensional and even the PF scale would be considered moderately to largely multidimensional. However, Bonifay and colleagues (2014) discussed that "the flaw of DETECT, in terms of predicting parameter bias, is that its values are based on the size of the conditional covariances. These conditional covariances are determined by the size of the loadings on the group factor, but they are, by definition, independent of the general factor." Bonifay and colleagues (2014) in the context of bifactor modeling suggested therefore to consider DETECT values in the context of the general factor strength. In a nonparametric context it is interesting to consider the Mokken results in relation to the DETECT results. Remember that the ratio between the first and second order factors equaled six for the Physical Function scale and that the Mokken analysis showed that the H_{ij} values were very high (roughly between 0.7–0.9). These results point at a strong general factor. Thus, because DETECT is aimed at maximizing the differences between the item clusters and because it does not take the general factor into account, it is very sensitive to classifying items into different clusters. And perhaps most importantly, content-wise the DETECT results also lead to very narrow-band subscales, namely a three-item "walking scale," a three-item "climbing flights of stairs scale," and a subscale with the other items. Thus, it seems rather absurd to consider the PF data as multidimensional.

These conclusions are in line with the results reported in Bonifay and colleagues (2014), who found in a simulation study that using the rules of thumb suggested by Roussos and Ozbek (2006) for DETECT leads to many classifications of "multidimensionality" whereas a strong common factor was present in the data. Like in the present study, this was due to strong group factors.

Person-Fit Results

To illustrate the usefulness of person-fit analysis, we investigated the score patterns of the PF scale in more detail. As shown earlier, the scale consists of 10 items that allow for IIO.

Given that we order the PF items from most popular to least popular, a simple and powerful person-fit statistic is the number of Guttman errors (Meijer, 1994). For dichotomous items, the number of Guttman errors equals the number of zero scores preceding a one score in a score pattern, thus, the pattern (10110010) contains five Guttman errors. A drawback of this statistic, however, is that it is confounded with the total score (Meijer, 1994). For polytomous items Emons (2008), therefore, proposed a normed version of the number of Guttman errors:

$$G_N^p = \frac{G^p}{\max\left(G^p \mid X_+\right)}.$$

In this statistic the number of Guttman errors (G^p) is weighted by its maximum value given the sum score (for details see Emons, 2008). G_N^p values ranged from zero (i.e., no misfit) through one (i.e., maximum misfit); for perfect response patterns the statistic is undefined.

We used the *R*-package *PerFit* (Tendeiro, 2014) to calculate G_N^p. The mean G_N^p equaled M = 0.05 (SD = 0.09). Most persons obtained low G_N^p values, indicating model conform behavior. However, there were outliers. One of the most extreme patterns was the pattern of person 535 with $G_N^p = 0.66$. It is instructive to compare the score pattern of person 535 with the score pattern of a randomly chosen person (person 165) with a low G_N^p value and a similar total score of $X_+ = 8$.

Person 165: [2 1 2 1 0 1 0 1 0 0] total score 8: $G_N^p = 0.06$.

Person 535: [0 0 1 2 0 1 0 0 2 2] total score 8: $G_N^p = 0.66$.

The items are ordered so that item 1 reflects the easiest tasks (*Bathing or dressing yourself*) and item 10 the most difficult tasks (*Vigorous activities*). Intriguing is that person 535 reports problems in bathing and dressing (item score 0), whereas there are no problems with "*Vigorous activities, such as running, lifting heavy objects, participating in strenuous sports*" (item score 2). This is rather unexpected and certainly deserves closer attention. It is also clear that the total score patterns of both persons do indicate different things about physical functioning.

Summary

Reise and Waller (2009) wrote: "the clinical measures we examined are characterized by relatively small samples of poorly defined mixtures of patient groups of convenience, highly skewed score distributions, poorly articulated content domains, constructs with a limited number of potential indicators, narrow band constructs (e.g., fatigue), quasi-traits, and high correlations among scales measuring different traits (e.g., due to the omnipresent negative affectivity dimension)." In this context, we hope to have shown that nonparametric IRT methods that explore data quality can be very useful before using more complex models or models that are based on more restrictive assumptions than nonparametric approaches. In contrast to the statistical tradition of data exploration, plotting data, looking for outliers, and carefully considering different models and approaches, the psychometric literature sometimes seems obsessed with all kinds of "model wars" and to formulate "do's" and "don'ts" to support a "Holy Grail" model. We do not endorse this. We see psychometric modeling more as a way to explore data quality than as a model fit contest (so researchers need to stop being fitidiots). Nonparametric approaches are excellent tools to decide whether parametric models are justified. Moreover, given the often not-so-easy-to-interpret fit statistics for parametric models, nonparametric tools provide a nice extension of the parametric toolkit to IRT modeling.

This is not to say that in some situations parametric models and even restrictive parametric models may be preferred over nonparametric models. For example, using θ scoring instead of total scores can reduce ceiling effects. Also the use of computer adaptive testing is much easier using parametric models than nonparametric approaches.

Finally and returning to the content of many outcome measures, our analyses once again showed that many clinical scales are simple instruments that require little or no understanding of psychological theory. This also makes it difficult, for example, to investigate IIO.[2] We seldom find detailed descriptions that made clear that the content of one item reflected a less severe type of the construct that is being measured than the content of another item. For example, we do not encounter many clinical or personality scales that a priori describe symptoms in order of severity. Perhaps this reflects the fact that many symptoms go together and that there is no real ordering in item severity. On the other hand we have the impression that not much thought is given to the theoretical underpinnings of many constructs.

References

Bonifay, W. E., Reise, S. P., Scheines, R., & Meijer, R. R. (In press). When are multidimensional data unidimensional enough for structural equation modeling? An evaluation of the DETECT multidimensionality index. *Structural Equation Modeling*.

Buss, A.H., & Perry, M. (1992). The aggression questionnaire. *Journal of Personality and Social Psychology*, *63*(3), 452–459.

Chalmers, R.P. (2012). Mirt: A multidimensional item response theory package for the R environment. *Journal of Statistical Software*, *48*(6), 1–29.

Chen, W., & Thissen, D. (1997). Local dependence indexes for item pairs using item response theory. *Journal of Educational and Behavioral Statistics*, *22*(3), 265–289.

Chernyshenko, O.S., Stark, S., Chan, K., Drasgow, F., & Williams, B. (2001). Fitting item response theory models to two personality inventories: Issues and insights. *Multivariate Behavioral Research*, *36*(4), 523–562.

2 Ligtvoet (2010) showed that very large samples (almost 3,000 persons) are needed to distinguish realistic numbers of ISRFs. Ligtvoet (2010) suggested that alternative approaches are needed to establish IIO in practice. One suggested approach was to form clusters of items that have similar adjacent IRFs and to establish IIO across different item clusters. A drawback of this approach may be that item clusters may consist of items that are redundant.

Derogatis, L. R. (1983). Brief Symptom Inventory: Administration, scoring, and procedures manual. Minneapolis, MN: National Computer Systems.

Egberink, I. L., & Meijer, R. R. (2011). An item response theory analysis of Harter's Self-Perception Profile for Children or why strong clinical scales should be distrusted. *Assessment, 18*(2), 201–212.

Emons, W. M. (2008). Nonparametric person-fit analysis of polytomous item scores. *Applied Psychological Measurement, 32*(3), 224–247.

Guttman, L. (1950). *The basis for scalogram analysis*. In: S. A. Stouffer, L. Guttman, E. A. Suchman, P. F. Lazersfeld, S. A. Star, & J. A. Clausen (Eds.), *Measurement and prediction* (pp. 60–90). Princeton, NJ: Princeton University Press.

Hemker, B. T., Sijtsma, K., Molenaar, I. W., & Junker, B. W. (1997). Stochastic ordering using the latent trait and the sum score in polytomous IRT models. *Psychometrika, 62*(3), 331–347.

Holland, P. W., & Rosenbaum, P. R. (1986). Conditional association and unidimensionality in monotone latent variable models. *Annals of Statistics, 14*(4), 1523–1543.

Ligtvoet, R. (2010). *Essays on invariant item ordering*. Unpublished doctoral dissertation, University of Tilburg.

Ligtvoet, R., van der Ark, L., te Marvelde, J. M., & Sijtsma, K. (2010). Investigating an invariant item ordering for polytomously scored items. *Educational and Psychological Measurement, 70*(4), 578–595.

Mazza, A., Punzo, A., & McGuire, B. (2012). KernSmoothIRT: An R package for kernel smoothing in item response theory. Retrieved from http://arxiv.org/pdf/1211.1183v1.pdf.

Meijer, R. R. (1994). The number of Guttman errors as a simple and powerful person-fit statistic. *Applied Psychological Measurement, 18*(4), 311–314.

Meijer, R. R. (2010). Watson, Deary, and Austin (2007) and Watson, Roberts, Gow, and Deary (2008): How to investigate whether personality items form a hierarchical scale?: Comment. *Personality and Individual Differences, 48*(4), 502–503.

Meijer, R. R., & Baneke, J. J. (2004). Analyzing psychopathology items: A case for nonparametric item response theory modeling. *Psychological Methods, 9*(3), 354–368.

Meijer, R. R., de Vries, R. M., & van Bruggen, V. (2011). An evaluation of the Brief Symptom Inventory–18 using item response theory: Which items are most strongly related to psychological distress? *Psychological Assessment, 23*(1), 193–202.

Meijer, R. R., & Egberink, I. L. (2012). Investigating invariant item ordering in personality and clinical scales: Some empirical findings and a discussion. *Educational and Psychological Measurement, 72*(4), 589–607.

Meijer, R. R., Egberink, I. L., Emons, W. M., & Sijtsma, K. (2008). Detection and validation of unscalable item score patterns using item response theory: An illustration with Harter's Self-Perception Profile for Children. *Journal of Personality Assessment, 90*(3), 227–238.

Meijer, R. R., Niessen, A. S. M., & Tendeiro, J. N. (2014). A practical guide to check the consistency of item response patterns in clinical research through person-fit statistics: Examples and a computer program.

Meijer, R. R., & Sijtsma, K. (2001). Methodology review: Evaluating person fit. *Applied Psychological Measurement, 25*(2), 107–135.

Mellenbergh, G. J. (2011). *A conceptual introduction to psychometrics: Development, analysis, and application of psychological and educational tests*. The Hague: Eleven International.

Mokken, R. J. (1971). *A theory and procedure of scale analysis*. The Hague: De Gruyter.

Molenaar, I. W. (1997). Nonparametric model for polytomous responses. In W. J. van der Linden & R. K. Hambleton (Eds.), *Handbook of modern item response theory* (pp. 369–380). New York: Springer-Verlag.

Molenaar, I. W. (2004). About handy, handmade and handsome models. *Statistica Neerlandica, 58*(1), 1–20.

Molenaar, I. W., & Sijtsma, K. (2000). *User's manual MSP5 for Windows*. IEC ProGAMMA, Groningen.

Mroch, A. A., & Bolt, D. M. (2006). A simulation comparison of parametric and nonparametric dimensionality detection procedures. *Applied Measurement in Education, 19*(1), 67–91.

Ones, D.S., Viswesvaran, C., & Reiss, A.D. (1996). Role of social desirability in personality testing for personnel selection: The red herring. *Journal of Applied Psychology*, *81*(6), 660–679.

Partchev, I. (2013). Package "irtoys": Simple interface to the estimation and plotting of IRT models. Retrieved from http://cran.r-project.org/web/packages/irtoys/irtoys.pdf.

Pinsoneault, T.B. (2007). Detecting random, partially random, and nonrandom Minnesota Multiphasic Personality Inventory-2 protocols. *Psychological Assessment*, *19*(1), 159–164.

Ramsay, J.O. (1991). Kernel smoothing approaches to nonparametric item characteristic curve estimation. *Psychometrika*, *56*(4), 611–630.

Ramsay, J.O. (2000). TestGraf: A program for the graphical analysis of multiple choice test and questionnaire data. Retrieved from www.psych.mcgill.ca/faculty/ramsay/TestGraf.html.

Rao, C.R., & Sinharay, S. (2007). *Handbook of Statistics 26. Psychometrics*. Amsterdam: Elsevier.

Reise, S.P. (2009). The emergence of item response theory models and the patient reported outcomes measurement information systems. *Austrian Journal of Statistics*, *38*(4), 211–220.

Reise, S.P., & Waller, N.G. (2009). Item response theory and clinical measurement. *Annual Review of Clinical Psychology*, *5*, 27–48.

Roussos, L.A., & Ozbek, O. (2006). Formulation of the DETECT population parameter and evaluation of DETECT estimator bias. *Journal of Educational Measurement*, *43*(3), 215–243.

Santor, D.A., & Ramsay, J.O. (1998). Progress in the technology of measurement: Applications of item response models. *Psychological Assessment*, *10*(4), 345–359.

Santor, D.A., Ramsay, J.O., & Zuroff, D.C. (1994). Nonparametric item analyses of the Beck Depression Inventory: Evaluating gender item bias and response option weights. *Psychological Assessment*, *6*(3), 255–270.

Sijtsma, K., & Junker, B.W. (1996). A survey of theory and methods of invariant item ordering. *British Journal of Mathematical and Statistical Psychology*, *49*(1), 79–105.

Sijtsma, K., & Meijer, R.R. (1992). A method for investigating the intersection of item response functions in Mokken's nonparametric IRT model. *Applied Psychological Measurement*, *16*(2), 149–157.

Sijtsma, K., & Meijer, R.R. (2007). *Nonparametric item response theory and special topics*. In C.R. Rao & S. Sinharay (Eds.), *Handbook of Statistics 26. Psychometrics* (pp. 719–746). Amsterdam: Elsevier.

Sijtsma, K., Meijer, R.R., & Andries van der Ark, L.L. (2011). Mokken scale analysis as time goes by: An update for scaling practitioners. *Personality and Individual Differences*, *50*(1), 31–37.

Sijtsma, K., & Molenaar, I.W. (2002). *Introduction to nonparametric item response theory*. Thousand Oaks, CA: Sage.

Smits, I.M., Timmerman, M.E., & Meijer, R.R. (2012). Exploratory Mokken scale analysis as a dimensionality assessment tool: Why scalability does not imply unidimensionality. *Applied Psychological Measurement*, *36*(6), 516–539.

Stout, W. (1987). A nonparametric approach for assessing latent trait unidimensionality. *Psychometrika*, *52*(4), 589–617.

Stout, W.F. (1990). A new item response theory modeling approach with applications to unidimensionality assessment and ability estimation. *Psychometrika*, *55*(2), 293–325.

Stout, W., Habing, B., Douglas, J., & Kim, H. (1996). Conditional covariance-based nonparametric multidimensionality assessment. *Applied Psychological Measurement*, *20*(4), 331–354.

Straat, J.H. (2012). *Using scalability coefficients and conditional association to assess monotone homogeneity* (Doctoral dissertation). Retrieved from http://arno.uvt.nl/show.cgi?fid=128094.

Straat, J.H., Van der Ark, L.A., & Sijtsma K. (2013). Comparing optimization algorithms for item selection in Mokken scale analysis. *Journal of Classification*, *30*, 75–99.

Tellegen, A. (1988). The analysis of consistency in personality assessment. *Journal of Personality*, *56*(3), 621–663.

Tendeiro, J.N. (2014). PerFit (version 1.2) [Computer software]. University of Groningen. Available from http://cran.r-project.org/web/packages/PerFit/.

van Abswoude, A.H., van der Ark, L., & Sijtsma, K. (2004). A comparative study of test data dimensionality assessment procedures under nonparametric IRT models. *Applied Psychological Measurement*, *28*(1), 3–24.

van der Ark, L. A. (2007). Mokken scale analysis in R. *Journal of Statistical Software*, *20*, 1–19.
van der Ark, L. A. (2012). New developments in Mokken scale analysis in R. *Journal of Statistical Software*, *48*, 1–27.
van der Linden, W. J., & Hambleton, R. K. (Eds.) (1997). *Handbook of modern item response theory*. New York: Springer-Verlag.
Wainer, H. (2005). *Graphic discovery. A trout in the milk and other visual adventures*. Princeton, NJ: Princeton University Press.
Ware, J. E., Jr., & Sherbourne, C. D. (1992). The MOS 36-item short-form health survey (SF-36): Conceptual framework and item selection. *Medical Care*, *30*, 473–483.
Watson, R., Deary, I., & Austin, E. (2007). Are personality trait items reliably more or less "difficult"? Mokken scaling of the NEO-FFI. *Personality and Individual Differences*, *43*(6), 1460–1469.
Zhang, J. (2007). Conditional covariance theory and detect for polytomous items. *Psychometrika*, *72*(1), 69–91.
Zhang, J., & Stout, W. (1999). The theoretical DETECT index of dimensionality and its application to approximate simple structure. *Psychometrika*, *64*(2), 213–249.
Zigmond, A. S., & Snaith, R. P. (1983). The Hospital Anxiety and Depression Scale. *Acta Psychiatrica Scandinavica*, *67*(6), 361–370.

6 Evaluating the Fit of IRT Models

Alberto Maydeu-Olivares[1]

Introduction

The goodness of fit (GOF) of a statistical model, such as an item response theory (IRT) model, describes how well the model matches a set of observations. It is useful to distinguish between goodness of fit *indices* and goodness of fit statistics. Goodness of fit indices summarize the discrepancy between the values observed in the data and the values expected under a statistical model. Goodness of fit *statistics* are GOF indices used in statistical hypothesis testing. In other words, GOF statistics are GOF indices with known sampling distributions usually obtained using asymptotic methods. Because p-values obtained using asymptotic methods may behave poorly in small samples, a great deal of research has been devoted to investigate using simulation studies under which conditions the asymptotic p-values of GOF statistics are accurate (e.g., Maydeu-Olivares & Montaño, 2013).

Assessing the absolute model fit of a model (i.e., the discrepancy between a model and the data) is critical in applications, as inferences drawn on poorly fitting models may be badly misleading. Applied researchers must examine not only the overall fit of their models, but they should also perform a piecewise assessment. It may well be that a model fits well overall but that it fits poorly some parts of the data, suggesting the use of an alternative model. Also, piecewise GOF assessment may reveal the source of misfit in poorly fitting models.

Assessing the absolute fit of a statistical model involves determining whether the model could have generated the observed data. In IRT applications, however, degrees of freedom are most often so large that no model can be expected to fit the data exactly. For example, an IRT model for 20 polytomous items, each one consisting of five response categories, involves modeling 5^{20} response patterns and it yields more than 95×10^{12} degrees of freedom. In models with so many degrees of freedom I recommend instead to assess whether the model approximately fits the data. By this we mean determining whether a goodness of fit statistic is smaller than some arbitrary nonzero value. In contrast, assessing whether the model fits exactly amounts to testing whether the value of a goodness of fit statistic equals zero.

This work is organized as follows: In this section, I review the classical statistics for assessing the overall fit of categorical data models (such as IRT models) and their limitations. In the next section, I review some new developments in this area. Thus, I describe the new limited information overall goodness of fit statistics that have been proposed in the literature as these overcome the limitations of classical statistics. I also briefly introduce

1 This research was supported by an ICREA-Academia Award and grant SGR 2009 74 from the Catalan Government and grants PSI2009–07726 and PR2010–0252 from the Spanish Ministry of Education.

methods for assessing approximate fit, as well as methods for piecewise assessment of fit. The next section includes an application to the PROMIS® depression short form (Pilkonis et al., 2011). This chapter concludes with a discussion and recommendations for applied users.

Classical Goodness of Fit Statistics

Consider the responses given by N individuals to n test items, each with K categories coded as $0,1,\ldots,K-1$. The resulting data can be gathered in a n-dimensional contingency table with $C = K^n$ cells. Within this setting, assessing the goodness of fit of a model involves assessing the discrepancy between the observed proportions and the probabilities expected under the model across all cells of the contingency table. More formally, let π_c be the probability of one such cell (i.e., a response pattern to the n test items) and let p_c be the observed proportion, $c = 1,\ldots,C$. Also, let $\pi(\theta)$ be the C-dimensional vector of model probabilities expressed as a function of the, say q, model parameters to be estimated from the data. Then, the null hypothesis to be tested is $H_0 : \pi = \pi(\theta)$ against $H_1 : \pi \neq \pi(\theta)$.

The two standard goodness of fit statistics for discrete data are Pearson's statistic $X^2 = N\sum_c (p_c - \hat{\pi}_c)^2 / \hat{\pi}_c$, and the likelihood ratio statistic $G^2 = 2N\sum_c p_c \ln(p_c / \hat{\pi}_c)$, where $\hat{\pi}_c = \pi_c\left(\hat{\theta}\right)$. Asymptotic p-values for both statistics can be obtained using a chi-square distribution with $C - q - 1$ degrees of freedom when maximum likelihood estimation is used. However, these asymptotic p-values are only correct when all expected frequencies are large (>5 is the usual rule of thumb). A practical way to evaluate whether the asymptotic p-values for X^2 and G^2 are valid is to compare them. If the p-values are similar, then both are likely to be correct. If they are very different, it is most likely that both p-values are incorrect.

Unfortunately as the number of cells in the table increases, the expected frequencies must be small because the sum of all C probabilities must be equal to one (Bartholomew & Tzamourani, 1999). As a result, in IRT modeling, most often the p-values for these statistics cannot be used (Thissen & Steinberg, 1997). In fact, when the number of categories is large (say > 4) the asymptotic p-values almost invariably become inaccurate as soon as $n > 5$. To overcome the problem of the inaccuracy of the asymptotic p-values for these statistics two general methods have been proposed: resampling methods (e.g., bootstrap), and pooling cells. Unfortunately, existing evidence suggests that resampling methods do not yield accurate p-values for the X^2 and G^2 statistics (Tollenaar & Mooijart, 2003).

Pooling cells results in statistics whose asymptotic distribution may be well approximated by asymptotic methods because pooled cells must have larger expected frequencies. However, pooling must be performed before the analysis is made to obtain a statistic with the appropriate asymptotic reference distribution. A straightforward way to pool cells a priori for goodness of fit testing is to use low order margins, that is, probabilities that are univariate, bivariate, and so forth. Goodness of fit statistics based on low order margins are referred to in the literature as limited information statistics because they do not use all the information available in the data for testing the overall goodness of fit of the model. Because they are based on pooled cells, the p-values of limited information statistics are accurate in very large models even with samples as small as $N = 100$ observations. Furthermore, because they "concentrate" the information available for testing, they are most often more powerful than full information statistics such as Pearson's X^2 to detect alternatives of interest.

Research Methods

Overall Goodness of Fit Testing Using Limited Information Statistics

To understand limited information methods consider the following 2 × 3 contingency table:

	$Y_2 = 0$	$Y_2 = 1$	$Y_2 = 2$
$Y_1 = 0$	π_{00}	π_{01}	π_{02}
$Y_1 = 1$	π_{11}	π_{11}	π_{12}

This table can be characterized using the cell probabilities $\pi' = (\pi_{00}, \cdots, \pi_{12})$. Alternatively, it can be characterized using the univariate $\dot{\pi}_1' = \left(\pi_1^{(1)}, \pi_2^{(1)}, \pi_2^{(2)}\right)$ and bivariate $\dot{\pi}_2' = \left(\pi_{1\,2}^{(1)(1)}, \pi_{1\,2}^{(1)(2)}\right)$ probabilities, where

	$Y_2 = 0$	$Y_2 = 1$	$Y_2 = 2$	
$Y_1 = 0$				
$Y_1 = 1$		$\pi_{1\,2}^{(1)(1)}$	$\pi_{1\,2}^{(1)(2)}$	$\pi_1^{(1)}$
		$\pi_2^{(1)}$	$\pi_2^{(2)}$	

and $\pi_2^{(2)} = \Pr(Y_2 = 2)$ and $\pi_{1\,2}^{(1)(2)} = \Pr(Y_1 = 1, Y_2 = 2)$. Both characterizations are equivalent, and the equivalence extends to contingency tables of any dimension. In other words, one can always transform the cell probabilities into the moments $\pi_2' = \left(\dot{\pi}_1', \dot{\pi}_2'\right)$ and vice versa. $\dot{\boldsymbol{\pi}}_1$ and $\dot{\boldsymbol{\pi}}_2$ are clearly univariate and bivariate moments if the variables are binary, and moments of indicator variables used to denote each category except the zero category if the variables are polytomous (Maydeu-Olivares & Joe, 2006). I use the term *moments* to distinguish $\dot{\boldsymbol{\pi}}_1$ and $\dot{\boldsymbol{\pi}}_2$ from the set of univariate and bivariate probabilities, $\tilde{\pi}_1' = \left(\pi_1^{(0)}, \pi_1^{(1)}, \pi_2^{(0)}, \pi_2^{(1)}, \pi_2^{(2)}\right)$ and $\tilde{\pi}_2 = \pi$ (in this example). Notice that the moments of order r simply consist of the r-way marginal probabilities that do not involve the category 0.

A limited information goodness of fit statistic uses only the moments up to order $r < n$ for testing. Thus, in the example cited earlier, a statistic that only involves univariate moments would be a limited information test statistic. In contrast, full information statistics use all moments (up to order n or $\boldsymbol{\pi}_n$). Pearson's X^2 statistic is a full information statistic and therefore it can be written as a function of the cell probabilities:

$$X^2 = N(\mathbf{p} - \hat{\pi})' \hat{\mathbf{D}}^{-1} (\mathbf{p} - \hat{\pi}) \tag{6.1}$$

where $\mathbf{p} - \hat{\pi}$ are the cell residuals, and $\hat{\mathbf{D}} = diag\left(\pi\left(\hat{\theta}\right)\right)$ is a diagonal matrix of estimated cell probabilities, or as a function of the moments:

$$X^2 = N(\mathbf{p}_n - \hat{\boldsymbol{\pi}}_n)' \hat{\boldsymbol{\Xi}}_n^{-1} (\mathbf{p}_n - \hat{\boldsymbol{\pi}}_n) \tag{6.2}$$

where $\mathbf{p}_n - \hat{\boldsymbol{\pi}}_n$ are the residual moments, and $N\hat{\boldsymbol{\Xi}}_n$ is the asymptotic covariance matrix of the sample moments up to order n, $\mathbf{p}_n$, evaluated at the parameter estimates.

For IRT applications Maydeu-Olivares and Joe (2005, 2006) suggested testing using $r = 2$, that is, using only univariate and bivariate moments because the lower the order of moments used the more accurate the p-values and (generally) the higher the power. More specifically, they suggested testing using the limited information test statistic:

$$M_2 = N(\mathbf{p}_2 - \hat{\boldsymbol{\pi}}_2)' \hat{\mathbf{C}}_2 (\mathbf{p}_2 - \hat{\boldsymbol{\pi}}_2), \qquad \mathbf{C}_2 = \boldsymbol{\Xi}_2^{-1} - \boldsymbol{\Xi}_2^{-1}\boldsymbol{\Delta}_2(\boldsymbol{\Delta}_2'\boldsymbol{\Xi}_2^{-1}\boldsymbol{\Delta}_2)^{-1}\boldsymbol{\Delta}_2'\boldsymbol{\Xi}_2^{-1}, \tag{6.3}$$

where $\boldsymbol{\Delta}_r$ denotes the matrix of derivatives of the univariate and bivariate moments with respect to the parameter vector $\boldsymbol{\theta}$, and $N\boldsymbol{\Xi}_2$ denotes the asymptotic covariance matrix of the univariate and bivariate sample moments. These matrices are evaluated at the parameter estimates, $\hat{\theta}$. When all items consist of the same number of categories, K, M_2 is asymptotically distributed as a chi-square with $df_2 = n(K-1) + \frac{n(n-1)}{2}(K-1)^2 - q$ degrees of freedom. M_2 is a member of the M_r class of test statistics ($M_1, M_2, M_3, \ldots, M_n$). The members of this class of statistics are of the form (6.3) and simply differ from M_2 in the amount of information used. Thus, in M_1 only univariate moments are used. IRT models cannot be tested using only univariate information as there are no degrees of freedom available for testing. In M_3, univariate, bivariate, and trivariate moments are used, whereas in M_n all moments (up to order n) are used. For maximum likelihood estimation, M_n equals X_2 algebraically (i.e., the second term in the weight matrix equals zero).

Testing Models for Large and Sparse Ordinal Data

When the number of categories per item is large M_2 suffers from two limitations. The first limitation is that if the number of items is also large, M_2 may not be computable because of the size of the matrices that need to be stored in memory. The second limitation is that the bivariate tables may be sparse, particularly in one or both extremes of the response scale. In this case, the asymptotic p-values of M_2 may not be accurate enough (Cai & Hansen, 2013).

If the number of variables and categories is large, or if the bivariate tables are sparse, one should assess the overall goodness of fit of the model using M_{ord},

$$M_{ord} = N(\mathbf{k} - \hat{\boldsymbol{\kappa}})' \hat{\mathbf{C}}_{ord} (\mathbf{k} - \hat{\boldsymbol{\kappa}}), \; \mathbf{C}_{ord} = \boldsymbol{\Xi}_{ord}^{-1} - \boldsymbol{\Xi}_{ord}^{-1}\boldsymbol{\Delta}_{ord}(\boldsymbol{\Delta}_r'\boldsymbol{\Xi}_{ord}^{-1}\boldsymbol{\Delta}_{ord})^{-1}\boldsymbol{\Delta}_{ord}'\boldsymbol{\Xi}_{ord}^{-1}, \tag{6.4}$$

which is a statistic for ordinal data only. This statistic has the same form as M_2 but the statistics in the quadratic form are now the sample means and cross-products $\mathbf{k}$. Thus, $N\boldsymbol{\Xi}_{ord}$ is their asymptotic covariance matrix, $\boldsymbol{\kappa}$ is the population counterpart of $\mathbf{k}$ (the population means and cross-products of the multinomial variables ignoring the multivariate nature of the multinomial variables), and $\boldsymbol{\Delta}_{ord}$ is the matrix of derivatives of $\boldsymbol{\kappa}$ with respect to the model parameters, $\boldsymbol{\theta}$. $\boldsymbol{\kappa}$, $\boldsymbol{\Xi}_{ord}$ and $\boldsymbol{\Delta}_{ord}$ are to be evaluated at the parameter estimates—that is, $\hat{\kappa}$ denotes $\kappa(\hat{\theta})$. More specifically the elements of $\boldsymbol{\kappa}$ are of the form:

$$\kappa_i = E[Y_i] = 0 \times \Pr(Y_i = 0) + \ldots + K_i \times \Pr(Y_i = K_i), \tag{6.5}$$

$$\kappa_{ij} = E\left[Y_i Y_j\right] = 0 \times 0 \times \Pr\left(Y_i = 0, Y_j = 0\right) + \ldots + K_i \times K_j \times \Pr\left(Y_i = K_i, Y_j = K_j\right), \tag{6.6}$$

with sample counterparts $k_i = \bar{y}_i$ (the sample mean), and $k_{ij} = \mathbf{y}_i'\mathbf{y}_j / N$ (the sample cross-product), respectively. In particular, for our previous example, the elements of $\boldsymbol{\kappa}$ are

$$\begin{aligned} \kappa_1 &= E[Y_1] = 1\Pr(Y_1 = 1) = \pi_1^{(1)} \\ \kappa_2 &= E[Y_2] = 1\Pr(Y_2 = 1) + 2\Pr(Y_2 = 1) = \pi_2^{(1)} + 2\pi_2^{(2)} \\ \kappa_{12} &= E[Y_1 Y_2] = 1 \times 1\Pr(Y_1 = 1, Y_2 = 1) + 1 \times 2\Pr(Y_1 = 1, Y_2 = 2) = \pi_{1\ 2}^{(1)(1)} + 2\pi_{1\ 2}^{(1)(2)}. \end{aligned} \tag{6.7}$$

Thus, for our 2 × 3 example, M_2 is a quadratic form in the sample counterparts of $\pi_2' = \left(\pi_1^{(1)}, \pi_2^{(1)}, \pi_2^{(2)}, \pi_{1\ 2}^{(1)(1)}, \pi_{1\ 2}^{(1)(2)}\right)$, and M_{ord} is a quadratic form in the sample counterparts of $\boldsymbol{\kappa}$ given in (6.7). Clearly, $\boldsymbol{\kappa}$ is obtained as a linear combination of $\boldsymbol{\varphi}_2$ where the weights are used as given by the coding of the categories. Thus, it only makes sense to use $\boldsymbol{\kappa}$ and their sample counterparts, and therefore M_{ord}, when the data is ordinal. When the data is binary, M_{ord} equals M_2. In general, M_{ord} is asymptotically distributed as a chi-square with $df_{ord} = \frac{n(n+1)}{2} - q$ degrees of freedom.

M_{ord} cannot be used if the number of categories is large and the number of items is small because of lack of degrees of freedom for testing. For instance, for a unidimensional logistic graded model (e.g., Samejima, 1969), the number of items must be larger than the number of categories plus two (i.e., $n \geq K + 2$) for the degrees of freedom M_{ord} to be positive.

To summarize this subsection, for ordinal data, if the model involves a large number of variables and categories one must resort to M_{ord} as M_2 cannot be computed. On the other hand, when the number of categories is large and the number of items is small, M_{ord} cannot be computed because of lack of degrees of freedom. In some medium-sized models for ordinal data, there is a choice between M_2 and M_{ord}. Because $\boldsymbol{\kappa}$ concentrates the information available in $\boldsymbol{\varphi}_2$, M_{ord} may be more powerful than M_2 (Joe & Maydeu-Olivares, 2010). On the other hand, if the concentration of the information is not along the alternative of interest, M_2 will be more powerful than M_{ord} along that direction.

Testing for Approximate Fit

In IRT applications to patient-reported outcomes, degrees of freedom are so large that it is unrealistic to expect that any model will fit the data. In other words, it is unrealistic to expect that the fitted IRT model is the data-generating mechanism. Hence, it is more reasonable to test for approximate fit than for exact fit. By this I simply mean testing whether some statistic is smaller than some cutoff. Drawing from work on the structural equations modeling literature by Browne and Cudeck (1993), Maydeu-Olivares and Joe (2014) have recently suggested the use of the sample bivariate root mean square error of approximation ($RMSEA_2$):

$$\hat{\varepsilon}_2 = \sqrt{\frac{M_2 - df_2}{N \times df_2}} \tag{6.8}$$

to estimate the corresponding population bivariate population RMSEA$_2$. They suggested that a cutoff of $\varepsilon_2 \leq 0.05$ indicates adequate fit. They show that this cutoff separates rather well mis-specified IRT models with correctly specified latent trait dimensionality from mis-specified IRT models with mis-specified latent trait dimensionality. They also show that the population RMSEA$_2$ is relatively unaffected by the number of variables being tested, but that it is strongly affected by the number of categories. The larger the number of categories, the smaller the value of the population RMSEA$_2$. They also showed that dividing the RMSEA$_2$ by the number of categories minus one, one obtains an RMSEA$_2$ relatively unaffected by the number of categories. Consequently, they suggest using $\varepsilon_2 \leq 0.05/(K-1)$ as a cutoff for good fit.

A RMSEA$_{ord}$ can be similarly constructed around M_{ord}:

$$\hat{\varepsilon}_{ord} = \sqrt{\frac{M_{ord} - df_{ord}}{N \times df_{ord}}}. \tag{6.9}$$

However, if M_{ord} is more powerful than M_2, then RMSEA$_{ord}$ must be larger than RMSEA$_2$ as the RMSEAs are simply a function of the estimated non-centrality parameters. Thus, a larger cutoff must be used for RMSEA$_{ord}$ than for RMSEA$_2$. Most importantly, RMSEA$_{ord}$ is strongly affected by the number of variables: the larger the number of variables the smaller the population RMSEA$_{ord}$, all other factors constant. For these reasons, to assess the approximate fit of large models for ordinal data I advocate instead the use of a Standardized Root Mean Square Residual (SRMSR) borrowed from the factor analysis literature (see for instance Hu & Bentler, 1999). For a pair of items i and j, the standardized residual is defined as the sample (product-moment or Pearson) correlation minus the expected correlation. In turn, the expected correlation simply equals the expected covariance divided by the expected standard deviations:

$$r_{ij} - \hat{\rho}_{ij} = \frac{s_{ij}}{\sqrt{s_{ii}}\sqrt{s_{jj}}} - \frac{\hat{\sigma}_{ij}}{\sqrt{\hat{\sigma}_{ii}}\sqrt{\hat{\sigma}_{jj}}} = r_{ij} - \frac{\hat{\kappa}_{ij} - \hat{\kappa}_i\hat{\kappa}_i}{\sqrt{\hat{\kappa}_{ii} - \hat{\kappa}_i^2}\sqrt{\hat{\kappa}_{jj} - \hat{\kappa}_j^2}}. \tag{6.10}$$

where the means (κ_i and κ_j) and the cross-product κ_{ij} were given in (6.5) and (6.6), and κ_{ii} is:

$$\kappa_{ii} = E\left[Y_i^2\right] = 0^2 \times \Pr(Y_i = 0) + \ldots + K_i^2 \times \Pr(Y_i = K_i). \tag{6.11}$$

The SRMSR is simply the squared root of the average of these squared correlation residuals:

$$SRMSR = \sqrt{\sum_{i<j} \frac{\left(r_{ij} - \hat{\rho}_{ij}\right)^2}{n(n-1)/2}}. \tag{6.12}$$

An advantage of the SRMSR over the RMSEAs is that because the SRMSR is an average of standardized residuals, its interpretation is straightforward. In contrast, the RMSEAs cannot be readily interpreted. An advantage of the RMSEAs (6.8) and (6.9) over the SRMSR is that it is straightforward to compute confidence intervals and hypothesis testing for them because they are simply transformations of the M_2 and M_{ord} statistics, which are chi-square distributed when the fitted model is correctly specified (Maydeu-Olivares & Joe, 2014). In contrast, computation of confidence intervals and hypothesis testing for the SRMSR is cumbersome as the asymptotic distribution of SRMSR is a mixture of independent chi-squares when the fitted model is correctly specified. Thus, the SRMSR is best used as a goodness of fit index with SRMSR ≤ 0.05 indicating adequate fit. Of course, another advantage of the RMSEA is that it takes model complexity into account, although this is only of interest when comparing different models fitted to a data set.

Piecewise Assessment of Fit

After examining the overall fit of a model, it is necessary to perform a piecewise goodness of fit assessment. If the overall fit is poor, a piecewise assessment of fit may suggest how to modify the model. Even if the model fits well overall, a piecewise goodness of fit assessment may reveal parts of the model that misfit. A useful starting point for our discussion of piecewise fit assessment is the bivariate Pearson's X^2 statistic. After the IRT model parameters have been estimated using the full data, a X^2 may be computed for each pair of variables:

$$X_{ij}^2 = N\left(\mathbf{p}_{ij} - \hat{\pi}_{ij}\right)' \hat{\mathbf{D}}_{ij}^{-1}\left(\mathbf{p}_{ij} - \hat{\pi}_{ij}\right). \tag{6.13}$$

This is just the standard X^2 statistic (6.1) applied to the bivariate table involving variables i and j. Thus, for a model fitted to K category items, $\mathbf{p}_{ij}$ is K^2 vector of observed bivariate proportions, $\hat{\pi}_{ij} = \pi_{ij}\left(\hat{\theta}_{ij}\right)$ is the vector of expected probabilities that depend only on the q_{ij} parameters involved in the bivariate table, $\hat{\theta}_{ij}$, and $\hat{\mathrm{D}}_{ij} = \mathrm{diag}(\hat{\boldsymbol{\pi}}_{ij})$. Suppose the model is unidimensional graded logistic, in this case, q_{ij} involves 2 slopes and $2 \times (K - 1)$ intercepts. It is tempting to refer X_{ij}^2 to a chi-square distribution degrees of freedom equal to the number of parameters in the unrestricted model $\boldsymbol{\pi}_{ij}$, $K^2 - 1$, minus the number of parameters in the restricted model $\pi_{ij}\left(\theta_{ij}\right)$, q_{ij}, so that $df_{ij} = K^2 \times q_{ij} - 1$. However, Maydeu-Olivares and Joe (2006) showed that the distribution of X_{ij}^2 is larger than this reference distribution. This means that referring X_{ij}^2 to this distribution leads to rejecting well-fitting items. They also showed that the M_2 statistic (6.3) applied to a bivariate subtable is asymptotically distributed as chi-square with df_{ij} degrees of freedom. Finally, they also showed that when applied to a single marginal subtable M_2 can be written in terms of the bivariate cell residuals as:

$$M_2^{(ij)} = X_{ij}^2 - N\left(\mathbf{p}_{ij} - \hat{\pi}_{ij}\right)' \hat{\mathbf{D}}_{ij}^{-1}\hat{\Delta}_{ij}\left(\hat{\Delta}_{ij}'\hat{\mathbf{D}}_{ij}^{-1}\hat{\Delta}_{ij}\right)^{-1}\hat{\Delta}_{ij}'\hat{\mathbf{D}}_{ij}^{-1}\left(\mathbf{p}_{ij} - \hat{\pi}_{ij}\right), \tag{6.14}$$

where $\boldsymbol{\Delta}_{ij}$ denotes the matrix of derivatives of the bivariate probabilities $\boldsymbol{\pi}_{ij}$ with respect to the parameters involved in the bivariate table, $\hat{\theta}_{ij}$. Unfortunately, Maydeu-Olivares and Liu (in press); see also Liu & Maydeu-Olivares, 2012) have recently shown that $M_2^{(ij)}$ does not have much power against certain alternatives. $M_2^{(ij)}$ is simply a correction to X_{ij}^2. Alternatively, X_{ij}^2 can be corrected by its asymptotic mean and variance:

$$\mathrm{MV}\left(X_{ij}^2\right) = X_{ij}^2\sqrt{\frac{df_{ij}}{tr_2}} + df_{ij} - \sqrt{\frac{df_{ij}tr_1^2}{tr_2}}, \tag{6.15}$$

which is referred to a chi-square distribution with $df_{ij} = K^2 \times q_{ij} - 1$ degrees of freedom. In (6.15):

$$tr_1 = \mathrm{tr}\left(\mathbf{D}_{ij}^{-1}\Omega_{ij}\right)$$

$$tr_2 = \mathrm{tr}\left(\mathbf{D}_{ij}^{-1}\Omega_{ij}\mathbf{D}_{ij}^{-1}\Omega_{ij}\right) \tag{6.16}$$

and:

$$N\hat{\Omega}_{ij} = \mathbf{D}_{ij} - \pi_{ij}\pi_{ij}' - \Delta_{ij}\left(\mathcal{I}^{-1}\right)_{ij}\Delta_{ij}' \tag{6.17}$$

is the asymptotic covariance matrix of the cell residuals for the pair of variables i and j when the model parameters have been estimated by maximum likelihood using the full table. In Equation (6.17), $\mathcal{I}^{-1}$ denotes the covariance matrix of the full set of item parameters and $\left(\mathcal{I}^{-1}\right)_{ij}$ denotes the rows and columns of this matrix corresponding to the item parameters involved in the subtable for variables i and j. The covariance matrix $\mathcal{I}^{-1}$ is generally estimated using the cross-products information matrix (e.g., Bock & Lieberman, 1970):

$$\mathcal{I}_O = \Delta_O' \mathbf{D}_O \Delta_O, \; \mathbf{D}_O = \mathrm{diag}\left(\mathbf{p}_O / \pi_O^2\right), \tag{6.18}$$

where $\mathbf{p}_O$ and $\boldsymbol{\pi}_O$ denote the proportions and probabilities of the C_O observed patterns, and $\boldsymbol{\Delta}_O$ is a $C_O \times q$ matrix of derivatives of the observed patterns with respect to the full set of q item parameters.

A drawback of using quadratic form statistics such as $\mathrm{MV}\left(X_{ij}^2\right)$ and $M_2^{(ij)}$ is that they do not convey information about the direction of misfit, as these statistics are necessarily positive. Thus, they are best combined with the residual correlations of Equation (6.10) as these indicate the direction of the misfit: A positive residual correlation implies a model expected correlation larger than the observed correlation, whereas a negative residual correlation implies an observed correlation larger than the model expected correlation.

Another drawback of quadratic form statistics such as $\mathrm{MV}\left(X_{ij}^2\right)$ and $M_2^{(ij)}$ is that they cannot be employed with binary data because of lack of degrees of freedom. For the same reason, they cannot be applied to assess the misfit of single items. Z-statistics for univariate and bivariate residual moments can be used instead to diagnose the fit of models for binary data (Maydeu-Olivares & Joe, 2005; Reiser, 1996). These z-statistics are simply:

$$z_i = \frac{p_i - \hat{\pi}_i}{\mathrm{SE}(p_i - \hat{\pi}_i)} = \frac{p_i - \hat{\pi}_i}{\sqrt{\hat{\omega}_{ii} / N}} \quad z_{ij} = \frac{p_{ij} - \hat{\pi}_{ij}}{\mathrm{SE}\left(p_{ij} - \hat{\pi}_{ij}\right)} = \frac{p_{ij} - \hat{\pi}_{ij}}{\sqrt{\hat{\omega}_{ij,ij} / N}}. \tag{6.19}$$

Here, $\pi_i = \Pr\left(Y_i = 1\right)$, $\pi_{ij} = \Pr\left(Y_i = 1, Y_j = 1\right)$, p_i and p_{ij} are their corresponding proportions and $\hat{\omega}_{ii}$ and $\hat{\omega}_{ij,ij}$ are the corresponding diagonal elements of $\hat{\Omega}_{ij}$ in (6.17).

In polytomous data, a z-statistic can also be easily computed for the bivariate residual cross-product:

$$z_{ord} = \frac{k_{ij} - \hat{\kappa}_{ij}}{\mathrm{SE}\left(k_{ij} - \hat{\kappa}_{ij}\right)} = \frac{k_{ij} - \hat{\kappa}_{ij}}{\sqrt{\hat{\omega}_{ord} / N}} \tag{6.20}$$

where κ_{ij} is given in (6.6) and:

$$N\hat{\omega}_{ord} = N\mathbf{v}'\hat{\Omega}_{ij}\mathbf{v} = \mathbf{v}'\left(\mathbf{D}_{ij} - \pi_{ij}\pi_{ij}' - \Delta_{ij}\left(\mathcal{I}^{-1}\right)_{ij}\Delta_{ij}'\right)\mathbf{v}, \tag{6.21}$$

with $\mathbf{v}' = (0, 1, \ldots, K-1)$. However, in some instances (6.21) becomes negative when the cross-products information (6.18) is used and z_{ord} cannot be computed. Univariate counterparts of (6.20) cannot be computed.

Application

To illustrate the described procedures I will use the $n = 8$ item PROMIS® depression short form (Pilkonis et al., 2011). Respondents are asked to report the frequency with which they experienced certain feelings in the past seven days using a $K = 5$ point rating scale ranging from "never" to "always." The responses were coded from 0 to 4 for the analyses. I used the $N = 768$ complete responses to these data kindly provided by the editors. A unidimensional logistic graded response model (Samejima, 1969) with a normally distributed latent trait was estimated by maximum likelihood using flexMIRT (Cai, 2012); 100 rectangular quadrature points between −8 and 8 were used and standard errors were computed using the cross-products information matrix (6.18). The item stems and the estimated intercepts and slopes are reported in Table 6.1 (in logistic metric). There are $q = 5 \times 8 = 40$ estimated parameters.

The model does not fit the data exactly as the value of the statistic M_2 in (6.3) is 767.58 on 440 degrees of freedom, $p < 0.01$. The bivariate RMSEA (6.8) estimate is $RMSEA_2 = 0.03$.[2] We can compute a 90 percent confidence interval around its true parameter (Maydeu-Olivares & Joe, 2014) obtaining (0.03; 0.03).[3] Thus, the fit of the model is adequate ($RMSEA_2 \leq 0.05$) but falls short of our criterion for excellent fit, $RMSEA_2 \leq (0.05 / (K - 1) = 0.0125$.

The residual correlations (6.10) provide us with an easy-to-interpret assessment of the magnitude of the misfit (the effect size of the misfit). The standardized squared root mean squared residual is low, SRMSR = 0.02, indicating that the average size of the misfit is very small. Examining the individual residual correlations shown in Table 6.2, we see that all of them are small. In fact, only three of them are larger than 5 percent in absolute value: those corresponding to the item pairs (5,1), (7,4), and (8,3). I have also included in this table the average of the absolute values of the residual correlations involving each item. Interestingly, the average residual correlation is similar for all items.

Table 6.1 PROMIS® Depression Short Form: Estimated Item Parameters and Standard Errors for a Logistic Graded Model

Item	*Stem*	*Slope*	*Intercept 1*	*Intercept 2*	*Intercept 3*	*Intercept 4*
1	I felt worthless	4.05(0.29)	-2.24(0.24)	-4.62(0.35)	-7.15(0.50)	-9.70(0.71)
2	I felt like a failure	3.35(0.22)	-1.40(0.19)	-3.26(0.25)	-5.73(0.39)	-8.60(0.72)
3	I felt depressed	3.66(0.28)	-1.70(0.21)	-3.92(0.30)	-6.74(0.44)	-9.51(0.72)
4	I felt hopeless	3.40(0.23)	1.36(0.18)	-1.60(0.19)	-4.88(0.33)	-8.39(0.58)
5	I felt that I had nothing to look forward to	3.71(0.27)	-1.11(0.20)	-3.11(0.26)	-6.50(0.45)	-8.48(0.61)
6	I felt helpless	3.63(0.24)	0.11(0.18)	-2.61(0.23)	-5.31(0.34)	-8.69(0.56)
7	I felt unhappy	4.08(0.29)	1.28(0.21)	-2.09(0.24)	-5.74(0.39)	-9.16(0.61)
8	I felt sad	4.65(0.39)	-2.25(0.27)	-5.15(0.45)	-8.01(0.65)	-11.70(1.18)

Notes: $N = 768$; maximum likelihood estimation was used; standard errors in parentheses.

2 FlexMIRT provides both M_2 and M_{ord} (as their associated RMSEAs) whereas IRTPRO currently only provides M_2.

3 The extremes of the confidence interval are equal to two decimal digits.

Table 6.2 Residual Correlations After Fitting a Graded Model

Item	*1*	*2*	*3*	*4*	*5*	*6*	*7*	*8*	*Average*
1		0.03	0.02	<–0.01	**0.06**	–0.01	–0.01	0.02	0.02
2	0.03		<–0.01	–0.01	0.03	–0.01	0.02	0.02	0.02
3	0.02	<–0.01		<–0.01	0.01	0.01	–0.02	**0.08**	0.02
4	<–0.01	–0.01	<–0.01		–0.03	0.04	**0.06**	<–0.01	0.02
5	**0.06**	0.03	0.01	–0.03		<–0.01	–0.01	0.02	0.02
6	–0.01	–0.01	0.01	0.04	<–0.01		0.04	<–0.01	0.02
7	–0.01	0.02	–0.02	**0.06**	–0.01	0.04		–0.01	0.02
8	0.02	0.02	**0.08**	<–0.01	0.02	<–0.01	–0.01		0.02

Notes: df = 14; I have marked in bold the correlations larger than $|0.05|$.

Table 6.3 Mean and Variance Adjusted Bivariate X^2_{ij} Statistics

Item	*1*	*2*	*3*	*4*	*5*	*6*	*7*	*8*	*Average*
1		24.36	22.52	**37.20**	23.58	26.10	**37.70**	19.30	27.25
2	24.36		17.30	23.16	**38.48**	22.16	30.45	23.55	25.64
3	22.52	17.30		**35.55**	33.61	19.35	17.76	27.13	24.75
4	**37.20**	23.16	**35.55**		32.83	33.67	33.14	**38.83**	33.48
5	23.58	**38.48**	33.61	32.83		21.16	**56.01**	23.77	32.78
6	26.10	22.16	19.35	33.67	21.16		23.27	17.55	23.32
7	**37.70**	30.45	17.76	33.14	**56.01**	23.27		25.68	32.00
8	19.30	23.55	27.13	**38.83**	23.77	17.55	25.68		25.12

Notes: df = 14; I have marked in bold the statistics statistically significant at the 5 percent significance level with a Bonferroni adjustment.

The mean and variance corrected X^2 statistics for each pair of variables (6.15) reported in Table 6.3 provide us with an alternative way to locate the source of the misfit. Because the tests are not independent, and to control for the multiple testing, I use a Bonferroni adjusted p-value. Because there are $(8 \times 7) / 2 = 28$ statistics the cut-off p-value used is $0.05 / 28 = 0.002$. The critical value for a chi-square distribution with $5^2 - 2 \times 5 - 1 = 14$ degrees of freedom yielding this p-value is 34.43. I have boldfaced all the values above this critical value in Table 6.3. Next to the statistic's value I could have indicated whether the corresponding residual is positive (+) or negative (–); this is not necessary, as I provide the residual correlations in the previous table. As we can see in this table, there are six statistically significant residuals, corresponding to the item pairs (4,1), (4,3), (5,2), (7,1), (7,5), and (8,4). Table 6.3 also reports the average of the values of these statistics for each item. An inspection of these averages suggests that the worst-fitting item in this short form is item 4.

Alternative Statistics for Piecewise Model Fit Assessment

At this time, I believe that the two statistics that show greatest promise for detecting the source of misfit in IRT models are the standardized residual correlations and the mean

Table 6.4 Bivariate X_{ij}^2 Statistics

Item	*1*	*2*	*3*	*4*	*5*	*6*	*7*	*8*	*Average*
1		24.63	23.33	**38.95**	24.02	27.33	**39.79**	18.99	28.15
2	24.63		17.30	23.50	**40.21**	22.54	31.58	24.48	26.32
3	23.33	17.30		**37.15**	**35.16**	20.32	18.51	28.05	25.69
4	**38.95**	23.50	**37.15**		34.09	**35.20**	**34.87**	**40.58**	34.91
5	24.02	**40.21**	**35.16**	34.09		21.83	**59.54**	23.85	34.10
6	27.33	22.54	20.32	**35.20**	21.83		24.03	17.57	24.12
7	**39.79**	31.58	18.51	**34.87**	**59.54**	24.03		26.18	33.50
8	18.99	24.48	28.05	**40.58**	23.85	17.57	26.18		25.67

Notes: I have marked in bold the statistics larger than 34.43, the critical point for a chi-square distribution with 14 *df* and 5 percent significance level with a Bonferroni adjustment.

Table 6.5 Bivariate $M_2^{(ij)}$ Statistics

Item	*1*	*2*	*3*	*4*	*5*	*6*	*7*	*8*	*Average*
1		22.26	20.83	30.99	13.50	19.18	23.16	16.77	20.96
2	22.26		15.33	22.30	**35.69**	16.42	25.54	22.27	22.83
3	20.83	15.33		**34.88**	33.23	16.07	9.42	12.89	20.38
4	30.99	22.30	**34.88**		17.13	30.72	20.83	32.29	27.02
5	13.50	**35.69**	33.23	17.13		20.09	**34.49**	20.01	24.88
6	19.18	16.42	16.07	30.72	20.09		14.27	16.15	18.99
7	23.16	25.54	9.42	20.83	**34.49**	14.27		14.90	20.37
8	16.77	22.27	12.89	32.29	20.01	16.15	14.90		19.33

Notes: $df = 14$; I have marked in bold the statistics statistically significant at the 5 percent significance level with a Bonferroni adjustment.

and variance-adjusted X_{ij}^2 statistics. In this subsection, I present the results obtained using the other statistics discussed in this chapter, X_{ij}^2 , $M_2^{(ij)}$, and z_{ord}, given in Equations (6.13), (6.14), and (6.20), respectively.[4] X_{ij}^2 must reject more often than expected under a reference a chi-square distribution with df_{ij} degrees of freedom as its distribution is larger than this reference distribution. Results for X_{ij}^2 are shown in Table 6.4. As we can see in this table, it incorrectly suggests that nine pairs of items show misfit even after applying a Bonferroni correction. In contrast, the use of $M_2^{(ij)}$ suggests that only three of these nine pairs are statistically significant using the same reference distribution (see Table 6.5). $M_2^{(ij)}$ may not be powerful enough to detect some misspecifications because the mean and variance-corrected X_{ij}^2 suggests that six out of the nine pairs items flagged by X_{ij}^2 are statistically significant.

4 All these statistics can be computed using *R* code provided in Liu and Maydeu-Olivares (2014).

Table 6.6 Chen and Thissen's Standardized LD X2 Statistics (CT X^2_{ij})

Item	*1*	*2*	*3*	*4*	*5*	*6*	*7*	*8*	*Average*
1		1.6	1.4	**4.1**	1.5	2.0	**4.3**	0.6	2.21
2	1.6		0.3	1.4	**4.4**	1.2	2.8	1.8	1.93
3	1.4	0.3		**3.8**	**3.4**	0.8	0.5	2.3	1.79
4	**4.1**	1.4	**3.8**		**3.2**	**3.4**	**3.5**	**4.4**	3.40
5	1.5	**4.4**	**3.4**	**3.2**		1.1	**7.8**	1.5	3.27
6	2.0	1.2	0.8	**3.4**	1.1		1.5	0.3	1.47
7	**4.3**	2.8	0.5	**3.5**	**7.8**	1.5		1.8	3.17
8	0.6	1.8	2.3	**4.4**	1.5	0.3	1.8		1.81

Notes: I have marked in bold the statistics statistically significant at the 5 percent significance level with a Bonferroni adjustment ($z > |2.91|$).

The X^2_{ij}, $M_2^{(ij)}$, and MV(X^2_{ij}) statistics are closely related to the standardized LD X^2 statistic introduced by Chen and Thissen (1997). When all items consist of the same number of categories, the LD X^2 statistic is:

$$\text{LD } X^2 = \frac{X^2_{ij} - (K-1)^2}{\sqrt{2(K-1)^2}} \,. \tag{6.22}$$

This statistic is conveniently printed as an option by the software used in this application, flexMIRT, and the results obtained using this statistic are shown in Table 6.6.[5] Given the lack of an appropriate reference distribution for X^2_{ij}, Chen and Thissen (1997) observed empirically that its distribution could be approximated when fitting a two-parameter logistic model for binary data using a chi-square degrees of freedom corresponding to an independence model. If a chi-square distribution with independence degrees of freedom closely matches the distribution of X^2_{ij}, then the statistic (6.22) should be approximately standard normal. Yet we see in Table 6.6 that standardized LD X^2 is even more liberal than X^2_{ij} : it rejects too often.

I now turn to the z_{ord} statistic given in Equation (6.20). Results for this statistic are presented in Table 6.7. It is simply the z-statistic for the cross-product of two item scores. I mentioned that this statistic may not be available for some pairs, particularly in small samples. We see in Table 6.9 that this is the case for three item pairs, none of which was flagged as misfitting by any of the previous procedures. Yet the z_{ord} statistics suggest that there is only one misfitting pair, that of items (5,4). This was only flagged by the LD X^2 statistic and it was not the pair with highest LD value.

In Table 6.8 I conveniently summarize the application of all these statistics for piecewise model fit to the Depression Short scale by listing the item pairs flagged by each procedure. This table shows a large degree of agreement between X^2_{ij}, $M_2^{(ij)}$, MV(X^2_{ij}), and Chen and Thissen's LD X^2. This is not surprising as all of them are based on the same statistic, Pearson's X^2 applied to a pair of variables, which I have denoted

5 In Cai (2012) *p* next to a bivariate local dependence (LD) statistic indicates positive LD—a negative residual correlation, whereas *n* indicates a negative LD—a positive residual correlation.

Table 6.7 Bivariate Standardized Cross-Products (z_{ord} statistics)

Item	*1*	*2*	*3*	*4*	*5*	*6*	*7*	*8*
1		0.59	0.76	−0.41	1.59	−0.49	−0.49	0.88
2	0.59		−0.25	−1.01	0.22	−1.26	0.28	0.31
3	0.76	−0.25		−0.32	0.32	0.33	*n.a.*	2.63
4	−0.41	−1.01	−0.32		**−4.23**	1.22	2.62	−0.17
5	1.59	0.22	0.32	**−4.23**		−0.63	−1.18	0.71
6	−0.49	−1.26	0.33	1.22	−0.63		*n.a.*	−0.06
7	−0.49	0.28	*n.a.*	2.62	−1.18	*n.a.*		*n.a.*
8	0.88	0.31	2.63	−0.17	0.71	−0.06	*n.a.*	

Notes: I have marked in bold the statistics statistically significant at the 5 percent significance level with a Bonferroni adjustment ($z > |2.91|$); *n.a.* = not available because the estimated variance of the residual cross-product is negative.

Table 6.8 Item Pairs That Show Misfit Using Different Procedures for Piecewise Model Fit Assessment

Item pair	X_{ij}^2	$MV(X_{ij}^2)$	$M_2^{(ij)}$	$CT\ X_{ij}^2$	z_{ord}	$r_{ij} - \hat{\rho}_{ij}$
4,1	√	√		√		
4,3	√	√	√	√		
5,1						√
5,2	√	√	√	√		
5,3	√			√		
5,4				√	√	
6,4	√			√		
7,1	√	√		√		
7,4	√			√		√
7,5	√	√	√	√		
8,3						√
8,4	√	√		√		

Notes: MV(X_{ij}^2) = mean and variance adjusted X_{ij}^2, $r_{ij} - \hat{\rho}_{ij}$ = residual correlation, CT X_{ij}^2 = Chen and Thissen's standardized LD X_{ij}^2.

by X_{ij}^2. The statistics differ in the extent to which they reject pairs. We know that X_{ij}^2 is too liberal (it rejects too often), $M_2^{(ij)}$ may be too conservative, and we see in this table that the mean and variance-corrected X_{ij}^2 lies in between. We also see in Table 6.8 that the results obtained using these statistics do not agree with results obtained using z-scores for residual cross-products, or with residual correlations. The latter do not agree with each other. More work is needed to gauge the performance of all these competing statistics.

Table 6.9 PROMIS® Depression Short Form: Estimated Item Parameters and Standard Errors for a Logistic Graded Model with Correlated Errors

Item	*Slope 1*	*Slope 2*	*Slope 3*	*Slope 4*	*Intercept 1*	*Intercept 2*	*Intercept 3*	*Intercept 4*
1	4.54(0.34)	1	0	0	−2.54(0.28)	−5.27(0.41)	−8.13(0.57)	−10.99(0.80)
2	3.43(0.24)	0	0	0	−1.43(0.20)	−3.33(0.26)	−5.86(0.41)	−8.78(0.75)
3	4.39(0.35)	0	1	0	−2.08(0.27)	−4.80(0.38)	−8.19(0.59)	−11.57(0.95)
4	3.97(0.26)	0	0	1	1.62(0.21)	−1.88(0.23)	−5.80(0.42)	−9.92(0.74)
5	4.26(0.34)	1	0	0	−1.28(0.23)	−3.60(0.33)	−7.54(0.59)	−9.82(0.79)
6	3.71(0.26)	0	0	0	0.12(0.18)	−2.65(0.24)	−5.42(0.36)	−8.84(0.59)
7	4.87(0.36)	0	0	1	1.58(0.25)	−2.46(0.29)	−6.93(0.52)	−11.03(0.81)
8	5.61(0.49)	0	1	0	−2.75(0.34)	−6.30(0.57)	−9.75(0.81)	−14.27(1.44)

Notes: Standard errors in parentheses. The latent dimensions are uncorrelated. The variances of the latent dimensions are 1, 1.20 (0.48), 2.11 (0.60), 1.82 (0.47).

Improving the Fit of the Model

The fitted model makes three assumptions: 1) depression as measured by these items is unidimensional, 2) the latent trait representing depression is normally distributed, and 3) the item response functions follow Samejima's graded response model. The fact that the model does not fit perfectly may be due to the violation of any combination of these three assumptions. Assumption 2) may be relaxed by estimating the latent trait nonparametrically (Mislevy, 1984). Assumption 1) may also be relaxed by using a nonparametric IRT model (Chernyshenko et al., 2001; Maydeu-Olivares, 2005) or an alternative parametric IRT model.[6]

In my opinion, in this example unidimensionality is the least-likely culprit, as an inspection of the item stems does not suggest any multidimensionality. However, violations of the unidimensionality assumption are most easily remedied. Within an ordinal factor analysis framework, all that is needed is adding a correlated residual parameter for each pair of items with an outstanding bivariate residual. Unfortunately, existing software for IRT estimation using full information maximum likelihood (e.g., Bock & Aitkin, 1981) do not have currently have capabilities for specifying correlated residual parameters. However, they can be tricked as follows: Specify an additional latent dimension for each correlated residual parameter to be added to the model. This latent dimension is defined to be uncorrelated with all existing "substantive" dimensions and it consists of only two nonzero slope parameters, one for each item in the outstanding residual pair. The slopes are to be fixed to (1,1) if the residual is positive and to (1,−1) if the residual is negative. The variance of the latent dimension is estimated. The estimated variance for this additional dimension is simply a reparameterization of the covariance of the residuals.

I used this method to add the three correlated residual parameters—corresponding to the item pairs (5,1), (7,4), and (8,3)—suggested by the residual correlation analysis. I obtained $M_2 = 697.86$ on 437 degrees of freedom, $p < 0.01$, $RMSEA_2 = 0.02$. Thus, the model appears to fit better. The estimated parameters are shown in Table 6.9. We see in this table that all three additional parameters added to the model to account for the correlated

6 However, there is evidence that the graded model is the best-fitting model for rating data among existing parametric models with monotonically increasing category trace lines (Maydeu-Olivares, 2005).

residuals are statistically significant. Also, slope estimates are reduced when these correlated errors are introduced in the model. However, the fit improvement obtained by relaxing the unidimensionality assumption is modest. I used the same method to add instead the six correlated residual parameters suggested by the mean and variance corrected X^2 statistics; those corresponding to the item pairs (4,1), (4,3), (5,2), (7,1), (7,5), and (8,4). The model did not converge, suggesting that it is an inappropriate model for these data. I conclude that, as expected, the unidimensionality assumption is the least likely culprit for the misfit of the graded model to these data. If a better fit is desired, an alternative model should be sought.

Summary

Researchers should always assess the overall GOF of their models using a GOF statistic to assess the magnitude of the discrepancy between the data and the model taking into account sampling variability. In IRT applications to patient-reported outcomes, degrees of freedom will generally be so large that no model will fit exactly. In other words, we should always expect to reject the null hypothesis that the fitted model is the data-generating model.

Having rejected the null hypothesis, we need to judge the magnitude of the misfit. If the data are ordinal the standardized residual correlations provide the most convenient way to gauge the effect size of the misfit. In particular, the Standardized Root Mean Square Residual (SRMSR) correlation provides the average effect size of the misfit. Of course, the average misfit may be small but some parts of the model may show a large misfit. Hence, it is necessary to inspect all standardized residual correlations, not just the SRMSR.

The standardized residual correlations are just one way to assess piecewise model fit. One alternative that I have offered here is the use of X^2 statistics applied to pairs of items adjusting them by their mean and variance so that their distribution is asymptotically chi-square. The use of unadjusted X^2_{ij} is incorrect. The statistic is too liberal and it rejects well-fitting items. An alternative is the $M_2^{(ij)}$ statistic. $M_2^{(ij)}$ works well when the model fits. However, when the model is mis-specified, it may lack power, rejecting too few items. The behavior of the mean and variance-adjusted X^2_{ij} lies between that of X^2_{ij} and $M_2^{(ij)}$: it is not as liberal as X^2_{ij} nor as conservative as $M_2^{(ij)}$.

The SRMSR and standardized residual correlations are probably best used as goodness-of-fit indices with some arbitrary cutoff, say 5 percent, as computing confidence intervals for them is cumbersome. Confidence intervals can be computed for RMSEA statistics based on M_2, or if the model is large and data is ordinal, based on M_{ord}. However, as our example illustrates, for IRT applications to patient-reported outcomes, confidence intervals for RMSEA statistics are generally very narrow. Also, because RMSEA statistics take not only model fit into account but also model parsimony, they will decrease (all other factors held constant) as the number of categories increases. An adjustment can be made to the cutoff for RMSEA_2 to accommodate this fact, but not to RMSEA_{ord}. Hence, when M_{ord} is used I recommend the use of the SRMSR instead of RMSEA_{ord}.

Because the RMSEA statistics take not only model fit into account but also model parsimony, their use is particularly indicated when several alternative models are being considered. However, model selection necessarily involves subjective judgment and it is wise to examine all the implications of the competing models under examination (latent trait estimates, measurement errors, etc.) in addition to goodness of fit statistics such as the RMSEA when selecting among competing models.

Future Directions

IRT modeling involves identifying a plausible process that individuals may have used to respond to items. From this point of view, it is important to assess how well the fitted IRT model reproduces the data at hand. However, IRT models are also fitted to serve some purpose (scoring, linking, etc.) and therefore it is important also to assess how well the model meets these purposes. IRT users should not be unnecessarily obsessed with the goodness of fit of their models. Rather, they need to take the necessary time and effort to evaluate whether their IRT model serves its intended purpose. By routinely reporting the fit of their fitted models, together with an assessment of how well the model serves its intended purpose, we may learn "how bad is this fit for this purpose" and establish reasonable fit criteria. Different fit criteria may be needed for different purposes. A model that shows a substantial degree of misfit may still prove useful for purpose A. But a model with the same degree of misfit may prove useless for purpose B. What degrees of misfit are acceptable for different purposes is what we ought to determine. Further research is needed to link the goodness-of-fit statistics described in this chapter to specific research questions.

References

Bartholomew, D.J., & Tzamourani, P. (1999). The goodness of fit of latent trait models in attitude measurement. *Sociological Methods and Research*, *27*, 525–546.

Bock, R.D., & Aitkin, M. (1981). Marginal maximum likelihood estimation of item parameters: Application of an EM algorithm. *Psychometrika*, *46*, 443–459.

Bock, R.D., & Lieberman, M. (1970). Fitting a response model for *n* dichotomously scored items. *Psychometrika*, *35*, 179–197.

Browne, M.W., & Cudeck, R. (1993). Alternative ways of assessing model fit. In K.A. Bollen & J.S. Long (Eds.), *Testing structural equation models* (pp. 136–162). Newbury Park, CA: Sage.

Cai, L. (2012). *flexMIRT: A numerical engine for multilevel item factor analysis and test scoring* [Computer software]. Seattle, WA: Vector Psychometric Group.

Cai, L., & Hansen, M. (2013). Limited-information goodness-of-fit testing of hierarchical item factor models. *British Journal of Mathematical and Statistical Psychology*, *66*, 245–276.

Chen, W.-H., & Thissen, D. (1997). Local dependence indexes for item pairs using item response theory. *Journal of Educational and Behavioral Statistics*, *22*, 265–289.

Chernyshenko, O.S., Stark, S., Chan, K.-Y., Drasgow, F., & Williams, B. (2001). Fitting item response theory models to two personality inventories: Issues and insights. *Multivariate Behavioral Research*, *36*, 523–562. doi:10.1207/S15327906MBR3604_03

Hu, L., & Bentler, P.M. (1999). Cutoff criteria for fit indexes in covariance structure analysis: Conventional criteria versus new alternatives. *Structural Equation Modeling*, *6*(1), 1–55.

Joe, H., & Maydeu-Olivares, A. (2010). A general family of limited information goodness-of-fit statistics for multinomial data. *Psychometrika*, *75*, 393–419.

Liu, Y., & Maydeu-Olivares, A. (2012). Local dependence diagnostics in IRT modeling of binary data. *Educational and Psychological Measurement*, *73*, 254–274.

Liu, Y., & Maydeu-Olivares, A. (2014). Identifying the source of misfit in item response theory models. *Multivariate Behavioral Research*, *49*(4), 354–371. doi:10.1080/00273171.2014.910744

Maydeu-Olivares, A. (2005). Further empirical results on parametric vs. non-parametric IRT modeling of Likert-type personality data. *Multivariate Behavioral Research*, *40*, 275–293.

Maydeu-Olivares, A., & Joe, H. (2005). Limited and full information estimation and goodness-of-fit testing in 2^n contingency tables: A unified framework. *Journal of the American Statistical Association*, *100*, 1009–1020.

Maydeu-Olivares, A., & Joe, H. (2006). Limited information goodness-of-fit testing in multidimensional contingency tables. *Psychometrika*, *71*, 713–732.

Maydeu-Olivares, A., & Joe, H. (2014). Assessing approximate fit in categorical data analysis. *Multivariate Behavioral Research*, *49*(4), 305–328. doi:10.1080/00273171.2014.911075

Maydeu-Olivares, A., & Liu, Y. (2012). Item diagnostics in multivariate discrete data. Manuscript under review.

Maydeu-Olivares, A., & Montaño, R. (2013). How should we assess the fit of Rasch-type models? Approximating the power of goodness-of-fit statistics in categorical data analysis. *Psychometrika*, *78*, 116–133.

Mislevy, R.J. (1984). Estimating latent distributions. *Psychometrika, 49*, 359–381.

Pilkonis, P.A., Choi, S.W., Reise, S.P., Stover, A.M., Riley, W.T., & Cella, D. (2011). Item banks for measuring emotional distress from the Patient-Reported Outcomes Measurement Information System (PROMIS®): Depression, anxiety, and anger. *Assessment*, *18*, 263–283.

Reiser, M. (1996). Analysis of residuals for the multinomial item response model. *Psychometrika*, *61*, 509–528.

Samejima, F. (1969). Calibration of latent ability using a response pattern of graded scores. *Psychometrika Monograph Supplement*, No. 17.

Thissen, D., & Steinberg, L. (1997). A response model for multiple-choice items. In W.J. van der Linden & R.K. Hambleton (Eds.), *Handbook of modern item response theory* (pp. 51–66). New York: Springer Verlag.

Tollenaar, N., & Mooijart, A. (2003). Type I errors and power of the parametric goodness-of-fit test. Full and limited information. *British Journal of Mathematical and Statistical Psychology*, *56*, 271–288.

7 Assessing Person Fit in Typical-Response Measures

Pere J. Ferrando

Introduction

The fit of an item response theory (IRT) model to the data is usually assessed by considering the entire sample of test respondents (Chapter 6). Overall model-data fit is assessed by jointly considering all the items × individuals responses. At a more specific level, item fit is assessed on an item-by-item basis by considering the item responses across the group of respondents.

Model-data fit can also be assessed at the level of each individual respondent (person fit) by considering the responses of the individual across the set of test items. Because each individual response pattern contributes to the overall fit of the model (e.g., Reise & Widaman, 1999), overall fit and person fit are necessarily related, and overall fit must be assessed before person fit. A reasonably good overall model-data fit is essential if the IRT model is to be regarded as appropriate. However, an acceptable fit is still compatible with a certain proportion of individuals whose response patterns cannot be adequately explained by the model (Levine & Drasgow, 1983). These patterns will be referred to as misfitting or inconsistent.

Assessing person fit is important for at least three reasons. First, as mentioned earlier, the existence of misfitting patterns can affect the overall fit of the model. And even if this fit is found to be acceptable, their presence might still result in biased estimates of some model parameters (Bollen & Arminger, 1991; Nering, 1997). Second, in validity assessment, scores based on inconsistent patterns could affect the estimated relations between trait levels and relevant external variables (Schmitt, Chan, Sacco, McFarland, & Jennings, 1999). The third and main reason, however, is that if a response pattern is not well explained by the model, there is no guarantee that the score assigned to this pattern adequately reflects the "true" trait level of the individual. If it does not, the invalid score can lead to erroneous decisions. The examples included in this chapter illustrate the importance of this problem in practical settings.

Consider an employment selection process that is (partly) based on a measure of emotional stability. Suppose next that an applicant gives honest answers to the most "neutral" items but deliberately distorts his responses to the most socially desirable items in order to appear more stable than he really is (i.e., faking good). As a result his trait estimate is upwardly biased. Finally, assume that the "true" trait level of this respondent would have placed him below the cutoff value but that the biased estimate places him above, so this applicant is hired. An erroneous decision has been made and the wrong person has probably been selected.

As a second example, consider a clinical scenario in which dysfunctional impulsivity is assessed by means of a test. Consider now: (a) a respondent who is not interested in the assessment and who answers many of the items randomly, and (b) a respondent who answers honestly but who tends to make a disproportionate use of the scale endpoints in many of the items (i.e., an extreme respondent). In both cases the trait estimate of the respondent is likely to be biased, and in case (a) it is probably meaningless. Now, if these estimates were interpreted as if they were valid trait indicators, the assessment of these individuals would probably be highly distorted.

In the examples just discussed, the response pattern of the individuals is expected to be inconsistent to some extent. In the first example, the respondent would give faked responses to some items and honest responses to the rest. In the second example, the respondent would answer some of the items consistently and others at random. In the final example, the respondent would give responses too extreme for her real trait level in some of the items. Now, if these inconsistencies could be detected by using person fit analysis, the flawed interpretations and wrong decisions caused by the blind use of the trait estimates might be avoided.

"Person fit" is a general term that includes all the procedures for assessing response inconsistency at the individual level (Meijer & Sijtsma, 2001). This chapter, however, takes a narrower view, and focuses on procedures that assume a particular parametric IRT model to fit the data. These procedures were initially developed within the maximum performance domain (Reise & Flannery, 1996).

Assessing Person Fit in Typical-Response Measures

Typical-response-based person fit assessment differs from maximum-performance-based assessment in several aspects. I shall discuss this issue in relation to three main points: (a) theoretical relevance, (b) sources of misfit, and (c) psychometric properties.

Theoretical relevance. Person fit procedures in maximum-performance tests have largely been developed for practical purposes, particularly to identify protocols that are invalid because of cheating, guessing, or for other reasons (Meijer, 1996). In typical-response measurement, on the other hand, inconsistent responding has often been linked to theory (Reise & Waller, 1993). In the personality domain in particular, there has been a rich debate on the meaning of intra-individual consistency (e.g., trait relevance or trait organization).

Sources of misfit. The sources of person misfit in typical-response measurement are different from those in maximum-performance measurement. The main sources described so far are: (a) idiosyncratic interpretation of the item content (including problems of understanding item meaning), (b) unmotivated or unsympathetic test responding, (c) multidimensionality, (d) person unreliability/untraitedness, (e) response biases, mainly acquiescence and faking/socially desirable responding, and (f) idiosyncratic response scale usage, including extreme and middle responding (Ferrando, 2010; Meijer, Egberink, Emons, & Sijtsma, 2008; Reise & Flannery, 1996; Reise & Waller, 1993; Waller & Reise, 1992; Zickar & Drasgow, 1996). These sources will be further discussed with regard to (a) the type of inconsistency that they are expected to produce, and (b) the potential effectiveness of the proposed procedures for detecting it.

Psychometric properties. In general, the psychometric requisites that are conducive to valid and statistically powerful person fit assessment are more difficult to attain in the case of personality and attitude measures than in the case of maximum-performance measures. This point is further discussed later in this chapter.

So far, person fit applications based on personality and attitude tests are scarce. There are early applications with an important methodological component, for example: Ferrando and Chico (2001), Reise (1995), Reise and Flannery (1996), Reise and Waller (1993), and Zickar and Drasgow (1996). At the purely applied level, however, it appears that this methodology has started to permeate the field only recently (Conrad et al., 2010; Dodeen & Darabi, 2009; Egberink & Meijer, 2011; Ferrando, 2012; Meijer et al., 2008; Woods, Oltmanns, & Turkheimer, 2008). This state of affairs might be partly due to the fact that most applied researchers remain either unaware or unconvinced of the value of person fit assessment. Person fit research that has been carried out to date has been far too technical and has focused mostly on statistical issues (Meijer, 2003; Meijer et al., 2008). Moreover, as we shall see, person fit procedures still have important practical limitations.

Emons, Sijtsma, and Meijer (2004, 2005) proposed that additional information should be obtained about (a) the type of inconsistency, (b) the type of item in which inconsistency occurs, and (c) the impact that inconsistency has on the trait estimates so that the assessment of individual misfit could be improved. Their proposal is based on a combined use of global scalar indices, graphical procedures, and indices at the level of items or subsets of items. In this chapter I shall propose a closely related approach.

The remainder of this chapter is organized as follows. First, the models on which the person fit procedures proposed here are based are reviewed. Second, the proposed global, graphical, and single-response procedures are discussed. Third, a series of examples based on real-data applications are presented and discussed. Finally, a general discussion is provided.

Review of the Models and Needed Results

The models reviewed in this section are dominance models. So, the expected item score (in the appropriate direction) is assumed to increase with trait level. They are intended for binary, graded, and (approximately) continuous item response formats. Binary items are still quite common in personality assessment (Reise, Waller, & Comrey, 2000). Graded-response items, particularly Likert scales, are the most commonly used in both personality and attitude tests. Finally, graded responses with a large number of points or continuous-limited formats are increasingly being used in computerized administration (Ferrando, 2002).

Consider a typical-response test, made up of n items, that aims to measure a trait θ and that is administered to a respondent i. Let X_{ij} be the observed score of respondent i on item j and assume that θ is scaled in a z-score metric (mean 0 and variance 1) in the population of respondents.

Assume first that the n items use a binary response format (0 or 1). The probability that respondent i will endorse item j is assumed to be given by:

$$P_j(\theta_i) = P(X_{ij} = 1 \mid \theta_i) = \frac{\exp\left[a_j(\theta_i - b_j)\right]}{1+\exp\left[a_j(\theta_i - b_j)\right]} = \Psi\left(a_j(\theta_i - b_j)\right). \tag{7.1}$$

Equation (7.1) is the logistic version of the two-parameter model (2PM). The location parameter b_j ("item difficulty" in ability measurement) indicates the trait level that is required to have a probability of 0.50 of endorsing this item. The discrimination parameter a_j indicates the quality of the item as a measure of the trait (Lord & Novick, 1968). The higher a_j is, the more precise the item and the more information it provides about the trait that is measured. Finally, the probability of item endorsement when viewed as a function of θ (i.e., $P_j(\theta)$), which is also the regression of the item scores on θ, is called the item characteristic function (ICF) of item j.

When a_j is set at the same value for all the items, the 2PM reduces to the one-parameter model (1PM). In some clinical instruments that measure narrow traits, substantial variations in item discriminating power have been observed (Reise & Waller, 2009). So in this case the 1PM would clearly be inappropriate. However, in many normal-range typical-response items that measure broad traits the variation in discriminating power is relatively modest (Ferrando, 2004; Hulin, Drasgow, & Parsons, 1983; Levy, 1973). If this is so, the 1PM is a model that should be considered.

Assume now that the items use a graded response format with $m + 1$ categories. In this case, item j has m fixed ordered locations or thresholds $b_{j1}<b_{j2}<b_{jr}\ldots<b_{jm}$. As a function of θ, the probability of endorsing category r, which is called the item category response function, is now:

$$P(X_{ij} = r \mid \theta) = \Psi(Da_j(\theta - b_{jr-1})) - \Psi(Da_j(\theta - b_{jr})) . \tag{7.2}$$

Equation (7.2) is the logistic version of Samejima's (1969) graded-response model (GRM). And the expected item score that corresponds to a given trait level—in other words, the regression of the item scores on θ—is given by (Chang & Mazzeo, 1994):

$$E(X_j \mid \theta) = \sum_r rP(X_j = r \mid \theta) . \tag{7.3}$$

Finally, assume that the items use a continuous response format. The conditional distribution of the item score for fixed θ is now assumed to be normal, with mean and variance given by:

$$E(X_j \mid \theta) = \mu_j + \lambda_j \theta_i \quad ; \quad Var(X_j \mid \theta) = \sigma^2_{\varepsilon j} , \tag{7.4}$$

where μ_j is the item intercept, λ_j the item loading, slope, or regression weight, and $\sigma^2{}_{\varepsilon j}$ the variance of the measurement error. The conditional mean in (7.4) is the linear ICF of the model. Model (7.4) is Spearman's Factor Analysis (FA) model, which in the psychometric literature is also known as the congeneric test (item) score model (Jöreskog, 1971). Ferrando (2009) proposed a re-expression of model (7.4) to make it closer to the 2PM in (7.1). To make the comparison even closer, the item scores can be rescaled to have values between zero and one so that 0.5 corresponds to the midpoint of the item response scale. By making the transformation:

$$\beta_j = \frac{1 - 2\mu_j}{2\lambda_j} , \tag{7.5}$$

the conditional expectation in (7.4) can be written as:

$$E(X_j \mid \theta) = 0.5 + \lambda_j(\theta - \beta_j). \tag{7.6}$$

The item parameter β_j is now defined on the same scale as θ and is a location index. It can be interpreted as the trait level that corresponds to an expected score of 0.5 (i.e., the response scale midpoint).The slope λ_j is interpreted as the item discrimination index (Mellenbergh, 1994).

Linear FA is by far the most used model for fitting graded or continuous typical-response items (Hofstee, Ten Berge, & Hendricks, 1998). In principle, it is a model intended for continuous-unlimited scores and, because item responses are bounded and to a greater or lesser extent discrete, it can only be approximately correct. As an approximation, however, both theoretical (Culpepper, 2013; Lord & Novick, 1968) and empirical (Muthén & Kaplan, 1985; Olsson, 1979) evidence suggests that the linear model works well with graded or more continuous items when (a) the discriminating power of the items is moderate or low, and (b) the items have no extreme locations. Typical-response items, which measure broad normal-range traits, tend to meet these conditions (Ferrando, 2004;

Levy, 1973). On the other hand, clinical items that measure narrow traits sometimes have both high discriminations and extreme distributions (Reise & Waller, 2009). The linear model is clearly inappropriate in this case.

It is assumed that all the models discussed so far are fitted by using a two-stage approach (i.e., calibration and scoring; see McDonald, 1999). During the calibration stage, the appropriateness of the model is first assessed by conducting an overall model-data fit investigation, and if it is judged to be appropriate, the item parameters are estimated. During the scoring stage, the item estimates obtained during the previous stage are taken as fixed and known and used to estimate the individual trait levels. Within this framework, the procedures considered in this chapter assess the extent to which a response pattern is consistent with the pattern that would be expected given (a) the item parameter estimates obtained during the calibration stage, and (b) the trait level estimate of the respondent obtained during the scoring stage.

Many scoring results that are now provided are directly linked to the procedures described in the following sections. The likelihood of a response vector $\mathbf{x}_i$ for each of the models is:

$$\text{1PM and 2PM: } L(\mathbf{x}_i \mid \theta) = \prod_j P_j(\theta)^{X_{ij}} (1 - P_j(\theta))^{1-X_{ij}}. \tag{7.7}$$

$$\text{GRM: } L(\mathbf{x}_i \mid \theta) = \prod_j \prod_r P_{jr}(\theta)^{u_{ijr}}, \tag{7.8}$$

where $u_{ijr} = 1$ if respondent i chooses category r for item j, and $u_{ijr} = 0$ otherwise. And:

$$\text{Congeneric model: } L(\mathbf{x}_i \mid \theta) = \prod_j \left[\frac{1}{\sigma_{\varepsilon j}\sqrt{2\pi}} \exp - \frac{1}{2}\left(\frac{x_{ij} - \mu_j - \lambda_j \theta}{\sigma_{\varepsilon j}} \right)^2 \right]. \tag{7.9}$$

Maximum likelihood (ML) estimates of the trait level of individual i in the three types of models are the values that maximize (7.7), (7.8), and (7.9). In the binary and graded response cases, these estimates must be obtained iteratively. In the congeneric model they can be obtained in closed form and are the well-known Bartlett's factor scores (e.g., McDonald, 1999; Mellenbergh, 1994).

$$\hat{\theta}_i = \frac{\sum_j \frac{\lambda_j (x_{ij} - \mu_j)}{\sigma^2_{\varepsilon j}}}{\sum_j \frac{\lambda^2_j}{\sigma^2_{\varepsilon j}}}. \tag{7.10}$$

Research Methods

Current Person Fit Methods

Global Person Fit Indices

Global indices will be discussed by making a distinction between practical and specific indices. From a hypothesis-testing point of view, practical indices test the null hypothesis of consistency against no specific alternative. So, even if the index is capable of detecting that a pattern is inconsistent, it provides no further information regarding the type of inconsistency. In contrast, specific indices test against specific types of misfit (e.g., faking or extreme responding) and so, in principle, they are more powerful and provide more information.

Practical Indices

Likelihood-Based Indices

Of the considerable number of practical indices (Karabatsos, 2003; Meijer & Sijtsma, 2001), some of the most popular are still the likelihood-based (L-B) indices initially proposed by Levine and Rubin (1979). They have a clear rationale, are easy to compute, and, although they have limitations, they generally perform equal to or better than alternative indices (Armstrong, Stoumbos, Kung, & Shi, 2007; Drasgow, Levine, & McLaughlin, 1987; Li & Olejnik, 1997; Meijer, 1996; Nering, 1997; Nering & Meijer, 1998; Reise & Due, 1991).

The basic rationale on which L-B indices are based is that that the likelihood function value of a particular item response pattern will be large for patterns that are consistent with the model and small for inconsistent patterns. Assuming that the item parameters are fixed and known, the unstandardized log-likelihood index l_0 is simply the logarithm of the likelihood function evaluated at the maximizing value of θ (i.e., the ML trait level estimate). According to (7.7) and (7.8), the indices corresponding to the binary and the graded response cases for respondent i, item j, and response category r are:

$$l_0(\theta_i) = \sum_j \{X_{ij} \ln P_j(\theta_i) + \left[(1 - X_j)\ln(1 - P_j(\theta_i))\right]\}. \tag{7.11}$$

And:

$$l^{(p)}{}_0(\theta_i) = \sum_j \sum_r u_{ijr} \ln P_{jr}(\theta_i). \tag{7.12}$$

Ideally, a person fit index should: (a) have reference values so that it can be interpreted, (b) be independent of test length, and (c) be independent of the trait level, and so detect misfitting patterns equally well at all levels (Drasgow, Levine, & Williams, 1985). However, l_o and $l_o^{(p)}$ do not comply with any of these requirements. To improve these limitations, Drasgow and colleagues (1985) derived the standardized lz versions:

$$l_z = \frac{l_0 - E(l_0)}{\sqrt{Var(l_0)}}; \; l_z^{(p)} = \frac{l^{(p)}{}_0 - E(l^{(p)}{}_0)}{\sqrt{Var(l^{(p)}{}_0)}}. \tag{7.13}$$

The formulas and rationale for the expectations and variances in (7.13) can be found in Drasgow and colleagues (1985) and Hulin, Drasgow, and Parsons (1983). If the "true" trait levels were known, then the standardized indices in (7.13) would be expected to asymptotically follow a standard normal distribution under the null hypothesis of consistency (Drasgow et al., 1985).

Ferrando (2007) derived two L-B global indices for the congeneric model. According to (7.9), the log-likelihood corresponding to this model is:

$$\ln L(\mathbf{x}_i \mid \theta_i) = \sum_j (\ln \frac{1}{\sigma_{\varepsilon j}\sqrt{2\pi}}) - \frac{1}{2}\sum_j z_{ij}^2, \tag{7.14}$$

where:

$$z_{ij} = \frac{X_{ij} - \mu_j - \lambda_j \theta_i}{\sigma_{\varepsilon j}}. \tag{7.15}$$

The first index proposed by Ferrando is:

$$lco(i) = -2(\ln(\mathbf{x}_i \mid \theta_i) - \sum_j^n (\ln \frac{1}{\sigma_j \sqrt{2\pi}})) = \sum_j^n z_{ij}^2(\theta_i), \tag{7.16}$$

where $\hat{\theta}_i$ is Bartlett's ML estimate (7.10). Ferrando (2007) showed that, under the model's assumptions the distribution of the individual *lco* values across respondents was χ^2 with $n - 1$ degrees of freedom.

The second index is a normal approximation computed as:

$$lcz_i = \sqrt{2lco_i} - \sqrt{2n-3}. \tag{7.17}$$

Conceptually, all the indices discussed so far essentially measure a type of misfit that can be named "violation to a Guttman pattern" (Armstrong et al., 2007; Meijer, 2003). Thus, in the binary case, which is the clearest, a well-fitting, scalable pattern is one in which the respondent tends to endorse the items whose difficulty index is below his/her estimated trait level but not endorse the items whose difficulty index is above this level. Indeed, at the extreme of this trend, the best-fitting patterns as measured by *lz* are those of a Guttman scale. Non-fitting patterns will be those in which the pattern of endorsement is not consistent with the ordering of items by their difficulty. As for interpretation, *lz* and $lz^{(p)}$ are interpreted as a standard normal *z*-score. A large negative value is an indicator that the pattern is inconsistent given the model and the estimated trait value. A large positive value indicates that the pattern is more deterministic than the stochastic model predicts. The *lcz* index is minimum chi-square, and functions in the opposite direction. So large positive values are indicators of misfit.

Limitations of the L-B Indices

The standard-normal reference distribution for *lz* and $lz^{(p)}$ is an asymptotic result obtained by assuming that the "true" trait level is known. Drasgow and colleagues (1985) found that using the true trait levels in tests of 80 or more items produced close agreements with the normal distribution. In practice, however, the true trait level is unknown and an estimate is used in its place. Furthermore, typical-response measures usually have considerably fewer than 80 items. Research suggests that the use of a trait estimate instead of the true level generally leads to a negatively skewed distribution of the statistic, the variance of which is smaller than expected if θ were known (Magis, Raîche, & Béland, 2012; Molenaar & Hoijtink, 1990; Nering, 1995, 1997; Reise, 1995). This second result leads to underdetection of the inconsistent patterns (van Krimpen-Stoop & Meijer, 2002). As expected, the shorter the test is, the more serious this problem becomes.

Corrections for improving these problems have been proposed for *lz*. Snijders (2001; see also Magis et al., 2012) studied the distribution of *lz* when the true θ is replaced by an estimate and proposed a corrected version of the index that asymptotically approaches the standard normal distribution as long as the trait estimate fulfills some restrictions. On the other hand, de la Torre and Deng (2008) proposed a method that (a) uses an improved expected a posteriori (EAP) trait estimate that is corrected for unreliability, and (b) constructs the distribution of the person fit statistic by using resampling methods. This second proposal can be easily extended to $lz^{(p)}$.

The *lcz* index is expected to behave better than *lz* and $lz^{(p)}$ as far as the two limitations discussed earlier are concerned. First, it explicitly takes into account that the ML trait estimate is used instead of the "true" trait level. Second, the distribution is not asymptotic but exact and so it is correct for any test length. However, the index is based on assumptions that can only be approximately correct (linearity, homoscedasticity, and conditional normality). So the χ^2 reference distribution must be considered as an approximation. Further research is clearly needed on the behavior of the index and potential improvements (Clark, 2010).

We turn now to the more general limitations. First, although the item parameters are taken as fixed and known, they are generally estimated in a sample that probably contains an unknown proportion of inconsistent respondents. Second, the same pattern is used to estimate the trait level and to compute the person fit index (e.g., Karabatsos, 2003). As for the first point, the presence of inconsistent respondents in the calibration sample is expected to affect the quality of item parameter estimates and this result, in turn, is expected to lead to poorly estimated or biased individual trait estimates (Nering, 1997). As for the second, when the estimate is used instead of θ, the result is a decrease in detection power, which, to a large extent, comes from the shift in the estimate due to the inconsistent responses (Armstrong et al., 2007). For the first problem, Nering (1997) suggested using a series of successive recalibrations in which the inconsistent patterns were removed from the sample in each step. As for the second, a potential solution is to use improved estimates that minimize the shift noted earlier. Estimates such as expected a posteriori (EAP) that use more information (in the form of a prior), or robust procedures such as the biweight that down-weights the most inconsistent scores are sound candidates (Meijer & Nering, 1997; Reise, 1995).

By far the most important practical shortcoming of unspecific indices is their low detection power. Research (Ferrando, 2004; Molenaar & Hoijtink, 1990; Reise & Due, 1991) clearly shows that the power of L-B indices (and many other person fit indices) depends on three main factors: (a) test length, (b) spread of item locations, and (c) amount of item discrimination. Many typical-response scales are short, too short in fact even to accurately estimate trait levels (Emons, Sijtsma, & Meijer, 2007). They are also made up of items with moderate or low discriminations and developed with little concern for the range of θ at which the test measures accurately. My opinion is that the quality of most typical-response measures needs to be improved. However, accepting the situation for what it is, a direct potential improvement can be made to point (a). Many personality and attitude measures are multidimensional tests made up of several short scales (Ferrando, 2009; Hulin, Drasgow, & Parsons, 1983; Reise & Flannery, 1996). So, provided that inconsistency generalizes over scales, the development of multidimensional indices that are based on all the items in the test might increase the power.

Parsons (see Hulin, Drasgow, & Parsons, 1983) proposed a first heuristic multidimensional extension for discrete-response models. If the dimensions measured by the questionnaire are highly correlated, then lz or $lz^{(p)}$ can be obtained from all of the items as if they formed a common scale. If this is not the case, a multidimensional lz index can be obtained as a weighted average of the unidimensional lz's, the weights being proportional to the number of items in the sub-scale.

Drasgow, Levine, and McLaughlin (1991) proposed a more rigorous extension of this type intended for what they termed a "multi-unidimensional" test (i.e., a test consisting of a series of unidimensional scales). They showed that in this type of test: (a) the multidimensional index l_0 was the sum of the unidimensional indices, and (b) the mean and variance of l_0 were the sum of the unidimensional means and variances, respectively. Next, they used these results to propose a multidimensional standardized index with the form (7.13).

Ferrando (2009) proposed multidimensional extensions of indices (7.16) and (7.17) intended for the FA model. For k common factors, the first index is:

$$M - lco_i = \sum_{j=1}^{n} \left[\frac{X_{ij} - \mu_j - \lambda_{j1}\hat{\theta}_{i1} \dots - \lambda_{jk}\hat{\theta}_{ik}}{\sigma_{\varepsilon j}} \right]^2 = -2\ln(\mathbf{X}_i \mid \hat{\theta}_i) + C\,, \tag{7.18}$$

where C is a constant value that does not depend on the trait levels. Under the same assumptions used in (7.16) the expected distribution of (7.18) is χ^2 with $n - k$ degrees of freedom. When $k = 1$, $M - lco$ reduces to the unidimensional index (7.16).

As in the unidimensional case, the second index is a normal approximation to the χ^2 distribution.

$$M - lcz = \sqrt{2M - lco} - \sqrt{2(n-k) - 1}\,. \tag{7.19}$$

Little research has been carried out on multidimensional L-B indices and applications are still scarce. Also, whether they make any improvement is not clear. As mentioned earlier, they should be more appropriate for sources of inconsistency that generalize across subtests. And the most likely source of this type is idiosyncratic scale usage (e.g., extreme responding; see Emons, 2009). Sources such as multidimensionality, person unreliability, or certain response biases, however, might well be (at least in part) scale specific. If they are, the multidimensional extensions might be insensitive to overall patterns that show inconsistency on few specific subscales (Schmitt et al., 1999).

In closing, a summary on L-B indices is provided. To start, they have clear limitations and can be improved. Potential lines of improvement are: (a) calibration schemas that take into account the presence of inconsistent patterns, (b) estimation procedures that are more robust and/or use more information, (c) development and use of more accurate reference distributions, possibly obtained via resampling, and (d) development of multidimensional extensions that use more information from the data.

In spite of their limitations, L-B indices are quite useful and the strong criticisms they have received may be largely due to unrealistic expectations. First, both the indices and the models on which they are based are (at best) approximations, and so the indices cannot be expected to closely adhere to a theoretical distribution. Second, inconsistency is a complex phenomenon that has multiple potential sources. So, classification solely based on these indices is a highly error-prone process and it cannot be expected to produce satisfactory results. However, L-B indices are useful as first-step, broad screening tools aimed at flagging potentially problematic patterns. As discussed earlier, once a pattern has been detected, further information must be obtained.

Relative-Variance Indices

L-B indices give an overall idea of the extent to which the observed item scores cannot be well predicted by the IRT model. However, knowing that a pattern is inconsistent does not provide sufficient information about how this inconsistent responding affects the trait level estimate of the respondent. A large negative value of lz, for example, is compatible with a small bias in the trait estimate that does not have too much practical relevance, and the opposite can also be true (Meijer & Nering, 1997).

On the basis of a previous proposal by Drasgow, Levine, and McLaughlin (1987), Ferrando (2010) proposed a person fit index for the congeneric model known as *JRV* (jackknife relative variance). This index, which can be used with any of the models considered in this chapter, is based on a deletion approach and uses jackknife estimation (Cook & Weisberg, 1982). Conceptually, the idea is to estimate θ based on different subsets of items, and assess the variance of the resulting estimates. If this variance is large, none of the estimates can be probably trusted. Furthermore, so as to make the index relative, *JRV* is defined as the ratio between the variance of the jackknife trait estimates and the asymptotic variance of the ML estimator (i.e., the model-expected variability; see Ferrando, 2010, for details).

$$JRV_i = \frac{Var(\theta_i^*)}{Var(\hat{\theta}_i(ML) \mid \theta_i)}. \tag{7.20}$$

The present proposal is not to use *JRV* as an alternative to the L-B indices but rather as an auxiliary measure that provides complementary information. High values of *JRV* suggest that the estimation of θ is unstable, in the sense that very different estimates might be obtained if certain responses are not considered. Therefore, the point estimate obtained cannot be trusted. On the other hand, small values of *JRV* would indicate that the trait level is consistently estimated by the different item scores.

Expected Behavior of Practical Indices with Different Types of Inconsistency

As a general reference, global indices assess the consistency of the complete pattern, so they are expected to function better with sources of inconsistency that have a global effect on the response vector (Emons, 2009). On the other hand, they are expected to show less sensitivity to sources that affect responses to individual items or small groups of items.

Person Unreliability (Ferrando, 2004; Lumsden, 1977)

Person unreliability can be conceptualized as an individual-differences dimension with two extremes. When going in the direction of high reliability, the response pattern becomes more deterministic or error free, and at the extreme, the pattern behaves according to Guttman's model. In the other direction, the pattern becomes more insensitive to the normative ordering of the items and, at the extreme, the item responses are totally random.

From a person fit point of view, person unreliability produces global observed-expected deviations and is generally well detected by L-B indices (Ferrando, 2004). Highly reliable respondents produce patterns that are too consistent given the stochastic assumptions of the IRT model and that tend to give rise to large and positive values of lz and $lz^{(p)}$ (large and negative for lcz). On the other hand, the insensitive patterns of unreliable respondents tend to give rise to large and negative values of lz and $lz^{(p)}$ (large and positive for lcz). The extreme of random responding, however, might be problematic because in this case the items do not provide model-based information for estimating θ so the power is likely to be low. As discussed later, graphical procedures are generally more suitable for detecting this extreme.

Multidimensionality and Idiosyncratic Responding

Waller and Reise (1992) consider that multidimensionality is mostly expected to arise when many items are weakly related to the measured trait. For these items, the influence of the individual's specific factor score outweighs that of his/her common score and this gives rise to idiosyncratic responses. This source of misfit affects specific items or groups of items. So it is difficult to predict whether L-B indices will have enough sensitivity to detect it. If omission of the outlying responses substantially changes the trait estimate, the *JRV* index is expected to be more sensitive.

Faking

Faking can be modeled by assuming a temporal change in the trait level of the individual intended to provide improved scores (Zickar & Drasgow, 1996). The basic point is whether the amount of change tends to remain essentially constant over the different items or whether it tends to vary as a function of the items (i.e., fakeable items vs.

faking-resistant items). In the first case, the faked pattern would be elevated but consistent, so faking would not be detected by standard indices. In the second case, provided that the inconsistency was strong enough, faking might be detected (Zickar & Drasgow, 1996).

Recent research (Ferrando & Anguiano-Carrasco, 2013; Zickar & Sliter, 2012) suggests that faking is expected to produce some intra-individual inconsistency in the response pattern. However, the degree of inconsistency is generally subtle and not large enough to be detected with a practical person fit index (Ferrando & Chico, 2001; Reise & Flannery, 1996; Reise & Waller, 2009). As discussed later in this chapter, optimal indices are thought to be more appropriate here.

Acquiescence

Several authors (Curtis, 2004; Reise & Flannery, 1996) have conjectured that acquiescence might be a detectable source of misfit. Ferrando and Lorenzo-Seva (2010) analytically derived some results and arrived at the following predictions. If a fully balanced scale can be obtained, and acquiescence is operating, then (a) the estimated trait level is expected to be essentially correct, but (b) both L-B and *JRV* indices are expected to flag this respondent as inconsistent given the overall large discrepancies between the observed and model-expected item scores. It is much harder to make predictions when a balanced scale is not available because in this case the trait estimate is expected to be biased. If the scale is not balanced at all, acquiescence will probably remain undetected. As discussed later, inconsistency in the case of partially balanced scales is better assessed by using graphical and single-response analyses.

Sabotaging/Malingering

Patterns that can be qualified as sabotaging or malingering have been identified in various data sets (Ferrando, 2012). The trend is that the respondents agree with the most extreme or "difficult" items and disagree with the "easier" items. The degree of inconsistency that this type of responding produces is global and strong and is generally well detected by L-B indices.

Extreme and Middle Responding

Both extreme and middle responding are global sources of misfit. Inconsistency due to extreme responding is expected to be well detected by unspecific indices (Emons, 2009; Ferrando, 2010).

Middle responding produces undifferentiated patterns that make it very difficult to obtain accurate trait estimates. The lack of information results in L-B indices with reduced power for detecting this source and not even the *JRV* is expected to detect instabilities. However, as discussed later, middle responding is easily detected by using graphical procedures.

Specific Indices: Optimal Indices

Levine and Drasgow (1983) proposed a general likelihood ratio test person fit procedure intended to be used to detect specific forms of misfit. The test is based on two likelihoods for a response pattern: (a) the likelihood given a certain model of inconsistent responding, and (b) the likelihood given a model of consistent responding. So the procedure requires a model-based profile of misfit to be specified and, as a result, it is (theoretically) more informative and powerful than the unspecific indices.

Consider the likelihoods (7.7), (7.8), and (7.9) for the different models in this chapter. They correspond to the normative model of consistent responding and will be denoted here generically as $L_C(x_i|\theta)$.

Assume now that an alternative likelihood can be specified for the same pattern based on an IRT modeling of the specific inconsistency to be assessed, and denote this likelihood by $L_{IC}(x_i|\theta)$. Finally, let $f(\theta)$ be the density of θ. The unconditional likelihoods are:

$$\begin{aligned} P_C(\mathbf{x}_i) &= \int_{-\infty}^{\infty} L_C(\mathbf{x}_i \mid \theta) f(\theta) d\theta \\ P_{IC}(\mathbf{x}_i) &= \int_{-\infty}^{\infty} L_{IC}(\mathbf{x}_i \mid \theta) f(\theta) d\theta, \end{aligned} \tag{7.21}$$

(in practice, the integrals in (7.21) can be approximated with the required precision by using numerical procedures).

The likelihood ratio (LR) is now obtained as:

$$LR = \frac{P_{IC}(\mathbf{x}_i)}{P_C(\mathbf{x}_i)}. \tag{7.22}$$

And the decision rule is to classify $\mathbf{x}_i$ as inconsistent if:

$$P_{IC}(\mathbf{x}_i) \geq \omega \, P_C(\mathbf{x}_i). \tag{7.23}$$

From a purely statistical point of view, test (7.23) is optimal in the Neyman-Pearson sense (hence the name): for a fixed error rate among consistent respondents, no other test has a greater probability of correctly classifying inconsistent respondents. The critical value ω can be interpreted as a cutoff value that controls the ratio between hit rates (proportion of inconsistent respondents classified as such) and false alarm rates (proportion of consistent respondents misclassified as consistent).

The main practical limitation of an optimal index is the specification of the alternative likelihood corresponding to the inconsistency model. For this reason, applications in typical-response measurement are rather scarce and have been limited to the identification of faking. Zickar and Drasgow (1996) modeled the alternative likelihood as a shift of +0.50 to the right of the θ scale for those items that were deemed fakeable while no shift occurred in the remaining items. Ferrando and Anguiano-Carrasco (2013) proposed to obtain both likelihoods in (7.21) by using a partially invariant factor-analytic model that is fitted simultaneously to two data sets: neutral and experimentally induced faking. This second proposal produced better detection rates than many of the procedures reported so far. Thus, further research about its behavior seems warranted.

Like L-B indices, multidimensional versions of the optimal index (7.22) have been proposed (Drasgow, Levine, & McLaughlin, 1991). In Ferrando and Anguiano-Carrasco's (2013) study, the use of the multidimensional extension resulted in a clear improvement in power with respect to the indices based on single scales. However, more research into its behavior is needed.

Graphical Procedures

Most of the procedures proposed so far for the graphical assessment of person misfit (a) are derived from a basic function that can be termed "Person Response Curve" (PRC; Weiss, 1973), and (b) are not intended to be used instead of the scalar-valued indices but rather as useful tools that complement the information provided by these indices (Emons, Sijtsma, & Meijer, 2005; Nering & Meijer, 1998; Sijtsma & Meijer, 2001).

The proposal by Weiss (1973) considered the PRC to be the expected score of person *i* as a function of some item difficulty or location scale δ. The two basic assumptions were (a) that the location parameter δ was continuous, and (b) that the PRC was decreasing in δ, so that the more difficult the item was, the lower the expected score of the person on this item.

The general approach proposed in this section is based on the PRC principles discussed earlier and consists of using a nonparametric curve to assess the fit of an expected curve. Both curves are obtained by plotting the item responses of the individual against the ordered item difficulty/location values that, in all the cases, are defined on the θ-continuum.

The graphical representation I propose has three elements: (a) the theoretical or expected person response curve (EPRC), (b) the observed responses, and (c) the empirical or observed person response curve (OPRC). The EPRC is the Weiss curve as defined earlier. The OPRC is the nonparametric smoothed curve that best fits the observed responses, and so does not impose any particular functional form for the curve. Of the several smoothing approaches that can be chosen to fit the OPRC, I propose to use kernel smoothing (KS). KS is widely used, relatively simple, and, when applied at the item level, works well even in comparison with more complex procedures (Härdle, 1990). In accordance with common terminology (Emons, Sijtsma, & Meijer, 2004), both curves will be denoted here generically by $E(S_i | \delta)$.

The appropriateness of the individual response pattern is graphically assessed by inspecting the discrepancies between the OPRC and the EPRC. Large discrepancies indicate person misfit. These discrepancies can be general (e.g., curves with opposite trends) or reflect local deviations in certain groups of items (Emons et al., 2004, 2005). Additionally, pointwise confidence intervals can be obtained at the evaluation points and then joined by a line to draw confidence bands on the estimated OPRCs. These confidence bands, which can be obtained via resampling (Emons et al., 2004) or analytically (see Härdle, 1990, section 4.2), provide two important pieces of information: (a) the extent to which the OPRC is well defined across the range of δ considered (which is assessed by the width of the bands), and (b) the regions at which there are significant discrepancies with respect to the EPRCs.

Graphical Procedures for Binary Responses

In the 1PM the EPRC is directly considered to be a function of the item location parameter b, so it is defined as:

$$E(S_i \mid b) = \Psi\left(a(\theta_i - b)\right). \tag{7.24}$$

And it is a decreasing one-parameter ogive in which the person trait level θ_i defines the point along the b difficulty continuum at which $E(S_i) = 0.5$.

The OPRC can be obtained by using the Nadaraya-Watson KS estimator (see Härdle, 1990):

$$E(S_i \mid b) = \frac{\sum_j^n K(\frac{b-b_j}{h})X_{ij}}{\sum_j^n K(\frac{b-b_j}{h})}, \tag{7.25}$$

where $K(x)$ is the KS function, a nonnegative, continuous, bounded, and (usually) symmetric function that assigns its highest values to points near 0.0 and decreases as it gets further away from 0.0. The parameter h is called the bandwidth; it is selected by the user, and controls the amount of smoothing.

The definition of the EPRC becomes more complex for the 2PM because in this case the expected item score depends on two parameters, so the *b* parameter does not order the items identically for each θ.

$$E(S_i \mid b) = \Psi\left(a_j(\theta_i - b)\right). \tag{7.26}$$

As discussed earlier, however, a common finding when the 2PM is fitted to normal-range measures is that the item discriminations do not differ greatly. If they do not, the expected points obtained by (7.26) will not exactly define a line, but they will be tightly clustered around a well-defined decreasing trend. Assuming that this is the case, it is proposed to define the EPRC in the 2PM case as the KS curve that best fits the scatter of expected points obtained by (7.26). So, in this case, the KS estimator (7.25) is used both with the observed points and with the expected points derived from the model predictions.

Graphical Procedures for Continuous Responses

When assessment is based on the congeneric model it is more convenient to work with parameterization (7.6) for two main reasons. First, the EPRC based on (7.6) is decreasing, as it should be. Second, it is more clearly interpretable and the interpretation is equivalent to that of the binary models.

As in the binary case, we shall first consider the τ-equivalent restricted case in which all the discriminations λ are equal. The EPRC in this case can be directly considered to be a function of the location parameter β, and it is defined as:

$$E(S_i \mid \beta) = \left[0.5 + \lambda\theta_i\right] - \lambda\beta. \tag{7.27}$$

Equation (7.27) describes a decreasing straight line in which, as in the 1PM case in (7.24), the person trait level θ_i defines the point along the β continuum at which $E(S_i) = 0.5$ (i.e., the scale midpoint). Note also that the negative slope $-\lambda$ reflects the common discriminating power of the items.

As occurs with the 2PM, in the general congeneric case with different item discriminations:

$$E(S_i \mid \beta) = 0.5 + \lambda_j(\theta_i - \beta), \tag{7.28}$$

the expected values in (7.28) as a function of β will no longer accurately define a line. However, in many applications, the same considerations discussed in the binary case lead us to expect the points to be tightly clustered around a well-defined linear decreasing trend. If this is the case, it is again proposed to define the EPRC as the KS curve that best fits the scatter of expected points.

Graphical Procedures for Graded Responses

In the GRM an item is no longer defined by a single location parameter but by *m* thresholds. So the graphical representation becomes more complex. In this chapter, attempts are made to obtain a single graphic for each respondent, which leads to the basic initial problem: How can the graded-response items be ordered by some single location value defined on the θ-continuum?

Consider the item-trait regression (7.3), which has been defined as the item response function for a graded-response item. I define the generalized difficulty index (GDI) of item *j* as the trait value at which the expected score in (7.3) is the response scale midpoint. The GDI is thus defined on the θ-continuum, and has a similar interpretation to the b_j and β_j location parameters in the binary and the congeneric models. Conceptually, GDI*j* is the point on the trait continuum that marks the transition from the tendency to disagree with the item to the tendency to agree with it, and so it can be interpreted as a generalized threshold. Overall, the graphical representation proposed for the GRM case is a single plot for each respondent that displays the item scores as a function of the ordered GDIs.

If the expected scores for an individual are obtained by using his/her trait estimate in Equations (7.2) and (7.3), and then plotted against the corresponding GDIs, the resulting points are not expected to fall onto a single line, not even if all the items have the same discrimination. This is because the spacing and distribution of the thresholds are generally different for different items. So, in the present proposal, the points will only accurately define a curve if, in addition to the restriction of equal discriminations, further restrictions such as those considered by Andrich (1978) are fulfilled (i.e., the thresholds remain invariantly spaced across items, so that they can be shifted left or right but their relative spacing remains the same). Experience suggests that most normal-range typical-response items do not greatly depart from Andrich's (1978) restrictions. For this reason, it is also proposed to define the EPRC in this case as the KS curve (7.25) that best fits the scatter of expected points just described.

These conditions may not be fulfilled in the case of clinical items that measure narrow traits. Reise and Waller (2009) noted that in many applications of this type discriminations varied considerably, the range of thresholds was limited, and threshold values were extreme. They also considered that these results were more likely to be obtained in scales that measure quasi-traits (i.e., traits that are relevant in only one direction). In contrast, the base results that justify our EPRC proposal (similar discriminations, equally spaced thresholds) are more plausible in medium-to-broad bandwidth scales that measure normal-range dimensional traits (as defined in Tellegen, 1988). In any case, the adequacy of the proposal is an empirical question. For the EPRC to be meaningful the scatter must clearly define a decreasing trend and this result must be checked by inspecting the data.

Graphical Assessment of Different Types of Inconsistency

Extreme and Middle Responding

Both extreme and middle responding are better assessed by inspecting the scatter of observed scores. As one of the illustrative examples later in this chapter shows, these sources are generally detected quite easily.

Person Unreliability and Random Responding

Person unreliability mainly affects the amount of dispersion of the observed points around the EPRC. So for over-consistency the observed points are tightly clustered around the EPRC, while for low reliability they are widely scattered. In the binary and graded-response models, person reliability also affects the shape of the OPRC, which becomes steeper for highly reliable respondents and flatter for unreliable respondents. In all the models the extreme of random responding gives rise to a flat OPRC that reflects the total insensitivity of the responses to the normative item ordering (Emons et al., 2005).

Acquiescence

No specific shape for the OPRC can be predicted in this case. However, in balanced and partially balanced scales, inspection of the observed points is expected to show unusually large distances between the two groups of items (positive and negative direction) and the EPRC.

Sabotaging/Malingering

As mentioned earlier, sabotaging/malingering tends to produce an OPRC with a trend that is opposite to that of the EPRC (i.e., increasing instead of decreasing) and that generally can be detected quite easily.

Multidimensionality and Idiosyncratic Responding

Because it is a specific source of misfit, this type of responding is better assessed by inspecting the distances of the individual points from the EPRC. When misfit affects small groups of items (e.g., lower-level facets), the OPRC is likely to show local deviations with respect to the EPRC that can be detected with the help of the confidence bands.

Faking

Faking is unlikely to be detected by graphical procedures. Both the OPRC and the EPRC are expected to be elevated with respect to the generally unknown "true" curves. However, they are expected to be essentially consistent with each other. These predictions are illustrated in one of the empirical examples later in this chapter.

Scalar Valued Item-Level Indices

Assessment of misfit at the level of single item response will be discussed by using a basic distinction from regression diagnostics: outliers and influential observations (Cook & Weisberg, 1982; Zijlstra, van der Ark, & Sijtsma, 2007). In the present context, outliers are item responses that are highly unlikely given the model parameters and the estimated trait level of the respondent. Influential observations, on the other hand, are item responses that have a disproportionate influence on the estimated trait level of the respondent. More operatively, an item response can be considered to be influential when the estimated trait level of the respondent changes substantially when this response is deleted from the data (Ferrando, 2010; Zijlstra, van der Ark, & Sijtsma, 2007). In general, outliers need not be influential observations (Cook & Weisberg, 1982; Meijer & Nering, 1997).

Outliers

The most immediate and well-known indices of this type are scaled residuals between the observed and the model-expected item response. And the most common way of scaling the residual is to divide the raw observed-expected difference by the expected conditional standard deviation given the person estimate (e.g., Smith, 1990). The scaled residual then takes a z-score form, and its values are interpreted with reference to the standard normal distribution (Karabatsos, 2000).

For the one- and two-parameter models, the best-known scaled residual is the individual standardized residual proposed initially by Wright (1977) for the Rasch model:

$$z_{ij(BINARY)} = \frac{X_{ij} - P_j(\hat{\theta}_i)}{\sqrt{P_j(\hat{\theta}_i)(1 - P_j(\hat{\theta}_i))}}. \tag{7.29}$$

For the GRM case, the corresponding index is that proposed by Wright and Masters (1982) for the Rating Scale Model:

$$z_{ij(GRADED)} = \frac{X_{ij} - E(X_{ij} \mid \hat{\theta}_i)}{\sqrt{Var(X_{ij} \mid \hat{\theta}_i)}}, \tag{7.30}$$

where the second term in the numerator is the expected score (7.3) evaluated with the person estimates, and the conditional variance is given by:

$$Var(X_j \mid \hat{\theta}_i) = \left[\sum_r r^2 P_{jr}(\hat{\theta}_i)\right] - \left[E(X_j \mid \hat{\theta}_i)\right]^2. \tag{7.31}$$

Finally, the linear counterpart of the residuals (7.29) and (7.30) is the statistic proposed by Bollen and Arminger (1991) and by Ferrando (2010):

$$zc\ e_{ij} = \left(\frac{X_{ij} - \mu_j - \lambda_j \hat{\theta}_i(ML)}{\sqrt{Var(e_{ij})}}\right) = \frac{e_{ij}}{\sqrt{Var(e_{ij})}}, \tag{7.32}$$

where:

$$Var(e_{ij}) = \sigma^2_{\varepsilon j} - \frac{\lambda_j^2}{\sum_j^n \frac{\lambda_j^2}{\sigma^2_{\varepsilon j}}}. \tag{7.33}$$

From a graphical point of view, indices (7.29), (7.30), and (7.32) are standardized distances between the observed item score and the EPRC. Therefore, they are expected to be particularly useful for those types of inconsistency that are assessed on the basis of inspection of the observed response points: acquiescence, multidimensionality, and idiosyncratic responding.

Indices of types (7.29) and (7.30) have been criticized for two main reasons (Karabatsos, 2000; Smith, 1990). The first is the same as that of the L-B indices: the same response pattern is used to estimate the person parameters and analyze the fit. The second concerns the chosen reference distribution. The indices are transformed discrete variables that cannot be well approximated by a continuous distribution such as the standard normal.

Index (7.32) explicitly takes into account that the ML trait estimate is used instead of the "true" trait level. Furthermore, the item response is assumed to be continuous. It then follows that, if the congeneric model is correct and the item parameters are known, index (7.32) should follow a standard normal distribution. As discussed earlier, however, the congeneric model is only an approximation, and so is the reference distribution.

While the theoretical limitations so far discussed are relevant, item-level indices are generally used in practice to trace unexpected item responses in patterns that have been detected as potentially inconsistent by a global index so that insight can be gained into the causes of the misfit. They are not intended to be used as strict inferential measures, and the reference distribution is only used as a useful reference. As Smith (1990) discussed, for these purposes, the indices are possibly useful enough as they are.

Influential Observations

The developments that are now discussed are general and apply to all the IRT models considered here. To start, according to the definition of influential observations, the most direct measure of the influence of item *j*'s score is:

$$D_i(j) = \theta_i(ML) - \theta_i^{(-j)}(ML), \tag{7.34}$$

that is, the change in the ML trait estimate when item *j*'s score is deleted from the data. While (7.34) is indeed direct, it is difficult to interpret because of the lack of reference values. This limitation can be improved by adopting a resampling procedure proposed by Zijlstra, van der Ark, and Sijtsma (2007). In our case it consists of (a) randomly deleting a single item score and obtaining the change estimate using (7.34), and (b) repeating the process 1,000 times and establishing a confidence interval for the change values. If the estimated change corresponding to item *j* lies outside the boundaries of the confidence interval, this score can be regarded as influential.

A second way of making (7.34) more interpretable is to transform it with an appropriate scaling. Ferrando (2010) proposed a pseudo-standardized scaled measure that he termed $Dz_i(j)$, and that is based on the properties of the ML estimator:

$$Dz_i(j) = \frac{\hat{\theta}_i(ML) - \theta_i^{(-j)}(ML)}{\sqrt{Var(\hat{\theta}_i(ML) \mid \theta_i)}}. \tag{7.35}$$

Conceptually, *Dz* is a modification of Cook's distance (Cook & Weisberg, 1982), which informs of the change that takes place in the estimated trait level with respect to the variability that is expected in the estimation based on this particular response pattern.

Researchers must know how to proceed when influential observations have been detected. One possibility is not to trust the trait estimate or to retest the respondent (Meijer & Sijtsma, 2001). A second possibility is to re-estimate the trait level. One option within this second approach (Meijer & Nering, 1997) is simply to eliminate the influential scores and estimate θ on the basis of the remaining item scores. A more elaborate option is to use a robust procedure such as the biweight that downsizes the impact of the influential points. This second approach should not be automatically applied. It is expected to work well and provide a more valid estimate when only a few scores are identified as both outlying and influential and in which a convincing rationale for the discrepancies can be found. In other cases the modified trait estimate will probably continue to be completely meaningless.

Application

The examples in this section are applications in the personality domain intended to illustrate some of the points discussed in this chapter. In all cases, and as recommended, overall model-data fit and item fit were assessed before person fit. However, given the illustrative purposes of the examples we shall only focus on person fit results.

Example 1: A comparison of GRM-based and congeneric-based person fit results

The CTAC (Spanish acronym for Tarragona Questionnaire of Anxiety for Blind People; Pallero et al., 1998) is intended for blind and visually impaired people. It contains 35 items with a five-point response format and attempts to measure anxiety related to visual loss in a range of everyday situations. The CTAC items are generally non-extreme and have moderate discriminating power. So, as expected, both the GRM and the congeneric model fit the data about equally well. Given this result, the first example will illustrate the comparability of the person fit results based on both models.

We shall first discuss some overall results. First, the product-moment correlation between both sets of ML trait estimates was $r = 0.99$. Second, the correlation between $lz^{(p)}$ and *lcz* was $r = -0.70$ (negative as expected). However, the agreement between both indices was considerably higher than the correlation indicates. The dispersion of points was considerably lower at the extreme of inconsistency where the respondents that are flagged as inconsistent by both indices are concentrated. So the most inconsistent respondents would be flagged with one index or the other.

The first individual illustration corresponds to respondent number 393, who was flagged as potentially inconsistent according to the L-B indices. The $lz^{(p)}$ estimate obtained under the GRM calibration was $lz^{(p)} = -3.01$ whereas the lcz based on the linear model was 1.70. In both cases, however, the relative variance measures suggested that the variability between the trait estimates was not excessive. The *JRV* estimates were 1.36 (GRM) and 1.38 (congeneric model).

Figure 7.1 shows the graphical assessment based on the GRM (panel a) and the congeneric model (panel b). The similarity between both graphics is remarkable and they both clearly lead to the same diagnosis. The EPRC is decreasing, as it should be. However, the OPRC is virtually flat, which suggests that the respondent is largely insensitive to the normative ordering of the items. This type of result might be caused by a high degree of person unreliability, inapplicability of the trait (i.e., low traitedness) or, in the extreme, random responding. Further analyses do not seem necessary in this case, and it seems reasonable to assume that the trait estimate corresponding to this respondent cannot be validly interpreted.

The second illustration corresponds to respondent number 628. The L-B estimates in this case were: $lz^{(p)} = -3.90$ (GRM) and $lcz = 3.59$ (congeneric model). The corresponding relative variance indices were $JRV = 2.84$ (GRM) and $JRV = 2.04$ (congeneric model). There is close agreement between the results obtained from both models, which suggests that: (a) the response pattern of number 628 is highly inconsistent and (b) the trait estimates are rather unstable.

The two panels in Figure 7.2 again show the graphical assessment based on both models, and, as in the previous illustration, they agree very closely. In spite of the large global estimates, it is clear that the OPRC and the EPRC do not greatly differ in this case (compare with the previous assessment). However, the inspection of the graphs reveals interesting results. Note first that individual number 628 is probably an extreme responder, as most of the responses are 1 or 5 (0 and 1 in the transformed congeneric scale). Second, note that there are three potential outliers at the top right of the graph. Item-level analysis clearly identified these points with standardized residual values of 3.07, 2.69, and 2.64 (GRM-based z), and 2.56, 2.43, and 2.38 (congeneric-model-based zc). They are marked with an asterisk in Figure 7.2.

Contrary to what would be expected given the relatively high *JRV* values, the three outliers were not influential observations (Dz estimates of around 0.30 for the three points). Overall, the pseudo-standardized influential estimates were moderate for most of the items and none of them exceeded 1.65. Given the results it is not clear how to proceed with the trait estimate of this respondent. The trait estimate based on the complete pattern was the same in both models (about 0.65) and the jackknife estimates ranged from 0.60 to 0.75. So, in spite of the large amount of potential inconsistency detected by the global indices, the trait estimate in this case might well be essentially valid and interpretable.

Example 2: Experimentally induced faking

The second example shows how difficult it is to detect faking in real data sets when unspecific person fit procedures are used. The measure in this case is the Psychoticism (P) scale of the Eysenck Personality Questionnaire revised (EPQ-R; Eysenck, Eysenck, & Barrett, 1985), which consists of 32 binary items. The EPQ-R was administered on two occasions. At Time 1 the participants were asked to respond under the standard instructions provided in the manuals. At Time 2 they received faking-inducing instructions (try to give a good impression so that they will be given a job they really want).

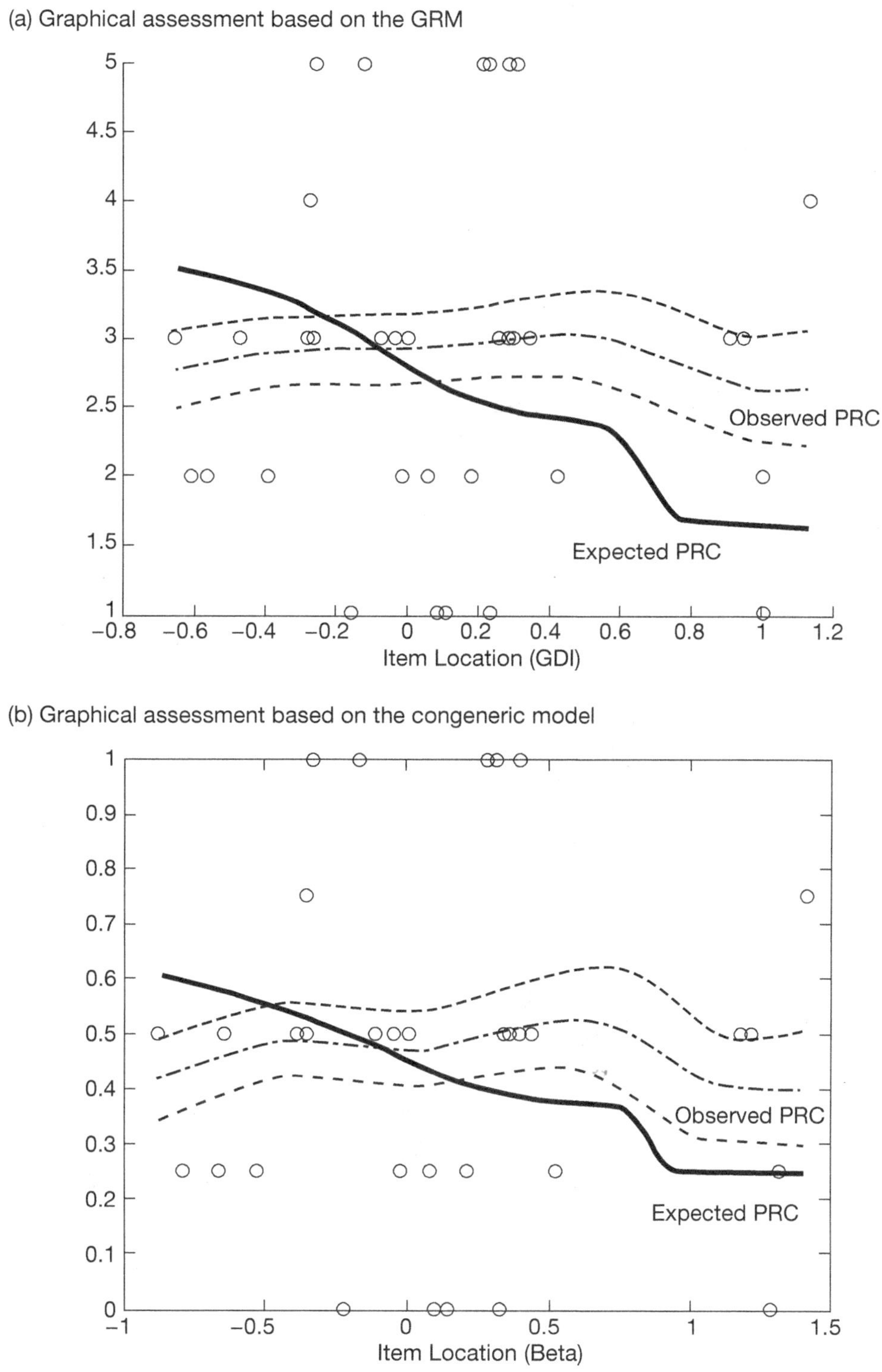

Figure 7.1 Graphical analysis of respondent number 393 based on the GRM (upper panel) and the congeneric model (lower panel). Example 1.

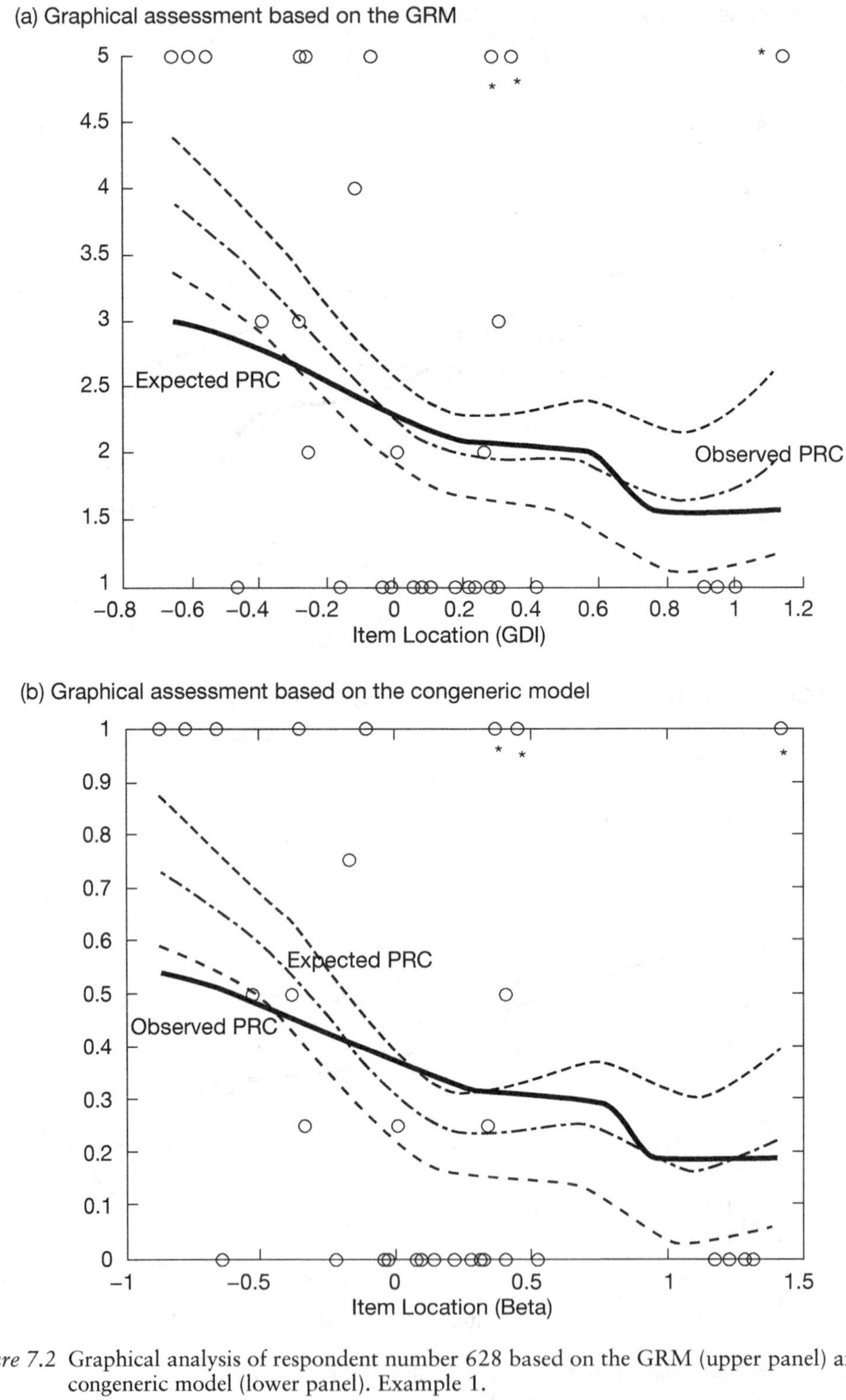

Figure 7.2 Graphical analysis of respondent number 628 based on the GRM (upper panel) and the congeneric model (lower panel). Example 1.

In the present illustration, the P items were calibrated using the data obtained in the neutral administration. The 2PM fit the data quite well, and so the estimated parameters were taken as fixed and known. Then on both occasions ML trait estimates were obtained from these item parameters.

For illustrative purposes, the response patterns given by respondent number 156 under both conditions are now assessed. First, a dramatic change in the ML trait estimate is observed. The estimate obtained in neutral conditions is $\hat{\theta}_{156} = 1.30$, which reflects a rather high level of P. However, the estimate obtained under faking good conditions is $\hat{\theta}_{156} = -3.68$, a very large decrease that goes in the expected direction: toward a lower P level (which is far more socially desirable). In spite of this decrease, however, the *lz* statistic was unable to detect the faking behavior of this respondent. The *lz* values were 1.57 (neutral condition) and 0.13 (faking condition), which would lead us to conclude that this participant responded quite consistently on both occasions.

The graphical assessment of these response patterns is shown in Figure 7.3 and helps to explain the result. The considerable difference in elevation between both sets of curves reflects the change in the estimated trait level. However, (a) the profile of both curves is similar, and (b) the OPRC and the EPRC generally agree in both cases. Overall, the results agree with the view that faking behavior generally produces a rather consistent elevation (a decrease in this case) of the scores that is unlikely to be detected by using practical indices. However, when the optimal person fit procedure discussed earlier was applied, the value of the *LR* statistic (7.22) was 1.52, a value that suggests that this respondent is a potential faker.

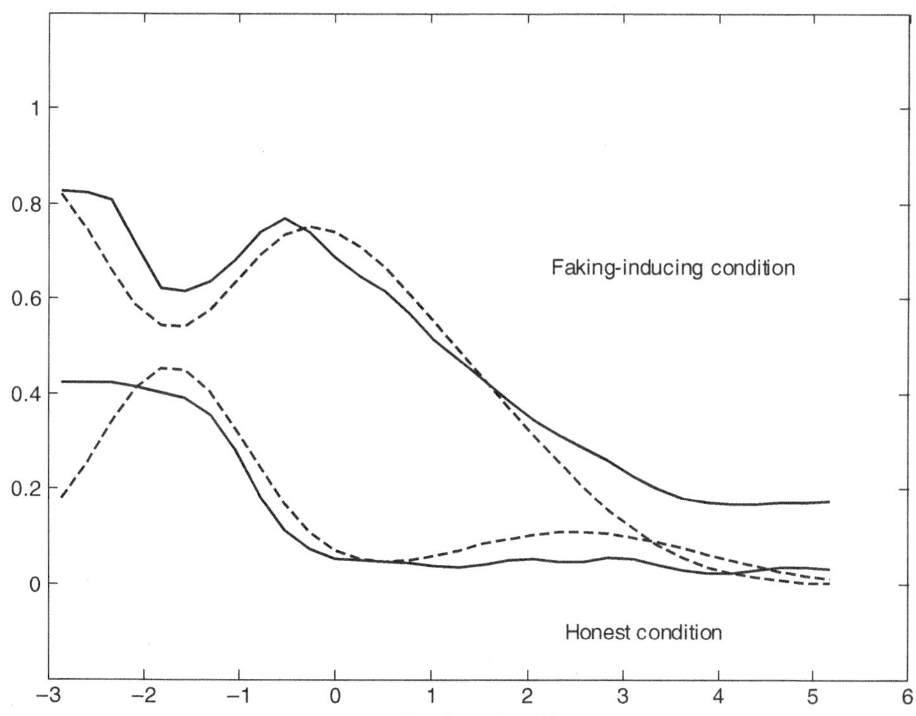

Figure 7.3 Graphical analysis of respondent number 156 based on the 2PM under faking-inducing and honest responding conditions. Example 2.

Example 3: Acquiescence on a partially balanced scale

The last example shows how the combined use of practical indices, graphical procedures, and item-level indices can detect acquiescence when the responses are based on a partially balanced scale. The measure in this case was a 35-item extraversion scale in which 25 items measured in the direction of the extraversion pole and the remaining 10 measured in the direction of the introversion pole. All the items were positively worded and used a five-point Likert format. The sample size was 480, and the data was well fitted by the GRM.

Response pattern 201 had a $lz^{(p)}$ estimate of –3.76, and the *JRV* estimate was 1.66. The first index suggests that this respondent answered inconsistently. However, the second suggests that the variability between the trait estimates is not much higher than the expected variability of the estimate based on the full response pattern. So no highly influential item scores are expected in this case.

As discussed earlier, acquiescence is thought to be better assessed when single-item discrepancies are used and the scatter of points is inspected. Inspection of the standardized residuals in Equation (7.30) showed large outliers (seven of which had an absolute value higher than 1.65) that closely corresponded to the 10 reverse items. Furthermore, all these residuals were negative. This is to be expected in the case of acquiescence: when the raw score in the introversion-worded items is reversed, the resulting score is lower than expected given the trait estimate of this respondent. As was also expected, inspection of the *Dz* influential indices in (7.35) showed that all the values corresponding to the reverse items were positive (when the lowered item score is omitted, the trait estimate based on

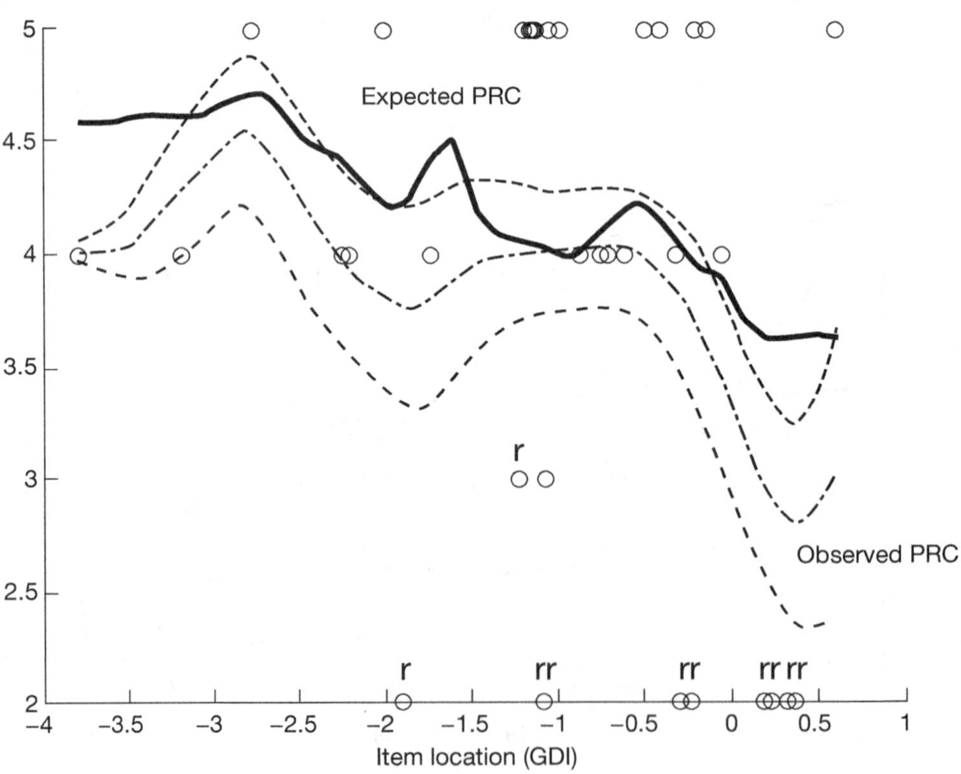

Figure 7.4 Graphical analysis of respondent number 201 based on the GRM. Example 3.

the remaining items increases). However, the *Dz* values were rather low, and none of them was higher than 0.5.

Figure 7.4 shows the graphical assessment of response pattern number 201 and, to help interpret the results, the items that were reversed are marked with an "r." The OPRC locally deviates from the OPRC at the right end of the graph, possibly because of the cluster of reversed items at the bottom right. Overall, however, what is most clearly seen in the graph are the large negative outliers, which correspond to the items that were reverse-scored.

It is hard to decide the extent to which the trait estimate of this respondent can be trusted. If the scale were fully balanced it would be assumed that the effects on the positive and the reverse set would cancel each other out, so the estimate based on the full pattern would have been reasonably correct (see Ferrando, 2010). However, the scale is only partially balanced, so it is likely that the trait estimate based on the full pattern is upwardly biased.

Future Directions

I begin the discussion with a caveat. This chapter has tried to provide a comprehensive approach to person fit in typical-response measures. However, in spite of its general purpose, this chapter reflects the views of the author, and part of the text is devoted to procedures the author himself has developed. So the chapter cannot be properly considered to be a review of existing person fit procedures. Person fit is a wide domain of research containing multiple approaches that reflect different views. So the interested reader is encouraged to explore alternative procedures and perspectives.

In recent decades typical-response psychometric applications have become more rigorous and, at present, most of them are model based. Therefore, an acceptable model-data fit is a basic requirement that has to be met before the test can be used to score individuals. However, in most applications at present, assessment of fit finishes once the test scores have been obtained: all the scores are then assumed to be valid indicators of the trait levels and, therefore, they are interpreted and/or used for selection purposes or in validity studies. In this chapter I have tried to make it clear that this assumption is not warranted. So my position is that person fit should always be assessed before the scores are interpreted or used. I have also made it clear that person fit procedures have considerable limitations and need to be improved in the future. Even so, they are useful, and the potential they have to improve measurement justifies their use in any typical-response application.

Experience suggests that recommendations such as this are only widely used if well-developed user-friendly software is readily available. So, in closing, I shall provide some discussion on noncommercial programs that implement the procedures discussed here.

WPerfit (Ferrando & Lorenzo-Seva, 2000) is a Windows program that computes L-B global indices based on the 1PM and the 2PM. It also implements graphical procedures, and obtains the PRCs corresponding to these models. L-B indices for the binary models can also be obtained with the R (http://cran.r-project.org) packages IRTOYS and MIRT. MIRT is able to compute both the unidimensional and multidimensional versions of the *lz* index.

For the GRM case, L-B indices can be obtained with the R program PERSONz (Choi, 2010), and again with MIRT. PERSONz allows cutoff values to be obtained via simulation. MIRT computes both the unidimensional and multidimensional versions of $lz^{(p)}$. Finally, the unidimensional and multidimensional indices proposed by Ferrando for the congeneric model can be obtained with the program FACTOR (Lorenzo-Seva & Ferrando, 2013).

The other indices and procedures discussed in this chapter are implemented in ad hoc programs that, at best, would be useful for methodologically oriented researchers. So a great deal of work is needed if the present proposal is to be widely used in applied research. And perhaps the best future line of action is to develop a comprehensive, user-friendly program that computes global and item-level indices together with clear and powerful graphical displays. In the meantime, the cited software allows applied researchers in the personality and attitude domains to undertake the most basic forms of person fit assessment. If this chapter convinces them to incorporate this assessment (albeit at the most basic level) in their applications, it will have fulfilled an important aim.

References

Andrich, D. (1978). Relationships between the Thurstone and Rasch approaches to item scaling. *Applied Psychological Measurement, 2*, 449–460.

Armstrong, R.D., Stoumbos, Z.G., Kung, M.T., & Shi, M. (2007). On the performance of lz statistic in person fit measurement. *Practical Assessment, Research & Evaluation, 12*.

Bollen, K.A., & Arminger, G. (1991). Observational residuals in factor analysis and structural equation models. In P.V. Marsden (Ed.), *Sociological methodology 1991* (pp. 235–262). New York: Basil Blackwell.

Chang, H., & Mazzeo, J. (1994). The unique correspondence of the item response function and item category response function in polytomously scored item response models. *Psychometrika, 59*, 391–404.

Choi, S.W. (2010). PERSONz: Person misfit detection using the lz statistic and Monte Carlo simulations. *Applied Psychological Measurement, 34*, 457–458.

Clark, J.M. (2010). *Aberrant response patterns as a multidimensional phenomenon: Using factor-analytic model comparison to detect cheating*. Doctoral dissertation, University of Kansas.

Conrad, K.J., Bezruczko, N., Chan, Y., Riley, B., Diamond, G., & Dennis, M.L. (2010). Screening for atypical suicide risk with person fit statistics among people presenting to alcohol and other drug treatment. *Drug and Alcohol Dependence, 106*, 92–100.

Cook, R.D., & Weisberg, S. (1982). *Residuals and influence in regression*. London: Chapman & Hall.

Culpepper, S.A. (2013). The reliability and precision of total scores and IRT estimates as a function of polytomous IRT parameters and latent trait distribution. *Applied Psychological Measurement, 37*, 201–225.

Curtis, D.D. (2004). Person misfit in attitude surveys: Influences, impacts and implications. *International Education Journal, 5*, 2125–2144.

de la Torre, J., & Deng, W. (2008). Improving person-fit assessment by correcting the ability estimate and its reference distribution. *Journal of Educational Measurement, 45*, 159–177.

Dodeen, H., & Darabi, M. (2009). Person-fit: Relationship with four personality tests in mathematics. *Research Papers in Education, 24*, 115–126.

Drasgow, F., Levine, M.V., & McLaughlin, M.E. (1987). Detecting inappropriate test scores with optimal and practical appropriateness indices. *Applied Psychological Measurement, 11*, 59–79.

Drasgow, F., Levine, M.V., & McLaughlin, M.E. (1991). Appropriateness measurement for some multidimensional test batteries. *Applied Psychological Measurement, 15*, 171–191.

Drasgow, F., Levine, M.V., & Williams, E.A. (1985). Appropriateness measurement with polychotomous item response models and standardized indices. *British Journal of Mathematical and Statistical Psychology, 38*, 67–86.

Egberink, I.J.L., & Meijer, R.R. (2011). An item response theory analysis of Harter's Self-Perception Profile for Children or why strong clinical scales should be distrusted. *Assessment, 18*, 201–212.

Emons, W.H.M. (2009). Detection and diagnosis of person misfit from patterns of summed polytomous item scores. *Applied Psychological Measurement, 33*, 599–619.

Emons, W. H. M., Sijtsma, K., & Meijer, R. R. (2004). Testing hypothesis about the person-response-function in person-fit analysis. *Multivariate Behavioral Research, 39*, 1–35.

Emons, W. H. M., Sijtsma, K., & Meijer, R. R. (2005). Global, local and graphical person-fit analysis using person-response functions. *Psychological Methods, 10*, 101–119.

Emons, W. H. M., Sijtsma, K., & Meijer, R. R. (2007). On the consistency of individual classification using short scales. *Psychological Methods, 12*, 105–120.

Eysenck, S. B. G., Eysenck, H. J., & Barrett, P. T. (1985). A revised version of the Psychoticism scale. *Personality and Individual Differences, 6*, 21–29.

Ferrando, P. J. (2002). Theoretical and empirical comparisons between two models for continuous item responses. *Multivariate Behavioral Research, 37*, 521–542.

Ferrando, P. J. (2004). Person reliability in personality measurement: An item response theory analysis. *Applied Psychological Measurement, 28*, 126–140.

Ferrando, P. J. (2007). Factor-analytic procedures for assessing response pattern scalability. *Multivariate Behavioral Research, 42*, 481–508.

Ferrando, P. J. (2009). Difficulty, discrimination and information indices in the linear factor-analytic model for continuous responses. *Applied Psychological Measurement, 33*, 9–24.

Ferrando, P. J. (2010). Some statistics for assessing person-fit based on continuous-response models. *Applied Psychological Measurement, 34*, 219–237.

Ferrando, P. J. (2012). Assessing inconsistent responding in E and N measures: An application of person-fit analysis in personality. *Personality and Individual Differences, 52*, 718–722.

Ferrando, P. J., & Anguiano-Carrasco, C. (2013). A structural model-based optimal person fit procedure for identifying faking. *Educational and Psychological Measurement, 73*, 173–190.

Ferrando, P. J., & Chico, E. (2001). Detecting dissimulation in personality test scores: A comparison between person-fit indices and detection scales. *Educational and Psychological Measurement, 61*, 997–1012.

Ferrando, P. J., & Lorenzo-Seva, U. (2000). WPerfit: A program for computing parametric person-fit statistics and plotting person response curves. *Educational and Psychological Measurement, 60*, 479–487. (Available at http://psico.fcep.urv.es/utilitats/wperfit/)

Ferrando, P. J., & Lorenzo-Seva, U. (2010). Acquiescence as a source of bias and model and person misfit: A theoretical and empirical analysis. *British Journal of Mathematical and Statistical Psychology, 63*, 427–448.

Härdle, W. (1990). *Applied nonparametric regression*. London: Chapman & Hall.

Hofstee, W. K. B., Ten Berge, J. M. F., & Hendricks, A. A. J. (1998). How to score questionnaires. *Personality and Individual Differences, 25*, 897–910.

Hulin, C. L., Drasgow, F., & Parsons, C. K. (1983). *Item response theory. Application to psychological measurement*. Homewood: Dow Jones-Irvin.

Jöreskog, K. G. (1971). Statistical analysis of sets of congeneric tests. *Psychometrika, 36*, 109–133.

Karabatsos, G. (2000). A critique of Rasch residual fit statistics. *Journal of Applied Measurement, 1*, 152–176.

Karabatsos, G. (2003). Comparing the aberrant response detection performance of thirty-six person-fit statistics. *Applied Measurement in Education, 16*, 277–298.

Levine, M. V., & Drasgow, F. (1983). Appropriateness measurement: Validating studies and variable ability models. In D. J. Weiss (Ed.), *New horizons in testing* (pp. 109–131). New York: Academic Press.

Levine, M. V., & Rubin, D. B. (1979). Measuring the appropriateness of multiple choice test scores. *Journal of Educational Statistics, 4*, 269–290.

Levy, P. (1973). On the relation between test theory and psychology. In P. Kline (Ed.), *New approaches in psychological measurement* (pp. 1–42). New York: Wiley.

Li, M. F., & Olejnik, S. (1997). The power of Rasch person-fit statistics in detecting unusual response patterns. *Applied Psychological Measurement, 21*, 215–231.

Lord, F. M., & Novick, M. R. (1968). *Statistical theories of mental test scores*. Reading, MA: Addison-Wesley.

Lorenzo-Seva, U., & Ferrando, P. J. (2013). FACTOR 9.2: A comprehensive program for fitting exploratory and semi-confirmatory factor analysis and IRT models. *Applied Psychological Measurement, 37*, 497–498. (Available at http://psico.fcep.urv.es/utilitats/factor/)

Lumsden, J. (1977). Person reliability. *Applied Psychological Measurement, 1*, 477–482.

Magis, D., Raîche, G., & Béland, S. (2012). A didactic presentation of Snijders's *lz** index of person fit with emphasis on response model selection and ability estimation. *Journal of Educational and Behavioral Statistics, 37*, 57–81.

McDonald, R.P. (1999). *Test theory: A unified treatment.* Mahwah, NJ: Lawrence Erlbaum Associates.

Meijer, R.R. (1996). Person-fit research: An introduction. *Applied Measurement in Education, 9*, 3–8.

Meijer, R.R. (2003). Diagnosing item score patterns on a test using item response theory-based person-fit statistics. *Psychological Methods, 8*, 72–87.

Meijer, R.R., Egberink, I.J.K., Emons, W.H.M., & Sijtsma, K. (2008). Detection and validation of unscalable item score patterns using item response theory: An illustration with Harter's Self-Perception Profile for Children. *Journal of Personality Assessment, 90*, 1–14.

Meijer, R.R., & Nering, M.L. (1997). Trait level estimation for nonfitting response vectors. *Applied Psychological Measurement, 21*, 321–336.

Meijer, R.R., & Sijtsma, K. (2001). Methodology review: Evaluating person fit. *Applied Psychological Measurement, 25*, 107–135.

Mellenbergh, G.J. (1994). A unidimensional latent trait model for continuous item responses. *Multivariate Behavioral Research, 29*(3), 223–237.

Molenaar, I.W., & Hoijtink, H. (1990). The many null distributions of person fit indices. *Psychometrika, 55*, 75–106.

Muthén, B., & Kaplan, D. (1985). A comparison of some methodologies for the factor analysis of non-normal Likert variables. *British Journal of Mathematical and Statistical Psychology, 38*, 171–189.

Nering, M.L. (1995). The distribution of person fit using true and estimated person parameters. *Applied Psychological Measurement, 19*, 121–129.

Nering, M.L. (1997). Trait level estimation for nonfitting response vectors. *Applied Psychological Measurement, 21*, 321–336.

Nering, M.L., & Meijer, R.R. (1998). A comparison of the person response function and the lz person-fit statistic. *Applied Psychological Measurement, 22*, 53–69.

Olsson, U. (1979). On the robustness of factor analysis against crude classification of observations. *Multivariate Behavioral Research, 14*, 485–500.

Pallero, R., Ferrando, P.J., & Lorenzo-Seva, U. (1998, July). *Questionnaire Tarragona of anxiety for blind people.* Paper presented at the IX International Mobility Conference, Atlanta.

Reise, S.P. (1995). Scoring method and the detection of person misfit in a personality assessment context. *Applied Psychological Measurement, 19*, 213–229.

Reise, S.P., & Due, A.M. (1991). The influence of test characteristics on the detection of aberrant response patterns. *Applied Psychological Measurement, 15*, 217–226.

Reise, S.P., & Flannery, W.P. (1996). Assessing person-fit on measures of typical performance. *Applied Measurement in Education, 9*, 9–26.

Reise, S.P., & Waller, N.G. (1993). Traitedness and the assessment of response pattern scalability. *Journal of Personality and Social Psychology, 65*, 143–151.

Reise, S.P., & Waller, N.G. (2009). Item response theory and clinical measurement. *Annual Review of Clinical Psychology, 5*, 27–48.

Reise, S.P., Waller, N.G., & Comrey, A.L. (2000). Factor analysis and scale revision. *Psychological Assessment, 12*, 287–297.

Reise, S.P., & Widaman, K.F. (1999). Assessing the fit of measurement models at the individual level: A comparison of item response theory and covariance structure approaches. *Psychological Methods, 4*, 3–21.

Samejima, F. (1969). *Estimation of latent ability using a response pattern of graded scores.* (Psychometrika Monograph No. 17). Iowa City: Psychometric Society.

Schmitt, N., Chan, D., Sacco, J.M., McFarland, L.A., & Jennings, D. (1999). Correlates of person-fit and effect of person-fit on test validity. *Applied Psychological Measurement, 23*, 41–53.

Sijtsma, K., & Meijer, R.R. (2001). The person response function as a tool in person-fit research. *Psychometrika, 66*, 191–207.

Smith, R.M. (1990).Theory and practice of fit. *Rasch Measurement Transactions, 3*, 78–80.

Snijders, T.A.B. (2001). Asymptotic null distribution of person fit statistics with estimated person parameter. *Psychometrika, 66*, 331–342.

Tellegen, A. (1988). The analysis of consistency in personality assessment. *Journal of Personality, 56*, 622–663.

van Krimpen-Stoop, E.M.L.A., & Meijer, R.R. (2002). Detection of person misfit in computerized adaptive tests with polytomous items. *Applied Psychological Measurement, 26*, 164–180.

Waller, N.G., & Reise, S.P. (1992). Genetic and environmental influences on item response pattern scalability. *Behavior Genetics, 22*, 135–152.

Weiss, D.J. (1973). *The stratified adaptive computerized ability test.* Research report 73-3. Minneapolis: University of Minnesota.

Woods, C., Oltmanns, T.F., & Turkheimer, E. (2008). Detection of aberrant responding on a personality scale in a military sample: An application of evaluating person fit with two-level logistic regression. *Psychological Assessment, 20*, 159–168.

Wright, B.D. (1977). Solving measurement problems with the Rasch model. *Journal of Educational Measurement, 14*, 97–116.

Wright, B.D., & Masters, G.N. (1982). *Rating scale analysis.* Chicago, IL: Mesa Press.

Zickar, M.J., & Drasgow, F. (1996). Detecting faking on a personality instrument using appropriateness measurement. *Applied Psychological Measurement, 20*, 71–87.

Zickar, M.J., & Sliter, K.A. (2012). Searching for unicorns: Item response theory-based solutions to the faking problem. In M. Ziegler, C. MacCann, & R.D. Roberts (Eds.), *New perspectives on faking in personality assessment* (pp. 113–130). New York: Oxford University Press.

Zijlstra, W.P., van der Ark, L.A., & Sijtsma, K. (2007). Outlier detection in test and questionnaire data. *Multivariate Behavioral Research, 42*, 531–555.

Part II

Classic and Emerging IRT Modeling Approaches

8 Three (or Four) Factors, Four (or Three) Models

Michael C. Edwards, R.J. Wirth, Carrie R. Houts, and Andrew J. Bodine

Introduction

Item response theory (IRT) models are some of the most widely used psychometric models. This is certainly the case in large-scale educational assessment. Over the past two decades these models have formed the core of many of the high-stakes assessments in K-12 education (and beyond). While there has always been some interest in applying these models to social science assessment beyond education, the progress on that front has lagged considerably. The project that is at the core of this book, the Patient Reported Outcomes Measurement Information System (PROMIS®, Cella et al., 2007), was a significant milestone in bringing the rigor of modern psychometric methods to the area of patient-reported outcomes (PROs). Not only did PROMIS® create a number of calibrated item banks and an adaptive testing system, the publications accompanying them laid out a blueprint for future researchers to incorporate these more advanced psychometric models into their own research (Cella et al., 2010).

While the work done under the auspices of the PROMIS® project has brought modern methods to the PRO space, it has only scratched the surface of the kinds of complex modeling of which IRT is capable. In this chapter we pick one particular aspect of model complexity, dimensionality, and describe the current state of the field with particular attention paid to what is accessible to users. After this, we focus on exploring the concepts underlying dimensionality and discuss some of the challenges researchers face when trying to choose between different models. We demonstrate these conceptual issues with both simulated and real data examples before turning to a broader discussion of how the issue of dimensionality may impact the PRO world.

RESEARCH METHODS

An Overview of Dimensionality

In this section, we hope to provide the reader with a general overview of the topic of dimensionality as it applies to modern psychometric methods. There is a vast literature on issues related to dimensionality in both the IRT and factor analysis frameworks (Chapter 2, this volume). As many authors have noted (Muthén & Lehman, 1985; Takane & de Leeuw, 1987; Thissen & Steinberg, 1988; Wirth & Edwards, 2007), there are strong ties between these two frameworks. Indeed, in many cases the differences are solely due to the choice of estimator used or implementation in software. There are two distinctions we would like to focus on that should help the reader better understand the issue of dimensionality. The first distinction is between conceptual and empirical dimensionality. The second is between within-item and between-item dimensionality.

Conceptual dimensionality refers to the implied or assumed number of common factors that are associated with a particular operationalization of a construct. For example, I may imagine depression is a single continuous construct or I may imagine that overall depression drives a factor related to affective symptoms and another related to somatic symptoms. I may believe quality of life is a single construct, or I may believe there are different kinds of quality of life (e.g., financial, health, social, etc.) that each exists as a separate construct. In these two cases (and in many others) there are competing conceptual models that suggest different dimensional structures. Note that we haven't collected or analyzed any data at this point—these are just ideas in the heads of researchers.

Empirical dimensionality relates to the observed statistical properties in a set of data. Both factor analysis and IRT have at their core assumptions about local independence—that once you control for the common factors the items are independent from one another. Stated another way, local independence implies that the only reason items correlate with one another is their relationship(s) to the common factor(s). A model's ability to capture empirical dimensionality is what is assessed (in part) by various indices of model fit. Researchers are often interested in the extent to which the empirical dimensionality reflects or supports their conceptual dimensionality. However, empirical dimensionality also must contend with "nuisance" factors that are perhaps not of primary interest to the researcher. For example, although it is common practice to reverse the valence of a subset of items on a scale, there is evidence that this can induce empirical dimensionality (Rodebaugh, Woods, & Heimberg, 2007; Woods, 2006). This is not necessarily dimensionality the researcher is interested in, but failure to model it can have ramifications for the parts of the model the researcher *is* interested in.

The between- versus within-item dimensionality distinction (Adams, Wilson, & Wang, 1997) is a straightforward one: Does an item[1] measure one construct or more than one construct? McDonald (1985) makes a similar distinction using the labels factorially simple and factorially complex. If an item measures one construct, then there is only one common factor influencing responses to that item. In such cases, even if there are multiple correlated factors being assessed, an independent clustering solution means that each dimension could be modeled separately without any bias (but sacrificing efficiency). In typical IRT parlance, such factors could be modeled using unidimensional IRT models. The three-factor model in Figure 8.1 (top right panel) is an example of between-item multidimensionality. If an item measures more than one construct, and there are at least two items measuring that construct in a particular set of items, then there are multiple common factors influencing responses to that item. In these cases, failing to model the influence of each of the common factors on the item response will result in bias/error in understanding the relationships that are modeled. The bifactor model in Figure 8.1 (bottom right panel) provides an example of within-item multidimensionality.

Multidimensional Models

To make this distinction more concrete, we present some standard IRT models to illustrate the differences. The one-dimensional, two-parameter logistic model (1D-2PLM) has historically been written as:

$$P\left(y_{ij} = 1|\theta_i\right) = \frac{1}{1 + \exp\left[-a_j\left(\theta_i - b_j\right)\right]}, \tag{8.1}$$

1 In the context of psychometrics, the measured variables are most commonly categorical responses to items, hence we will use the term "items" throughout this chapter as a generic indicator of categorical responses.

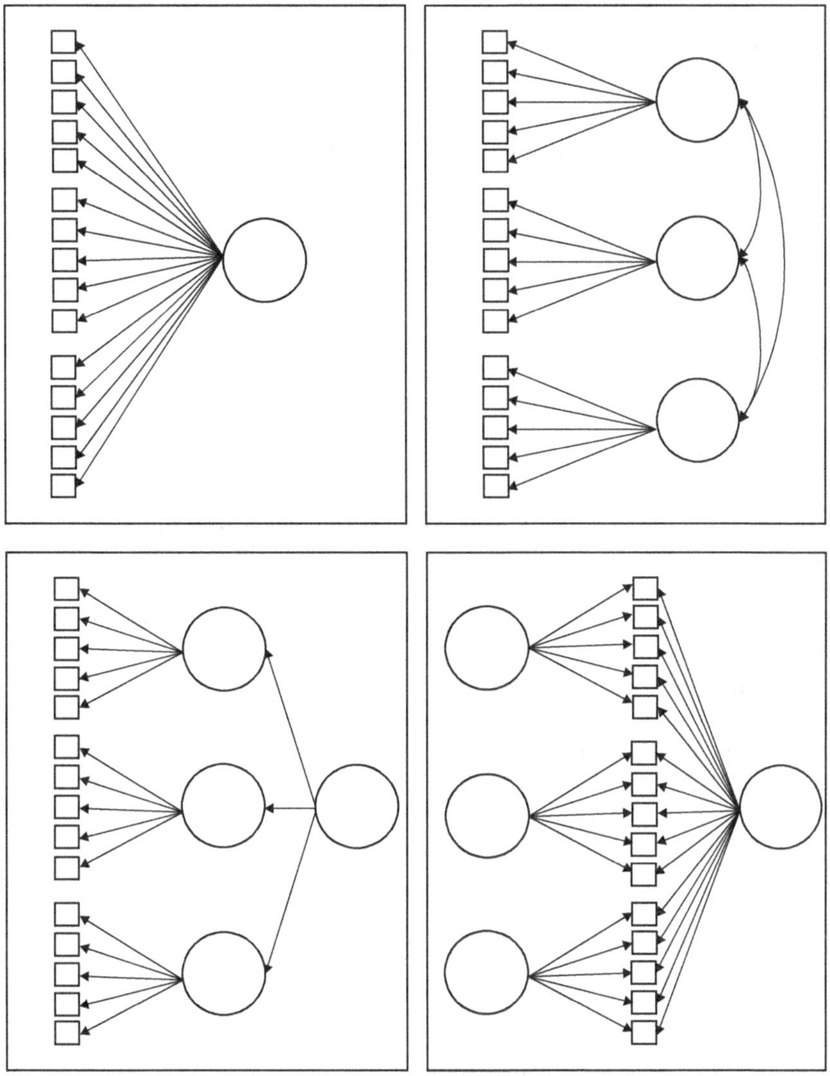

Figure 8.1 Four different factor models that could be used to conceptually model three empirical common factors: top left: Single factor model where all items load on single factor, top right: Three factor-independent clustering solutions where each item is an indicator of separate, but correlated, factors, bottom left: Higher-order factor model where the three factors are explained by a single higher-order factor, and bottom right: A bifactor model with one general and three specific factors.

where y_{ij} is the observed response from individual i to item j, a_j is a slope parameter for item j, b_j is a difficulty/severity parameter for item j, and θ_i represents individual i's level of the latent construct (singular, in this case) being assessed. Slopes in the 1D-2PLM reflect the strength of association between an item and the construct being measured—they are analogous to item-total correlations and factor loadings. The severity parameters reflect the point along the latent continuum where an individual has a 50 percent chance of endorsing a particular question. To estimate parameters for this model we assume that it is correctly specified in number of common factors (one) and functional form (logistic). We also assume that the construct follows a standard normal distribution. There are variants of this model that do not assume a logistic function (Duncan & MacEachern, 2008;

Junker & Sijtsma, 2001) and other variants that do not assume a normally distributed construct (Woods & Thissen, 2006). However, in the remainder of this chapter we will focus solely on the dimensionality aspect while retaining the logistic shape and normality assumption on the construct(s).

While Equation (8.1) is a common way to write the 1D-2PLM, it does not extend easily to cases where there are multiple common factors that impact an item response (i.e., within-item multidimensionality). Cai, Yang, and Hansen (2011) have suggested the following parameterization:

$$P\left(y_{ij} = 1 \mid \eta_{ij}\right) = \frac{1}{1 + \exp\left[-\left(d_j + \eta_{ij}\right)\right]}, \tag{8.2}$$

where d_j is an intercept parameter, $\eta_{ij} = \mathbf{a}_j \boldsymbol{\theta}_i$ (bold terms indicating matrices), and all other parameters are as previously defined. When there is only one common factor, this simplifies to the 1D-2PLM. If there is more than one common factor impacting an item, then this is a multidimensional 2PLM (MD-2PLM). The η term is used for mathematical convenience. It denotes a term that sums over all the $a * \theta$ combinations that are available in a given situation. The interpretation of the intercept is not as convenient as the historical *b*-parameter, but once we depart from unidimensional models this interpretability is lost anyway (but see Reckase, 2009, chapter 5, for examples of how to find interpretable parameters in multidimensional models).

Imagine an item that measures both depression and anxiety. An individual's response to this item (which is dichotomous in this example) will depend on both their level of depression and their level of anxiety. If we write out Equation (8.2) and substitute more descriptive terms we get:

$$P\left(y_{ij} = 1 \mid \theta_{i(dep)} \theta_{i(anx)}\right) = \frac{1}{1 + \exp\left[-\left(d_j + a_{j(dep)}\theta_{i(dep)} + a_{j(anx)}\theta_{i(anx)}\right)\right]}, \tag{8.3}$$

where item *j* has a unique relationship to depression ($a_{j(dep)}$) and a unique relationship to anxiety ($a_{j(anx)}$) and individual *i* has a particular level of depression ($\theta_{i(dep)}$) and a particular level of anxiety ($\theta_{i(anx)}$). These all come together, along with the item's intercept (d_j), to determine the model-predicted probability that this individual will endorse this item. This particular kind of multidimensional model is known as compensatory. Compensatory models allow for high standing in one dimension to "compensate" for low standing in another. There are other kinds of models (see Bolt & Lall, 2003, for some examples), but compensatory models are currently the most commonly used.

The 1D- and MD-2PLM are appropriate for dichotomous responses. While these are not uncommon in assessment, there are many items that use an ordered Likert-type response format with more than two categories. One such widely used response scale is agreement based, with options: *strongly disagree, disagree, neither, agree, strongly agree.* In such instances the graded response model (GRM) is a natural choice among IRT models. The multidimensional GRM (MD-GRM) can be written (using the same notation as earlier) as:

$$P(y_{ji} = k \mid \eta_{ij}) = \frac{1}{1 + \exp\left[-\left(d_{j(k-1)} + \eta_{ij}\right)\right]} - \frac{1}{1 + \exp\left[-\left(d_{jk} + \eta_{ij}\right)\right]}, \tag{8.4}$$

where *k* is the observed response category and all other parameters are as previously defined. Just as there are multiple severity parameters in the historical unidimensional formulation of the GRM there are multiple intercept parameters in this parameterization of the MD-GRM. For the model to function we must further specify that the probability of observing a response greater than or equal to zero is one and that the probability of observing a response greater than the largest possible response is zero. Despite the additional complexity of having multiple common factors, any existing intuitions the reader has about the functioning of the GRM should carry over to the MD-GRM.

Parameter Estimation

A brief detour is in order before addressing the topic of parameter estimation to clear up some confusion between what is factor analysis and what is IRT. More specifically, what is the difference between a factor analysis (conducted using methods to address the categorical nature of the data) and an IRT analysis? In many cases, the answer is: Not much. The most common difference until quite recently was which estimator was more common in software used to estimate parameters for factor analysis models versus software used to estimate parameters for IRT models. Although the models can look very different, especially when different estimators are used in specialized software packages, at the end of the day *IRT is a kind of factor analysis*. The θ parameter used in IRT equations is undeniably a common factor. A different term is needed to distinguish factor analysis of item-level data (which is very often categorical in nature) from the "usual" factor analysis assuming linear relationships between the latent variables and the manifest indicators. Suggestions have included categorical factor analysis (or categorical confirmatory factor analysis, as appropriate), nonlinear factor analysis, and item factor analysis. In this way, IRT can be viewed simply as an informative label telling the reader what kind of factor analytic techniques are likely being employed.

Full information estimation of multidimensional item response theory (MIRT) models began with maximum marginal likelihood using the expectation-maximization algorithm (MML-EM; Bock & Aitkin, 1981). The objective of this method was to provide model parameter estimates for tests containing many factors while using all available response pattern data. In rather general terms, MML-EM functions by using provisional parameter values to estimate the proportions of expected responses for different levels of each factor (expectation), computing parameter estimates from these proportions (maximization), then using these newly obtained estimates in the subsequent expectation step (see Rubin, 1991, for an excellent and accessible overview of the EM algorithm). This process repeats until little change is present in successive iterations. A more detailed description is available in Bock, Gibbons, and Muraki (1988).

Though MML-EM provides asymptotically consistent estimates with small variances, Gauss-Hermite quadrature, the method traditionally used to approximate integration in the expectation step, presents a few limitations. Namely, as the number of factors increases linearly, the computational burden increases exponentially. Because integration in MML-EM is performed over the number of factors being estimated, even with limits to the quadrature points used, the maximum number of factors that can be reliably and efficiently estimated by MML-EM with Gauss-Hermite quadrature is about five. Luckily, solutions developed both during and after the advent of MML-EM provide researchers with tools to circumvent problems related to dimensionality.

Limited information estimation represents one such tool. Rather than relying on entire response patterns to derive parameter estimates, limited information methods make use of (usually) univariate and bivariate summaries of the item responses. Two common limited information procedures include weighted least squares (WLS) and modified or diagonally weighted least squares (MWLS or DWLS). WLS and MWLS differ in terms of the type of weight matrix used in parameter estimation. While WLS employs a full asymptotic covariance matrix, MWLS uses only the diagonal elements of that matrix. Retaining only the diagonal elements gives MWLS a distinct computational advantage due to the necessary inversion of the weight matrix. Flora and Curran (2004), who provide a more in-depth exploration of these methods and a comparison of their performance, find the MWLS variants typically outperform their WLS counterpart.

Full information estimation may also be performed in a Bayesian framework using Markov chain Monte Carlo (MCMC) estimation. MCMC is an iterative method that produces samples ("chains") that are drawn from each parameter's posterior distribution. Estimates of these parameters and their standard errors may be easily computed from the posterior samples. Research in MCMC has become popular in recent years, and several studies are available for those interested in applying the method to IRT (Albert, 1992; Béguin & Glas, 2001; Edwards, 2010). While the availability of this method has expanded greatly in the past decade, it is still more difficult to implement compared to MML-EM or MWLS.

Another avenue of development has sought to retain MML-EM, but replace Gauss-Hermite quadrature as the method of integral approximation. Adaptive quadrature (Rabe-Hesketh, Skrondal, & Pickles, 2002) is one such method. Instead of using quadrature points at pre-specified values along the continuum, this method determines the ideal location of each quadrature point as part of its integration process. This modification results in more efficient use of quadrature points for each dimension. However, the number of points used still grows exponentially as the number of factors increases. Another way to improve integration in MML-EM is stochastic EM (Diebolt & Ip, 1996). Essentially, stochastic EM functions by replacing the usual expectation step with MCMC to facilitate integration. While this method requires more research in the context of IRT, it suggests a promising possible solution to the dimensionality problem. A third integration procedure recently applied to MML-EM, and available in commercial software, is the Metropolis-Hastings Robbins-Monro (MHRM) algorithms method (Cai, 2010a). It increases the number of dimensions that can be practically modeled with other integration methods by using the Robbins-Monro approximation (Robbins & Monro, 1951) and the Metropolis-Hastings algorithm (Hastings, 1970). This method is notable for its computational efficiency that results in speedy estimation.

A wide array of statistical software is available for estimating the IRT models described earlier. MML-EM and other full-information estimators are included in the programs flexMIRT® (Cai, 2012), IRTPRO (Cai, Du Toit, & Thissen, 2011), EQSIRT (Wu & Bentler, 2011), and the ltm package in R (Rizopoulos, 2006). Limited information estimation may be performed using structural equation modeling software like LISREL (Jöreskog & Sörbom, 2003), Mplus (Muthén & Muthén, 2008), and the lavaan package in R (Rosseel, 2012). Finally, a few programs are available for MCMC estimation of IRT models such as WinBUGS (Lunn, Thomas, Best, & Spiegelhalter, 2000), MultiNorm (Edwards, 2005), and MCMCpack in R (Martin, Quinn, & Park, 2011).

In the next section, we explore how users can go about choosing a particular model and parameter configuration.

APPLICATION

Choosing a Model

The issues of model fit and model selection have a rich history in psychometrics. While omnibus model fit has historically been associated with factor analytic approaches to measurement, recent developments (e.g., Cai & Hansen, 2013; Maydeu-Olivares & Joe,

2005; Orlando & Thissen, 2000) have extended their reach to modern implementations of item factor models (aka IRT). Model fit and model selection are complementary but distinct aspects of the psychometric modeling process. Model fit indices tell the user if the proposed model provides an adequate representation of the observed data. There are as many variations to "adequate representation of the observed data" as there are different ways to assess model fit. In general, though, model fit indices compare observed quantities with quantities predicted by a model with certain estimated parameters. To the extent that the proposed model matches the conceptual model, model fit can provide a way to assess the agreement between the conceptual dimensionality and the empirical dimensionality. However, it is important to remember that there are many other possible models/estimates that would yield similar (in some cases identical) fit despite having very different conceptual underpinnings.

Consider, for example, the four models displayed in the four panels in Figure 8.1. These are four different conceptual models one could propose to understand the process driving responses to items from a scale. In this example, there are a total of 15 items. The top left panel posits a single common factor underlying all the responses. In the top right panel, the conceptual model posits three related, but distinct, factors with each item relating to only one of the three factors (often called an independent cluster structure). In the bottom left panel we have the same item-to-construct structure as the three-factor model, but we are now hypothesizing a single higher-order factor giving rise to the three lower-order factors. The bottom right panel depicts a bifactor model (e.g., Cai, 2010b; Holzinger & Swineford, 1937; Reise, 2012), where every item is related to a general factor and one additional specific/group factor. In the bifactor model the specific factors are uncorrelated with one another and with the general factor.

It is useful to acknowledge some known analytic relationships between these models before continuing. These relationships have been noted by many researchers, including Lee and Hershberger (1990) and MacCallum, Wegener, Uchino, and Fabrigar (1993). The three-factor and higher-order models are mathematically equivalent. This means they will have identical log likelihood values and explain the data equally well as gauged by most commonly used fit measures. This is a special case that holds only with three common factors. In the event that there are more than three common factors the higher-order model is an approximation for the corresponding independent clustering model (Thissen, 2012). As the inter-factor correlations increase, the three-factor model will become more similar to the one-factor model. If the inter-factor correlations are one, the one- and three-factor models are essentially equivalent. For a given bifactor model, there is a corresponding higher-order model representation that is nested within the bifactor model (Rindskopf & Rose, 1988; Yung, Thissen, & McLeod, 1999). Finally, a bifactor model with additional constraints can be shown to be equivalent (Li, Bolt, & Fu, 2006; Thissen, 2012) to the testlet response model of Wainer and colleagues (e.g., Bradlow, Wainer, & Wang, 1999; Wang, Bradlow, & Wainer, 2002).

As we hope the preceding paragraph made clear, there are many strong analytic relationships between these four models. As a result, there are some predictable patterns to expect with regards to how these various models fit data. In the case of three factors, the independent-cluster three-factor model and the corresponding higher-order model are equivalent and will yield the same model fit. In general, freeing constraints to go from the higher-order to the bifactor model will result in an improvement in model fit. The size of the improvement will depend on the data at hand. The three-factor, higher-order, and bifactor models will all be expected to provide similar (or identical) levels of fit to a given data set. Despite this, the conceptual models look quite different. How is one to choose between them when model fit is removed as a distinguishing characteristic? A common answer is that, when choosing between models that have equivalent (or nearly equivalent) model fit, the more parsimonious model should be selected. As the three-factor and higher-order models have exactly the same number of parameters, parsimony is not an aid. Parsimony would lead us to choose the three-factor or higher-order over a bifactor model, but, as we will argue, relying on parsimony alone may not be the best solution.

One of the insights researchers in IRT can bring to the world of factor analysis is that one very important consequence of the model you choose is what can legitimately be inferred from the scores that are produced. Factor scores have a long and somewhat turbulent history in the factor analysis literature (e.g., Green, 1976), but much less so in the IRT literature. In fact, IRT scores are used commonly in high-stakes testing throughout the world. This more applied focus on using the scores produced by the models has likely influenced some of the different thinking in the IRT literature as compared to the factor analytic literature. To some extent, the differences in outlook on factor scores stem from the primary objectives of performing a factor analysis versus an IRT analysis. In factor analysis, the motivating question is often one of structure: How many factors are there? Which items relate to which factors? How related are the factors? Additionally, if one wants to further extend the models to predict the factors (or use the factors as predictors) it is often quite simple to extend a restricted factor analysis model to a full structural equation model. In many of these cases, the primary goal is *scientific*. A particular theory is being tested or particular sets of relationships are being explored. This differs from many common applications of IRT, where the primary goal is to produce reliable scores that can be used to make valid, actionable inferences about the test takers.

In the next section, we use simulated data to explore the impact of fitting different kinds of models to the same data. We examine available fit indices as well as discuss potential differences between interpretations of the resulting scores.

Simulated Applications

Method

All simulations and calibrations were conducted in flexMIRT® version 1.88 (Cai, 2012). Three data sets of $N = 3000$ each were generated. The multidimensional structure of the generating model was three correlated factors, consistent with the upper right panel in Figure 8.1, with five items serving as indicators for each factor. Generating item parameter values were selected from item parameters reported for the PROMIS® depression bank (i.e., Pilkonis et al., 2011). Actual values used are reported in Table 8.1. As indicated by the four intercept parameters for each item, all items were generated to resemble a five-point Likert-type response scale. The latent traits were simulated from a multivariate normal distribution with zero means and unit variances. The inter-factor correlation value was constant within a simulation, but varied across the simulations, taking values of r = 0.4, 0.6, and 0.8.

For each of the three data sets, three models were fit: a unidimensional model (top left in Figure 8.1), a multidimensional model with three correlated factors exhibiting independent clustering (top right in Figure 8.1), and a multidimensional bifactor model, with one general factor and three specific factors (bottom right in Figure 8.1). The three models fit to each of the three data sets resulted in a total of nine estimated models. The fit of each model was then considered.

In terms of assessing model fit, four fit indices were used: the Akaike information criterion (AIC; Akaike, 1974), the Bayesian information criterion (BIC; Schwarz, 1978), M_2^* (Cai & Hansen, 2013), and the root mean square error of approximation (RMSEA; Steiger & Lind, 1980). The AIC and BIC are fit indices calculated using the log-likelihood

Table 8.1 Generating Item Parameters for Simulated Data

Item	*Slope 1*	*Slope 2*	*Slope 3*	*Intercept 1*	*Intercept 2*	*Intercept 3*	*Intercept 4*
1	3.13	0	0	−2.66	−4.41	−6.54	−8.70
2	2.84	0	0	−0.20	−2.36	−5.03	−7.95
3	2.55	0	0	−0.31	−2.40	−4.95	−7.78
4	3.11	0	0	0.09	−2.02	−4.88	−7.46
5	2.74	0	0	0.00	−2.03	−4.74	−7.12
6	0	2.62	0	0.24	−2.10	−4.69	−7.20
7	0	3.19	0	−0.41	−2.26	−4.63	−7.18
8	0	2.92	0	−0.38	−2.39	−4.61	−7.18
9	0	2.80	0	−0.22	−1.96	−4.28	−6.89
10	0	3.10	0	1.33	−1.05	−4.12	−6.67
11	0	0	2.57	0.29	−1.59	−4.06	−6.45
12	0	0	3.19	1.05	−1.05	−3.92	−6.57
13	0	0	2.59	0.39	−1.45	−3.65	−5.83
14	0	0	2.38	1.26	−0.98	−3.50	−6.09
15	0	0	2.69	1.00	−0.94	−3.47	−6.00

value obtained from the fitted model. They both incorporate penalties for model complexity, with the BIC imposing a stronger penalty. For both the AIC and the BIC, lower values indicate the statistically preferred model.

Maydeu-Olivares and Joe (2005) introduced a framework for limited-information fit indices and proposed a limited-information fit statistic that they called M_2. Cai and Hansen (2013), building on the M_2 framework, introduced M_2^* for ordinal data,[2] in an attempt to address shortcomings of M_2 when applied to items with polytomous responses. The M_2^* statistic is asymptotically chi-square distributed with degrees of freedom equal to $n(n+1)/2$ (where n is the number of items) minus the number of unconstrained parameters in the model. This recently introduced statistic has been shown to have a well-calibrated Type I error rate and is more sensitive to model misspecification than the original M_2 when applied to polytomous items (Cai & Hansen, 2013).

Finally, the RMSEA, as calculated from the M_2^* values (see Maydeu-Olivares, Cai, & Hernandez, 2011), was also used. RMSEA values < 0.08 are generally taken to indicate adequate fit, while values < 0.05 indicate close fit (Browne & Cudeck, 1993). Although there is evidence that these cutoffs are not directly transferable to the RMSEA computed for IRT (Cai & Hanson, 2013), we use them here as very rough guidelines. We encourage researchers interested in using RMSEA to evaluate IRT models to consult the literature on this topic as it is evolving rapidly (Edwards, 2013).

Results

The fit results for the nine models can be found in Table 8.2. Several trends are obvious. First, as the inter-factor correlations increase, the fit of the one-factor model improves. In

2 Note that Maydeu-Olivares (2013) refers to this as M_{ord} and the RMSEA computed using it as $RMSEA_{ord}$.

Table 8.2 Model Fit for Simulated Examples

R	*Model*	*AIC*	*BIC*	M_2	*DF*	*RMSEA*
0.4	1-Factor	101718.8	102169.3	3426.69	45	0.16
0.4	3-Factor	90948.31	91416.81	33.67	42	0.00
0.4	Bifactor	90955.79	91496.36	23.35	30	0.00
0.6	1-Factor	96761.33	97211.81	2219.04	45	0.13
0.6	3-Factor	89696.43	90164.92	37.94	42	0.00
0.6	Bifactor	89706.53	90247.11	24.59	30	0.00
0.8	1-Factor	90709.33	91159.8	1002.65	45	0.08
0.8	3-Factor	87755.88	88224.38	39.81	42	0.00
0.8	Bifactor	87765.57	88306.15	30.09	30	0.00

Note: R is the inter-factor correlation level specified for all three correlations in model B, the generating model. AIC is the Akaike information criterion, BIC is the Bayesian information criterion, M_2 is the M_2^* statistic, DF is degrees of freedom of M_2^*, and RMSEA is the root mean square error of approximation computed using M_2^*.

fact, when the inter-factor correlations reach 0.8, the RMSEA for this model (0.08) suggests that it could be a viable model. Second, the generating model has better fit than the one-factor model across the board. This is not surprising. Also unsurprising is that the bifactor model, with more parameters than the generating model, also fits the data very well. Both the three-factor and bifactor models achieve RMSEA values of 0.00 in all six cases.

Posterior mean estimates (often called *expected a posteriori* scores, or EAPs) were computed for each of the nine models. Figures 8.2 through 8.4 provide summaries of how these different scores relate to one another and to the generating values in each of the three correlation conditions (0.4, 0.6, and 0.8, respectively). The contents of a row/column correspond to a particular set of EAPs. They correspond to, in order of their appearance in these figures: generating thetas from factor 1, generating thetas from factor 2, generating thetas from factor 3, estimated EAPs from the one-factor model, estimated EAPs from the first factor of the three-factor model, estimated EAPs from the second factor of the three-factor model, estimated EAPs from the third factor of the three-factor model, estimated EAPs from the general factor of the bifactor model, estimated EAPs from the first specific factor of the bifactor model, estimated EAPs from the second specific factor of the bifactor model, and estimated EAPs from the third specific factor of the bifactor model. The diagonals are histograms of the corresponding set of generating values/estimates. The upper triangle holds correlations between corresponding sets of generating values/estimates and the lower triangle provides scatter plots of those same sets.

The first three rows/columns provide a check on whether the simulated data behave as expected. In all three cases the observed correlations are close to the generating correlations and the resulting empirical histograms look approximately normal. We can also examine, in rows/columns 5–7, how well the generating parameters were recovered when the generating model was fit. The correlations between the estimated θ values and generating θ values are all high (> 0.92 in all cases), indicating good recovery of generating values.[3]

3 The theta estimates are based on the observed data and the item parameter estimates. If the generating theta values are well recovered, it seems reasonable to assume that the generating item parameters were also well recovered.

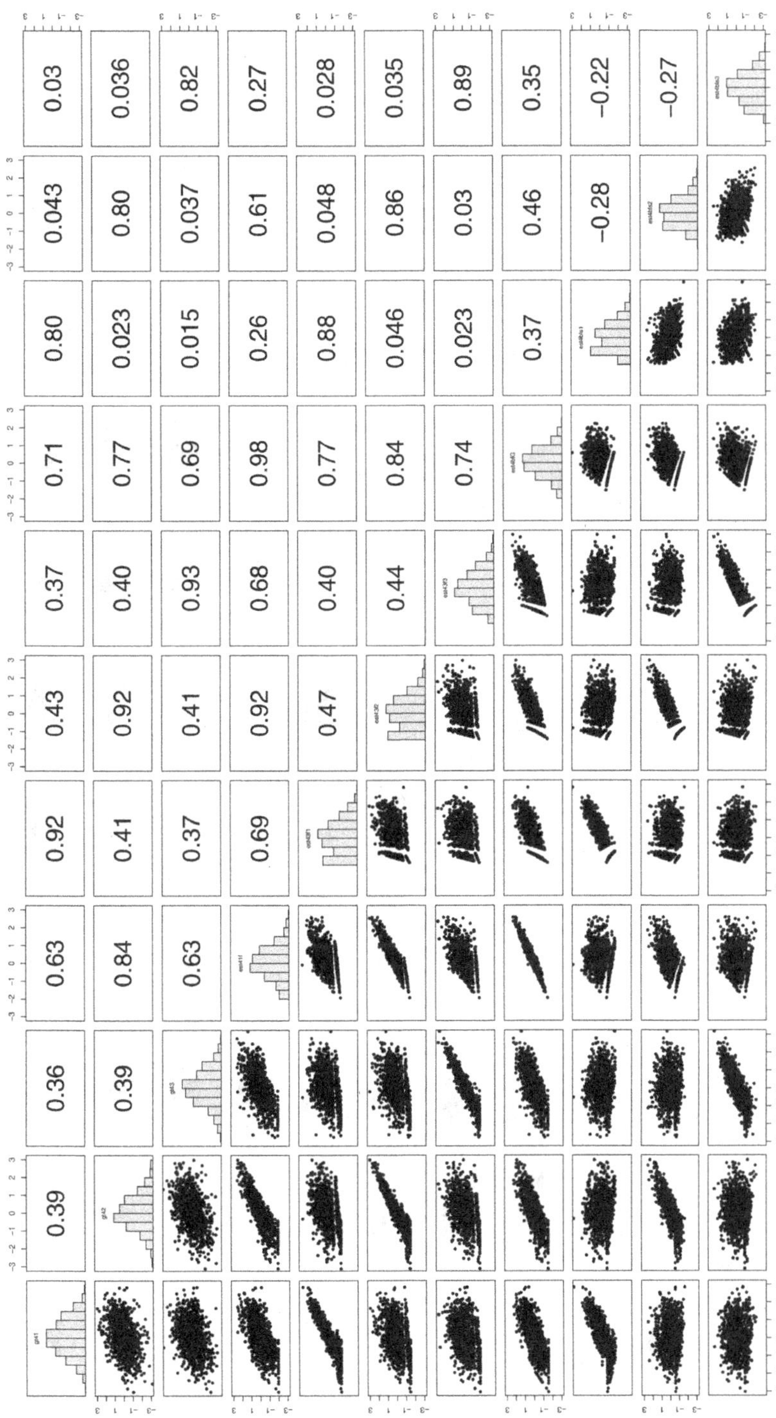

Figure 8.2 A matrix plot detailing results from the three-factor simulated example with inter-factor correlations of 0.4. Variable layout is described on p. 168. Elements in the upper triangle of the matrix are Pearson product moment correlations between the two corresponding variables. Elements in the lower triangle of the matrix are scatterplots between the two corresponding variables. Elements on the diagonal are histograms of the corresponding variables. This figure describes a 1,000-person random subsample of the 3,000 generated data points used in the analyses.

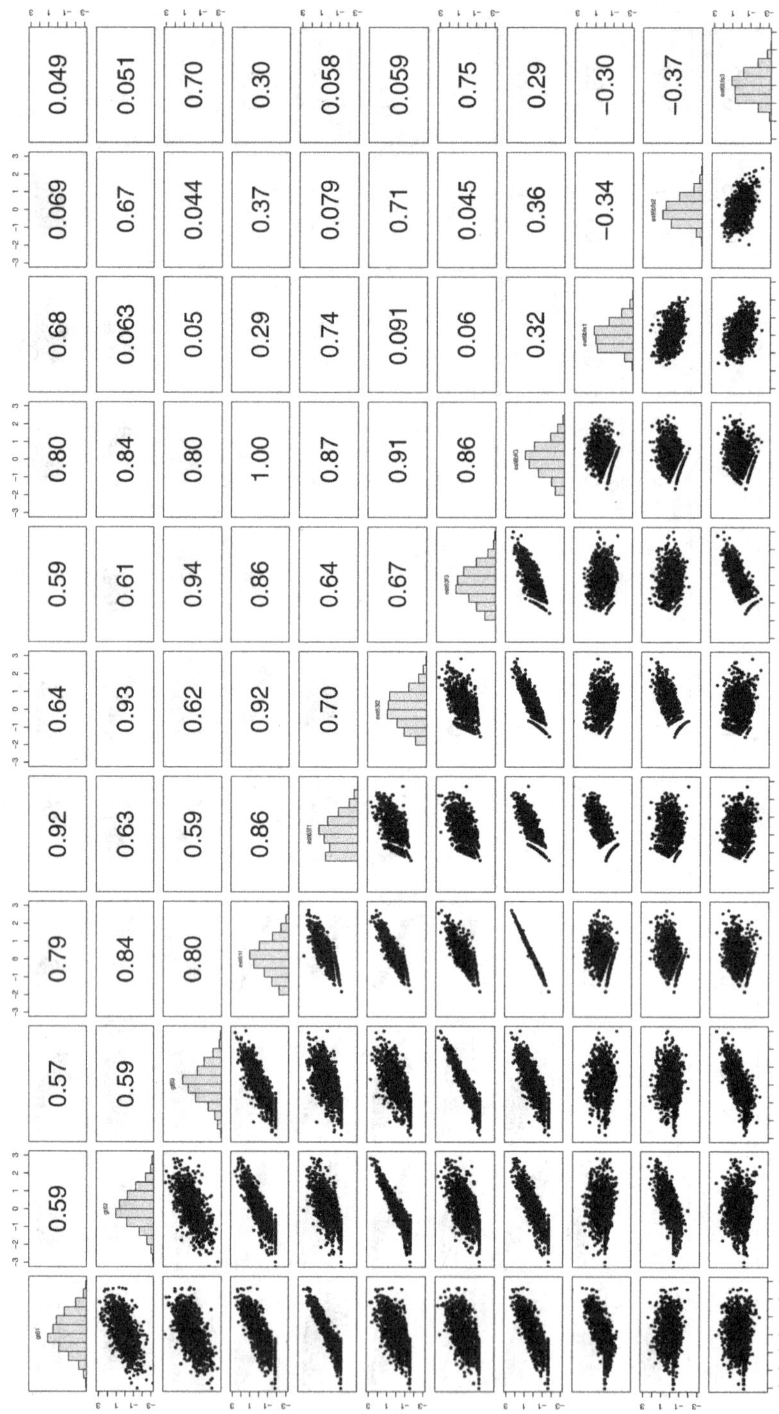

Figure 8.3 A matrix plot detailing results from the three-factor simulated example with inter-factor correlations of 0.6. Variable labels appear in the diagonal of the matrix. Elements in the upper triangle of the matrix are Pearson product moment correlations between the two corresponding variables. Elements in the lower triangle of the matrix are scatterplots between the two corresponding variables. Elements on the diagonal are histograms of the corresponding variables. This figure describes a 1,000-person random subsample of the 3,000 generated data points used in the analyses.

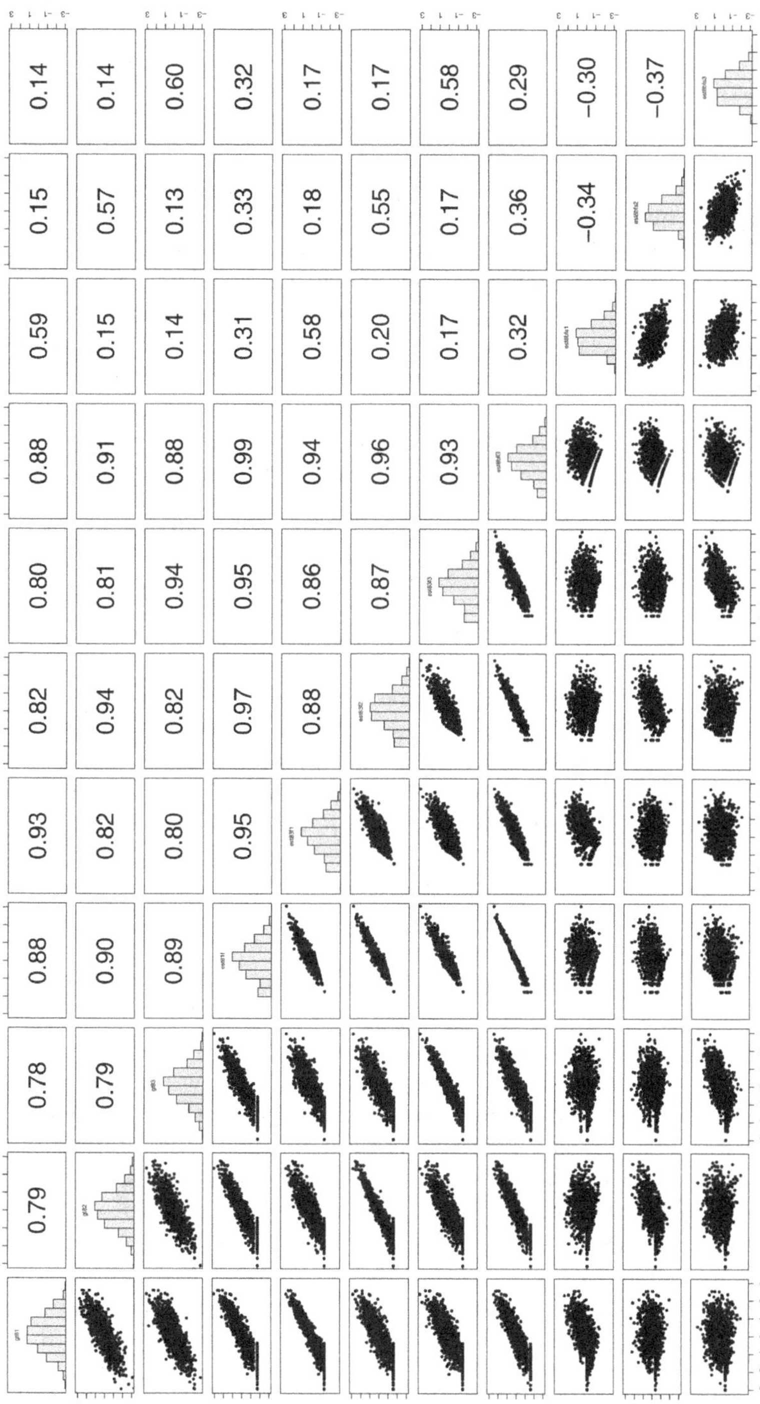

Figure 8.4 A matrix plot detailing results from the three-factor simulated example with inter-factor correlations of 0.8. Variable layout is described on p. 168. Elements in the upper triangle of the matrix are Pearson product moment correlations between the two corresponding variables. Elements in the lower triangle of the matrix are scatterplots between the two corresponding variables. Elements on the diagonal are histograms of the corresponding variables. This figure describes a 1,000-person random subsample of the 3,000 generated data points used in the analyses.

There is a large amount of information in each of these figures, but we will focus on a few particularly interesting pieces in this section. First, the overall trends are fairly similar across the three correlation conditions, so we focus our attention on Figure 8.3, which provides information on the model where the inter-factor correlations are 0.6. The most notable feature among the correlations is a 1.00 correlation between estimated θs from a single factor model and the general factor in a bifactor model. This suggests that, at least in this case, the θ specified by the mis-specified one-factor model and the θ specified by the over-specified bifactor model are, for most practical purposes, identical. The last four rows/columns display the relationships among the four latent scores estimated as part of the bifactor model. Although the bifactor model estimates the parameters with the imposed constraint that all of the factors are uncorrelated, it is interesting to see how correlated the resulting EAP estimates are.[4] These are not huge values, ranging from 0.29 to 0.37 in absolute magnitude, but they are quite far from zero. The scatterplots clearly demonstrate floor effects in a number of places. This is not unexpected given that the items in this particular item bank were not meant to provide particularly reliable scores below the population average.

Simulated Data Summary

With the exception of the $r = 0.8$ condition, the one-factor model would likely be rejected as a competing model when compared with the three-factor or bifactor models. If one were choosing between three-factor and bifactor models, parsimony (and the AIC and BIC) would suggest a preference for the three-factor model. As previously mentioned, though, one thing to keep in mind when choosing between models is the intended use of the results. In an IRT context, "results" usually refers to factor scores/θ estimates that are used to make some sort of decision regarding an individual. In some cases, the distinction between the three factors could be tremendously important and the pattern of θs for each person could be very useful/informative. However, in other cases, a single number summary may be more desirable for a certain purpose. In these cases, the general factor might be a more useful score, even if the model is somewhat over-fit.

This raises an interesting question: How do we reconcile the fact that the general factor score from the bifactor model is nearly perfectly correlated with the scores from the one-factor model, despite its superior fit?[5] For starters, bear in mind that the bifactor model produces four scores in this example, not just one. While the scores from the general factor may contain no more information than the scores from the one-factor model, the package of four scores (one general and three specific) does. This may provide a warning to researchers who would use a bifactor model to achieve adequate fit, but then only use the general factor scores subsequently. There are many similar instances in the literature where the model used to evaluate fit is not the eventual model used to produce scores. One common example is when a factor model is used to establish dimensionality, but then a summed score approach is used to create scores. In such a case, the scoring model has never been directly evaluated for fit and may or may not fit the data well.

Another thing to bear in mind is that model fit statistics are quite narrow in the question they are meant to address: How well does the specified model and the estimated parameters recreate the observed data? This is certainly an important question, as a model

4 In fact, we were surprised enough by these results that we reran everything using WLSmv in Mplus. The resulting estimates showed similar magnitudes and patterns.

5 A similar discussion can be found in Reise, Scheines, Widaman, and Haviland (2013) regarding the issue of when data are "unidimensional enough" to fit a single-dimension factor analysis model.

that fails to explain the observed data is unlikely to be of much use. Most of null hypothesis testing that exists for fit statistics, which test the fundamentally uninteresting question of whether the model we fit is an exact replication of the mechanism generating the data, do not necessarily tell us what we want to know. In this case, for example, we cannot reject the bifactor model as the generating mechanism, but we know it was not. Because the bifactor model is a more general version of the higher-order model, and we know that the three-factor model is equivalent to the higher-order model, this result should perhaps not be surprising. Simulated data represent an anomalous case where we know what the right answer is—indeed, it may be the only time in factor analysis *where there is a right answer at all.* The four scores of the bifactor model in this case are not the right answer, but they are able to reproduce the important aspects of the right answer as evaluated by the various model fit statistics. In the real world, with real data, fit statistics don't tell us what is true (or not), simply what is able to reproduce what we see (or not).

A Real Data Example

Method

In this example we use data from Brodey and colleagues' (under review) development of the Brodey Depression Scale (BDS).[6] A total of 915 participants were recruited from both private (n = 401) and public (n = 514) mental health clinics. More than half of the sample was female (72.4%) and a majority of the sample self-identified as either Caucasian/white (57.2%) or African American (35.1%). All participants were older than the age of 18. Four participants did not complete any of the 34 BDS[7] items, reducing the sample size for this example to 911.

As can be seen in Table 8.3, each of the 34 items was hypothesized to map directly onto one of the DSM-IV-TR (APA, 2000) criteria for Major Depressive Episode (MDE). Each item had five response categories ranging from "strongly disagree" to "strongly agree." The substantive goal of the original project was to identify an appropriate statistical model for the BDS. Two specific models were examined: a one-factor graded response model and a DSM-consistent bifactor[8] graded response model.

The one-factor model consisted of a single latent variable (MDE) that was hypothesized to account for the common variance among all of the items. The bifactor model allowed all items to load onto a single latent variable (MDE) and one of 10 specific factors (criterion 1–5, 7–10, & C in Table 8.3). Each specific factor corresponded to either the MDE symptoms in Criterion A or the distress/impairment identified in Criterion C. Only a single item was available for the psychomotor criterion, so this item was allowed to load only on the general MDE factor. When a specific factor had only two items associated with it (e.g., loss of energy), the slopes relating those items to their specific factor were constrained

6 The original BDS development found varying levels of differential item functioning depending on the type of clinic, gender, and race. We ignore these differences here for ease of presentation but note that the pattern of the results presented here reflects those discussed in the original paper.

7 The original manuscript examines 35 items. However, the models discussed in the original paper include multiple group, bifactor models accounting for differential item functioning. Because these complexities are ignored in this example, one item (Q1482 "I had a hard time getting things done") was removed from this example.

8 Technically, as one of the items only has a relationship to the general factor, this model is not a bifactor model. However, it is very close to a bifactor model in specification and identical in purpose, so we refer to it as such in the remainder.

Table 8.3 Item Content and DSM-IV-TR Criterion for the 35 BDS Items

Item #	*Wording*	*DSM-IV-TR Criterion*
Q1213	I felt sad.	1: Depressed Mood
Q1217	I felt like nothing went right for me.	1: Depressed Mood
Q1270	I felt happy.	1: Depressed Mood
Q1275	I felt hopeless about the future.	1: Depressed Mood
Q1460	Sadness interfered with my life.	1: Depressed Mood
Q1328	I felt irritated.	2: Irritation (Depression)
Q1329	I was easily irritated.	2: Irritation (Depression)
Q1215	I had fun.	3: Anhedonia
Q1299	I was interested in doing things.	3: Anhedonia
Q1302	I enjoyed doing things in my free time.	3: Anhedonia
Q1303	I enjoyed life.	3: Anhedonia
Q1375	The things I usually enjoy bored me.	3: Anhedonia
Q1305	I had no appetite.	4: Weight/appetite
Q1475	I ate too much.	4: Weight/appetite
Q1288	I fell asleep easily at night.	5: Insomnia/hypersomnia
Q1292	I slept well in the middle of the night.	5: Insomnia/hypersomnia
Q1293	I slept too much.	5: Insomnia/hypersomnia
Q1333	I slept well.	5: Insomnia/hypersomnia
Q1461	I woke up too early and could not fall back to sleep.	5: Insomnia/hypersomnia
Q1219	I felt tense.	6: Psychomotor
Q1295	I got tired quickly.	7: Loss of energy
Q1334	I got tired easily.	7: Loss of energy
Q1278	I felt successful.	8: Worthlessness/Inappropriate Guilt
Q1281	I felt guilty.	8: Worthlessness/Inappropriate Guilt
Q1304	I felt worthless.	8: Worthlessness/Inappropriate Guilt
Q1228	I had a hard time concentrating.	9: Cognition
Q1283	I had a hard time making decisions.	9: Cognition
Q1285	I had a hard time remembering things.	9: Cognition
Q1286	I was able to think clearly.	9: Cognition
Q1276	I felt like ending my life.	10: Suicidal ideation
Q1277	I had thoughts of ending my life.	10: Suicidal ideation
Q1394	I had difficulty taking care of my household responsibilities.	C: Functional Impairment
Q1462	I felt out of control.	C: Functional Impairment
Q1463	I felt like my life was out of control.	C: Functional Impairment
Q1482	I had a hard time getting things done.	C: Functional Impairment

Note: Question Q1219 is the only psychomotor item used on the BDS, thus it was not associated with any specific factor in the bifactor model.

to be equal. This is necessary for identification of a specific factor with two items and is functionally equivalent to a residual correlation commonly seen in the SEM framework. It was hypothesized that the bifactor model would better account for the observed responses given its greater fidelity to the clinical/conceptual model of MDE.

Both the one-factor and bifactor models were evaluated using flexMIRT® v. 1.88 (Cai, 2012). The models were compared using the AIC, BIC, M_2, and RMSEA using the criteria outlined in the simulated example. The scores and their standard errors were also compared across models.

Results

The hypothesized bifactor model had 10 specific factors. Early model evaluation found that the Appetite specific factor was not needed in the model (both appetite items had slopes of zero on the specific factor). This specific factor was removed from the final bifactor model. Both models (the one-factor and modified bifactor) converged without issue.

Table 8.4 provides the model fit for the one-factor and bifactor models. As can be seen in Table 8.4, the bifactor model was found to fit the data better than the one-factor model. As the bifactor model has many more parameters (roughly equal to the number of items) than the one-factor model, its superior performance was not surprising. However, both the AIC and BIC suggested that even when accounting for the additional parameters, the bifactor model was the preferred model.

The fit indices clearly support the bifactor model, but how do things look when we examine the estimated parameters? Table 8.5 contains the estimated IRT slopes for both the one-factor and bifactor models. Many of the slope parameters (a_1 for the one-factor and bifactor models) appear to differ substantially between the models. For example, the item Q1213 "I felt sad" was found to have a slope of 2.5 in the one-factor model and a slope of 3.5 in the bifactor model. In other cases, some of the parameter estimates appeared unrealistically high (see Q1276 in Table 8.5). For example, slope estimates higher than four in a 2PLM have been reported to be a sign of trouble in unidimensional models (Wirth & Edwards, 2007).

Although there are a number of rules of thumb about when slope values in IRT are high enough to cause concern, these were all derived *for unidimensional models*. When there is only one latent dimension to consider we can develop simple rules of thumb for the slopes (and intercepts to some degree) that generalize across most models. However, in MIRT models the magnitude of the slope estimates and whether such a magnitude is problematic is a function of other slopes/factors in the model. Standardizing the slopes, such as converting the IRT slopes to standardized factor loadings (see Table 8.6) allows for further evaluation of the parameter estimates. As can be seen in Table 8.6, once the

Table 8.4 Model Fit for Empirical Examples

Model	*AIC*	*BIC*	M_2	*DF*	*RMSEA*
1-factor	75209.2	76027.7	4583.1	425	0.10
Bifactor	71625.1	72578.4	1545.8	397	0.06

Note: AIC is the Akaike information criterion, BIC is the Bayesian information criterion, M_2 is the M_2^* statistic, DF is degrees of freedom of M_2^*, and RMSEA is the root mean square error of approximation computed using M_2^*.

Table 8.5 Real Data Example Model Parameter Estimates and Standard Errors in Parentheses

		Bifactor Model		
		General Factor	*Specific Factor*	*Specific Factor*
Item	*1-Factor Slope (se)*	*Slope (se)*	*Slope (se)*	
Q1213	2.46 (0.14)	3.51 (0.44)	1.63 (0.46)	2
Q1217	2.33 (0.12)	2.50 (0.14)	0.22 (0.12)	2
Q1270	2.36 (0.13)	2.35 (0.15)	0.09 (0.13)	2
Q1275	2.48 (0.13)	2.75 (0.15)	0.16 (0.12)	2
Q1460	2.53 (0.13)	3.22 (0.30)	1.28 (0.32)	2
Q1328	1.74 (0.11)	3.02 (0.20)	2.51 (0.15)	3
Q1329	1.74 (0.12)	3.15 (0.22)	2.51 (0.15)	3
Q1215	1.82 (0.10)	2.22 (0.15)	1.38 (0.14)	4
Q1299	1.91 (0.10)	2.47 (0.15)	1.56 (0.15)	4
Q1302	1.63 (0.10)	2.35 (0.19)	2.02 (0.22)	4
Q1303	2.31 (0.13)	2.81 (0.18)	1.29 (0.13)	4
Q1375	1.58 (0.10)	1.68 (0.11)	0.47 (0.09)	4
Q1305	0.92 (0.08)	0.96 (0.09)		
Q1475	0.32 (0.07)	0.36 (0.07)		
Q1288	1.12 (0.10)	1.69 (0.14)	2.10 (0.14)	5
Q1292	1.18 (0.10)	2.04 (0.16)	2.62 (0.18)	5
Q1293	0.30 (0.07)	0.42 (0.08)	-0.77 (0.09)	5
Q1333	1.34 (0.12)	3.48 (0.42)	4.49 (0.52)	5
Q1461	1.04 (0.09)	1.23 (0.11)	1.19 (0.10)	5
Q1219	1.81 (0.11)	1.94 (0.12)		
Q1295	1.16 (0.10)	2.38 (0.18)	3.00 (0.15)	6
Q1334	1.17 (0.10)	2.37 (0.19)	3.00 (0.15)	6
Q1278	1.77 (0.10)	1.89 (0.12)	0.47 (0.21)	7
Q1281	1.65 (0.10)	1.80 (0.12)	-0.13 (0.12)	7
Q1304	3.06 (0.17)	5.00 (1.85)	1.86 (1.35)	7
Q1228	1.84 (0.11)	2.98 (0.28)	2.17 (0.31)	8
Q1283	1.91 (0.11)	2.24 (0.14)	0.96 (0.11)	8
Q1285	1.34 (0.09)	1.67 (0.13)	1.32 (0.15)	8
Q1286	1.88 (0.11)	2.04 (0.13)	0.72 (0.11)	8
Q1276	1.89 (0.20)	5.91 (0.50)	5.01 (0.33)	9
Q1277	1.77 (0.19)	5.57 (0.44)	5.01 (0.33)	9
Q1394	1.00 (0.08)	1.06 (0.09)	0.04 (0.12)	10
Q1462	2.29 (0.13)	2.93 (0.34)	1.15 (0.41)	10
Q1463	2.56 (0.14)	3.53 (0.51)	1.34 (0.53)	10

Note: (se) indicates standard errors. "Specific Factor" indicates which specific factor a given item is related to.

Table 8.6 Real Data Example Factor Loading Estimates and Standard Errors in Parentheses

		Bifactor model		
		General Factor	*Specific Factor*	*Specific Factor*
Item	*1-Factor λ (se)*	*λ (se)*	*λ (se)*	
Q1213	0.82 (0.03)	0.83 (0.03)	0.39 (0.11)	2
Q1217	0.81 (0.02)	0.82 (0.02)	0.07 (0.07)	2
Q1270	0.81 (0.03)	0.81 (0.03)	0.03 (0.07)	2
Q1275	0.82 (0.02)	0.85 (0.02)	0.05 (0.06)	2
Q1460	0.83 (0.02)	0.83 (0.02)	0.33 (0.10)	2
Q1328	0.71 (0.04)	0.71 (0.04)	0.59 (0.04)	3
Q1329	0.72 (0.04)	0.72 (0.04)	0.57 (0.04)	3
Q1215	0.73 (0.03)	0.71 (0.04)	0.44 (0.06)	4
Q1299	0.75 (0.03)	0.73 (0.03)	0.46 (0.05)	4
Q1302	0.69 (0.04)	0.67 (0.04)	0.57 (0.06)	4
Q1303	0.81 (0.03)	0.80 (0.03)	0.37 (0.05)	4
Q1375	0.68 (0.04)	0.69 (0.04)	0.19 (0.06)	4
Q1305	0.48 (0.05)	0.49 (0.06)		
Q1475	0.19 (0.07)	0.21 (0.07)		
Q1288	0.55 (0.06)	0.53 (0.05)	0.66 (0.04)	5
Q1292	0.57 (0.06)	0.55 (0.05)	0.70 (0.04)	5
Q1293	0.17 (0.07)	0.22 (0.07)	-0.40 (0.07)	5
Q1333	0.62 (0.06)	0.59 (0.05)	0.76 (0.04)	5
Q1461	0.52 (0.05)	0.51 (0.06)	0.49 (0.05)	5
Q1219	0.73 (0.03)	0.75 (0.04)		
Q1295	0.56 (0.06)	0.57 (0.05)	0.72 (0.04)	6
Q1334	0.57 (0.06)	0.57 (0.05)	0.72 (0.03)	6
Q1278	0.72 (0.03)	0.73 (0.04)	0.18 (0.13)	7
Q1281	0.70 (0.04)	0.73 (0.04)	0.05 (0.08)	7
Q1304	0.87 (0.02)	0.89 (0.02)	0.33 (0.20)	7
Q1228	0.73 (0.03)	0.73 (0.03)	0.53 (0.06)	8
Q1283	0.75 (0.03)	0.75 (0.03)	0.32 (0.05)	8
Q1285	0.62 (0.05)	0.61 (0.04)	0.49 (0.06)	8
Q1286	0.74 (0.03)	0.74 (0.03)	0.26 (0.06)	8
Q1276	0.74 (0.06)	0.75 (0.04)	0.63 (0.04)	9
Q1277	0.72 (0.06)	0.73 (0.04)	0.65 (0.04)	9
Q1394	0.51 (0.05)	0.53 (0.06)	-0.02 (0.10)	10
Q1462	0.80 (0.03)	0.82 (0.03)	0.32 (0.14)	10
Q1463	0.83 (0.02)	0.85 (0.02)	0.32 (0.14)	10

Note: (se) indicates standard errors. “Specific Factor” indicates which specific factor a given item is related to.

slopes are converted to standardized factor loadings, very few differences (e.g., see λ_1 for Q1213 in both models) remain between the one-factor and bifactor (general factor) models. Moreover, what appeared to be extremely high parameter estimates using traditional cutoffs ($a_1 = 5.9$ for Q1276) were found to be within the acceptable parameter range ($\lambda_1 = 0.8$).

The similarity in standardized parameter estimates for the one-factor and bifactor general factor would suggest that the scores should also be similar (see Chapter 2, this volume). This was indeed found to be the case. EAP scores estimated using the parameter estimates for the one-factor model and the general factor from the bifactor model were found to be almost perfectly correlated ($r = 0.996$). While the point estimates were nearly redundant, the standard errors can still be quite different. In fact, the standard errors from these two sets of scores correlated only 0.7. The difference in the standard errors (bifactor minus one-factor) range from −0.11 to 0.17 with an average difference of 0.03 (SD = 0.002). As can be seen in Figure 8.5, while the two models may produce similar scores, failing to account for multiple sources of variance (if multiple sources do in fact exist) can result in inaccurate standard errors. In this particular instance, the researcher would conclude from the one-factor results that the scores were (in general) more reliable than they actually are. This can lead to several negative consequences including an adaptive test terminating early, incorrect conclusions regarding relative scale performance, and overconfidence in individual scores or in conclusions based on aggregation of scores.

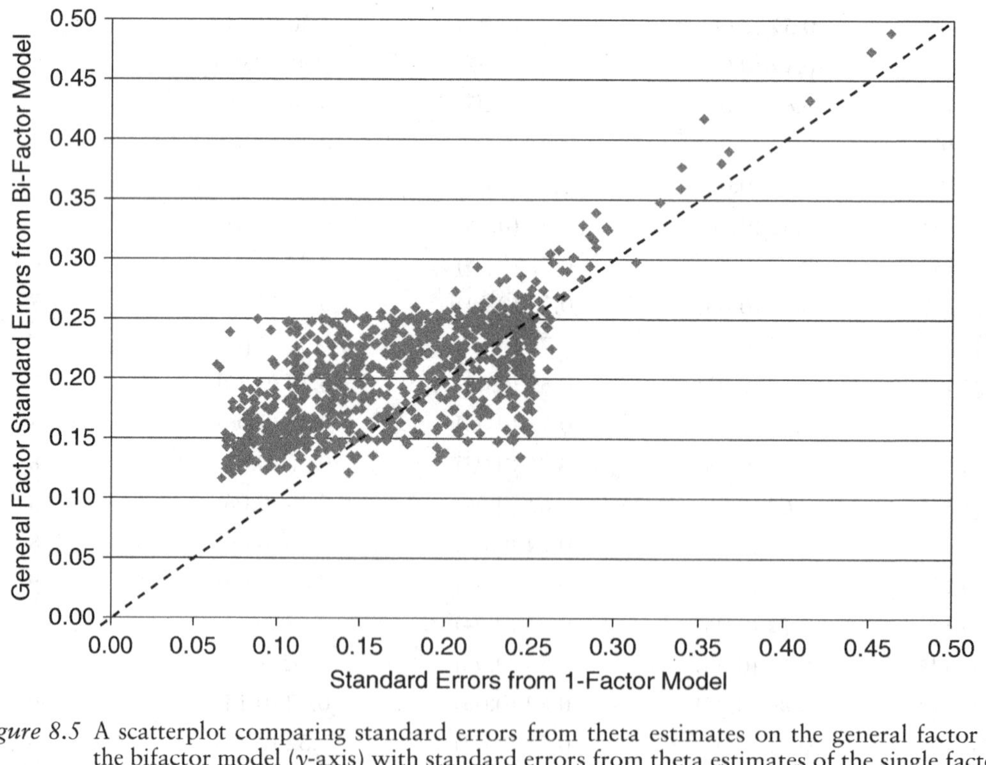

Figure 8.5 A scatterplot comparing standard errors from theta estimates on the general factor in the bifactor model (y-axis) with standard errors from theta estimates of the single factor from the one-factor model (x-axis).

Real Data Summary

The substantive goal of these analyses was to compare two competing models: a one-factor model and a bifactor model where the specific factors were hypothesized to correspond to the DSM-IV-TR criterion for MDE. Comparing the fit of the two models supports our hypothesis that the bifactor model was better able to reproduce the observed data.

Beyond the substantive conclusions, there are some interesting methodological lessons here. First, as we discussed earlier, existing rules of thumb in the IRT literature regarding reasonable values for slope estimates do not necessarily make sense when using multidimensional models. This underlines the value of having easy access to the results in the standardized factor loading metric. These data also highlight the tension between ideas of model fit and utility of results. In this case, if our intent was to use a single score to rank individuals, or select people for treatment, or as an outcome/predictor in subsequent models, there may be little practical benefit to adopting the more complex bifactor model. However, if part of our intent is to assess the reliability of a measure, or if the standard errors come into play in the subsequent use of scores, then the bifactor model's impact on results becomes more important. This example further serves to highlight that, even though one model may be far superior as judged by model fit statistics, in practice there may be less to recommend one model over another.

SUMMARY

The PROMIS® project has made great strides in making the advantages of IRT more widely available to those interested in measuring health outcomes. As people begin to use IRT more frequently, they will undoubtedly encounter situations that require the use of more complex models than the traditional unidimensional models. The tremendous advances in estimation have provided a number of methods capable of providing estimates for models with large numbers of factors. These methods have fairly quickly made their way into available software, which is a crucial step in making statistical advances in estimation available to researchers.

As the existing capabilities expand, researchers are pushing models, including IRT, into relatively new areas. The history of IRT provides an interesting example of this process. Notice that in IRT, there are actually two different phrases used (IRT and MIRT) to describe models with one factor or more than one factor. How odd would it be for there to be "unidimensional factor analysis" and "multidimensional factor analysis"? Indeed, despite the long-standing separation, this is exactly what we are describing when we use phrases like MIRT. As the barriers separating factor analysis and IRT are removed, we find interesting parallels and differences between how the two methods are used in practice. In this chapter, we have illustrated a few of the model selection problems facing MIRT users and provided some of the existing knowledge regarding these problems from a factor analytic perspective. We have also explored, from the perspective of scores, how fairly different models can have surprising levels of overlap.

Latent variable modeling is an inherently difficult process. In addition to very substantial problems of estimation, we face additional problems regarding validity. We not only have to prove our models are reasonable from a fit perspective, we have to support our claims that we are measuring what we say we are. Validity is an inherent challenge to all measurement, but it is a significant part of what brings value to the enterprise. When choosing between different possible statistical models, we must learn to rely both on statistical guidance in the form of model fit statistics and on the impact of model differences on the validity of the resulting inferences. Our efforts will be valuable to the extent that the scores we use are based on models that approximate reality and do so in a way that advances our substantive theory and understanding.

References

Adams, R.J., Wilson, M., & Wang, W. (1997). The multidimensional random coefficients multinomial logit model. *Applied Psychological Measurement, 21*, 1–23.

Akaike, H. (1974). A new look at the statistical model identification. *IEEE Transactions on Automatic Control*, 19, 716–723.

Albert, J.H. (1992). Bayesian estimation of normal ogive item response curves using Gibbs sampling. *Journal of Educational and Behavioral Statistics*, *17*(3), 251–269.

American Psychiatric Association. (2000). *Diagnostic and statistical manual of mental disorder* (4th ed., text rev.). Washington, DC: American Psychiatric Association.

Béguin, A.A., & Glas, C.A.W. (2001). MCMC estimation and some model-fit analysis of multidimensional IRT models. *Psychometrika, 66*, 541–562.

Bock, R.D., & Aitkin, M. (1981). Marginal maximum likelihood estimation of item parameters: Application of an EM algorithm. *Psychometrika, 46*, 443–459.

Bock, R.D., Gibbons, R., & Muraki, E. (1988). Full-information item factor analysis. *Applied Psychological Measurement*, *12*(3), 261–280.

Bolt, D.M., & Lall, V.F. (2003). Estimation of compensatory and noncompensatory multidimensional item response models using Markov chain Monte Carlo. *Applied Psychological Measurement, 27*, 395–414.

Bradlow, E.T., Wainer, H., & Wang, X. (1999). A Bayesian random effects model for testlets. *Psychometrika, 64*, 153–168.

Brodey, B., Wirth, R.J., Wilson, M.E., Goodman, S.H., Baldasaro, R.E., Brooks-DeWeese, A., Houts, C.R., Brodey I.S.B., & Doyle, N.M. (under review). Development of the Brodey Perinatal Depression Scale using item response theory.

Browne, M.W., & Cudeck, R. (1993). Alternative ways of assessing model fit. In K.A. Bollen and J.S. Long (Eds.), *Testing structural equation models* (pp. 136–162). Newbury Park, CA: Sage.

Cai, L. (2010a). High-dimensional exploratory item factor analysis by a Metropolis-Hastings Robbins-Monro algorithm. *Psychometrica, 75*(1), 33–57.

Cai, L. (2010b). A two-tier full-information item factor analysis model with applications. *Psychometrika, 75*, 581–612.

Cai, L. (2012). flexMIRT® version 1.88: A numerical engine for multilevel item factor analysis and test scoring. [Computer software]. Seattle, WA: Vector Psychometric Group, LLC.

Cai, L., Du Toit, S.H.C., & Thissen, D. (2011). IRTPRO: Flexible, multidimensional, multiple categorical IRT modeling [Computer software]. Chicago, IL: Scientific Software International.

Cai, L., & Hansen, M. (2013). Limited-information goodness-of-fit testing of hierarchical item factor models. *British Journal of Mathematical and Statistical Psychology, 66*, 245–273.

Cai, L., Yang, J.S., & Hansen, M. (2011). Generalized full-information item bifactor analysis. *Psychological Methods, 16*, 221–248.

Cella, D., Riley, W., Stone, A., Rothrock, N., Reeve, B., Yount, S., . . . the PROMIS Cooperative Group. (2010). The Patient Reported Outcomes Measurement Information System (PROMIS) developed and tested its first wave of adult self–reported health outcome item banks: 2005–2008. *Journal of Clinical Epidemiology, 63*, 1179–1194.

Cella, D., Yount, S., Rothrock, N., Gershon, R., Cook, K., Reeve, B., . . . the PROMIS Cooperative Group. (2007). The Patient Reported Outcomes Measurement Information System (PROMIS): Progress of an NIH Roadmap Cooperative Group during its first two years. *Medical Care, 45*, S3–11.

Diebolt, J., & Ip, E.H.S. (1996). Stochastic EM: Method and application. In W.R. Gilks, S. Richardson, & D.J. Spiegelhalter (Eds.), *Markov chain Monte Carlo in practice* (pp. 259–273). London: Chapman & Hall.

Duncan, K.A., & MacEachern, S.N. (2008). Nonparametric Bayesian modelling for item response. *Statistical Modeling, 8*, 41–66.

Edwards, M.C. (2005). MultiNorm: Multidimensional normal ogive item response theory analysis [Computer software].

Edwards, M.C. (2010). A Markov chain Monte Carlo approach to confirmatory item factor analysis. *Psychometrika, 75*(3), 474–497.

Edwards, M.C. (2013). Purple unicorns, true models, and other things I've never seen. *Measurement: Interdisciplinary Research and Perspectives, 11*, 107–111.

Flora, D.B., & Curran, P.J. (2004). An empirical evaluation of alternative methods of estimation for confirmatory factor analysis with ordinal data. *Psychological Methods, 9*(4), 466–491.

Green, B.F. (1976). On the factor score controversy. *Psychometrika, 41*, 263–266.

Hastings, W.K. (1970). Monte Carlo sampling methods using Markov chains and their applications. *Biometrika, 57*(1), 97–109.

Holzinger, K.J., & Swineford, F. (1937). The bi-factor method. *Psychometrika, 2*, 41–54.

Jöreskog, K.G., & Sörbom, D. (2003). LISREL 8.54 [Computer software]. Chicago, IL: Scientific Software International.

Junker, B.W., & Sijtsma, K. (2001). Nonparametric item response theory in action: An overview of the special issue. *Applied Psychological Measurement, 25*, 211–220.

Lee, S., & Herschberger, S. (1990). A simple rule for generating equivalent models in structural equation modeling. *Multivariate Behavioral Research, 25*, 313–334.

Li, Y., Bolt, D.M., & Fu, J. (2006). A comparison of alternative models for testlets. *Applied Psychological Measurement, 30*, 3–21.

Lunn, D.J., Thomas, A., Best, N., & Spiegelhalter, D. (2000). WinBUGS—a Bayesian modelling framework: Concepts, structure, and extensibility. *Statistics and Computing, 10*, 325–337.

MacCallum, R.C., Wegener, D.T., Uchino, B.N., & Fabrigar, L.R. (1993). The problem of equivalent models in applications of covariance structure analysis. *Psychological Bulletin, 114*, 185–199.

Martin, A.D., Quinn, K.M., & Park, J.H. (2011). MCMCpack: Markov chain Monte Carlo in R. *Journal of Statistical Software, 42*(9), 1–21.

Maydeu-Olivares, A. (2013). Goodness-of-fit assessment in item response theory models. *Measurement: Interdisciplinary Research and Perspectives, 11*, 71–101.

Maydeu-Olivares, A., Cai, L., & Hernandez, A. (2011). Comparing the fit of IRT and factor analysis models. *Structural Equation Modeling, 18*, 333–356.

Maydeu-Olivares, A., & Joe, H. (2005). Limited and full information estimation and testing in 2^n contingency tables: A unified framework. *Journal of the American Statistical Association, 100*, 1009–1020.

McDonald, R.P. (1985). *Factor analysis and related methods.* Hillsdale, NJ: Lawrence Erlbaum Associates.

Muthén, B., & Lehman, J. (1985). Multiple group IRT modeling: Applications to item bias analysis. *Journal of Educational Statistics, 10*, 133–142.

Muthén, L.K., & Muthén, B.O. (2008). Mplus version 5.1 [Computer software]. Los Angeles, CA: Muthén & Muthén.

Orlando, M., & Thissen, D. (2000). Likelihood-based item-fit indices for dichotomous item response theory models. *Applied Psychological Measurement, 24*, 50–64.

Pilkonis, P.A., Choi, S.W., Reise, S.P., Stover, A.M., Riley, W.T., & Cella, D. (2011). Item banks for measuring emotional distress from the Patient-Reported Outcomes Measurement Information System (PROMIS®): Depression, anxiety, and anger. *Assessment, 18*, 263–283.

Rabe-Hesketh, S., Skrondal, A., & Pickles, A. (2002). Reliable estimation of generalized linear mixed models using adaptive quadrature. *Stata Journal, 2*(1), 1–21.

Reckase, M.D. (2009). *Multidimensional item response theory.* New York: Springer.

Reise, S.P. (2012). The rediscovery of bifactor measurement models. *Multivariate Behavioral Research, 47*, 667–696.

Reise, S.P., Scheines, R., Widaman, K.F., & Haviland, M.G. (2013). Multidimensionality and structural coefficient bias in structural equation modeling: A bifactor perspective. *Educational and Psychological Measurement, 73*, 5–26.

Rindskopf, D., & Rose, T. (1988). Some theory and applications of confirmatory second-order factor analysis. *Multivariate Behavioral Research, 23*, 51–67.

Rizopoulos, D. (2006). ltm: An R package for latent variable modelling and item response theory analyses, *Journal of Statistical Software, 17*(5), 1–25.

Robbins, H., & Monro, S. (1951). A stochastic approximation method. *Annals of Mathematical Statistics*, 22(3), 400–407.

Rodebaugh, T.L., Woods, C.M., & Heimberg, R.G. (2007). The reverse of social anxiety is not always the opposite: The reverse-scored items of the social interaction anxiety scale do not belong. *Behavior Therapy, 38*, 192–206.

Rosseel, Y. (2012). lavaan: An R package for structural equation modeling. *Journal of Statistical Software*, *48*(2), 1–36.

Rubin, D.B. (1991). EM and beyond. *Psychometrika, 56*, 241–254.

Schwarz, G.E. (1978). Estimating the dimension of a model. *Annals of Statistics, 6*, 461–464.

Steiger, J.H., & Lind, J.M. (1980). Statistically based tests for the number of common factors. Paper presented at the annual meeting of the Psychometric Society, Iowa City, IA.

Takane, Y., & de Leeuw, J. (1987). On the relationship between item response theory and factor analysis of discretized variables. *Psychometrika, 52*, 393–408.

Thissen, D. (2012). *Using the testlet response model as a shortcut to multidimensional item response theory subscore computation.* Paper presented at the International Meeting of the Psychometric Society, Lincoln, NE.

Thissen, D., & Steinberg, L. (1988). Data analysis using item response theory. *Psychological Bulletin, 104*, 385–395.

Wang, X., Bradlow, E.T., & Wainer, H. (2002). A general Bayesian model for testlets: theory and applications. *Applied Psychological Measurement, 26*, 109–128.

Wirth, R.J., & Edwards, M.C. (2007). Item factor analysis: Current approaches and future directions. *Psychological Methods, 12*, 58–79.

Woods, C.M. (2006). Careless responding to reverse-worded items: Implications for confirmatory factor analysis. *Journal of Psychopathology and Behavioral Assessment, 3*, 189–194.

Woods, C.M., & Thissen, D. (2006). Item response theory with estimation of the latent population distribution using spline-based densities. *Psychometrika, 71*, 281–301.

Wu, E.J.C., & Bentler, P.M. (2011). EQSIRT: A user-friendly IRT program. [Computer Software]. Encino, CA: Multivariate Software, Inc.

Yung, Y.-F., Thissen, D., & McLeod, L.D. (1999). On the relationship between the higher-order factor model and the hierarchical factor model. *Psychometrika, 64*, 113–128.

9 Using Hierarchical IRT Models to Create Unidimensional Measures From Multidimensional Data

Brian D. Stucky and Maria Orlando Edelen

Introduction

Approaching the measurement of psychological constructs from an item analysis tradition (e.g., item response theory (IRT)) often reveals the inadequacy of single-factor or simple structure models in describing complex psychological phenomena. When test analysts closely evaluate the interrelationships among a collection of item responses it is not uncommon to find that a more complex measurement model is needed. For example, consider the seemingly well-known mental health construct of depression. Though responses to scales measuring depression are routinely treated as though there is only a single latent trait accounting for their covariance, item analysis often uncovers the presence of a single *general* dimension common to all the items, but additional *specific* dimensions that account for the uniqueness of content clusters (e.g., somatic symptoms; Irwin et al., 2010). In these modeling scenarios, some type of general hierarchical IRT model (e.g., bifactor or two-tier) may be appropriate.

This chapter reviews the structure of traditional bifactor models along with more recent advances in generalizations of bifactor model structure in the form of two-tier models that are being increasingly utilized to account for the covariance among items assessing psychological constructs. We begin by briefly reviewing the historical development of hierarchical item analysis. We then present the analytic structure of various multidimensional measurement models (for example, multidimensional IRT (MIRT; see Reckase, 2009), traditional bifactor IRT (Gibbons & Hedeker, 1992), and two-tier IRT models (Cai, 2010)) in an effort to highlight the utility and computational challenges of various modeling approaches. Next, using data from the Patient Reported Outcomes Measurement Information System (PROMIS®) adult anger, anxiety, and depression short forms (Pilkonis et al., 2011), we present a brief application of a bifactor IRT modeling process.

Finally, a general framework is offered that describes how unidimensional item subsets can be selected from a larger bifactor model (i.e., item-level dimensionality assessment). This framework may be useful in scale development scenarios where a unidimensional representation of a construct is desired, yet the data suggest multidimensionality. These item selection techniques are demonstrated by developing a hypothetical unidimensional *emotional distress* short form based on a bifactor IRT model representation of the three PROMIS® short forms. These techniques are developed as a response to the alternative of fitting unidimensional models to multidimensional data that is described in Chapter 2 of this volume.

Traditional and Restricted Bifactor Models

Holzinger and Swineford (1937) describe a bifactor pattern of loadings in which each item has a nonzero loading on exactly two factors: a general (i.e., primary) factor and a specific (i.e., secondary) factor. The item responses are conditionally independent after accounting for the general and specific dimensions. The general factor "runs through" all the items, effectively capturing their shared content with the unifying concept. The specific factors, of which there are at least two, account for response variation that is unique or particular to item subsets. For example, the uniqueness of the specific factors may be due to content, item formatting, or other conceptual influences that result in the item responses being correlated above and beyond their association with the general dimension. Consider, for example, the PROMIS® adult anger, anxiety, and depression item banks. Though these banks were developed to measure separate constructs, the interrelationships among the items suggest the possibility of a relatively strong general dimension representative of emotional distress. In this scenario, the bifactor IRT model allows for the measurement of a unifying emotional distress dimension, along with the specific dimensions in the fashion of subscales representing distinct underlying concepts (i.e., anger, anxiety, depression). In this manner IRT conceptualizations of bifactor models have been used in psychological (Thissen & Steinberg, 2010), health (Gibbons, Rush, & Immekus, 2009; Reeve et al., 2007; Reise, Morizot, & Hays, 2007), and educational research settings (Bradlow, Wainer, & Wang, 1999; Wainer, Bradlow, & Du, 2000; Wang, Bradlow, & Wainer, 2002).

While traditional bifactor models are useful in situations where a prominent (i.e., general) dimension is comprised of multiple subscales that are of interest in their own right, *restricted* bifactor models are useful in situations where a collection of items are generally unidimensional but small clusters of items (e.g., so-called item doublets or triplets) demonstrate unintended excess covariance. Unlike traditional bifactor models, when modeling restricted bifactor models the general dimension is usually of most concern and the specific dimensions are of less interest (hence they are commonly referred to as "nuisance" dimensions). The model is *restricted* in the sense that, in addition to the general dimension, items will only have an additional specific factor loading when necessary to account for excess local dependence (LD) that is not accounted for by the single dimension. LD, which refers to a violation of the IRT assumption of unidimensionality (i.e., local independence of items), often results from clusters of items having overly similar meaning or phrasing (Steinberg, 1994). By introducing specific dimension(s) for unwanted covariation formed by item clusters, doublets, or triplets, the restricted bifactor measurement model reestablishes the IRT assumption of conditional independence.

Historical Developments in Hierarchical IRT

Bifactor models have traditionally been estimated in a confirmatory factor analytic framework. This is due in part to the bifactor's historical roots in factor analysis (see Thurstone, 1947), and in part due to the computational ease of the factor analytic approach. For ordered-categorical responses, limited-information factor analysis of the polychoric correlation matrix is relatively straightforward and additional specific factors can be added to the model without burdening the estimation. Among the advantages of this method is the abundance of model fit indices available with mean and variance adjusted weighted least squares estimation (WLSMV; Muthén, du Toit, & Spisic, 1997) or diagonally weighted least squares estimation (DWLS; Jöreskog & Sörbom, 1988) (e.g., CFI, TLI, RMSEA). However, this approach requires a complete pairwise correlation matrix, and estimates may be unstable as the sample proportions become small in the two-way frequency tables. The information is "limited" in this sense because the only available information is contained in the pairwise correlations.

In contrast to limited information factor analysis, hierarchical IRT models (including bifactor IRT models) have their roots in the full-information item analysis framework for categorical response items. Bock and Aitken (1981) first describe the relationships among item responses in a single-dimension IRT framework using marginal maximum likelihood estimation with the expectation maximization algorithm (MML-EM), which was then extended by Bock, Gibbons, and Muraki (1988) to allow for the estimation of multiple dimensions. Following these advancements, Gibbons and Hedeker (1992) then provided a bifactor IRT model with an approach to item parameter estimation consistent with the methodology of Bock and Aitken (1981). The Gibbons and Hedeker approach capitalized on the within-item two-dimensional structure of the bifactor model to allow for the routine estimation of high-dimensional bifactor IRT models.[1]

Research Methods

The differences between various multidimensional hierarchical IRT approaches are best described by examining them in some analytic detail. In this section we review the relative advantages and disadvantages of traditional MIRT, bifactor, and two-tier IRT models. To aid in the presentation of the structure of these models we adopt a consistent notation that will be used throughout the remainder of this chapter. To begin we assume there are $i = 1, \ldots, N$ respondents and $j = 1, \ldots, n$ items with K_j response categories such that y_{ij} represents the response y from person i to item j and $\mathbf{y}$ is a $n \times 1$ response pattern vector of person i, for simplicity we will assume i and j subscripts are implicit in the $\mathbf{y}$ response vector. For now we use Cai's (2010) notation and assume that the responses $\mathbf{y}$ are accounted for by an IRT model with an $S \times 1$ vector of latent variables for the specific dimensions $\xi_i = (\xi_{i1},\ldots,\xi_{is})'$ and a $G \times 1$ vector of latent variables for the general dimensions $\eta_i = (\eta_{i1},\ldots,\eta_{iG})'$. Considering a vector of general dimensions is a departure from the traditional bifactor model but will enable analytic comparisons to more recent, generalized versions of the bifactor model.

The following marginal likelihood computations assume that specific dimensions $\boldsymbol{\xi}$ and general dimensions $\boldsymbol{\eta}$ are orthogonal to one another, and the joint probability density is simply the product of the separate univariate distributions for the general and specific dimensions:

$$f(\mathbf{y} \mid \eta_i, \xi_i) = f(\mathbf{y} \mid \eta_i) f(\mathbf{y} \mid \xi_i). \tag{9.1}$$

Otherwise known in the IRT literature as conditional independence, Equation (9.1) indicates that the joint likelihood of all general and specific dimensions can be computed from the product of the dimensions. The assumption is that the correlation between the item responses is due entirely to the presence of the general and specific dimensions, and that after these dimensions are accounted for the item responses should be uncorrelated. There is a large literature on the impact of violating the assumption of conditional independence in the IRT literature (Ackerman, 1989; Ansley & Forsyth, 1985; De Ayala, 1994; Drasgow & Parsons, 1983; Harrison, 1986; Luecht & Miller, 1992; Reckase, 1979; Tuerlinckx & De Boeck, 2001; Way, Ansley, & Forsyth, 1988); however, the topic is much less frequently addressed in regards to bifactor IRT and other MIRT models, primarily because these models are specifically fit in order to account for violations of the unidimensionality assumption.

1 It is worth noting that the development of hierarchical IRT models evolved alongside several other related methodologies. In particular the correlated-traits MIRT model shares many similarities with hierarchical IRT (for review, see Reckase, 2009). Likewise, item factor analytic approaches serve as a bridge between analytic approaches that are sometimes seen as strictly factor analytic or item response theory based. In particular, see Reise (2012) for a comparison of IRT and factor analytic approaches to the bifactor model, and Takane and de Leeuw (1987), Bartholomew and Knott (1999), Bolt (2005), and Wirth and Edwards (2007) for general reviews of the relationship between IRT and factor analytic models.

Multidimensional IRT Likelihoods

The marginal distribution of a standard multidimensional IRT model is comprised of a number of correlated dimensions that are commonly referred to in the MIRT literature simply as a vector of latent variables $\boldsymbol{\theta}$. However, to maintain a constant notation and to aid in later comparisons to the bifactor model we refer to the set of dimensions as $\boldsymbol{\eta}$ and $\boldsymbol{\xi}$, noting that this temporarily results in some unnecessary notational clutter. Assuming this arrangement the marginal distribution of the unrestricted MIRT model is:

$$f(\mathbf{y}) = \int_{-\infty}^{\infty}\cdots\int_{-\infty}^{\infty} f(\mathbf{y}_i \mid \eta_1 \ldots \eta_G, \xi_1 \ldots \xi_S)\, d\eta_1 \ldots d\eta_G, d\xi_1 \ldots d\xi_S. \tag{9.2}$$

The integrand containing the complete set of latent variables is typically approximated with computationally intensive Gaussian rectangular quadrature across a range of equally spaced nodes Q with corresponding weights (or heights) W given by the normal densities for the latent dimensions X_q:

$$L(\mathbf{y}) \approx \sum_{qG=1}^{Q}\cdots\sum_{q1=1}^{Q},\sum_{qS=1}^{Q}\cdots\sum_{q1=1}^{Q} f(\mathbf{y} \mid X_{q1}\ldots X_{qS}, X_{q1}\ldots X_{qG}) W(X_{q1})\ldots W(X_{qS}), W(X_{q1})\ldots W(X_{qG}). \tag{9.3}$$

The "challenge of dimensionality," as Wirth and Edwards (2007) note, is that in this arrangement of the marginal likelihood the number of quadrature nodes evaluated grows exponentially with increases in the number of dimensions. That is, the joint likelihood function is constructed from Q^{G+S} quadrature nodes, and each node must be evaluated with a call to the likelihood function. As the size of the model grows (i.e., the number of dimensions), fitting an IRT model becomes computationally prohibitive. It is in part for this reason that MIRT models have been slow to make inroads in many substantive research contexts. This challenge is especially central to many scale development scenarios or initial item analyses when multiple subfactors, triplets, or doublets need to be specified to achieve conditional independence among the item responses. In these situations even if one chooses to construct the joint-likelihood from a modest number of the quadrature nodes, the high-dimensional structure means that the number of computations needed to integrate across $G+S$ dimensions is beyond even the speed and memory capacities of modern computers.

Full-Information Bifactor IRT Model Likelihoods

To address this computational challenge, Gibbons and Hedeker (1992) developed a full-information estimation technique based on bifactor model restrictions that reduces the integration needed by transforming the unwieldy multidimensional likelihood function into a series of more manageable two-dimensional functions. Cai, Yang, and Hansen (2011) refer to the process of integral evaluations as iterated integration:

$$f(\mathbf{y}) = \int_{-\infty}^{\infty}\left\{\prod_{s=1}^{S}\int_{-\infty}^{\infty}\left[\prod_{j=1}^{n} f(\mathbf{y} \mid \eta_1, \xi_s)\right] f(\xi_s)\, d\xi_s\right\} f(\eta_1)\, d\eta_1. \tag{9.4}$$

In this presentation of the traditional bifactor joint-likelihood, the bifactor model assumes only a single general dimension (η_1) and S possible specific dimensions. In the Gibbons and Hedeker (1992) arrangement of the likelihood function, the two-dimensional η_1 and ξ_S integral is repeatedly evaluated for each specific dimension. Again the integrals can be evaluated with numeric quadrature:

$$f(\mathrm{y}) = \sum_{q_{G=1}}^{Q} \left\{ \prod_{S=1}^{S} \sum_{q=1}^{Q} \left[\prod_{j=1}^{n} f(\mathrm{y} \mid X_{G=1,} X_s) \right] W(X_s) \right\} W(X_{G=1}). \tag{9.5}$$

As can be seen, the number of two-dimensional integrations needed increases in multiples of the specific dimensions (i.e., $S \times Q^2$). This so-called dimensionality reduction allows even complex measurement models to be estimated with relative ease. For example, consider evaluating a six-dimensional bifactor measurement model with one general dimension and five specific dimensions and 21 quadrature nodes evenly spaced from –5 to 5 in multiples of 0.25, a reasonable number of points for many full-information analyses. Without the reduction in dimensionality inherent in bifactor model structure, using Equation (9.2) the number of evaluations needed for such a model is more than 85 million (21^6). Even with adaptive quadrature, which is useful in greatly reducing the number of necessary quadrature points and allows for the routine estimation of low-dimensional MIRT models (Schilling & Bock, 2005), the problem remains computationally intractable (Gibbons & Hedeker, 1992). However, using the dimensionality reduction technique (i.e., repeatedly integrating out the general dimension per specific dimension as in Equation (9.5)) the number of evaluations needed is reduced from Q^{G+S} in the unrestricted MIRT model to $S \times Q^2$ for the bifactor model, or in the present case to (5×21^2), a little more than 2,000.

Two-Tier Model Likelihoods

Application of the traditional bifactor model is limited to situations in which there is exactly one general dimension. This necessary restriction, although allowing for a computationally efficient algorithm, somewhat limits its applicability. Recently Cai (2010) has extended the earlier bifactor model work of Bock, Gibbons, and Muraki (1988) and Gibbons and Hedeker (1992) by developing the two-tier model (i.e., one tier for the general dimension(s) and one tier for the specific dimensions). The two-tier model may be viewed as a blending of traditional MIRT models and more restricted bifactor models: the model may include multiple correlated general dimensions, items may only load on one specific dimension, general and specific dimensions are orthogonal (and all specific dimensions are jointly orthogonal). Importantly, the added computational complexity of the model only occurs as the number of general dimensions increases:

$$f(\mathrm{y}_i) = \int_{-\infty \Re G}^{\infty} \prod_{s=1}^{S} \int_{-\infty}^{\infty} \left[\prod_{j \in I_s} f(\mathrm{y} \mid \eta, \xi_s) f(\xi_s) d(\xi_s) \right] f(\eta) d(\eta). \tag{9.6}$$

The difference between the bifactor model Equation (9.4) and the two-tier model Equation (9.6) is that the two-tier model iterates the simultaneous integration of all general dimensions G and each specific dimension (only for those items pertaining to the specific dimension as indexed by I_S) across the number of specific dimensions. The conditional independence assumption in Equation (9.1) may be updated to incorporate two-tier model efficiency:

$$f(\mathrm{y} \mid \eta, \xi) = \prod_{S=1}^{S} \prod_{j \in I_s} f(y_j \mid \eta, \xi_s). \tag{9.7}$$

Cai (2010) restates the conditional independence assumption in Equation (9.1) for general MIRT models as the joint likelihood of the product of the general dimensions and each specific dimension across the set of specific dimensions. Using two-tier model restrictions the number of function calls needed is now $S \times Q^{G+1}$ as per the general two-tier model, as opposed to Q^{G+S} calls for the standard MIRT model and $S \times Q^2$ calls for the traditional bifactor models:

$$f(\mathbf{y}) = \sum_{q_{G=1}}^{Q} \cdots \sum_{q_1}^{Q} \left\{ \prod_{S=1}^{S} \sum_{q=1}^{Q} \left[\prod_{j \in I_s}^{n} f(y \mid (X_1, \ldots, X_G)', X_q) W_q \right] \right\} W_{q_1} \ldots W_{q_G}. \tag{9.8}$$

This model extends the possible applications of hierarchical IRT by allowing for a variety of factor patterns. However, the two-tier model is still somewhat more restrictive than a general multidimensional IRT model. For example, the two-tier specific factors are uncorrelated with each other and with the general factors, and only one specific factor loading may be estimated per item. Nonetheless, the two-tier model is less restrictive than the standard bifactor IRT model given that multiple correlated general factors are permitted. With the same restrictions, other multidimensional IRT models like correlated MIRT models (Reckase, 2009), testlet IRT models (Wainer et al., 2007), and bifactor IRT models (Gibbons & Hedeker, 1992) conform to the two-tier model structure (see Cai, 2010 for more details).

Consider Tables 9.1 and 9.2 that present hypothetical bifactor-like models with multiple general dimensions, which we may now call two-tier models. Table 9.1 presents a model with two general dimensions each with a *doublet* item pair identified by their specific dimension slopes constrained to equality to identify the model (i.e., analogous to a one-degree of freedom residual correlation in factor analysis). A two-tier model of this variety is useful when the data suggest two *nearly* unidimensional factors, but with the presence of LD. Modeled as such, the two-tier algorithm can estimate a specific dimension within each general dimension and the correlation between the general dimensions.

Similarly, Table 9.2 presents a model that very nearly conforms to the traditional bifactor structure; however, in this case there is a doublet involving two items (4 and 5) that load on separate specific dimensions (item 4 loads on the first specific dimension, item 5 loads on the second). To satisfy the two-tier restrictions, this doublet is specified as a separate general dimension so that each item loads on no more than a single specific dimension. Specified in this manner the likelihoods for models in Tables 9.1 and 9.2 both require $2 \times Q^3$ function evaluations, still easily manageable by modern computing standards. In

Table 9.1 Example of Two-Tier Structure: Two General Dimensions, Each With a Doublet

Item	η_1	η_2	ξ_1	ξ_2
1	a_{11}		a_{11}	
2	a_{21}		a_{21}	
3	a_{31}			
4	a_{41}			
5		a_{52}		a_{52}
6		a_{62}		a_{62}
7		a_{72}		
8		a_{82}		

Note: For the purpose of identification the slope parameters in each specific dimension are constrained to equality.

Table 9.2 Example of Two-Tier Structure: Traditional Bifactor Model With a Doublet Across Both Specific Dimensions

Item	η_1	η_2	ξ_1	ξ_2
1	a_{11}		a_{11}	
2	a_{21}		a_{21}	
3	a_{31}		a_{31}	
4	a_{41}	a_{42}	a_{41}	
5	a_{51}	a_{52}		a_{52}
6	a_{61}			a_{62}
7	a_{71}			a_{72}
8	a_{81}			a_{82}

Note: For the purpose of identification the slope parameters in η_2 are constrained to equality.

fact, it seems that the two-tier reduction in integration demands makes possible all but the most complex models that could be envisioned in item and scale analysis scenarios.

Multidimensional IRT Models

Thus far our presentation of the hierarchical IRT model joint-likelihood estimation has left the item response model implicit. In this section we fill in that gap by briefly discussing item parameter interpretation when using multidimensional IRT models (Muraki & Carlson, 1993; Reckase, 2009). Although this discussion is applicable to any IRT model, we use Samejima's (1969) graded response model (GRM) as generalized to be applicable for MIRT. Later in this chapter we describe the multidimensional GRM and discuss how to interpret the dimensionality based on the (now conditional) slope parameters. This model describes the probability of responding in item response category k or higher, where $k = 0, 1, \ldots, m$. Using general two-tier structure, the multidimensional GRM for the two-tier model describes the cumulative response category probabilities as:

$$p^*(y = 1 \mid \eta, \xi_s) = \frac{1}{1 + \exp\left[-(a'\eta + a_s\xi_s + c_1)\right]}, \tag{9.9}$$

for responses in the first category. Response probabilities in the last category m are defined as:

$$p^*(y = m \mid \eta, \xi_s) = \frac{1}{1 + \exp\left[-(a'\eta + a_s\xi_s + c_m)\right]}. \tag{9.10}$$

P^* traces the probability that an item response is in category k or higher conditional on the vector of general dimensions (η) and at most one specific dimension (ξ_s) with corresponding slope parameters (**a**) that describe the strength of the relationship of the item response with each latent dimension, and $m - 1$ intercept parameters (c_k). The probability of responding in a particular category, k, is the difference between the probability of responding in category k or higher and the higher response, $k + 1$, or higher:

$$p(\eta, \xi_s) = p^*(k \mid \eta, \xi_s) - p^*(k + 1 \mid \eta, \xi_s). \tag{9.11}$$

Interpreting Conditional Parameter Estimates From MIRT Models

In practice using the slope parameters to interpret the dimensionality of hierarchical models is challenging because the interpretation is limited to assessing the probability of response on one dimension conditional on the model's other dimension(s). The difficulty is that unlike unidimensional models in which a slope on a general factor indicates the marginal item response relationship, a slope parameter in a multidimensional model indicates the relation of an item response with the given dimension conditional on all other dimensions for which the item loads. Hence, using the general dimension slope parameter to interpret the relation between the item and the general dimension may be confusing or misleading, because its magnitude depends on the magnitudes of the item's other slopes (on a specific dimension and any other general dimensions that may be present).

Stucky, Thissen, and Edelen (2013) use the following example to illustrate this challenge: consider two items with the following general and specific dimension slope parameters: item 1 with $a_{general} = 3$ and $a_{specific} = 2$, and item 2 with $a_{general} = 4$ and $a_{specific} = 3$. Though the conditional general dimension slope is higher in magnitude for item 2, the marginal relationship between this item and the general dimension is reduced given the item's relatively high conditional relationship with the specific dimension; as we will see shortly for this example, the net effect is that the strength of the relationship of both items with the general dimension is nearly identical. Such occurrences are not infrequent and clearly present an interpretive challenge even for those familiar with bifactor IRT models.

Marginal IRT Response Functions for Multidimensional Models

As a response to the challenge of interpreting the strength of the relationship between an item response and the general dimension in hierarchical IRT models, Ip (2010a, 2010b) and Stucky and colleagues (2013) developed marginal trace lines (i.e., the IRT response function; Lazarsfeld, 1950) for the general dimension that allow unidimensional-equivalent trace line interpretation. Generalized here for two-tier IRT models, to obtain the marginal trace line for the first general dimension η_1, one must integrate over the remaining general dimensions $(\eta_2 \ldots \eta_G)$ as well as the single specific dimension ξ_s on which the item loads. For example, in a two-tier IRT model, the marginal trace line for the first general dimension is:

$$p_{\text{Marginal}}(y \mid \eta_1) = \int f(\eta, \xi_s)\phi(\eta_2 \ldots \eta_G)\phi(\xi_s)d\eta_2 \ldots d\eta_G d\xi_s. \qquad (9.12)$$

In this example, the product of the conditional trace surface and the normal distribution density functions ϕ, integrated across the specific dimension ξ_2 and additional general dimensions $(\eta_2 \ldots \eta_G)$ is the marginal trace line for η_1, P_{Marginal}.[2] In other words, the marginal trace line is obtained by weighting the MIRT model response function by the normal distribution(s) and integrating out the specific (i.e., *nuisance*) dimension and other general dimensions. In practice this integral may be approximated computationally using quadrature.

Logistic Approximations of Marginal Trace Lines for Multidimensional Graded Response Models

After obtaining the marginal trace lines from the general hierarchical IRT model, it is useful to obtain their logistic approximations. For these logistic functions one can obtain IRT

2 Though we demonstrate the marginal trace line for the first general dimension, in practice it could be computed for any general dimension of interest.

item parameters that result in computationally tractable approximations to the marginal trace lines.[3] As an extension of methods proposed by Ip (2010a) for 2-PL and 3-PL models, for the graded response model the technique for obtaining the discrimination parameter estimate for the marginal trace line, a_1^*, from the conditional slope parameter a_1 is to transform the MIRT slope parameters into the bifactor loading metric (λ_1), and then reverse the transformation for the general dimension to arrive at the marginal slopes (Stucky et al., 2013). In other words, for the dimension of interest, in this case the general dimension θ_l:

$$\lambda_1 = \frac{a_1 / D}{\sqrt{1 + \sum (a/D)^2}}, \tag{9.13}$$

where λ_1 is the general dimension loading in factor analytic notation and D is the commonly used scaling constant 1.7. To simplify the notation, we use the square root of the item variance unexplained by the general latent dimension:

$$\sigma_1 = \sqrt{1 - \lambda_1^2}, \tag{9.14}$$

then the slope parameter estimate for the marginal trace line is:

$$a_1^* = \left(\frac{\lambda_1}{\sigma_1}\right) D \cdot \tag{9.15}$$

Because of the weighting process in Equation (9.12), the slope of the marginal trace line (a_1^*) is never greater in magnitude than the slope of conditional trace lines for θ_l given values of θ_2 (that is, the trace lines described by a_1) and depending on the relationship between the conditional slopes (a_1 and a_2) the marginal slope may be much smaller.

To obtain the marginal threshold estimates for the logistic approximations of the marginal trace line for the general dimension, the GRM intercept parameters are transformed for each dimension of interest after accounting for all other dimensions. Generalized from unidimensional IRT, for the multidimensional model the marginal threshold for the general dimension is the location on θ_1 where the probability of endorsing a particular response category is 0.5 given that all specific dimensions are fixed at zero. To obtain the threshold for the general dimension the exponents in Equations (9.9) and (9.10) are set to zero (because 1/ [1 + exp (0)] = 0.5), and all specific dimensions are then fixed to be zero so that the exponent is $a_1^* \ \theta_1 - c_{ik} = 0$, or rearranged for simplicity:

$$b_{ik}^* = {}^{-c_{ik}}\!\big/_{a_{1i}} \cdot \tag{9.16}$$

Here b_{ik}^* is the location on the general dimension where the probability of endorsing a particular response category is 0.5, averaged over the specific dimensions. Repeating this process for the specific dimension yields a different set of location parameters and may be helpful in understanding the compensatory nature of the model.

3 Regarding the use of the logistic distribution to approximate the normal CDF, Haley (1952) notes that the two never differ by probability values greater than 0.01. Further, Ip (2010a) provides a graphical illustration comparing marginal and logistic approximations that suggests close correspondence. In our experience, across a wide range of marginals the maximum difference in probability between the marginal and logistic approximation of the trace line is never more than about ±0.01. Given this close correspondence, it appears a logistic approximation is sufficiently accurate for most uses.

Application

In this final section we demonstrate the utility of the hierarchical IRT model as a means of describing dimensionality, but also as a way of informing the potential selection of unidimensional item subsets from a larger, multidimensional model. Using the item responses from three PROMIS® short forms (Anger, Anxiety, and Depression, as described later in this chapter), we first demonstrate that despite the high intercorrelations among the three short forms a violation of local independence occurs when the three scales are fit to a single underlying dimension. Next, we evaluate the resulting matrix of LD indices from the unidimensional model to inform the structure of a subsequent bifactor IRT model. Similar to Chapter 2 of this volume, we then consider the extent of the multidimensionality and provide some techniques for assessing the bias in parameter estimates that result from fitting a mis-specified unidimensional IRT model to multidimensional data. Finally, based on recently developed techniques for bifactor models, we explore the potential for selecting a subset of items from the bifactor model that may adequately fit a unidimensional model. As will be demonstrated, this technique serves to identify the items that are both closely representative of the general dimension and not overly influenced by the specific dimensions.

The data used in this application were collected as part of the development and evaluation of the emotional distress item banks from the PROMIS® initiative. PROMIS® is a multi-site research initiative designed to develop, evaluate, and standardize item banks for use in health outcomes research, and its framework includes calibrated item banks covering many domains of health outcomes. For the purposes of our example, we focus on the short form items from the adult emotional distress item bank domains of anger (8 items), anxiety (7 items), and depression (8 items) (Pilkonis et al., 2011). The data collection procedures used a randomized block design that assigned a subset of items to participants in order to maximize response coverage ($N = 15{,}725$). All items had the same five-point response scale with the options 0 = *never*, 1 = *rarely*, 2 = *sometimes*, 3 = *often*, and 4 = *always*.

Prior analyses of the PROMIS® anger, anxiety, and depression short forms by Pilkonis and colleagues revealed that distinct unidimensional models closely represent each short form. However, the somewhat strong factor score correlations (depression and anxiety $r = 0.81$, depression and anger $r = 0.60$, anxiety and anger $r = 0.59$; Pilkonis et al., 2011) led Pilkonis and colleagues to suggest that a single construct perhaps labeled "internalized distress" could potentially underlie all three domains. The purpose of this application is to explore the extent to which a bifactor IRT model may best reflect the relationship among the responses to these short forms, and then subsequently to use recently developed psychometric techniques to inform the selection of a unidimensional subset of items. The concept of a unidimensional set of item responses is clearly plausible when considering anxiety and depressive symptoms. Indeed, the idea of a single construct underlying both anxiety and depression has been widely studied and various authors have suggested a range of hierarchical theories each in an attempt to conceptually merge anxiety and depressive symptoms, including "general distress" (Clark & Watson, 1991; Watson et al., 1995a, 1995b), "internalizing spectrum" (Krueger, 1999; Krueger & Finger, 2001; Krueger, McGue, & Iacono, 2001), and "anxious apprehension" (Gray, 1987). In this tradition we propose that a single general underlying dimension, *emotional distress*, may best reflect the shared variance among a subset of anxiety and depression items. The relationship of the anger items with this general emotional distress dimension will also be considered.

Initial Unidimensional IRT Model

It is often informative to begin the item analysis process by fitting a parsimonious unidimensional model in a factor analytic framework. In this approach model fit indices and LD information (e.g., modification indices (Sörbom, 1989) in LISREL or *Mplus*) are often used to determine the appropriateness of a single-factor model or the need for a more complex hierarchical model. However, for our particular application the use of limited-information estimators (like WLSMV (Muthén, du Toit, & Spisic, 1997) in *Mplus* or DWLS (Jöreskog & Sörbom, 1988) in LISREL) is not possible because the data collection procedures used a randomized block design that resulted in bivariate missingness, predominately between anger and both anxiety and depression items.

Instead we began the model fitting process in an IRT framework by fitting the data to a unidimensional IRT model using marginal maximum likelihood in IRTPRO (Cai, du Toit, & Thissen, 2011). While the full-information model makes use of the complete individual response patterns, one loses access to traditional model fit indices that are helpful in establishing whether the item responses are characterized by a single or multidimensional model (for some recent IRT-based model fit indices, see Maydeu-Olivares & Joe (2005, 2006) and Maydeu (this volume). However, there are several IRT-based indices of LD (e.g., Chen & Thissen, 1997; Liu & Maydeu-Olivares, 2013; Liu & Thissen, 2012; Yen, 1984) that serve the same purpose as the more commonly used factor analytic-based modification indices. As will be shown, IRTPRO provides a matrix of standardized LD χ^2 indices based on differences between the unidimensional model-implied and model-observed bivariate response frequencies (Chen & Thissen, 1997) that provide a means of identifying unmodeled multidimensionality. These indices can be very useful in evaluating the appropriateness of the unidimensional model and correspondingly the need for additional dimensions.

Evaluating Slope Parameter Magnitude

After fitting the PROMIS® anger, anxiety, and depression short form responses with a single unidimensional IRT model, it is useful to first evaluate the magnitude of the slope parameters to establish any potentially dominant item content. Table 9.3 lists the unidimensional IRT parameters sorted by magnitude of the slope parameter within each short form. Clearly the depressive symptoms items dominate the factor structure (average slope = 3.37), followed to a somewhat lesser extent by anxiety (average slope = 2.87), with the anger items being less representative of the dimension (average slope = 2.23). Taken together these results provide the first indication that a possible general dimension may be more representative of feelings of depression and anxiety than feelings of anger (i.e., irritation/annoyance).

Evaluating LD Indices

Next, to understand the residual relationships among item responses that are not accounted for by the unidimensional model, we use the previously mentioned Chen-Thissen LD χ^2 to identify LD as implemented in IRTPRO. The matrix of LD indices provided in HTML format is arranged in deepening shades of red to reflect increasingly large positive LD or deepening shades of blue to reflect increasingly negative LD (which is often ignorable). For demonstration purposes, in Table 9.4 we simplify the resulting LD matrix by merely labeling positive LD as "+", negative LD as "-", and blank values in cells for which there is no bivariate response coverage.[4] To provide some contrast in the LD matrix, positive values greater than nine are in boldface. If the model were sufficiently unidimensional, then we would expect the standardized χ^2 from each item pair to randomly deviate between a

4 As a result of data collection procedures that used a randomized block design, the pairwise response coverage was particularly weak between anger items and both depression and anxiety items, resulting in noticeably more blank values in the anger—depression and anger—anxiety blocks of Table 9.4.

Table 9.3 Unidimensional Item Parameter Estimates for the PROMIS® Anger, Anxiety, and Depression Short Forms

		a	b_1	b_2	b_3	b_4
Anger 1	I felt like I was ready to explode	2.51	0.35	1.18	2.17	3.35
Anger 2	I stayed angry for hours	2.44	0.45	1.39	2.35	3.35
Anger 3	I was grouchy	2.44	-0.91	0.28	1.66	3.04
Anger 4	I felt angrier than I thought I should	2.38	-0.05	0.80	1.94	2.74
Anger 5	I felt annoyed	2.27	-1.24	-0.06	1.27	2.86
Anger 6	I felt angry	2.21	-0.91	0.39	1.85	3.16
Anger 7	I was irritated more than people knew	1.81	-0.93	0.03	1.29	2.48
Anger 8	I made myself angry about something just by thinking about it	1.75	-0.50	0.61	1.93	3.11
Depr 1	I felt helpless	4.21	0.36	0.90	1.62	2.34
Depr 2	I felt worthless	4.11	0.42	0.97	1.65	2.32
Depr 3	I felt hopeless	3.96	0.47	0.97	1.66	2.4
Depr 4	I felt that I had nothing to look forward to	3.38	0.34	0.93	1.60	2.37
Depr 5	I felt unhappy	3.29	-0.68	0.22	1.19	2.14
Depr 6	I felt depressed	2.94	-0.17	0.61	1.48	2.38
Depr 7	I felt sad	2.74	-0.55	0.43	1.45	2.42
Depr 8	I felt like a failure	2.36	0.21	0.88	1.82	2.57
Anx 1	I felt uneasy	3.93	-0.27	0.58	1.54	2.47
Anx 2	I felt tense	3.06	-0.57	0.30	1.27	2.35
Anx 3	I felt nervous	2.82	-0.29	0.64	1.67	2.78
Anx 4	I found it hard to focus on anything other than my anxiety	2.64	0.43	1.23	2.13	2.96
Anx 5	I felt worried	2.61	-0.60	0.28	1.37	2.37
Anx 6	I felt anxious	2.51	-0.18	0.67	1.72	2.67
Anx 7	I felt fearful	2.49	0.38	1.21	2.16	2.99

(small) positive or negative value. Taken as a whole, then, the matrix would show no pattern or clustering of positive or negative values, but rather a random arrangement of "+" or "-" symbols. So, while it is the case that a more nuanced level of detail is lost in this "+/-" display of the matrix, this particular presentation, just by virtue of the pattern of "+" and "-" symbols, shows a clear violation of the IRT assumption of unidimensionality.

Table 9.4 LD Indices for a Unidimensional Model

		Anger								*Depression*								*Anxiety*						
	Item	1	2	3	4	5	6	7	8	9	10	11	12	13	14	15	16	17	18	19	20	21	22	23
Anger	1		+	+	+	+	+	+	+	-	-	-						-	+				-	-
	2	+		+	+	+	+	+	+	-	-	-						-	-					
	3	+	+		+	+	+	+	+	-	-	-							-					
	4	+	+	+		+	+	-	+				-											
	5	+	+	+	+		+	-	-					-	-					-				
	6	+	+	+	+	+		-	-					-	-					-				
	7	+	+	+	-	-	-		+						-					-				
	8	+	+	+	+	-	-	+							-	+				+				
Depression	9	-	-	-							+	+	+	+	+	+	+	-	-	-	-	-	-	-
	10	-	-	-						+		+	+	+	+	+	+	-	-	-	-	-	-	-
	11	-	-	-						+	+		+	+	+	+	+	-	-	-	-	-	-	-
	12				-					+	+	+		+	+	+	+	+	-	+	-	-	-	-
	13					-	-			+	+	+	+		+	+	+	+	+	+	-	-	-	-
	14					-	-	-	-	+	+	+	+	+		+	+	+	+	+	-	-	-	-
	15								+	+	+	+	+	+	+		-	-	-	-	-	-	-	-
	16									+	+	+	+	+	+	-		-	-	-	-	-	-	-
Anxiety	17	-	-							-	-	-	+	+	+	-	-		+	+	+	+	+	+
	18	+	-	-						-	-	-	-	+	+	-	-	+		+	+	+	+	+
	19					-	-	-	+	-	-	-	+	+	+	-	-	+	+		+	+	+	+
	20									-	-	-	-	-	-	-	-	+	+	+		+	+	-
	21									-	-	-	-	-	-	-	-	+	+	+	+		+	+
	22	-								-	-	-	-	-	-	-	-	+	+	+	+	+		+
	23	-								-	-	-	-	-	-	-	-	+	+	+	-	+	+	

Note: Positive LD values are noted by "+"; positive values greater than nine in bold; and negative values are noted by "-".

That is, the covariance within each short form domain is stronger than predicted by a unidimensional model, which is indicated by predominantly bolded "+" cells in these quadrants of the table. Likewise, the item covariance across short form domains is weaker than expected by the model (indicated by predominantly "-" cells in the corresponding quadrants). Thus, in this particular case the pattern of LD neatly illustrates that anger, anxiety, and depression may comprise specific dimensions in a bifactor model.

A Bifactor IRT Model for the PROMIS® Emotional Distress Short Forms

To account for the unique variance among the anger, anxiety, and depression short form items as suggested by the LD indices in Table 9.4, and in order to evaluate the shared variance across these content clusters, we next fit a traditional bifactor model (see Table 9.5). We first note that the threshold estimates appearing in Table 9.5 are presented with respect

Table 9.5 Bifactor IRT Parameter Estimates for the PROMIS® Anger, Anxiety, and Depression Short Forms

	a_1	a_2	a_3	a_4	b_1	b_2	b_3	b_4
Anger 1	2.41	2.1	0	0	0.43	1.45	2.67	4.08
Anger 2	1.98	1.84	0	0	0.61	1.84	3.08	4.36
Anger 3	2.41	1.32	0	0	-1.00	0.29	1.79	3.30
Anger 4	2.07	1.9	0	0	-0.05	1.03	2.48	3.49
Anger 5	2.42	1.24	0	0	-1.30	-0.07	1.33	3.00
Anger 6	2.42	2.01	0	0	-1.05	0.46	2.16	3.67
Anger 7	2.17	1.05	0	0	-0.89	0.04	1.28	2.42
Anger 8	2.01	1.57	0	0	-0.52	0.68	2.12	3.37
Depr 1	4.18	0	1.81	0	0.41	1.01	1.79	2.58
Depr 2	4.44	0	2.22	0	0.48	1.09	1.85	2.61
Depr 3	4.71	0	1.93	0	0.50	1.03	1.75	2.54
Depr 4	3.71	0	2.13	0	0.40	1.07	1.81	2.69
Depr 5	3.63	0	0.56	0	-0.66	0.23	1.18	2.13
Depr 6	3.66	0	0.64	0	-0.18	0.58	1.43	2.28
Depr 7	3.74	0	0.35	0	-0.55	0.38	1.36	2.25
Depr 8	3.46	0	1.71	0	0.24	0.90	1.82	2.53
Anx 1	4.31	0	0	1.79	-0.29	0.58	1.57	2.55
Anx 2	3.15	0	0	1.43	-0.62	0.30	1.32	2.45
Anx 3	3.62	0	0	1.93	-0.31	0.65	1.73	2.88
Anx 4	3.16	0	0	1.29	0.43	1.26	2.17	3.00
Anx 5	3.35	0	0	1.22	-0.61	0.27	1.34	2.32
Anx 6	3.32	0	0	1.48	-0.20	0.66	1.70	2.62
Anx 7	2.65	0	0	1.16	0.37	1.23	2.22	3.06

Note: Threshold parameters were computed with respect to the general dimension.

to the general dimension using Equation (9.16). As Way, Ansley, and Forsyth (1988) noted, threshold estimates should not be expected to be sensitive to dimensionality because they are essentially transformations of the relative proportions of endorsed response categories. Indeed, in this example, there is little difference in these estimates relative to the thresholds from the unidimensional model in Table 9.3, which ignores local dependence. The average absolute difference between the unidimensional and bifactor model item thresholds is 0.04 (SD = 0.04), 0.08 (SD = 0.11), 0.16 (SD = 0.19), and 0.24 (SD = 0.27) for the first through fourth thresholds, respectively. The increasing discrepancy for the higher thresholds merely indicates a loss of estimation precision at the more extreme end of the distribution.

Next, we consider the challenge of interpreting conditional slope parameters in bifactor IRT models. Comparing the general dimension slope estimates in Table 9.5 to the unidimensional estimates in Table 9.3, we note that, without exception, the slope parameters for the general dimension of the bifactor model are larger in magnitude than those from the

Table 9.6 Factor Loadings and Marginal Slope Parameters Based on a Bifactor IRT Analysis

	Factor loadings					*Marginal slopes*			
	λ_1	λ_2	λ_3	λ_4	I-ECV	a_1	a_2	a_3	a_4
Anger 1	0.66	0.58	0	0	0.56	1.49	1.21		
Anger 2	0.62	0.58	0	0	0.53	1.34	1.21		
Anger 3	0.75	0.41	0	0	0.77	1.93	0.76		
Anger 4	0.63	0.58	0	0	0.54	1.38	1.21		
Anger 5	0.75	0.39	0	0	0.79	1.93	0.72		
Anger 6	0.68	0.56	0	0	0.60	1.58	1.15		
Anger 7	0.73	0.36	0	0	0.80	1.82	0.66		
Anger 8	0.66	0.51	0	0	0.63	1.49	1.01		
Depr 1	0.86	0	0.37	0	0.84	2.87		0.68	
Depr 2	0.85	0	0.42	0	0.80	2.74		0.79	
Depr 3	0.88	0	0.36	0	0.86	3.15		0.66	
Depr 4	0.81	0	0.46	0	0.76	2.35		0.88	
Depr 5	0.90	0	0.14	0	0.98	3.51		0.24	
Depr 6	0.90	0	0.16	0	0.97	3.51		0.28	
Depr 7	0.91	0	0.08	0	0.99	3.73		0.14	
Depr 8	0.82	0	0.41	0	0.80	2.44		0.76	
Anx 1	0.87	0	0	0.36	0.85	3.00			0.66
Anx 2	0.82	0	0	0.37	0.83	2.44			0.68
Anx 3	0.81	0	0	0.44	0.77	2.35			0.83
Anx 4	0.83	0	0	0.34	0.86	2.53			0.61
Anx 5	0.85	0	0	0.31	0.88	2.74			0.55
Anx 6	0.83	0	0	0.37	0.83	2.53			0.68
Anx 7	0.79	0	0	0.35	0.84	2.19			0.64
ECV	0.79	0.11	0.05	0.05					

unidimensional model. This apparent slope inflation is a (misleading) result of the estimates from the bifactor IRT model reflecting the conditional relationships among the dimensions. Note that the factor analytic parameterization of this structure may be advantageous in certain situations as it results in somewhat simpler interpretations of parameter estimates. For this reason, evaluating the strength of the general dimension in bifactor models using standard rules of thumb based on experience with unidimensional models will inevitably lead to misinterpretation. For example, depression items 3 and 2 (*I felt hopeless* and *I felt worthless*) have the two largest slopes on the general dimension in the bifactor model (4.71 and 4.44, respectively); however, interpreting the strength of their association with the general dimension must be made given their relationship with the specific dimension. To ease this interpretational challenge, the columns to the right in Table 9.6 provide the marginal trace line slope parameters for the general and specific dimensions that were computed from the conditional bifactor parameter estimates using Equation (9.15).

Evaluating the marginal slope parameters in Table 9.6 provides a new, perhaps simplified interpretation of the bifactor results. Because the conditional parameter estimates have been transformed, the values in Table 9.6 can be evaluated as if they are in the metric of the univariate IRT model. In doing so, our perspective on the items' structure may need adjustment. Returning to depression items 3 and 2, the slope parameters for these items reflect a reduced association with the general dimension when going from the conditional to marginal estimates (the item 3 slope is reduced from 4.71 to 3.15, and the item 2 slope is reduced from 4.44 to 2.74). In fact, after evaluating the marginal slope parameters it is clear that the general dimension is most closely represented by depression items 7, 6, and 5 (*I felt sad* (3.73), *I felt depressed* (3.51), and *I felt unhappy* (3.51), respectively). This shift in content emphasis suggests that the unidimensional model, which ignored LD, was oriented toward items measuring more severe aspects of depression (for example, the items reflecting feeling "helpless" and "worthless" had the highest unidimensional IRT slope parameter magnitudes).[5] In contrast, the bifactor IRT model, as hypothesized, accounts for each short form's unique content (i.e., the more severe symptom aspects) via the specific dimensions and accounts for information shared across short forms via the general dimension, which appears to be representative of a less severe symptom expression akin to emotional distress (for example, feeling "unhappy" or "sad").

Evaluating the Magnitude of Multidimensionality in the PROMIS® Emotional Distress Bifactor IRT Model

When fitting bifactor IRT models it is often useful to consider the relative strength or weakness of the general dimension with respect to the specific dimensions. These comparisons not only aid in the interpretation of the general dimension, but also indicate sets of items for which the multidimensionality is relatively weak and possibly ignorable. In particular we find the Explained Common Variance (ECV) index to be a useful indicator of unidimensionality (Reise, Moore, & Haviland, 2010; ten Berge & Socan, 2004). When computed based on the percentage of common variance across all items that is explained by the general dimension, the ECV serves as an index of unidimensionality:

$$\text{ECV} = \frac{\sum \lambda^2_{\text{Gen}}}{\left(\sum \lambda^2_{\text{Gen}}\right) + \left(\sum \lambda^2_{\text{Spec}_K}\right)}. \tag{9.17}$$

5 Chapter 2 of this volume deals exclusively with the degree to which multidimensionality impacts or distorts the estimation of unidimensional IRT parameter estimates.

Using the factor loadings in Table 9.6, the ECV for the general dimension is 0.79. Our experience suggests that ECV values of approximately 0.85 or higher are needed to consider a set of items sufficiently unidimensional to warrant a one-factor model (Stucky et al., 2013; Stucky et al., 2014).[6] The ECV index may also be computed for each specific dimension in the bifactor model to establish the uniqueness of each, simply by replacing the numerator in Equation (9.17) with the specific dimension of interest. In this example, the ECVs are low for the depression and anxiety item sets (specific-dimension ECVs = 0.05 for both, see Table 9.6), as these items largely dominate the general dimension, leaving little remaining unique variance for the specific dimensions. Notice, however, that the anger items represent a somewhat unique construct as evidenced by their low loadings on the general dimension and somewhat higher specific-dimension loadings (ECV = 0.11).

The Impact of Ignoring Multidimensionality

Despite the telltale pattern of LD indices from the unidimensional model that was initially fit, the ECV for the general dimension of the bifactor specification does indicate the presence of a strong dimension underlying this group of items. This naturally leads one to consider the consequences of ignoring the multidimensionality that is present in these items. Is it in fact true that a unidimensional model cannot sufficiently account for the covariances among these items? While it is well known that ignoring the specific dimensions leads to artificially inflated estimates of score reliability (Sireci, Thissen, & Wainer, 1991; Thissen, Steinberg, & Mooney, 1989), the severity of the local independence violations necessary to affect score reliability remains largely unknown, and in this particular example, the severity of the violation is very much in the "gray area."

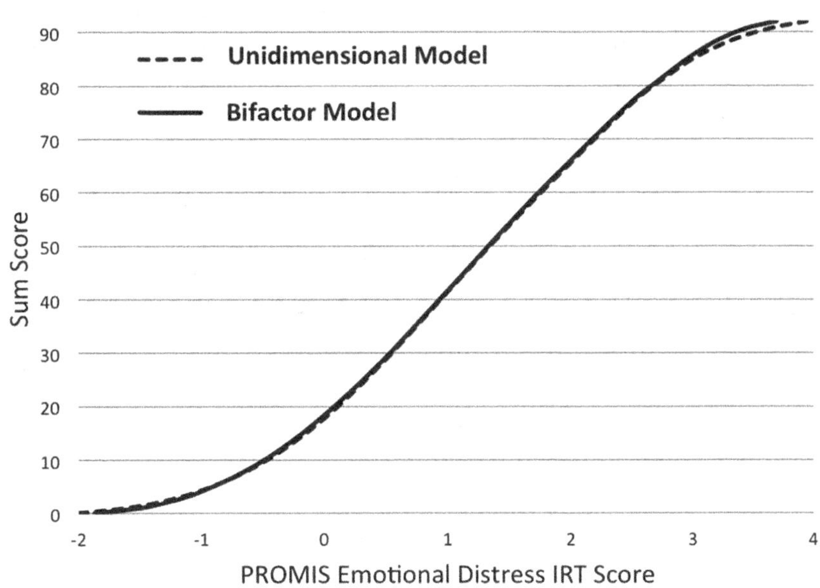

Figure 9.1 Ignored (minor) multidimensionality has negligible impact on score estimates.

6 In studies investigating the effects of fitting unidimensional models to multidimensional data Reise and colleagues (Reise, Scheines, Widaman, & Haviland, 2013; Bonifay et al., under review) evaluate the relationship between the ECV index and various other model fit and factor strength indices (e.g., the Dimensionality Evaluation to Enumerate Contributing Traits index (DETECT; Kim, 1994; Zhang & Stout, 1999), the Percentage of Uncontaminated Correlations (PUC; Reise et al., 2013), and *omegaH* (McDonald, 1999)). Note that coefficient omega and the ECV index are available in the *psych* package for the statistical software R (Revelle, 2013).

One way of identifying the practical impact of ignored multidimensionality on scoring is to compare IRT score and standard error estimates based on the univariate IRT model that ignores multidimensionality with those from the general dimension of the bifactor IRT model that accounts for multidimensionality (i.e., the general dimension from the bifactor model scores will be compared against the single dimension scores from the univariate IRT model). We did this by computing IRT scores (i.e., *expected a posteriori* (EAP)) from summed scores using the recursive algorithm for unidimensional (Thissen, Nelson, Rosa, & McLeod, 2001; Thissen, Pommerich, Billeaud, & Williams, 1995) and bifactor models (Cai, 2010) as implemented in the scoring module of the computer software IRTPRO.[7] Figure 9.1 presents these EAPs in the form of (overlapping) test characteristic curves. Similar to findings by Yen (1993), it appears that minor violations of the assumption of local independence produce mostly negligible differences in scaled score estimates. To further evaluate the impact on scoring we computed the absolute value of the average difference in IRT scores between the univariate and bifactor general dimension model-based summed scores weighted by the probability of obtaining a given summed score. Based on this approach the average EAP difference between the two scores across the underlying continuum is 0.03, confirming the relatively minor impact of ignoring multidimensionality on scoring.

However, when evaluating the impact of ignored multidimensionality on score precision, the effects are more pronounced. Figure 9.2 shows the inflated score precision of the unidimensional model across the summed scores of the underlying dimension. The difference in marginal reliability is 0.07, which indicates that even when violations of the univariate IRT model's assumption of local independence appear minor by most accounts, the resulting bias in score precision can be large enough to potentially mischaracterize the utility of the scale. Because IRT estimates of score precision are based on the model parameters, the bias in score precision is the result of the unidimensional model's overestimation of the strength of the relationship between (at least some) items and the underlying

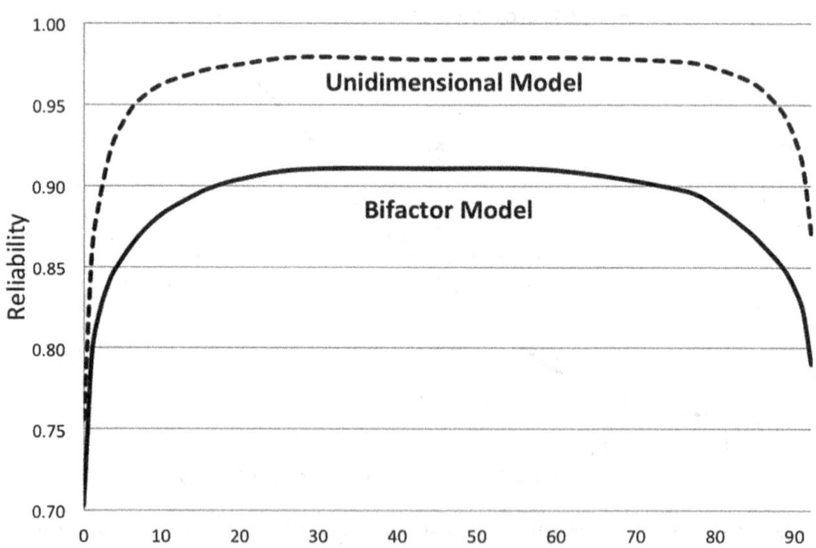

Figure 9.2 Ignored multidimensionality leads to inflated score precision.

7 A DOS-based computer program that computes IRT scores from summed scores is also freely available from the second author (orlando@rand.org).

dimension. In other words, the magnitudes of some of the slope parameters in the unidimensional model are exaggerated.

Identifying a Unidimensional Subset of Items

While our analyses thus far have shown the problematic effects of ignored multidimensionality, the results have also demonstrated the prominence of the general dimension (high ECV value for bifactor general dimension) in comparison to relatively weak specific dimensions. This leads to the question: Is there a unidimensional subset of items that represent the general dimension, emotional distress? While the high ECV value obtained earlier indicates that *some* subset of items may be fit with a unidimensional model, it does not indicate which items should be selected or which short form content domains should be represented in the unidimensional item subset. To inform the extent to which items from a given short form are likely to contribute to this unidimensional subset, it is useful to return to the ECV index. However, instead of computing a single ECV using the full collection of items, we compute separate *within-domain* ECVs for each short form. That is, Equation (9.17) is used to compute an ECV based only on the general and specific factor loadings for the items in a given short form (e.g., the within-domain ECV for anger is computed using only the eight anger items' general and specific factor loadings from the original bifactor model).

In this context the *within-domain* ECVs have the same interpretation as before, but now their relative magnitudes indicate which particular content domains are most representative of the general dimension, and indeed which short forms should contribute most to the unidimensional subset of items (i.e., short forms with higher within-domain ECVs). Moreover, it may not be appropriate to include items in the unidimensional item subset from content domains with low within-domain ECVs, as the combination of these items with items from other dimensions is unlikely to result in a unidimensional set of item responses. In this example, the within-domain ECV values for the anger, anxiety, and depression domain subsets are 0.65, 0.87, and 0.84, respectively. Noting that ECV values > 0.85 generally reflect a sufficiently unidimensional item set, the within-domain ECV values in this example indicate that covariance among items selected from the depression and anxiety domains may form an emotional distress construct that can be adequately represented by a unidimensional model.[8]

After establishing that the general dimension is most representative of the depression and anxiety domains, we now take a closer look at the items within these domains in an effort to select a unidimensional subset of items that maximizes the strength of the general dimension (emotional distress) while minimizing the impact of the specific dimensions. To aid in the selection of items we have recently used another variation of the ECV that is defined for each item (I-ECV). The I-ECV is calculated as the ratio of the item-level variance accounted for by the general factor to the total item-level variance accounted for by the general and specific dimensions (i.e., the numerator and denominator of Equation (9.17) use only the general and specific factor loadings from a single item). The I-ECV indicates the extent to which an item is representative of the general dimension alone—values near one indicate an item that only reflects the general dimension whereas increasingly smaller values reflect stronger associations with the specific dimension (Stucky, Thissen, & Edelen, 2013).

However, note that the magnitudes of the I-ECVs are entirely dependent on the content of the other items included in the specific dimension. Therefore, in a sense the I-ECV is a way to identify mostly general content items among a set of items with similar specific

8 The possibility of merging depression and anxiety item content to form an emotional distress unidimensional subset of items is somewhat further justified given the strong correlation between the anxiety and depression dimensions ($r = 0.87$).

content of various valence. In other words, the I-ECV provides the same indication of unidimensionality at the individual item level as the ECV does at the scale level. In practice the I-ECV is a useful aid in the selection of unidimensional subsets of items. Our experience using this index to select unidimensional items from bifactor IRT models suggests that choosing items with relatively high general factor loadings and I-ECV values greater than 0.80 or 0.85 will typically yield a fairly unidimensional item set that reflects the content of the general dimension.

Item Selection and Results for the Seven-Item Emotional Distress Short Form

Based on this criterion we selected the seven items from Table 9.6 (in boldface) with I-ECVs greater than 0.85. This item selection process resulted in a subset of items not overly dominated by either depression or anxiety, but rather balance a strong relation with the general dimension and weak relations with their respective specific dimensions, making them an ideal set to represent emotional distress. Note that, as suggested by the low within-domain ECV for anger, the eight anger items' I-ECVs indicated they would not be suitable for inclusion in this unidimensional subset.

To evaluate the appropriateness of this unidimensional model to characterize the covariance among the selected subset of item responses, we fit a one-factor model in *Mplus* using the limited information estimator WLSMV. The results suggest the subset of items is unidimensional, $\chi^2 = 205$, $df = 14$, $p < 0.01$, CFI = 0.995, TLI = 0.992, RMSEA = 0.039. In addition we note that while the initial bifactor model had an ECV of 0.79, indicative of a non-unidimensional model, the ECV of 0.91 computed from only the revised seven emotional distress dimension items clearly indicates a unidimensional item set.

Finally, it is important to ensure that the seven selected items appropriately reflect the reliability of scores for the emotional distress dimension as defined by the general factor of the original bifactor model. To evaluate the bias in scores that may have resulted in treating the seven items as a single dimension, we compared two separate estimates of the

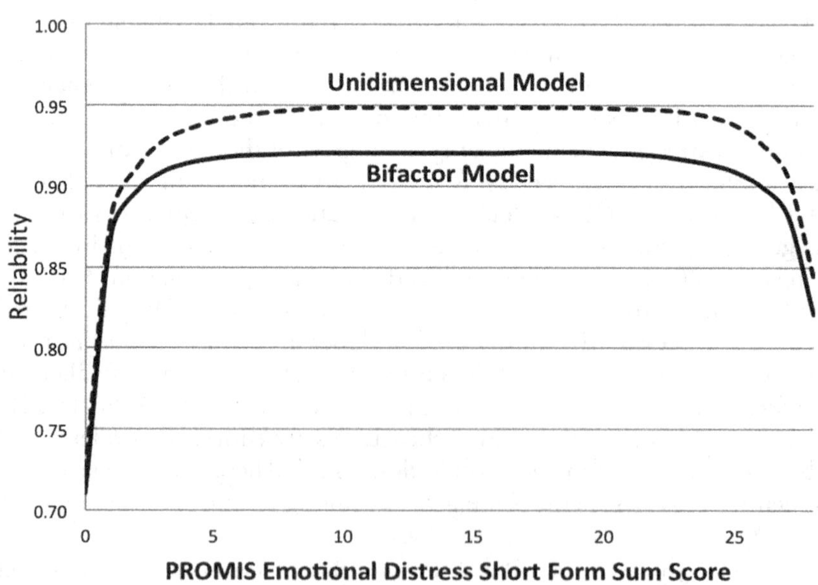

Figure 9.3 Score reliability for the seven-item emotional distress short form.

reliability of IRT scores computed from summed scores: 1) "bifactor-based" reliabilities computed for the general dimension using the item parameters from the original bifactor model (see Table 9.5), and 2) "IRT-based" reliabilities computed from a unidimensional seven-item IRT item calibration (see Figure 9.3). Because fitting unidimensional models to multidimensional data results in both biased parameter estimates (see Chapter 2 of this volume) and biased estimates of score precision, as previously discussed in this chapter, we would expect that a severe violation in unidimensionality would result in inflated estimates of score precision (as seen in Figure 9.2). Note that while Figure 9.3 indicates modest differences in score reliability, indicating some inflation in score precision, the average difference in short form score reliability for the two approaches is only 0.02 (in contrast to a difference of 0.07 obtained in the full item set), which is negligible for most scoring purposes.

Summary

The first part of this chapter reviewed a number of issues regarding the use of hierarchical IRT measurement models along with more recent generalizations (namely the two-tier model) that, with little added complexity, can accommodate less restrictive measurement models with multiple general and specific dimensions. We note that though informative, these hierarchical measurement models are challenging to interpret unless the estimated conditional parameters are transformed into the more familiar metric of the univariate IRT model (i.e., marginal trace lines).

Following this background, the second part of this chapter illustrates the versatility of the hierarchical model both as a means of describing the measurement properties of a set of items, and as a means of aiding in the selection of unidimensional subsets of items from multidimensional data. Following Chapter 2 of this volume, which describes how multidimensionality affects the parameter estimation of unidimensional IRT models, we conclude by presenting some novel psychometric techniques that may be useful in minimizing these well-known problems. We note that when used carefully these techniques do not result in (serious) biases in estimates of unidimensional item parameters or score reliabilities, though further work is needed to establish general guidelines. Taken together the marginal trace line item parameters ECV and I-ECV indices serve as useful tools for the test analyst with the goal of establishing a unidimensional scale, when faced with multidimensional data. We hope we have effectively demonstrated the utility of the general hierarchical model both as a means of describing the dimensionality of an item set and also as a way of gaining insight into the potential for alternative measurement structures.

References

Ackerman, T. A. (1989). Unidimensional IRT calibration of compensatory and noncompensatory multidimensional items. *Applied Psychological Measurement, 13*, 113–127.

Ansley, T. M., & Forsyth, R. A. (1985). An examination of the characteristics of unidimensional IRT parameter estimates derived from two-dimensional data. *Applied Psychological Measurement, 9*, 39–48.

Bartholomew, D. J., & Knott, M. (1999). *Latent variable models and factor analysis* (2nd ed.). London: Arnold.

Bock, R. D., & Aitkin, M. (1981). Marginal maximum likelihood estimation of item parameters: An application of the EM algorithm. *Psychometrika, 46*, 443–459.

Bock, R. D., Gibbons, R., & Muraki, E. (1988). Full-information item factor analysis. *Applied Psychological Measurement, 12*, 261–280.

Bolt, D. (2005). Limited vs. full information estimation in IRT modeling. In A. Maydeu-Olivares & J. McArdle (Eds.), *Contemporary psychometrics: A festschrift to Roderick P. McDonald* (pp. 27–72). Mahwah, NJ: Lawrence Erlbaum Associates.

Bonifay, W.E., Reise, S.P., Scheines, R., & Meijer, R.R. (under review). When are multidimensional data unidimensional enough for structural equation modeling? An evaluation of the *DETECT* Multidimensionality Index.

Bradlow, E., Wainer, H., & Wang, X. (1999). A Bayesian random effects model for testlets. *Psychometrika, 64*, 153–168.

Cai, L. (2010). A two-tier full-information item factor analysis model with applications. *Psychometrika, 75*, 581–612.

Cai, L., du Toit, S.H.C., & Thissen, D. (2011). IRTPRO Version 2: Flexible, multidimensional, multiple categorical IRT modeling [Computer software]. Chicago, IL: Scientific Software International.

Cai, L., Yang, J., & Hansen, M. (2011). Generalized full-information item bifactor analysis. *Psychological Methods, 16*, 221–248.

Chen, W.H., & Thissen, D. (1997). Local dependence indices for item pairs using item response theory. *Journal of Educational and Behavioral Statistics, 22*, 265–289.

Clark, L.A., & Watson, D. (1991). Tripartite model of anxiety and depression: Psychometric evidence and taxonomic implications. *Journal of Abnormal Psychology, 100*, 316–336.

De Ayala, R.J. (1994). The influence of multidimensionality on the graded response model. *Applied Psychological Measurement, 18*, 155–170.

Drasgow, F., & Parsons, C.K. (1983). Application of unidimensional item response theory models to multidimensional data. *Applied Psychological Measurement, 7*, 189–199.

Gibbons, R.D., & Hedeker, D.R. (1992). Full-information item bi-factor analysis. *Psychometrika, 57*, 3, 423–436.

Gibbons, R.D., Rush, A.J., & Immekus, J.C. (2009). On the psychometric validity of the domains of the PDSQ: An illustration of the bi-factor item response theory model. *Journal of Psychiatric Research, 43*, 401–410.

Gray, J.A. (1987). *The psychology of fear and stress* (2nd ed.). Cambridge, UK: Cambridge University Press.

Haley, D.C. (1952). *Estimation of the dosage mortality relationship when the dose is subject to error Technical Report No. 15* (Office of Naval Research Contract No. 25140, NR-342-022). Stanford University: Applied Mathematics and Statistics Laboratory.

Harrison, D.A. (1986). Robustness of IRT parameter estimation to violations of the unidimensionality assumption. *Journal of Educational Statistics, 11*, 91–115.

Holzinger, K.J., & Swineford, F. (1937). The bi-factor method. *Psychometrika, 2*, 41–54.

Ip, E.H. (2010a). Interpretation of the three-parameter testlet response model and information function. *Applied Psychological Measurement, 34*, 467–482.

Ip, E.H. (2010b). Empirically indistinguishable multidimensional IRT and locally dependent unidimensional item response models. *British Journal of Mathematical and Statistical Psychology, 63*, 395–416.

Irwin, D.E., Stucky, B.D., Langer, M.L., Thissen, D., DeWitt, E.M., Lai, J.S., Varni, J., Yeatts, K., & DeWalt, D.D. (2010). An item response analysis of the pediatric PROMIS anxiety and depressive symptoms scales. *Quality of Life Research, 19*, 595–607.

Jöreskog, K.G., & Sörbom, D. (1988). *PRELIS: A program for multivariate data screening and data summarization. A pre-processor for LISREL* (2nd ed.). Mooresville, IN: Scientific Software.

Kim, H. (1994). New techniques for the dimensionality assessment of standardized test data. (Doctoral dissertation. University of Illinois at Urbana-Champaign). *Dissertation Abstracts International, 55–12B*, 5598. Retrieved from: http://hdl.handle.net/2142/19110.

Krueger, R.F. (1999). The structure of common mental disorders. *Archives of General Psychiatry, 56*, 921–926.

Krueger, R.F., & Finger, M.S. (2001). Using item response theory to understand comorbidity among anxiety and unipolar mood disorders. *Psychological Assessment, 13*, 140–151.

Krueger, R. F., McGue, M., & Iacono, W. G. (2001). The higher order structure of common DSM mental disorders: Internalization, externalization, and their connections to personality. *Personality and Individual Differences, 30*, 1245–1259.

Lazarsfeld, P. F. (1950). The logical and mathematical foundation of latent structure analysis. In S. A. Stouffer et al. (Eds.), *Measurement and prediction*. Princeton NJ: Princeton University Press.

Liu, Y., & Maydeu-Olivares, A. (2013). Local dependence diagnostics in IRT modeling of binary data. *Educational and Psychological Measurement, 73*, 254–274.

Liu, Y., & Thissen, D. (2012). Identifying local dependence with a score test statistic based on the bifactor logistic model. *Applied Psychological Measurement, 36*, 670–688.

Luecht, R. M., & Miller, T. R. (1992). Unidimensional calibrations and interpretations of composite traits for multidimensional tests. *Applied Psychological Measurement, 16*, 279–293.

Maydeu-Olivares, A., & Joe, H. (2005). Limited and full information estimation and testing in 2^n contingency tables: A unified framework. *Journal of the American Statistical Association, 100*, 1009–1020.

Maydeu-Olivares, A., & Joe, H. (2006). Limited information goodness-of-fit testing in multidimensional contingency tables. *Psychometrika, 71*, 713–732.

McDonald, R. P. (1999) *Test theory: A unified approach*. Mahwah, NJ: Lawrence Erlbaum Associates.

Muraki, E., & Carlson, J. E. (1993). *Full-information factor analysis for polytomous item responses*. Paper presented at the annual meeting of the American Educational Research Association, Atlanta.

Muthén, B., du Toit, S. H. C., & Spisic, D. (1997). Robust inference using weighted least squares and quadratic estimating equations in latent variable modeling with categorical and continuous outcomes. Conditionally accepted for publication in *Psychometrika*.

Pilkonis, P. A., Choi, S. W., Reise, S. P., Stover, A. M., Riley, W. T., Cella, D., & PROMIS Cooperative Group (2011). Item banks for measuring emotional distress from the Patient-Reported Outcomes Measurement Information System (PROMIS®): Depression, Anxiety, and Anger, *18*, 263–283.

Reckase, M. D. (1979). Unifactor latent trait models applied to multifactor tests: Results and implications. *Journal of Educational Statistics, 4*, 207–230.

Reckase, M. D. (2009). *Multidimensional item response theory*. New York: Springer.

Reeve, B. B., Hays, R. D., Bjorner, J. B., Cook, K. F., Crane, P. K., Teresi, J. A., . . . Cella, D (2007). Psychometric evaluation and calibration of health-related quality of life items banks: Plans for the patient-reported outcome measurement information system (PROMIS). *Medical Care, 45*, S22–31.

Reise, S. P. (2012). The rediscovery of the bifactor measurement model. *Multivariate Behavioral Research, 47*, 667–696.

Reise, S. P., Moore, T. M., & Haviland, M. G. (2010). Bifactor models and rotations: Exploring the extent to which multidimensional data yield univocal scale scores. *Journal of Personality Assessment, 92*, 544–559.

Reise, S. P., Morizot, J., & Hays, R. D. (2007). The role of the bifactor model in resolving dimensionality issues in health outcomes measures. *Quality of Life Research, 16*, 19–31.

Reise, S. P., Scheines, R., Widaman, K. F., & Haviland, M. G. (2013). The effects of multidimensionality on structural coefficients in structural equation modeling: A bifactor perspective. *Educational and Psychological Measurement, 73*, 5–26.

Revelle, W. (2013). *Package "psych."* Retrieved from https://personality-project.org/r/psych.manual.pdf.

Samejima, F. (1969). Estimation of latent ability using a response pattern of graded scores. *Psychometrika Monograph Supplement*.

Schilling, S., & Bock, R. D. (2005). High-dimensional maximum marginal likelihood item factor analysis by adaptive quadrature. *Psychometrika, 70*, 533–555.

Sireci, S. G., Thissen, D., & Wainer, H. (1991). On the reliability of testlet-based tests. *Journal of Educational Measurement, 28*, 237–247.

Sörbom, D. (1989). Model modification. *Psychometrika, 54*, 371–384.

Steinberg, L. (1994). Context and serial order effects in personality measurement: Limits on the generality of "measuring changes the measure." *Journal of Personality and Social Psychology, 66*, 341–349.

Stucky, B. D., Edelen, M. O., Vaughan, C. A., Tucker, J. S., & Butler, J. (2014). The psychometric development and initial validation of the DCI-A Short Form for adolescent therapeutic community treatment process. *Journal of Substance Abuse and Treatment, 46*, 516–52.

Stucky, B. D., Thissen, D., & Edelen, M. O. (2013). Using logistic approximations of marginal trace lines to develop short assessments. *Applied Psychological Measurement, 37*, 23–39.

Takane, Y., & de Leeuw, J. (1987). On the relationship between item response theory and factor analysis of discretized variables. *Psychometrika, 52*, 393–408.

ten Berge, J. M. F., & Socan, G. (2004). The greatest lower bound to the reliability of a test and the hypothesis of unidimensionality. *Psychometrika, 69*, 613–625.

Thissen, D., Nelson, L., Rosa, K., & McLeod, L. D. (2001). Item response theory for items scored in more than two categories. In D. Thissen & H. Wainer (Eds.), *Test scoring* (pp. 141–186). Mahwah, NJ: Lawrence Erlbaum Associates.

Thissen, D., Pommerich, M., Billeaud, K., & Williams, V. S. L. (1995). Item response theory for scores on tests including polytomous items with ordered responses. *Applied Psychological Measurement, 19*, 39–49.

Thissen, D., & Steinberg, L. (2010). Using item response theory to disentangle constructs at different levels of generality. In S. Embretson (Ed.), *Measuring psychological constructs: Advances in model-based approaches* (pp. 123–144). Washington, DC: American Psychological Association.

Thissen, D., Steinberg, L., & Mooney, J. A. (1989). Trace Lines for Testlets: A use of multiple-categorical-response models. *Journal for Educational Measurement, 26*, 247–260.

Thurstone, L. L. (1947). *Multiple factor analysis*. Chicago: University of Chicago Press.

Tuerlinckx, F., & De Boeck, P. (2001). The effect of ignoring item interactions on the estimated discrimination parameters in item response theory. *Psychological Methods, 6*, 181–195.

Wainer, H., Bradlow, E. T., & Du, Z. (2000). Testlet response theory. An analog for the 3-PL useful in testlet-based adaptive testing. In W. J. van der Linden & C. A. W. Glas (Eds.), *Computerized adaptive testing: Theory and practice*. Kluwer-Nijhoff, 245–270.

Wainer, H., Bradlow, E. T., & Wang, X. (2007). *Testlet response theory and its applications*. Cambridge, UK: Cambridge University Press.

Wang, X., Bradlow, E. T., & Wainer, H. (2002). A general Bayesian model for testlets: Theory and applications. *ETS Research Report 02–02*.

Watson, D., Clark, L. A., Weber, K., Assenheimer, J. A., Strauss, M. E., & McCormick, R. A. (1995a). Testing a tripartite model: I. Evaluating the convergent and discriminant validity of anxiety and depression symptoms. *Journal of Abnormal Psychology, 104*, 3–14.

Watson, D., Clark, L. A., Weber, K., Assenheimer, J. S., Strauss, M. E., & McCormick, R. A. (1995b). Testing a tripartite model: II. Exploring the symptom structure of anxiety and depression in student, adult, and patient samples. *Journal of Abnormal Psychology, 104*, 15–25.

Way, W. D., Ansley, T. N., & Forsyth, R. A. (1988). The comparative effects of compensatory and noncompensatory two-dimensional data on unidimensional IRT estimates. *Applied Psychological Measurement, 12*, 239–252.

Wirth, R. J., & Edwards, M. C. (2007). Item factor analysis: Current approaches and future directions. *Psychological Methods, 12*, 58–79.

Yen, W. M. (1984). Effects of local item dependence on the fit and equating performance of the three-parameter logistic model. *Applied Psychological Measurement, 8*, 125–145.

Yen, W. M. (1993). Scaling performance assessments: Strategies for managing local item dependence. *Journal of Educational Measurement, 30*, 187–213.

Zhang, J., & Stout, W. (1999). The theoretical DETECT index of dimensionality and its application to approximate simple structure. *Psychometrika, 64*(2), 213–249.

10 An Illustration of the Two-Tier Item Factor Analysis Model

Wes E. Bonifay

Introduction

Multidimensional item response theory (IRT) presumes that the items on a test measure multiple underlying latent constructs. Thanks to the introduction of item factor analysis (IFA; Bock, Gibbons, & Muraki, 1988) and recent advances in efficient estimation of complex latent variable models (e.g., Rijmen, Vansteelandt, & De Boeck, 2008), multidimensional IRT has become increasingly popular in the modeling of item responses. Specifically, the standard (correlated-traits) multidimensional IRT model (see Reckase, 2009) and more sophisticated models such as the item bifactor model (Gibbons & Hedeker, 1992) and the testlet response model (Bradlow, Wainer, & Wang, 1999) have seen widespread use in psychological and educational measurement.

The bifactor IFA model and the testlet response model both utilize a factor structure that includes a single primary (or general) factor and multiple specific factors. The primary factor accounts for the latent dimension underlying all items in a test instrument, while the specific factors are designed to account for the residual dependence that exists after extracting this primary factor. Of course, addressing this residual dependence tends to result in models that provide superior goodness-of-fit to the data. Accordingly, these primary factor approaches to multidimensional item response analysis have seen a rise in popularity in recent years (the bifactor IRT model, in particular, has enjoyed a resurgence as of late; see Reise, 2012).

Although the testlet and bifactor IRT approaches are certainly bolstered by their ability to model residual dependence among test items, permitting just a solitary primary dimension may be an unnecessary restriction. To overcome this limitation, Cai (2010a) proposed the two-tier IFA model, which includes a Thurstonian simple structure among the primary dimensions while retaining the specific factors. The two-tier model positions the latent variables into two classes, or tiers: primary dimensions and specific dimensions. As in the testlet response and (confirmatory) bifactor IRT models, the primary tier dimensions and the specific tier dimensions are not correlated, and all specific dimensions are mutually orthogonal. Certain restrictions are then imposed on the factor pattern such that each item can be influenced by multiple primary factors and a single specific factor. Of course, the feature that distinguishes the two-tier model from previous multidimensional IRT models is the presence of *multiple* primary (or general) dimensions. Moreover, as discussed later in this chapter, the correlated-traits, bifactor IRT, and testlet response models are all subsumed by the more general two-tier model.

Cai (2010a) explores multiple uses for such a structure. First, the inclusion of multiple primary dimensions results in a superior measurement model, both in terms of measurement reliability and goodness-of-fit. This chapter will present a real data analysis that showcases the psychometric advantages of the two-tier IFA model. Second, the model can be adapted, quite easily, for longitudinal modeling (and in fact, the longitudinal bifactor IRT model (Hill, 2006) can be understood as a special case of the two-tier model). In the longitudinal case, the estimated correlation between the primary dimensions in the model represents the degree to which the latent trait is stable over time. The two-tier approach to longitudinal measurement improves upon standard longitudinal factor analytic models (e.g., Tisak & Meredith, 1989), which are not designed for item-level data. Third, the two-tier model can be used to model individual idiosyncrasies in response style by extending the random intercept IFA model introduced by Maydeu-Olivares and Coffman (2006). The longitudinal and response style applications of the two-tier model will not be discussed in this chapter; see Cai (2010a) for further information.

Research Methods

The Two-Tier Structure

As an illustration of the structure of a two-tier IFA model, suppose a test instrument includes 18 items and that the factor structure underlying the test includes three primary dimensions in the first tier and two specific dimensions per primary dimension (for a total of six specific latent factors) in the second tier. For this hypothetical model, the standard factor analytic measurement model $y = \Lambda\eta + \epsilon$ can be written as:

$$
\begin{pmatrix} y_1 \\ y_2 \\ y_3 \\ y_4 \\ y_5 \\ y_6 \\ y_7 \\ y_8 \\ y_9 \\ y_{10} \\ y_{11} \\ y_{12} \\ y_{13} \\ y_{14} \\ y_{15} \\ y_{16} \\ y_{17} \\ y_{18} \end{pmatrix}
=
\left(\begin{array}{ccc|cccccc}
\lambda_{1,1} & & & \lambda_{1,4} & & & & & \\
\lambda_{2,1} & & & \lambda_{2,4} & & & & & \\
\lambda_{3,1} & & \lambda_{3,3} & \lambda_{3,4} & & & & & \\
\lambda_{4,1} & & & & \lambda_{4,5} & & & & \\
\lambda_{5,1} & & & & \lambda_{5,5} & & & & \\
\lambda_{6,1} & & & & \lambda_{6,5} & & & & \\
 & \lambda_{7,2} & & & & \lambda_{7,6} & & & \\
 & \lambda_{8,2} & & & & \lambda_{8,6} & & & \\
 & \lambda_{9,2} & & & & \lambda_{9,6} & & & \\
 & \lambda_{10,2} & & & & & \lambda_{10,7} & & \\
 & \lambda_{11,2} & & & & & \lambda_{11,7} & & \\
 & \lambda_{12,2} & & & & & \lambda_{12,7} & & \\
 & & \lambda_{13,3} & & & & & \lambda_{13,8} & \\
 & & \lambda_{14,3} & & & & & \lambda_{14,8} & \\
 & & \lambda_{15,3} & & & & & \lambda_{15,8} & \\
 & & \lambda_{16,3} & & & & & & \lambda_{16,9} \\
 & \lambda_{17,2} & \lambda_{17,3} & & & & & & \lambda_{17,9} \\
 & & \lambda_{18,3} & & & & & & \lambda_{18,9}
\end{array}\right)
\begin{pmatrix} \eta_1 \\ \eta_2 \\ \eta_3 \\ \hdashline \xi_1 \\ \xi_2 \\ \xi_3 \\ \xi_4 \\ \xi_5 \\ \xi_6 \end{pmatrix}
+
\begin{pmatrix} \epsilon_1 \\ \epsilon_2 \\ \epsilon_3 \\ \epsilon_4 \\ \epsilon_5 \\ \epsilon_6 \\ \epsilon_7 \\ \epsilon_8 \\ \epsilon_9 \\ \epsilon_{10} \\ \epsilon_{11} \\ \epsilon_{12} \\ \epsilon_{13} \\ \epsilon_{14} \\ \epsilon_{15} \\ \epsilon_{16} \\ \epsilon_{17} \\ \epsilon_{18} \end{pmatrix},
\quad (10.1)
$$

where the dashed lines in the $\mathbf{\Lambda}$ (factor pattern) matrix and the $\boldsymbol{\eta}$ (latent variable) vector are included simply to delineate the first and second tiers. Notice that the two-tier model allows for cross-loadings among the primary (first-tier) dimensions; the $\mathbf{\Lambda}$ matrix clearly shows that item y_3 is free to load on primary factors η_1 and η_3, while item y_{17} is free to load on primary factors η_2 and η_3. In fact, the two-tier model permits any primary tier factor pattern (subject to identification) to be specified and tested. This ability to include primary dimension cross-loadings is the central feature that makes the two-tier model more flexible than the item bifactor or testlet response models. The $\boldsymbol{\Lambda}$ matrix also displays each specific factor ξ; as in the bifactor IRT and testlet models, cross-loadings between specific factors are prohibited in the two-tier IFA model.

The two-tier model also requires certain constraints on the factor covariance matrix such that the covariances among the $\boldsymbol{\eta}$ primary dimensions are freely estimated while the covariances among the $\boldsymbol{\xi}$ specific dimensions are fixed at zero. These specifications result in the following factor covariance matrix structure:

$$\begin{pmatrix} \Sigma & \\ 0 & \operatorname{diag}(\tau) \end{pmatrix}, \tag{10.2}$$

where $\boldsymbol{\Sigma}$ is the portion of the covariance matrix that is associated with the first tier dimensions and diag(τ) is the portion associated with the second tier dimensions. $\boldsymbol{\Sigma}$ can be of any type (subject to identification), thereby allowing any pattern of correlations among the primary factors, while the τ quadrant is necessarily diagonal, thereby ensuring that all specific factors are mutually orthogonal. Further, both the primary dimensions and the specific dimensions have unit variances.

To continue our illustration, let us consider the factor variance/covariance matrix of the hypothetical model:

$$\left(\begin{array}{ccc|cccccc}
\sigma_{11} & & & & & & & & \\
\sigma_{21} & \sigma_{22} & & & & & & & \\
\sigma_{31} & \sigma_{32} & \sigma_{32} & & & & & & \\
\hdashline
 & & & \tau_{44} & & & & & \\
 & & & & \tau_{55} & & & & \\
 & & & & & \tau_{66} & & & \\
 & & & & & & \tau_{77} & & \\
 & & & & & & & \tau_{88} & \\
 & & & & & & & & \tau_{99}
\end{array}\right) \tag{10.3}$$

Again, the dashed lines are included in order to differentiate between the (correlated) first-tier dimensions and the (orthogonal) second-tier dimensions. The off-diagonal σ_{ij} elements in the upper-left quadrant indicate that all three primary dimensions in our example model are allowed to mutually covary. However, the off-diagonal τ_{ij} elements in the lower-right quadrant are constrained to zero because, just as in the bifactor and testlet models, all specific dimensions are mutually orthogonal in the two-tier model.

Figure 10.1 is a visual representation of the example model. By using the diagrammatic conventions of square indicators and circular latent variables, Figure 10.1 clearly displays the two-tier structure of the model. The first tier is represented by the three primary latent variables in the top portion of the figure, while the second tier is represented by the six specific latent factors in the bottom portion. The cross-loadings between primary dimensions are also evident in this figure. The covariances between the primary dimensions are, of course, represented by the double-headed arrows between the first tier factors.

Figure 10.1 also enables one to visualize the relationships between the two-tier model and the correlated-traits, bifactor IRT, and testlet response models. Specifically, a standard

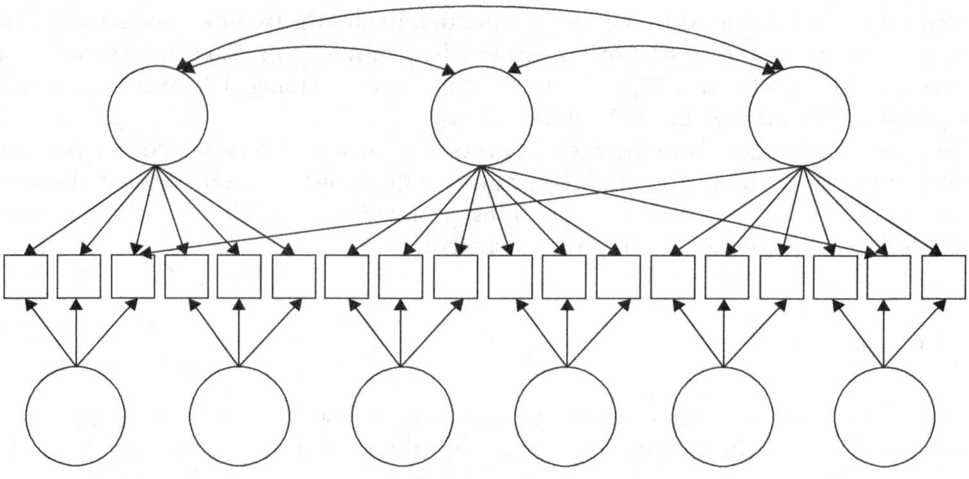

Figure 10.1 The two-tier factor structure of the hypothetical model.

correlated-traits IRT model, which does not account for residual dependence, would be produced by completely eliminating the second tier latent dimensions and all associated paths. Removing the covariances between the primary dimensions in the first tier would result in three separate bifactor IRT models. The testlet response model would be found by removing the primary dimension covariances, specifying equality constraints between the primary and specific slopes of each item, and freely estimating the specific factor variances. In sum, the two-tier IFA model incorporates the most common multidimensional IRT models and is therefore a more general and flexible structure.

The Two-Tier Model

The data analysis presented later in this chapter is based on a psychiatric symptom checklist of binary response (*presence* vs. *absence*) items. Accordingly, we will briefly discuss the two-tier formulation of the classical two-parameter logistic (2PL) IRT model. Although the 2PL model shown in Equation (10.4) is strictly for use with dichotomously scored items, the two-tier IFA model can also be implemented using polytomous items. See Cai (2010a) for two-tier adaptations of the graded response model (Samejima, 1969, 1997) and the nominal categories model (Thissen, Cai, & Bock, 2010).

Let there be p underlying primary dimensions and S specific dimensions. The conditional probability of correct/endorsement response for a dichotomously scored item y_{ij} is then defined by:

$$P_j\left(y_{ij}=1\mid\eta_i,\xi_{is},\theta\right)=\frac{1}{1+\exp\left\{-\left[\alpha_i(\theta)+\left[\beta_i(\theta)\right]'\eta_i+\beta_{is}(\theta)\xi_{is}\right]\right\}},\tag{10.4}$$

where α_i is the intercept, $\boldsymbol{\beta}_i$ is the $p \times 1$ vector of item slopes on the primary factor vector $\boldsymbol{\eta}_i$, β_{is} is the item slope on specific factor ξ_{is}, and $\boldsymbol{\theta}$ is a vector of all estimable and/or structural parameters in the two-tier model. Note that $\boldsymbol{\theta}$ is not interpreted according to traditional IRT conventions; rather, Equation (10.4) adopts the standard statistical usage of $\boldsymbol{\theta}$ as the parameter vector, which is necessary because of the confirmatory quality of the (potentially complex) two-tier model. The logit term in the denominator clearly highlights the dependence of the item parameters on the parameter vector $\boldsymbol{\theta}$. Finally, the conditional probability for the incorrect/non-endorsement response is simply $P_j(y_{ij} = 0 \mid \eta_i, \xi_{is}, \boldsymbol{\theta}) = 1 - P_j(y_{ij} = 1 \mid \eta_i, \xi_{is}, \boldsymbol{\theta})$.

Application

We turn now to a real data application of the two-tier IFA model. The analysis discussed in this chapter is based on the item responses of 3,999 individuals who participated in the Sequenced Treatment Alternatives to Relieve Depression (STAR*D; Fava et al., 2003; Rush et al., 2004) trial.[1] All participants satisfied DSM-IV criteria for nonpsychotic major depressive disorder, as indicated by a Hamilton Rating Scale for Depression (HAM-D) score of at least 14. The STAR*D studies were sponsored by the National Institute of Mental Health and conducted at 41 clinical outpatient facilities throughout the United States. Further information on the STAR*D trial and several publically available data sets can be found at www.star-d.org.

The Psychiatric Diagnostic Screening Questionnaire (PDSQ; Zimmerman & Mattia, 2001) is a 139-item[2] self-report scale that was designed to measure the 15 most common Axis I psychiatric disorders that are encountered in outpatient mental health settings: major depressive disorder (MDD), dysthymia (DYS), post-traumatic stress disorder (PTS), bulimia (BUL), obsessive-compulsive disorder (OCD), panic disorder (PAN), mania (MAN), psychosis (PSY), agoraphobia (AGO), social phobia (SOC), alcohol abuse (ALC), drug abuse (DRUG), generalized anxiety disorder (GAD), somatoform disorder (SOM), and hypochondria (HYPO). Zimmerman and Mattia (2001) reported that the PDSQ subscales had an average alpha coefficient of 0.86, with 14 of the 15 subdomains producing alpha values greater than 0.80. The authors also found an average test-retest reliability coefficient of 0.83, with nine of the subdomains producing test-retest coefficients that exceeded 0.80. Further, tests of convergent and discriminant validity indicated that each subscale was more highly correlated with other measures of the same constructs than with other measures of different symptoms (e.g., scores from the MDD subscale of the PDSQ were more highly correlated with scores from an alternate measure of depression than they were with scores from a measure of panic disorder). The developers of this instrument concluded that the strong diagnostic performance of these subscales allows for accurate classification of patients (Zimmerman & Mattia, 2001). Accordingly, the PDSQ is intended to be used as a screening instrument that incoming patients should complete prior to receiving a formal diagnostic evaluation.

When administering such a screening questionnaire, it is important to note that the factor structure of an instrument can impact its diagnostic properties. If, for example, the PDSQ has a unidimensional structure, then each of the 15 subscales can be thought of as representing a different threshold along a single underlying continuum. At the opposite extreme, the PDSQ may be a composite of 15 qualitatively distinct, psychometrically unrelated subdomains. Between these two alternatives exists the item bifactor model (Gibbons & Hedeker, 1992), wherein the structure of an instrument includes an overall

1 I would like to thank Waguih IsHak, Ph.D., for providing the PDSQ data set.

2 Two items were removed from the analyses in this chapter. Items 5 and 6 asked conflicting questions about appetite decrease and increase, respectively, while items 7 and 8 asked conflicting questions about sleep excess and deprivation, respectively. These contradictory items were eliminated, resulting in 137 items.

latent dimension (the "general factor") as well as several smaller, distinct dimensions (or "specific factors"). In the case of the PDSQ, a bifactor model would include an overall "psychiatric impairment" factor as well as 15 orthogonal specific factors, each of which represents one of the psychiatric disorders listed earlier. A practitioner could then ascertain, simultaneously, a patient's overall psychiatric impairment as well as the extent to which the patient conveys the symptoms of MDD, bulimia, and so on. Such a structure would thereby give added support to the practice of making diagnostic inferences based on PDSQ responses.

Gibbons, Rush, and Immekus (2009) fit the PDSQ data to several IRT models, including a bifactor model. The authors presented their bifactor results in terms of item factor loadings and showed that most of the items had acceptable loadings on both a general factor as well as a domain-specific factor. However, the MDD items produced relatively lower item factor loadings on the primary dimension (ranging from –0.04 to 0.34, with an average loading of 0.23) and quite heterogeneous specific factor loadings (ranging from 0.03 to 0.90). Non-MDD items, on the other hand, had higher average loadings on the primary dimension and more homogeneous loadings within each domain (see Table 1 in Gibbons, Rush, & Immekus, 2009).

A replication of this analysis (in terms of standard IRT parameters rather than item factor loadings) revealed that, although the bifactor model does explain the multidimensionality inherent in the PDSQ, many of the parameter estimates related to the MDD items were inadequate relative to the estimates of the other (non-MDD) domains. Regarding the IRT parameter estimates of the primary dimension, we found that the slope estimates of the MDD items ranged from 0.31 to 0.89 (M = 0.57) while the slope estimates of the non-MDD items ranged from 0.53 to 2.83 (M = 1.60). As for the domain-specific factors, the mean MDD slope estimate was 1.15 while the average slope estimate of each non-MDD domain ranged from 1.33 to 2.49 (with an overall mean of 1.88). In sum, the MDD items had lower primary and specific dimension discrimination parameter estimates than the other 14 domains on the PDSQ. Clearly, this discrepancy suggests that, in a bifactor structure, the MDD items are not as aligned with the general factor as well as the non-MDD items.

Two implications can be drawn from these results. First, the broad range of item factor loadings on the MDD specific factor suggests the presence of multidimensionality within this domain. Exploratory factor analyses (EFA) revealed that all of the PDSQ subdomains except MDD were sufficiently unidimensional. MDD was found to be composed of seven distinct factors, which aligned to item content related to general sadness, lack of interest, physical effects of depression, self-loathing, difficulty concentrating, suicidal ideation, and suicidal intent. However, because all 19 items were certainly indicative of an overall depression dimension, it was logical to fit a bifactor model to the MDD items. Thus, we conducted a confirmatory bifactor item factor analysis based on the optimal (7-factor) EFA solution.[3] The results of this analysis are displayed in Table 10.1. The pattern of loadings supports the multidimensionality of the MDD subscale—a modeling concern that was not addressed by Gibbons, Rush, and Immekus (2009) in their bifactor model of the PDSQ.

The second implication of the bifactor results is that the MDD items, relative to the other 14 PDSQ domains, appear to have a distinct relationship with the overall

3 MDD items 17 and 21 were causing estimation problems, so they were removed from this and all subsequent analyses.

Table 10.1 Confirmatory Bifactor Item Factor Analysis of the Major Depressive Disorder (MDD) Subdomain Items of the Psychiatric Diagnostic Screening Questionnaire

	General Factor	*Specific Factors*						
		1	2	3	4	5	6	7
MDD_01	.71	.46						
MDD_02	.66	.49						
MDD_03	.56		.67					
MDD_04	.55		.67					
MDD_10	.41		.28					
MDD_05	.25			.45				
MDD_07	.22			.63				
MDD_09	.30			.39				
MDD_11	.48				.43			
MDD_12	.64				.69			
MDD_13	.71				.47			
MDD_14	.48					.66		
MDD_15	.54					.64		
MDD_16	.67						.54	
MDD_18	.66						.54	
MDD_19	.62							.62
MDD_20	.60							.64

Note: N = 3999. RMSEA based on the M2 statistic = 0.05.

"psychiatric impairment" dimension. That is, the lower discrimination parameter estimates of the MDD subscale indicate that the depression items are not sufficiently explained by the general factor. One solution would be to model two separate bifactor solutions—one for the MDD items and one for the non-MDD items. Although this may suffice, Cai's (2010a) two-tier approach would allow all PDSQ items to be analyzed in a single model that would account for the multidimensionality of the MDD subscale while permitting the MDD items to load on a separate primary dimension from the other 14 subdomains. Moreover, the two-tier model draws on the covariance between the primary dimensions to provide more precise parameter estimates (i.e., lower standard errors) (Cai, 2010a).

The proposed two-tier item factor analysis model of the PDSQ is visually represented in Figure 10.2. Note that the alcohol abuse and drug abuse domains were not included in the model; as Gibbons, Rush, and Immekus noted, "ALC and DRUG domains were relatively independent of the primary dimension that the PDSQ measures, and represent 'independent' factors" (Gibbons, Rush, & Immekus, 2009, p. 408). Further, two MDD items (MDD_17 and MDD_21), several bulimia items (BUL_01 through BUL_04, BUL_06,

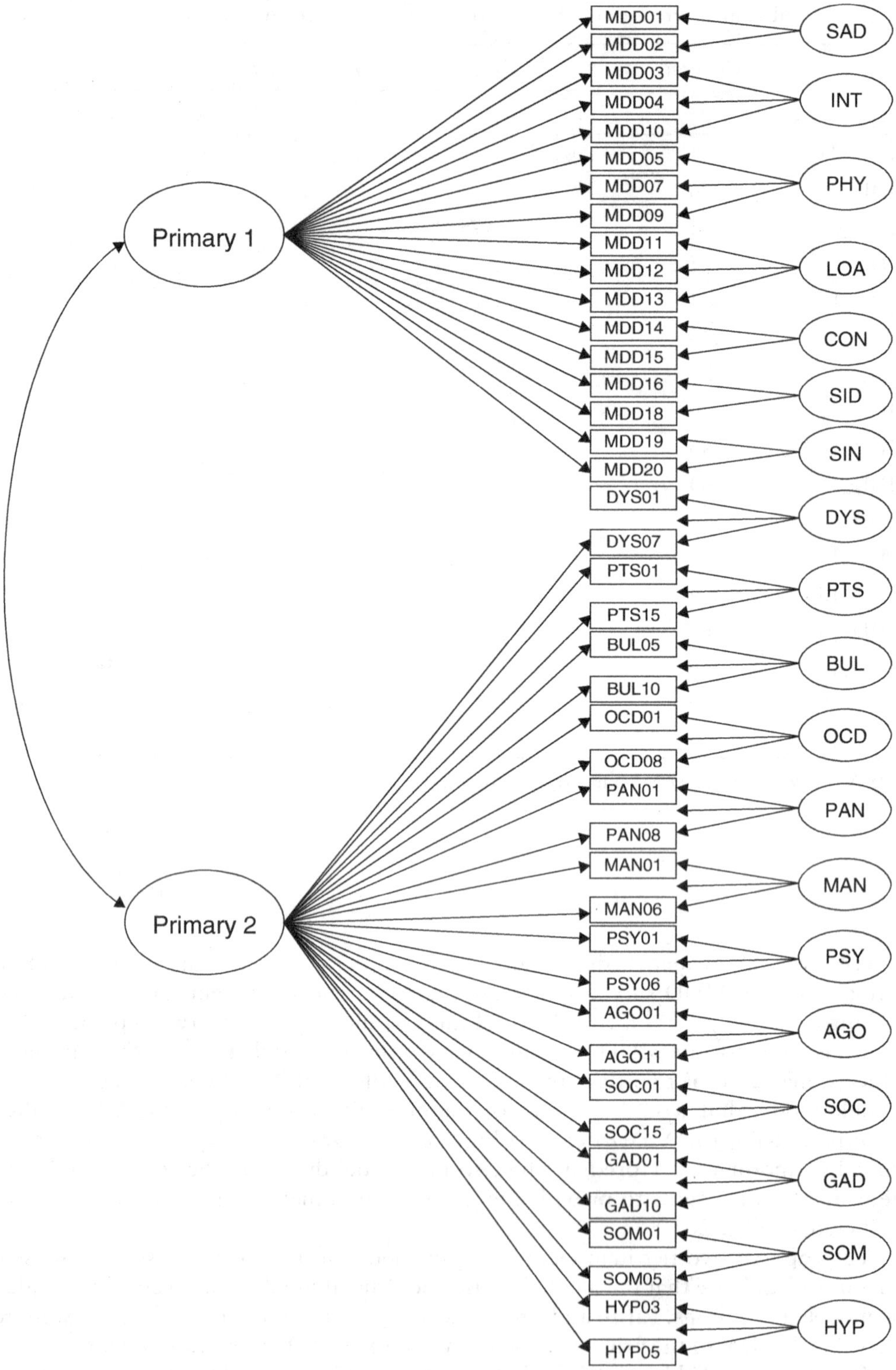

Figure 10.2 A two-tier model of the Psychiatric Diagnostic Screening Questionnaire.

and BUL_07), and a pair of hypochondria items (HYP_01 and HYP_02) were eliminated because of estimation problems. The final model included two correlated primary dimensions (MDD and non-MDD domains) in the first tier, 19 orthogonal specific dimensions (7 MDD specific factors + 12 non-MDD specific factors) in the second tier, and a total of 115 items (17 MDD items + 98 non-MDD items).

Results

Cai (2010a) proposed the two-tier full-information item factor analysis model to address data structures wherein there are multiple correlated primary factors rather than the single underlying dimension that characterizes the bifactor IRT and testlet response models. Rather than fitting separate bifactor models for each primary dimension, the two-tier model utilizes the correlation between primary dimensions to improve the accuracy of the parameter estimates. A two-tier model was therefore fit to the PDSQ data by specifying that the first primary dimension accounted for the MDD items and the second primary dimension accounted for the remaining items/subdomains.

This model was evaluated using the flexMIRT (version 2.00; Cai, 2013) multidimensional item analysis software. The PDSQ utilizes a binary response scale, so each item was fit to the two-parameter logistic (2PL) model shown earlier (Equation (10.4)). Parameter estimates were computed using the Metropolis-Hastings Robbins-Monro (MH-RM; Cai, 2010b) algorithm. The MH-RM estimation algorithm is ideal for the type of high-dimensionality factor structure that is present in the PDSQ, especially when computational burden is a concern. To further aid in the estimation process, a beta prior of (2,1) was specified for each of the 115 items. Finally, for identification purposes, an equality constraint was set for each of the specific dimension doublets among the MDD items.

Item Analysis

Table 10.2 displays the item parameter estimates of the first primary dimension (MDD) and Table 10.3 presents the estimates of the second primary dimension (non-MDD subdomains). These results are presented in separate tables for the sake of clarity, but the parameter estimates were produced by the same (two-tier) model. It is important to note that the covariance between the two primary dimensions was estimated at 0.45. This value indicates that the MDD subdomain is not completely unrelated to the other subdomains, nor are the two primary dimensions so strongly correlated that they can be thought of as measuring the exact same construct. In other words, the two primary dimensions in this model are related, but not identical.

Although the results in Tables 10.2 and 10.3 are too extensive to discuss in detail here, there are a few broad conclusions that can be drawn. First, the vast majority of the items were quite discriminating with regard to their respective primary and specific dimensions. Of the 230 estimated slope parameters (115 primary dimension estimates + 115 specific dimension estimates), 196 were at least 1.0 and the lowest slope overall was estimated at 0.49. On the first primary dimension, the least discriminating item was MDD_05, which asked about a decrease in appetite, and the most discriminating item was MDD_12, which addressed feeling negatively about oneself. On the second primary dimension, the least discriminating item was MAN_01 ("During the past six months, did you feel excessively cheerful and happy, much more than usual, and the good mood lasted most of the day for at least several days?"); the most discriminating item was AGO_11 ("Did you avoid [certain] situations because they make you feel anxious or fearful?"). Overall, the most discriminating subdomains of the second primary dimension were agoraphobia, panic disorder, and post-traumatic stress disorder.

Table 10.2 Slope and Intercept Parameter Estimates of the First Primary Dimension

	Item	*Primary Slope*	*Specific Slope*	*Threshold*
General Sadness	MDD_01	2.18	1.60	−2.55
	MDD_02	2.03	1.60	−.87
Lack of Interest	MDD_03	1.96	2.68	−1.27
	MDD_04	1.71	2.17	−1.33
	MDD_10	.79	.56	.32
Physical Effects	MDD_05	.53	.88	−.23
	MDD_07	.58	1.43	.26
	MDD_09	.70	.70	−2.34
Self-Loathing	MDD_11	1.16	.87	−.91
	MDD_12	3.73	4.18	−.71
	MDD_13	2.29	1.46	−.45
Poor Concentration	MDD_14	1.51	1.90	−1.02
	MDD_15	1.74	1.90	−.62
Suicidal Ideation	MDD_16	2.15	1.86	.25
	MDD_18	2.09	1.86	.38
Suicidal Intent	MDD_19	2.13	2.33	.30
	MDD_20	2.04	2.33	1.41

Note: $N = 3999$. All estimates are significant at $p < 0.05$.

Tables 10.2 and 10.3 also present the thresholds for each item. These values were found by taking the intercept parameter estimates provided by flexMIRT and transforming them to threshold values using the equation:

$$B_i = \frac{-c_i}{\sqrt{\sum_{k=1}^{m} a_{ik}^2}}, \qquad (10.5)$$

Table 10.3 Slope and Intercept Parameter Estimates of the Second Primary Dimension

	Item	Primary Slope	Specific Slope	Threshold		Item	Primary Slope	Specific Slope	Threshold
Dysthymia	DYS_01	1.28	2.79	–.42	*Psychosis*	PSY_01	1.35	1.20	1.60
	DYS_02	.87	1.38	–.08		PSY_02	1.77	1.63	1.01
	DYS_03	.99	1.88	–.66		PSY_03	1.79	1.27	1.91
	DYS_04	1.18	2.85	–.57		PSY_04	1.24	1.26	2.82
	DYS_05	1.27	2.24	–.24		PSY_05	1.63	1.40	2.43
	DYS_06	1.19	1.88	–.69		PSY_06	1.39	1.17	2.22
	DYS_07	1.23	1.75	–.33					
					Agoraphobia	AGO_01	2.00	.73	.82
Post-traumatic Stress	PTS_01	.69	1.09	.12		AGO_02	2.05	1.38	1.21
	PTS_02	.64	.85	.64		AGO_03	2.80	2.13	.55
	PTS_03	1.81	3.00	.20		AGO_04	2.40	1.58	.87
	PTS_04	2.00	3.21	.39		AGO_05	1.49	1.17	1.44
	PTS_05	2.39	3.77	.24		AGO_06	1.57	1.44	1.34
	PTS_06	2.47	3.59	.30		AGO_07	1.56	1.11	1.44
	PTS_07	2.01	3.09	.13		AGO_08	1.30	.49	1.52
	PTS_08	1.85	2.37	.48		AGO_09	2.19	1.45	1.93
	PTS_09	1.91	2.27	.66		AGO_10	2.78	2.18	.62
	PTS_10	2.17	2.16	.73		AGO_11	2.81	2.27	.45
	PTS_11	2.01	2.98	.53					
	PTS_12	1.61	2.39	.57	*Social Phobia*	SOC_01	1.84	2.15	.08
	PTS_13	1.49	1.90	.88		SOC_02	1.77	2.25	–.03
	PTS_14	1.70	2.42	.26		SOC_03	1.65	2.27	–.14
	PTS_15	1.92	2.15	.72		SOC_04	1.92	2.19	.11
						SOC_05	2.30	2.45	.36
Bulimia	BUL_05	.61	1.54	1.28		SOC_06	1.12	1.73	.14
	BUL_08	.87	2.05	1.53		SOC_07	1.27	1.27	1.12
	BUL_09	1.00	2.34	1.95		SOC_08	1.16	.83	1.95
	BUL_10	.58	1.92	.19		SOC_09	1.07	.95	1.64
						SOC_10	2.14	3.38	.15
Obsessive-Compulsive	OCD_01	1.23	1.03	1.80		SOC_11	1.63	2.53	.29
	OCD_02	1.46	.97	.72		SOC_12	.96	1.47	.97
	OCD_03	1.52	.70	.76		SOC_13	1.86	2.78	.40
	OCD_04	1.79	2.19	1.39		SOC_14	2.01	2.30	.25
	OCD_05	1.59	2.04	1.16		SOC_15	1.92	1.99	.22
	OCD_06	1.47	1.68	1.52					
	OCD_07	1.92	2.27	1.03		GAD_01	1.52	1.03	–.07
	OCD_08	1.34	1.36	1.74		GAD_02	1.53	.84	–.11

(*Continued*)

Table 10.3 (*Continued*)

					Generalized Anxiety	GAD_03	1.32	.95	–.39
Panic	PAN_01	1.81	2.51	.59		GAD_04	1.88	2.21	–.54
	PAN_02	1.95	2.54	.75		GAD_05	2.36	2.51	–.57
	PAN_03	1.90	2.14	.66		GAD_06	1.22	1.12	–.66
	PAN_04	1.87	1.18	.25		GAD_07	1.34	.97	–.81
	PAN_05	2.08	1.13	.49		GAD_08	1.95	1.82	–.84
	PAN_06	2.37	1.97	.34		GAD_09	1.07	.94	–1.12
	PAN_07	2.09	1.07	.83		GAD_10	2.17	2.49	–.57
	PAN_08	1.89	.58	.58					
					Somatoform	SOM_01	.78	.95	.32
Mania	MAN_01	.52	2.84	1.30		SOM_02	.99	1.25	–.20
	MAN_02	.57	3.45	1.32		SOM_03	1.18	2.33	1.01
	MAN_03	.64	3.22	1.58		SOM_04	1.01	1.70	1.63
	MAN_04	.96	1.52	1.44		SOM_05	.90	1.04	1.61
	MAN_05	.60	1.48	1.48					
	MAN_06	.77	1.08	1.66	*Hypochondria*	HYP_01	1.62	1.89	1.33
						HYP_02	2.44	2.76	1.18
						HYP_03	1.85	2.74	1.39

Note: $N = 3999$. All estimates are significant at $p < 0.05$.

where c_i is the intercept parameter for item *i*, *m* is the number of dimensions, and a_{ik}^2 is the squared slope parameter of item *i* on dimension *k* (Reckase, 2009). B_i is a multidimensional analog to the standard *b* ("difficulty" or "severity") parameter in unidimensional IRT. Whereas *b* indicates the steepest point on an item's trace line, *B* indicates the steepest point on a multidimensional surface. The interpretation, however, is identical: items with low *B* values are "easier" or "less severe," meaning there is a high probability of endorsement even when the vector of θ estimates is low, and items with high *B* values are "more difficult" or "more severe," meaning there is a high probability of endorsement only when the vector of θ estimates is high.

The threshold values in Table 10.2 reveal that the least severe depression item was MDD_01 ($B = -2.55$), which dealt with general feelings of sadness, while the most severe, by far, was MDD_20 ($B = 1.41$), which directly addressed suicidal intent. Regarding the non-MDD primary dimension shown in Table 10.3, the least severe item was GAD_09 ($B = -1.12$), which asked about stress-induced irritability, and the most severe was PSY_04 ($B = 2.85$), which inquired about the perception of special powers. Overall, the least severe subdomains of the second primary dimension were dysthymia and generalized anxiety disorder, while the most severe subdomains were psychosis and mania.

Although these results support the application of a two-tier model to the PDSQ data, it is useful to examine this model relative to an alternative structure. By reparameterizing the IRT estimates in factor analytic terms (see Wirth & Edwards, 2007), we can make a more direct comparison of the two-tier model with the bifactor results reported by Gibbons, Rush, and Immekus (2009). Table 10.4 displays the improvement in item factor loadings that is provided by the two-tier model. Clearly, allowing the depression items to load on a separate primary dimension drastically increases the item factor loadings. There is not a single item that loads higher on the primary dimension in the bifactor solution, and many items go from having negligible loadings in the bifactor model to quite strong loadings in the two-tier model. To be more precise, the mean loading of the MDD items on the primary dimension in the bifactor model was just 0.26; the mean loading on the primary dimension in the two-tier model was 0.53. Furthermore, we found that the loadings on the second primary dimension were quite similar to the non-MDD general factor loadings of the bifactor model. Hence, the two-tier model was able to boost the relatively weak loadings of the MDD items while preserving the strong loadings of the non-MDD items.

Regarding the specific dimensions, although some loadings were higher in the bifactor model (particularly the suicide items—MDD_16 through MDD_20), there was a marked lack of uniformity among these loadings; of the 17 MDD items in Table 10.4, six of the specific loadings in the bifactor model were below 0.30 while four were above 0.70

Table 10.4 A Comparison of the Item Factor Loadings of the PDSQ Major Depressive Disorder (MDD) Subscale in a Bifactor Model (as reported by Gibbons, Rush, & Immekus (2009)) and a Two-Tier Item Factor Model

	Primary loadings		*Specific loadings*							
	Bifactor	*Two-tier*	*Bifactor*	*Two-tier*						
				1	2	3	4	5	6	7
MDD_01	.17	.68	.52	.50						
MDD_02	.26	.66	.43	.52						
MDD_03	.17	.53	.39		.72					
MDD_04	.20	.53	.35		.67					
MDD_10	.18	.27	.24		.29					
MDD_05	.19	.25	.13			.44				
MDD_07	.25	.35	.08			.62				
MDD_09	.39	.40	.09			.35				
MDD_11	.36	.52	.33				.39			
MDD_12	.30	.64	.49				.71			
MDD_13	.34	.71	.54				.46			
MDD_14	.34	.51	.22					.64		
MDD_15	.33	.56	.28					.62		
MDD_16	.26	.65	.73						.56	
MDD_18	.22	.64	.85						.57	
MDD_19	.26	.59	.75							.65
MDD_20	.23	.58	.77							.66

Note: N = 3999. Bifactor item factor loadings were reported in Gibbons, Rush, and Immekus (2009).

(range = 0.77). The two-tier model addresses this issue by explicitly modeling the multidimensionality inherent in the MDD subscale. The two-tier specific loadings in Table 10.4 are therefore much more homogeneous: the smallest specific loading (MDD_10) is 0.29 and the largest (MDD_12) is 0.71, resulting in a narrower range of 0.42. Further, the mean specific dimension loading increased from 0.42 in the bifactor model to 0.55 in the two-tier model.

Scoring

In addition to improving the parameter estimates of the MDD items, the two-tier model also provides more accurate IRT-scaled scores. Posterior expectations can be computed for each of the $\boldsymbol{\eta}$ primary dimensions and $\boldsymbol{\xi}$ specific dimensions for every individual item response pattern. Estimation of these expected *a posteriori* (EAP) scores requires numerical integration of each latent variable (see Thissen & Wainer, 2001), and the restrictions of the two-tier model provide greater computational efficiency. The mathematical specifics of two-tier EAP estimation will not be discussed in this chapter; see Appendix B in Cai (2010a) for further details regarding EAP estimation in the two-tier IFA model (and Chapter 15 in this volume for scoring in commonly applied multidimensional models).

Cai (2010a) demonstrated that the EAP scores obtained from a two-tier model are almost identical to scores obtained from fitting two separate bifactor models, and that the two-tier scores are more precise and reliable. Specifically, he fit item responses from a combined math/reading test to both models and then compared just the math IRT-scaled scores from a two-tier model against the IRT-scaled scores found by treating the math items as a separate bifactor structure from the reading items. The EAPs were strongly correlated (r = 0.96), but the average standard error of measurement in the two-tier model was 20 percent lower than in the bifactor model (0.38 versus 0.49, respectively). Further, the standard deviation of the individual standard errors of measurement was lower in the two-tier model (0.05) than in the bifactor model (0.07). This improvement in precision is attributed to the "borrowing of strength" that characterizes the two-tier model; by utilizing information from one primary dimension, the two-tier model is better able to differentiate individuals along the other primary dimension (Cai, 2010a).

For the PDSQ analysis, EAPs were computed for each individual across all 21 dimensions, thereby allowing us to rank individuals according to their relative latent trait levels. Once these IRT-scaled scores have been calculated, it becomes possible to estimate an individual's EAP from his or her raw summed score. Table 10.5 displays the summed score to IRT-scaled score conversion for the MDD and non-MDD dimensions in the two-tier model. Using this table, a practitioner could simply sum a patient's score on the (reduced) PDSQ,[4] look up the value in the "Summed Score" column, and locate the corresponding IRT-scaled EAP score on each primary dimension. For example, a summed score of 59 is associated with an EAP score of 0.42 (SD = 0.86) on the first primary dimension and 0.75 (SD = 0.41) on the second primary dimension. The posterior standard deviations shown in Table 10.5 indicate that the EAPs associated with the non-MDD primary dimension are more precise than those associated with the MDD primary dimension (which was expected because of the longer test length of the non-MDD dimension). Although not

4 It should be noted once again that this conversion table is based on our truncated version of the PDSQ. The IRT-scaled scores can only be used if the summed score is calculated *without* including items MDD_06, 08, 17, and 21, BUL_01, 02, 03, 04, 06, and 07, HYP_01 and 02, or any of the ALC and DRUG items.

Table 10.5 Summed Score to IRT-Scaled Score Conversion for the Primary Dimensions

Summed Score	Primary 1		Primary 2		Summed Score	Primary 1		Primary 2	
	EAP	SD	EAP	SD		EAP	SD	EAP	SD
0	−3.09	.63	−2.92	.66	59	.42	.86	.75	.41
1	−2.84	.64	−2.78	.65	60	.44	.86	.79	.41
2	−2.62	.64	−2.65	.64	61	.46	.86	.83	.41
3	−2.43	.64	−2.53	.63	62	.48	.86	.87	.41
4	−2.26	.65	−2.42	.62	63	.50	.86	.92	.41
5	−2.10	.65	−2.33	.62	64	.52	.86	.96	.41
6	−1.95	.66	−2.23	.61	65	.55	.86	1.00	.41
7	−1.81	.67	−2.14	.60	66	.57	.86	1.04	.41
8	−1.68	.68	−2.05	.60	67	.59	.86	1.08	.41
9	−1.56	.69	−1.97	.59	68	.61	.86	1.13	.41
10	−1.45	.71	−1.89	.58	69	.63	.86	1.17	.41
11	−1.34	.72	−1.81	.58	70	.65	.86	1.21	.41
12	−1.24	.74	−1.73	.57	71	.68	.86	1.26	.41
13	−1.15	.75	−1.65	.56	72	.70	.86	1.30	.41
14	−1.06	.77	−1.58	.56	73	.72	.86	1.34	.40
15	−.98	.78	−1.50	.55	74	.75	.85	1.39	.40
16	−.91	.79	−1.43	.54	75	.77	.85	1.43	.40
17	−.84	.80	−1.36	.53	76	.79	.85	1.48	.40
18	−.78	.81	−1.29	.53	77	.82	.85	1.52	.40
19	−.72	.82	−1.22	.52	78	.84	.85	1.57	.40
20	−.67	.82	−1.15	.51	79	.87	.85	1.62	.40
21	−.62	.83	−1.08	.51	80	.90	.85	1.67	.40
22	−.57	.83	−1.02	.50	81	.92	.84	1.71	.40
23	−.52	.84	−.95	.50	82	.95	.84	1.76	.41
24	−.48	.84	−.89	.49	83	.98	.84	1.81	.41
25	−.44	.84	−.83	.49	84	1.01	.84	1.87	.41
26	−.40	.85	−.77	.48	85	1.04	.84	1.92	.41
27	−.36	.85	−.72	.48	86	1.07	.84	1.97	.41
28	−.33	.85	−.66	.48	87	1.10	.83	2.03	.41
29	−.29	.85	−.61	.47	88	1.14	.83	2.08	.41
30	−.26	.86	−.55	.47	89	1.17	.83	2.14	.41
31	−.23	.86	−.50	.47	90	1.20	.83	2.20	.42
32	−.20	.86	−.45	.46	91	1.24	.83	2.26	.42
33	−.17	.86	−.40	.46	92	1.28	.82	2.32	.42
34	−.15	.86	−.35	.46	93	1.31	.82	2.38	.42
35	−.12	.86	−.30	.46	94	1.35	.82	2.44	.43

(Continued)

Table 10.5 (Continued)

Summed Score	*Primary 1*		*Primary 2*		*Summed Score*	*Primary 1*		*Primary 2*	
	EAP	*SD*	*EAP*	*SD*		*EAP*	*SD*	*EAP*	*SD*
36	−.09	.86	−.25	.45	95	1.39	.82	2.51	.43
37	−.07	.86	−.20	.45	96	1.44	.81	2.58	.44
38	−.04	.86	−.16	.45	97	1.48	.81	2.64	.44
39	−.02	.86	−.11	.45	98	1.52	.81	2.71	.44
40	.01	.86	−.06	.44	99	1.57	.81	2.79	.45
41	.03	.87	−.02	.44	100	1.62	.80	2.86	.46
42	.05	.87	.03	.44	101	1.67	.80	2.93	.46
43	.08	.87	.07	.44	102	1.72	.80	3.01	.47
44	.10	.87	.12	.44	103	1.77	.80	3.09	.47
45	.12	.87	.16	.43	104	1.82	.79	3.17	.48
46	.15	.87	.20	.43	105	1.88	.79	3.25	.49
47	.17	.87	.25	.43	106	1.94	.79	3.33	.49
48	.19	.87	.29	.43	107	2.00	.78	3.41	.50
49	.21	.87	.33	.43	108	2.06	.78	3.50	.51
50	.23	.87	.38	.43	109	2.12	.78	3.58	.51
51	.25	.87	.42	.42	110	2.19	.77	3.67	.52
52	.27	.87	.46	.42	111	2.27	.76	3.76	.52
53	.30	.87	.50	.42	112	2.35	.76	3.86	.53
54	.32	.87	.54	.42	113	2.44	.75	3.97	.53
55	.34	.87	.58	.42	114	2.55	.75	4.10	.54
56	.36	.87	.63	.42	115	2.68	.74	4.23	.55
57	.38	.86	.67	.42					

Note: EAP = Expected *a posteriori* IRT-scaled score.

displayed here, the flexMIRT software program also provides summed score-to-EAP conversion tables for every combination of primary and specific dimensions.

Goodness of Fit

The validity of any measurement model is dependent on the degree to which the model fits the data. Unfortunately, the global goodness-of-fit of a full-information item factor analytic model is difficult to evaluate. Bock and Aitkin (1981) showed that the marginal maximum likelihood estimation of item parameters is based on an underlying contingency table of the fully cross-classified item responses. As the number of test items increases, this contingency table can become sparse (see Bartholomew & Tzamourani, 1999), and this sparseness disallows the use of the asymptotic chi-square approximation on which full-information fit statistics are based. Thus, evaluating full-information goodness-of-fit is especially problematic with regard to a scale as lengthy as the PDSQ.

Table 10.6 Relative Fit Statistics of the Bifactor and Two-Tier Item Factor Analysis Models

	Bifactor model	*Two-tier model*
–2LL	379,155.59	377,568.97
AIC	379,837.59	378,252.97
BIC	381,983.77	380,405.45

Note: Statistics are based on the 115-item revised PDSQ. –2LL = –2loglikelihood; AIC = Akaike information criterion; BIC = Bayesian information criterion.

Fortunately, the sparseness of the underlying contingency table does not invalidate the use of the likelihood ratio difference statistic for assessing the relative fit between nested models with similar dimensionality (see Haberman, 1977; Maydeu-Olivares & Cai, 2006). Gibbons, Rush, and Immekus (2009) investigated the relative fit of the (full 139-item) PDSQ by comparing the –2loglikelihood (–2LL) values derived from three competing IFA models: a unidimensional model, a simple structure model with 15 uncorrelated traits (to account for each of the 15 psychiatric subdomains), and a bifactor model. They then conducted a chi-square difference test (based on the –2LL value) for each pair of models (see Gibbons et al., 2007 for a discussion of model comparison tests). The authors concluded that the bifactor model produced significantly improved fit over both the unidimensional model, which ignored the specific subdomain factors, and the simple structure model, which ignored the primary psychiatric impairment factor.

We cannot directly compare our results with those reported by Gibbons, Rush, and Immekus (2009) because the MH-RM estimation of the two-tier model required the deletion of several items. However, fitting a bifactor model to the truncated (115-item) PDSQ data would facilitate a relative fit comparison with the two-tier model. The results of this comparison are displayed in Table 10.6, which reports the –2LL value as well as the Akaike information criterion (AIC; Akaike, 1973) and the Bayesian information criterion (BIC; Schwarz, 1978). For all three statistics, lower values indicate a better-fitting model. Not only does the –2LL statistic indicate that the two-tier model fits the data better than the bifactor model, but the AIC and BIC, which are specifically designed to penalize for model complexity, also indicate that the two-tier model achieves better fit.

The difference in degrees of freedom between a bifactor model and a two-tier model is equal to the number of covariances between primary dimensions. The proposed PDSQ two-tier structure includes two primary dimensions, and thus a single covariance; the likelihood ratio difference test between the bifactor and two-tier representations of the PDSQ was therefore based on a single degree of freedom. In terms of relative fit, the two-tier model provided a significant improvement over the bifactor model, $\chi^2_{LR}(1) = 379{,}155.59 - 377{,}568.97 = 1{,}586.62$, $p < 0.001$.

Although full-information fit measures have not yet been developed for two-tier models, Cai (2010a) notes that recent advances in limited-information goodness-of-fit assessment (e.g., Cai et al., 2006; Maydeu-Olivares, Chapter 6 of this volume; Maydeu-Olivares & Joe, 2005, 2006; Orlando & Thissen, 2000) can be used in the development of new global fit statistics for the two-tier model. Further, model misfit diagnostic statistics such as Chen and Thissen's (1997) local dependence index and the $S - X^2$ item fit statistic (Orlando & Thissen, 2000) may be extended for use with the two-tier model. Until such tools are introduced, applications of the two-tier IFA model must rely on relative, rather than absolute, fit statistics.

Summary

The two-tier full-information item factor analysis model is a notable development in the modeling of item response patterns for a number of reasons. First, the two-tier IFA structure encompasses the standard correlated-traits multidimensional IRT model, the testlet response model, and the item bifactor model. Second, the two-tier model is flexible; the ability to specify correlated primary dimensions results in more accurate measurement models (as demonstrated by the PDSQ analysis) and allows for longitudinal IRT modeling and analyses of idiosyncratic response style. Third, the two-tier model provides EAP scores that are more precise and reliable than those computed from a bifactor IRT model. Further, user specification of the two-tier model constraints is relatively straightforward in statistical software programs such as flexMIRT (version 2.00). In fact, the seemingly complex two-tier model of the PDSQ only differed from a bifactor IRT model in two basic ways; (1) by specifying a second primary dimension, and (2) by estimating the covariance between the primary dimensions. Overall, the data analysis presented in this chapter demonstrates that the two-tier full-information item factor analysis model is a powerful and flexible model that is particularly well equipped to handle complex data.[5]

REFERENCES

Akaike, H. (1973). Information theory and an extension of the maximum likelihood principle. In *Second international symposium on information theory* (pp. 267–281). Akademinai Kiado.

Bartholomew, D.J., & Tzamourani, P. (1999). The goodness of fit of latent trait models in attitude measurement. *Sociological Methods & Research*, *27*(4), 525–546.

Bock, R.D., & Aitkin, M. (1981). Marginal maximum likelihood estimation of item parameters: Application of an EM algorithm. *Psychometrika*, *46*(4), 443–459.

Bock, R.D., Gibbons, R., & Muraki, E. (1988). Full-information item factor analysis. *Applied Psychological Measurement*, *12*(3), 261–280.

Bradlow, E.T., Wainer, H., & Wang, X. (1999). A Bayesian random effects model for testlets. *Psychometrika*, *64*(2), 153–168.

Cai, L. (2010a). A two-tier full-information item factor analysis model with applications. *Psychometrika*, *75*(4), 581–612.

Cai, L. (2010b). High-dimensional exploratory item factor analysis by a Metropolis-Hastings Robbins-Monro algorithm. *Psychometrika*, *75*(1), 33–57.

Cai, L. (2013). flexMIRT® version 2.00: A numerical engine for flexible multilevel multidimensional item analysis and test scoring. [Computer software]. Chapel Hill, NC: Psychometric Group.

Cai, L., Maydeu-Olivares, A., Coffman, D.L., & Thissen, D. (2006). Limited-information goodness-of-fit testing of item response theory models for sparse 2^p tables. *British Journal of Mathematical and Statistical Psychology*, *59*, 173–194.

Chen, W.H., & Thissen, D. (1997). Local dependence indexes for item pairs using item response theory. *Journal of Educational and Behavioral Statistics*, *22*(3), 265–289.

Fava, M., Rush, A.J., Trivedi, M.H., Nierenberg, A.A., Thase, M.E., Sackeim, H.A., . . . Kupfer, D.J. (2003). Background and rationale for the Sequenced Treatment Alternatives to Relieve Depression (STAR* D) study. *Psychiatric Clinics of North America*, *26*(2), 457–494.

5 Acknowledgments: I would like to thank Scott Monroe for assistance with tuning the Metropolis-Hastings Robbins-Monro estimation algorithm and Li Cai for his valuable input and advice. The research reported here was supported by the Institute of Education Sciences, U.S. Department of Education, through Grant R305B080016 to the University of California, Los Angeles. The opinions expressed are those of the author and do not represent views of the Institute or the U.S. Department of Education.

Gibbons, R.D., Bock, R.D., Hedeker, D., Weiss, D.J., Segawa, E., Bhaumik, D.K., . . . Stover, A. (2007). Full-information item bifactor analysis of graded response data. *Applied Psychological Measurement*, *31*, 4–19.

Gibbons, R.D., & Hedeker, D.R. (1992). Full-information item bi-factor analysis. *Psychometrika*, *57*(3), 423–436.

Gibbons, R.D., Rush, A.J., & Immekus, J.C. (2009). On the psychometric validity of the domains of the PDSQ: An illustration of the bi-factor item response theory model. *Journal of Psychiatric Research*, *43*(4), 401–410.

Haberman, S.J. (1977). Log-linear models and frequency tables with small expected cell counts. *Annals of Statistics*, 1148–1169.

Hill, C.D. (2006). *Two models for longitudinal item response data*. Unpublished doctoral dissertation, Department of Psychology, University of North Carolina at Chapel Hill.

Maydeu-Olivares, A., & Cai, L. (2006). A cautionary note on using G2 (dif) to assess relative model fit in categorical data analysis. *Multivariate Behavioral Research*, *41*(1), 55–64.

Maydeu-Olivares, A., & Coffman, D.L. (2006). Random intercept item factor analysis. *Psychological methods*, *11*(4), 344.

Maydeu-Olivares, A., & Joe, H. (2005). Limited- and full-information estimation and goodness-of-fit testing in 2^n contingency tables: A unified framework. *Journal of the American Statistical Association*, *100*(471), 1009–1020.

Maydeu-Olivares, A., & Joe, H. (2006). Limited information goodness-of-fit testing in multidimensional contingency tables. *Psychometrika*, *71*(4), 713–732.

Orlando, M., & Thissen, D. (2000). Likelihood-based item-fit indices for dichotomous item response theory models. *Applied Psychological Measurement*, *24*(1), 50–64.

Reckase, M. (2009). *Multidimensional item response theory*. Springer.

Reise, S.P. (2012). The rediscovery of bifactor measurement models. *Multivariate Behavioral Research*, *47*(5), 667–696.

Rijmen, F., Vansteelandt, K., & De Boeck, P. (2008). Latent class models for diary method data: Parameter estimation by local computations. *Psychometrika*, *73*(2), 167–182.

Rush, A.J., Fava, M., Wisniewski, S.R., Lavori, P.W., Trivedi, M.H., Sackeim, H.A., . . . Niederehe, G. (2004). Sequenced treatment alternatives to relieve depression (STAR* D): Rationale and design. *Controlled Clinical Trials*, *25*(1), 119–142.

Samejima, F. (1969). Estimation of latent trait ability using a response pattern of graded scores. *Psychometrika Monograph, 17*.

Samejima, F. (1997). Graded response model. In W.J. van der Linden & R.K. Hambleton (Eds.), *Handbook of modern item response theory* (pp. 85–100). New York: Springer.

Schwarz, G. (1978). Estimating the dimension of a model. *Annals of Statistics*, *6*(2), 461–464.

Thissen, D., Cai, L., & Bock, R.D. (2010). The nominal categories item response model. In M.L. Nering & R. Ostini (Eds.), *Handbook of polytomous item response theory models* (pp. 43–75). New York: Routledge.

Thissen, D., & Wainer, H. (Eds.) (2001). *Test scoring*. New York: Routledge.

Tisak, J., & Meredith, W. (1989). Exploratory longitudinal factor analysis in multiple populations. *Psychometrika*, *54*(2), 261–281.

Wirth, R.J., & Edwards, M.C. (2007). Item factor analysis: Current approaches and future directions. *Psychological Methods*, *12*(1), 58.

Zimmerman, M., & Mattia, J.I. (2001). A self-report scale to help make psychiatric diagnoses: The Psychiatric Diagnostic Screening Questionnaire. *Archives of General Psychiatry*, *58*(8), 787.

11 Using Projected Locally Dependent Unidimensional Models to Measure Multidimensional Response Data

Edward H. Ip and Shyh-Huei Chen

Introduction

This chapter describes a measurement approach for scaling individuals on a single dimension in the presence of multidimensionality. The approach, which we call the projective item response model, uses a unidimensional model for assessing multidimensional response data that contain a dominant dimension of interest. The novel approach is motivated by several observations: (1) that while scale development efforts always strive for unidimensional constructs (e.g., mathematical ability, anxiety, or botherness due to a disease and its treatment), tests require content validity and such a requirement often leads to a conflation of constructs from multiple dimensions; (2) that while multidimensional models are, logically, tools of choice for handling multidimensional data, they are not well equipped for the purpose of direct comparison of specific latent constructs across studies; and (3) that while complex multidimensional models are now computationally feasible, estimations for high dimensions using generally available sample sizes—especially in psychological and health sciences—are often sensitive to model misspecification and that some components of the estimated model could exhibit a high level of error. The most "vulnerable" parts are dimensions that are relatively weak and not well represented across items.

The projective item response model offers a solution to the problem of handling multidimensional response data by using a robust class of item response theory (IRT) models—the unidimensional models (Lord, 1980). Briefly, the idea behind projective IRT, which term will be used interchangeably with the term *projective item response model*, can be summarized as follows: (1) Fit a provisional multidimensional IRT (MIRT) model to the response data, (2) "Project" the MIRT model such that an "equivalent" unidimensional IRT model is derived, and (3) Adjust the standard error (SE) of the latent trait estimate using proven robust estimation methods. We pay a "price" for the reduction in dimensionality: The "equivalent" unidimensional model in (2) does not satisfy the locally independent assumption, which states that given the target latent construct, the item responses are all conditionally independent of one another. In other words, a dependency model is required for fully characterizing the "equivalent" unidimensional IRT model. Step (3) is a way to compensate for the induced dependency.

Despite the additional complexity of having to deal with a dependency model, there are several key advantages of the projective IRT approach. First, the projected model allows direct assessment of a target construct in different multidimensional spaces. As a result, the method allows direct comparison between different test forms or even different instruments for which multidimensional data were collected. Two data sets measuring the same construct (e.g., self-efficacy in physical competency in older adults) but that are "contaminated" by different secondary dimensions within the data (e.g., positive emotions and negative feelings) still can have the same target construct accurately measured and compared. The point will be further elaborated after the theoretical basis for projective IRT is described. Second, projective IRT, as we shall see from our preliminary data, are generally robust to possible misspecification of the provisional "underlying" MIRT model. Third, the unidimensional IRT parameters are invariant with respect to how the dependency model is specified—the second-order dependency component and the first-order mean item response component are orthogonal and can be separately estimated. Finally, the family of unidimensional models is robust to data issues such as sample size variation; it is a well-tested and proven class of models. Furthermore, for unidimensional IRT, many powerful unidimensional procedures including differential item functioning (DIF), test equating, and models for item response time have reached a level of maturity that can be implemented using industry-strength software. Finally, compared to other methods such as MIRT, the projective IRT generally has a higher level of interpretability, which may be especially important in applications that involve experts from other substantive fields such as medical sciences.

The remainder of this chapter is structured as follows. First, we discuss the so-called dimensionality-versus-validity dilemma—that is, the tension between developing a purely unidimensional construct and the need to attend to scope and content for enhancing test validity. We then introduce the theoretical foundation of projective IRT, and describe a step-by-step implementation of the method. Results from simulation experiments for evaluating the validity of such a procedure are reported in summarized form. Subsequently, several examples are used to illustrate the properties of projective IRT. We conclude with some thoughts for future directions.

Background

The Unidimensionality-Versus-Validity Dilemma

The notion of parsimonious dimensionality, particularly unidimensionality, by which a single putative construct is to be measured, is implicit in both classical testing theory (CTT) and item response models. Thurstone, for example, insisted that all measurements in psychology should only measure a single construct, and he called it a universal characteristic of all measurements (Thurstone, 1931, p. 257). Stout (1987), in a conceptualization of the notion of essential unidimensionality, argued that a test for individual differences should always be designed to measure a "unified trait." On the other hand, test designers have exerted momentous and sometimes overzealous efforts to integrate every conceivable attribute into a test so that the targeted construct that the test purportedly measures will be meaningful, useful, and defensible.

Consider the measurement of emotional distress as a form of patient-reported outcome (PRO). The construct comprises at least several domains of distress: anxiety, depression, and anger. An item that measures depression (e.g., "My sleep was restless" from the CES-D) could also contain overlapping elements of anxiety. It is of course possible to only include strictly depression items and eliminate items that suggest even a hint of involving other dimensions. However, for a scale developer the risk involved in only allowing questions that directly and equivocally follow a narrow clinical definition of depression would appear to be even greater—it limits the richness of the scale and results in an instrument too narrow to function in a meaningful way for assessing the purported construct of depression. Thus, a purely unidimensional test could be highly restrictive and lacks the "psychological width" or in the words of Reise, Cook, & Moore (Chapter 1, this volume)—"clinical content"—to be valid.

The omnipresence of multidimensionality in psychological measures, quality of life, and other PRO measures is well recognized in the literature. Continuing the emotional distress example, Pilkonis and colleagues (2011) remarked: "the conventional wisdom is that traditional tests of ability in the educational literature (e.g., measures of verbal and mathematical proficiency with which the use of IRT has been most common) are more likely to fit unidimensional models than scales of emotional distress (Gibbons et al., 2007). Instruments assessing emotional distress often sample items from multiple domains (e.g., mood, cognition, behavior, somatic symptoms) to capture a comprehensive set of manifest indicators of the latent construct. Therefore, it is common to observe higher correlations within domains than is expected under the conditional independence assumption of a unidimensional IRT model (Bjorner et al., 2007; Steinberg & Thissen, 1996)." In other words, a valid instrument for assessing emotional distress is likely to contain item clusters each measuring one single dominant dimension (e.g., mood) that is "jumbled" together with a mix of other related dimensions (cognition, behavior, and so on).

Practically, instruments for assessing human psychological constructs and cognition are, to various extents, multidimensional. The tension between dimensionality and validity was acknowledged in work on factor methods dating from as early as the 1920s and 1930s (Holzinger & Swineford, 1937; Kelley, 1928; Spearman, 1933). Kelley (1928, chapter 1) maintained that the designation of a trait as a category of mental life requires the inclusion of all measurements that are "definable and verifiable." Humphreys (1986) highlighted the tension between unidimensionality and validity by going as far as to suggest that tests should be deliberately constructed to include numerous minor factors in addition to the dominant dimension. Ozer (2001) contended that in personality assessment it is "exceedingly difficult" to achieve structural validity of unidimensionality because "most constructs are theoretically defined as unidimensional, but item responses, as individual behaviors in their own right, are usually multiply determined." In fact, it is hard to argue that truly valid unidimensional tests exist in any subject matter area. Therefore, it may even be fair to assert that (to the credit of Milton Friedman) multidimensionality is *always* and *everywhere* a validity phenomenon.

Because maintaining the psychological width of a test is so critical to psychological, educational, and health measurement, some researchers have begun to question the utility of models of parsimonious dimensions, the case in point being the unidimensional item response model. We contend that, in reality, purely unidimensional tests, while being a welcomed convenience for psychometricians, are rare. A more common situation is that a test has good face validity of unidimensionality (e.g., as judged by content experts) but empirically exhibits evidence of a single, strong dimension and a few smaller and perhaps detectable dimensions (Embretson & Reise, 2000, p. 230; Hulin, Drasgow, & Parsons, 1983, p. 40). In that case, the researcher is left to grapple with a range of options such as removing or rewriting items, clustering items (Luecht & Miller, 1992), checking subsets of items using factor strength indexes (Reise, Bonifay, & Haviland, 2013), using multidimensional models including bifactor models, or simply conveniently ignoring the minor dimensions by fitting a unidimensional model to the data.

The MIRT approach is perhaps the most logical approach to solving this unidimensionality-versus-validity dilemma. There are several commonly used classes of MIRT models. To illustrate these ideas, consider the two-dimensional (2-D) IRT model (Reckase, 1997):

$$P(Y_{ij} = 1 \mid \theta_{j1}, \theta_{j2}) = \frac{\exp(a_{i1}\theta_{j1} + a_{i2}\theta_{j2} - d_i)}{1 + \exp(a_{i1}\theta_{j1} + a_{i2}\theta_{j2} - d_i)}, \tag{11.1}$$

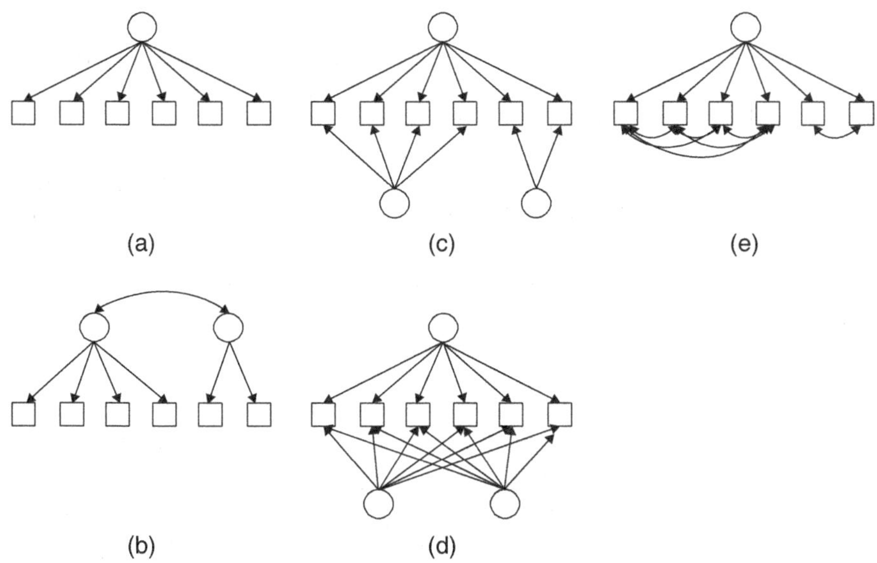

Figure 11.1 (a) traditional IRT model, (b) between-item multidimensional IRT (MIRT), (c) bifactor MIRT, (d) general MIRT, (e) locally dependent (LD)-IRT.

where $Y_{ij}, i = 1, \cdots, I, j = 1, \cdots, J$ is the binary response of the individual j to item i; a_{i1}, a_{i2} are the discrimination parameters; $(\theta_{j1}, \theta_{j2})$ is a vector of latent traits of dimension 2, distributed as bivariate normal with covariance matrix Σ that contains respective variances σ_1^2 and σ_2^2, and correlation ρ; and d_i is an intercept (difficulty) parameter. Constraints are routinely placed on the parameters to render the model identifiable. For a general MIRT with latent variable Θ of dimension p, the response surface $P\left(Y_{ij} = 1|\Theta\right)$ is a p-dimensional surface, as opposed to the one-dimensional item characteristic curve (ICC) in IRT.

Figures 11.1(b) and (c) show two such MIRT structures, as opposed to the traditional unidimensional IRT (Figure 11.1(a)) and the general MIRT (Figure 11.1(d)). Figure 11.1(b) shows a so-called between-item MIRT (Adams, Wilson, & Wang, 1997; Rijmen & De Boeck, 2005) or "simple structure" (Ackerman, Gierl, & Walker, 2003; Zhang, 2007). The leftmost four items (squares) belong to one dimension (represented by a latent variable, which is depicted as an oval in the graph), while the remaining two belong to another distinct dimension. The two dimensions can be correlated (indicated by double arrow). Compared with Figure 11.1(a), which shows that item responses are conditionally independent (no link between squares) given the latent variable (the oval), Figure 11.1(b) essentially consists of two unidimensional IRT models.

Alternatively, Figure 11.1(c) shows a bifactor model (Gibbons & Hedeker, 1992; Reise, Morizot, & Hays, 2007) in which a general factor underlies all items, together with two group factors. In contrast to the general MIRT model, in which each item is loaded on all three dimensions (Figure 11.1(d)), in the bifactor model each item has at most two dimensions—a generic factor and one of many group factors that correspond to specified, mutually exclusive subsets of items (here the terms *dimension* and *factor* are used interchangeably). As a special case of the MIRT, this kind of item-level bifactor pattern (Muthén, 1989) can be especially useful for tests that contain a general underlying factor (e.g., general reading ability) and clearly identifiable domains (e.g., comprehension and vocabulary). To facilitate our subsequent discussion, we call the group factors *domain-specific factors*. For example, in Figure 11.1(c), there are two domain-specific factors besides the general factor. It needs to be pointed out that a domain-specific score in a bifactor model only reflects the *residual* variance after partialing out the general factor. This will be an important distinction between a bifactor domain-specific score and a domain-projected IRT score, which does not involve a general factor.

While the MIRT approach is an apparent and logical solution to the unidimensionality-versus-validity dilemma, practical reasons limit the applications of MIRT. The first limitation is the lack of comparability across items and tests—different tests measuring the same construct (e.g., emotional distress) may contain different mixes of minor dimensions (e.g., anger, anxiety), and scores cannot be directly compared across different tests. For example, two independent bifactor models are fitted to data collected from two different tests that are designed to measure the same target construct. Consider the scenario in which one analysis results in one general factor and two domain-specific factors while the other results in one general and three domain-specific factors. Furthermore, checking for important measurement properties such as parameter invariance for MIRT is more challenging than for IRT.

Second, weaker dimensions in MIRT are often estimated with large variance and require large sample size for calibration. This is especially true for high-dimensional models. Our experience using simulated data suggested that even with state-of-the-art software programs, estimated minor dimensions in an MIRT were often not stable and had large root mean square errors (RMSEs), although the strong dimension was generally robust (Ip & Chen, 2012; Ip, Molenberghs, Chen, Goegebeur, & De Boeck, 2013). In general, fitting high-dimensional MIRT models could be a tricky endeavor. Currently, procedures for checking assumptions in MIRTs, which are typically strong statistical conditions, are not well developed, if they exist at all. Finally, another limitation of MIRTs is that these complex models are often difficult to interpret. Questions such as "Can the parameters on the same dimension be interpreted the same way across two tests?" often arise and potentially create confusion among users. The aforementioned comparability and interpretation issues are especially pertinent in health and medical sciences. For example, because of historical reasons, there often exist multiple commonly used PRO instruments for measuring the same health construct (e.g., depression). Comparability across measurements, or the lack thereof, has hindered research such as in the synthesis of results across studies (e.g., see Forrest et al., 2012).

Interestingly, the MIRT, as it turns out, is "equivalent" to a unidimensional IRT, provided that one is willing to relax the local independence assumption in the IRT model. Figure 11.1(e) shows an LD-IRT model that is "equivalent" to the bifactor model depicted in Figure 11.1(c). We further provide background for the "equivalence."

Equivalence of the MIRT and LD-IRT

Equivalence is formally defined in Ip (2010) using the concept of empirical indistinguishability. Two models are said to be empirically indistinguishable (EI) if their first two marginal moments match up. With this definition, Ip (2010) showed that a compensatory MIRT model is EI from a locally dependent (LD), unidimensional IRT model. Using the MIRT in Equation (11.1) as an example, the ICC of the corresponding EI unidimensional IRT model is given by:

$$P(Y_{ij} = 1 \mid \theta_j) = \frac{\exp(a_i^* \theta_i - d_i^*)}{1 + \exp(a_i^* \theta_i - d_i^*)}, \tag{11.2}$$

where:

$$a_i^* = \lambda_{logit}(a_{i1} + \frac{a_{i2}\rho\sigma_2}{\sigma_1}),\ d_i^* = \lambda_{logit}d_i, \tag{11.3}$$

with $\lambda_{logit} = \left[k^2a_2^2\left(1-\rho^2\right)\sigma_2^2+1\right]^{-1/2}$, $k = \frac{16\sqrt{3}}{15\pi} \cong 0.588$. Equation (11.2) actually suggests a specific projective model,[1] or a projection, of the MIRT, in this case onto the first dimension θ_1. The projected IRT model is not locally independent; the conditional correlation between item u and item $v\left(u \neq v\right)$ is approximately given by:

$$corr(Y_u, Y_v \mid \theta_1) = \frac{s_{uv}(\theta_1)}{\sqrt{\upsilon_u(\theta_1)\upsilon_u(\theta_1)}}, \tag{11.4}$$

where $s_{uv}\left(\theta_1\right)$ is given by:

$$\begin{aligned} s_{uv}(\theta_1) &= \frac{a_{u2}a_{v2}\sigma_2^2(1-\rho^2)[\exp(a_{u1}\theta_1 + a_{v1}\theta_1 - d_u - d_v)]}{[1+\exp(a_{u1}\theta_1 - d_u)]^2[1+\exp(a_{v1}\theta_1 - d_v)]^2} \\ &= a_{u2}a_{v2}\sigma_2^2(1-\rho^2)p_u^*q_u^*p_v^*q_v^*,\ if\ u \neq v, \end{aligned} \tag{11.5}$$

and $p_i^* = \exp\left(a_{i1}\theta_1 - d_i\right)/\left[1+\exp\left(a_{i1}\theta_1 - d_i\right)\right]$, $q_i^* = 1 - p_i^*$, $k_1 = a_{i2}^2\sigma_2^2\left(1-\rho^2\right)$, $k_2 = a_{i2}\rho\sigma_2 / \sigma_1, \sigma_1 > 0, \sigma_2 \geq 0, h'\left(u\right) = \exp\left(u\right) - [\exp\left(u\right)]^2 / \left[1+\exp\left(u\right)\right]^3$,

$$\begin{aligned} \upsilon_i(\theta_1) &= \mathrm{var}(Y_i \mid \theta_1) \\ &\approx \frac{[\exp(a_{i1}\theta_1 - d_i)]}{[1+\exp(a_{i1}\theta_1 - d_i)]^2} + \frac{a_{i2}^2\sigma_2^2(1-\rho^2)[\exp(a_{i1}\theta_1 - d_i)]^2}{[1+\exp(a_{i1}\theta_1 - d_i)]^4} + \frac{a_{i2}\rho\theta_1\sigma_2}{\sigma_1}h'(a_{i1}\theta_1 - d_i) \\ &= p_i^*q_i^*[1 + k_1p_i^*q_i^* + k_2\theta_1(q_i^* - p_i^*)]. \end{aligned} \tag{11.6}$$

Equations (11.2)–(11.6) lay out the explicit structure of the LD-IRT that is equivalent to a given MIRT. The derivation shows pure mathematical equivalence and does not involve identifiability constraints. Without loss of generality, the derivation focuses on a model that picks the first dimension in MIRT as the "projected" direction. Figure 11.2 shows the item response surface for a 2-D MIRT of given parameters and the projected item characteristic curve (solid line) on the dominant dimension.

The result for projection onto a fixed dimension can be extended to other directions of projection as well as directions that involve linear combination of several dimensions. Here we use the term *projective IRT* to describe the collection of methods for measuring multidimensional data using a single dimension through projection of the multidimensional space onto a target unidimensional space.

How the Results Can Be Used

An important implication of the result described earlier is that multidimensionality does not necessitate the use of multidimensional models. In other words, a collection of LD

1 Technically, the peripheral dimensions are integrated out, or marginalized. We have considered the term *marginal* to replace the term *projective* but decided against it because the term is likely to confuse with the commonly used term *marginal IRT model*, which integrates out all the latent dimensions. Furthermore, by calling it *projection*, it will be easier to set up comparison of the current method to other approaches such as empirical projection (directly fitting unidimensional model to response data). See Kahraman and Thompson (2009).

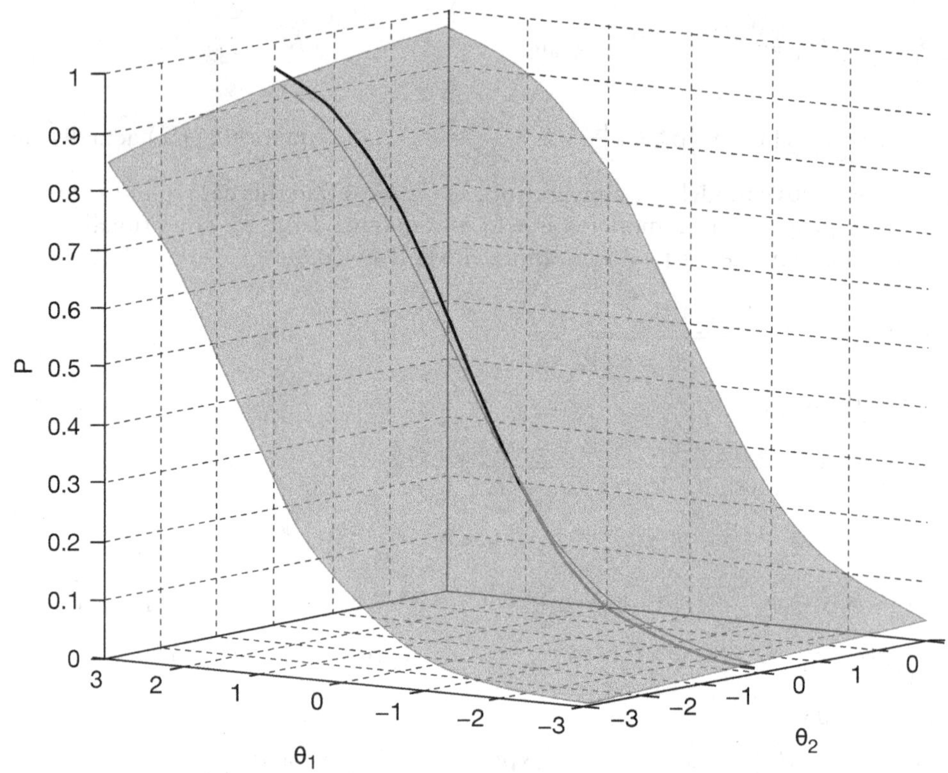

Figure 11.2 Projected item characteristic curve (solid line) from a 2-D MIRT with $a_1 = 1.15$, $a_2 = 0.27$, $d = 0.88$.

unidimensional IRT models can be used, with proper adjustment, as an alternative to MIRT for modeling multidimensional response data.

There are many benefits of using projective unidimensional IRT for psychometric analysis. Some of the advantages have also been discussed in the Introduction to this volume (see also van Abswoude, van der Ark, & Sijtsma, 2004). Yet perhaps the most salient feature of projective IRT is its preservation of an invariance property of IRT that is inherent in its conceptualization: that the item and person parameters are sample-independent. As Hambleton, Swaminathan, and Rogers (1991) forcibly argued, the invariance property represents a tremendous advantage of IRT over CTT, and the consequences of this property are: (a) those parameters that characterize an examinee are independent of the test items from which they are calibrated and (b) those parameters that characterize an item are independent of the ability distribution of the set of examinees.

The presence of multidimensionality poses a serious challenge to this notion of sample independence. Different test forms, for example, even when they are designed to assess the same construct within the same target population, may contain different mixes of multiple dimensions. Two fifth-grade math test forms—say Form A and Form B—may contain different mixes of math problems. For example, Form A contains a stronger component of verbal comprehension, while Form B contains a stronger spatial/geometric component. Assume that the same scaling procedure is applied to both tests. Because Form A and Form B measure slightly different mixes of math (the dominant trait), verbal and spatial abilities, their scores, even after standardizations, can still not be directly compared.

In other words, the latent trait estimated from one test is a function of the content of the test and does not lend itself to universal interpretation.

One of the reasons that IRT has become such a powerful tool, in contrast to CTT, is that it segregates the effect of item and the effect of person on item response, and that it can be used to estimate ability with different representative subsets of items sampled from the same universe of items. The presence of idiosyncratic or nuisance dimensions across different tests renders the sample-independent assumption invalid. The projective IRT can be used as a means to obtain "purified" dimensions. Because of its ability to project latent scores onto single identifiable dimensions (e.g., mathematical skill) and to rid of peripheral dimensions (e.g., verbal skill for word problems in math), projected test scores have the promise to be made directly comparable across different test forms. This is an important advantage over MIRT because, like regression coefficient estimates across different multiple regression models, latent trait estimates from different MIRTs are generally not comparable. For example, for two regression models: $Y = \beta_0 + \beta_1 x_1 + \beta_2 x_2$, and $Y = \gamma_0 + \gamma_1 x_1 + \gamma_2 x_2 + \gamma_3 x_3$, which are respectively analogous to the 2-D and 3-D MIRT, the coefficients of β_1 and γ_1 cannot be directly compared. The same statement is true when x_1 and x_2 are random effects.

Research Methods

Description of the Projective IRT Procedure

To operationalize the theoretical results described in the previous section, we need methods for the following two purposes: (1) obtaining point estimates for item parameters and ability scores for a projected IRT, and (2) obtaining the correct standard errors for the item parameters and ability estimates for a projected IRT.

Estimates for the Projected IRT Model

The results reported in Ip (2010) only prove the probabilistic equivalence of the MIRT and LD-IRT models—that is, if the item parameters of an MIRT model are known, then the equivalent LD-IRT model can be solved. However, in reality both the MIRT dimensionality and item parameters are unknown. Dimensionality determination often involves both substantive knowledge and empirical methods. There is a rather extensive literature on the determination of dimensionality (practical tools including Mplus and DIMTEST produce a broad array of goodness-of-fit indexes for models of different dimensions; see, for example, Muthén & Muthén, 2012; Stout, Froelich, & Gao, 2001); the topic is beyond the scope of this chapter. Assuming that the dimensionality of the test, say p, can be determined with reasonable accuracy, a p-dimensional MIRT/bifactor model still needs to be fitted to the response data prior to any projection activity.

To illustrate, consider an assessment of physical functioning in which some items measure upper extremity functioning and others measure lower extremity functioning, and that the dimensionality of the test has been determined to be $p = 2$. There are several options for projection: (1) project onto the dominant dimension (physical functioning), (2) project onto a pre-specified linear combination of the lower- and upper-extremity functioning dimensions, or (3) use the unidimensional IRT model and naively apply it to all the response data. It can be shown that fitting a unidimensional model to multidimensional response data is essentially finding the closest projected IRT model to the underlying MIRT from which data are generated (Ip et al., 2013; Kim, 1994). The ability score estimate from a projection method (3) is different from that obtained via the projection onto a coordinate (e.g., the dominant dimension in method (1)). In other words, naively fitting a unidimensional IRT model to empirical response data will not accomplish the goal of projecting on a pre-specified dimension.

Paradoxically, the route to operationalizing projective IRT goes through MIRT and bifactor models. This appears to be an unbecoming solution, but there is no "free lunch"—the underlying multidimensional structure needs to be first estimated before any projection onto a predetermined direction can take place. However, two points should be made here. First, there is some preliminary evidence that the projected unidimensional model is generally not very sensitive to whether the provisional (or "mother") MIRT model in the preceding estimation step to projection is correctly specified. In fact, we recommend using $p = 2$ (i.e., a 2-D MIRT), or a parsimonious bifactor model, for most purposes. We will show in this chapter evidence of robustness of such projective models. The second point is that once the projected IRT is obtained, all the benefits of the parsimonious projected IRT model can be reaped.

The operationalization of projective unidimensional IRT involves the following steps:

- Define the projected direction of interest.
- Estimate from the data the underlying MIRT/bifactor model, possibly with help from substantive analysis and the identification of anchoring items for the specific dimensions.
- Apply the empirical indistinguishability results for computing the equivalent projected unidimensional IRT and rescale the estimates if needed (the marginal distribution of projected θ could be different from the marginal distribution of the same θ from an MIRT).
- Adjust the standard error estimate using a proposed robust estimation procedure (to be discussed in the next section).
- Proceed with other psychometric routines (e.g., individual item analysis, DIF, test equating, or item selection in computerized adaptive test) as if the items were unidimensional in the defined direction of interest but adjust for LD.

Two common testing situations need to be distinguished: (a) the test is supposed to measure a well-defined construct, but a few nuisance dimensions are included because items need to maintain "psychological width"; and (b) the test measures a multidimensional construct whose structure can be determined through other means such as confirmatory factor analysis and bifactor modeling. However, "purified" dimensional scores are needed for special purposes such as comparison with other tests.

For (a), the "substantive dimension" is singular, whereas the "statistical dimension" is greater than one (Walker, Azen, & Schmitt, 2006). Under this situation, it is often sufficient to fit a 2-D MIRT and then find the projection on the dominant dimension. The nuisance dimensions are not of interest and are often well captured by a single additional dimension in MIRT.

For situation (b), one solution is to create a collection of low-dimensional (1- or 2-dimensional) projective IRT models for the bifactor analysis. While the bifactor model is simpler than the general MIRT, things can still get quite complicated when items in a test share a hierarchical structure. For a test with two domains and three subdomains within each domain, creating a bifactor model would require fitting a nine-dimensional MIRT model to the data. Model fitting may not be an issue given the recent advance in bifactor technology. However, the derivation of dimensional scores for new response data for the nine-dimensional model and the interpretation of the scores are more complex than those obtained from the projective IRT. Individually projected IRT models could be helpful for interpreting truly multidimensional data.

With some modifications, the operationalization of p-dimensional ($p > 2$) bifactor projective IRT onto 2-D MIRT models is similar to the procedure for projection onto a single dimension. Because of space limitations, we shall not further discuss the procedure here.

Estimation of Standard Errors for the Latent Trait Estimate

Because of the induced LD from the projection, items from the projected IRT in general do not satisfy the local independence assumption. The conditional correlation between items induced by the projection is always positive (assuming that item discrimination parameters in MIRT are all positive). As a result, the information derived from two distinctive items is no longer the sum of their information functions. In a certain sense, information from the two items "overlaps." In order to avoid "double counting" information, adjustment needs to be made to the sum of information functions, or alternatively, to the standard error estimate of ability (Bradlow, Wainer, & Wang, 1999; Braeken, Tuerlinckx, & De Boeck, 2007; Ip, 2000, 2001, 2002; Ip, Wang, De Boeck, & Meulders, 2004).

To illustrate this phenomenon of bias in SE estimate due to LD, we use as an example a data set that was generated from an MIRT model specified in Equation (11.1), and we used the following specifications: number of items $I = 40$, number of persons $J = 2000$. The discrimination parameter a_{i1} of the dominant dimension was sampled from a uniform distribution, Uniform(1, 4), whereas the discrimination parameter a_{i2} of the minor dimension was sampled from Uniform(1, 2), representing a moderate level of multidimensionality. The intercept parameter d was sampled from Uniform(−5, 5), and a standard bivariate normal distribution was used to generate the pair $(\theta_{j1}, \theta_{j2})$ with the correlation ρ between the dominant dimension θ_1 and the minor dimension θ_2 set to zero. After calibrating the items using a projected IRT model, we computed the projected person estimates (rescaled to line up with the original scale of the true ability) and the standard SEs. The performance of the 95 percent confidence interval, evaluated using a standard IRT method, was then assessed by calculating the percentage of times that confidence intervals bracket the true θ_1. Figure 11.3 shows the result of one such simulation experiment. The 95 percent coverage using standard IRT SE estimate is only 51.2 percent.

To handle the potential problem of overly optimistic confidence interval for the ability score, we propose the use of a robust sandwich estimate for the SE. Unlike the traditional sandwich estimate, which contains two identical components (the breads) and a middle component (the meat) that are uniform across individuals, the proposed sandwich estimate contains individualized breads and a common meat. We call the estimate the individual-bread-common-meat (IBCM) sandwich estimate for the standard error of the latent trait estimate. The IBCM sandwich estimator is a modified version of the Huber-White robust estimator in the statistics and econometrics literature (Fitzmaurice, Laird, & Ware, 2004, p. 303; Huber, 1964, 1981; Liang & Zeger, 1986; White, 1980; Zeger, Liang, & Albert, 1988). The robust estimate was popularized, in the context of generalized linear mixed models, to handle clustered responses such as repeated measurements taken from the same individual over time. In a sense, the proposed IBCM estimate is an extension of the Huber-White estimate for standard error from a regression setting to IRT. The basic idea here is that given item parameters, the estimation of individual ability and the associated standard error in LD-IRT can be solved using proven methods developed for generalized linear models for clustered responses.

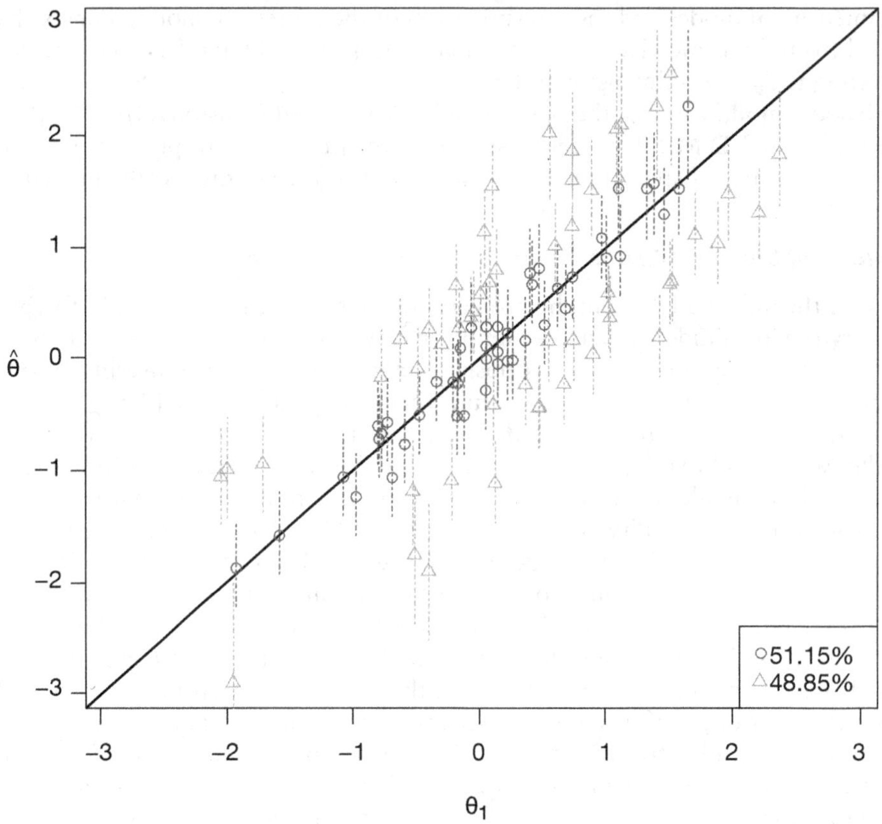

Figure 11.3 The coverage probability for the true ability using the conventional IRT estimate of standard error as shown by a random sample of 100 simulated subjects from a larger sample of 2,000. Each line represents the confidence limits of the point estimate, triangle indicates a "miss," and circle indicates a "hit."

To describe the IBCM estimate, we treat, for each individual, the "predictor" $\underline{X}_i$ as the vector of (assumed known) item parameter (d_i, a_i), and $\underline{\theta} = (-1, \theta_j)$ as the vector of (unknown) parameters. Furthermore, let, Y_{ij} denote the item response (0 or 1) from the jth individual on the ith item and $\mu_{ij} = E(Y_{ij} | \theta_j) = P(Y_{ij} = 1 | \theta_j)$ be specified by the two-parameter logistic (2-PL) model:

$$P(Y_{ij} = 1 \mid \theta_j) = g^{-1}(\underline{X}_i^T \underline{\theta}) = \frac{\exp(a_i\theta_j - d_i)}{1 + \exp(a_i\theta_j - d_i)}, \tag{11.7}$$

where a_i and d_i are, respectively, the discrimination and intercept parameters, and g(·), is the link function. Let $\hat{\theta}$ denote the ability estimate. Our proposed IBCM robust estimate for $Var(\hat{\theta}_j)$ takes the form:

$$Var_{robust}(\theta_j) = \left(D_j^T V_j^{-1} D_j\right)^{-1} \left(\frac{1}{J}\sum_{k=1}^{J}[D_k^T V_k^{-1}(\underline{Y}_k - \underline{\mu}_k)]^2\right)\left(D_j^T V_j^{-1} D_j\right)^{-1}, \tag{11.8}$$

where $D_j = \left[\frac{\partial\mu_{1j}}{\partial\theta_j}\frac{\partial\mu_{2j}}{\partial\theta_j}\cdots\frac{\partial\mu_{Ij}}{\partial\theta_j}\right]^T$, $V_j = A_j^{1/2}RA_j^{1/2}$, $A_j = \text{diag}\{\text{Var}(Y_{ij})\}$, and R is a correlation matrix indicating the conditional pairwise correlation between item responses. For a 2-PL model, the partial derivative term $\frac{\partial\mu_{ij}}{\partial\theta_j} = a_i\mu_{ij}(\theta_j)\bar{\mu}_{ij}(\theta_j)$, and $Var(Y_{ij}) = \mu_{ij}(\theta_j)\bar{\mu}_{ij}(\theta_j)$, where $\bar{\mu} = 1-\mu$. Because the true value of θ_j is not known, the values of $\mu_{ij}(\theta_j)$ in $D_j(\theta_j)$, $V_j^{-1}(\theta_j)$, and θ_j, in (11.8) have to be estimated. A common practice is to use an IRT estimate in the place of $r_k = \underbrace{D_k^T}_{1\times I}\underbrace{V_k^{-1}}_{I\times I}\underbrace{(\underline{Y}_k - \underline{\mu}_k)}_{I\times 1}$. It could be the maximum likelihood estimate, the maximum *a posteriori* estimate, or the expected *a posteriori* estimate. Note that in (11.8) both the "bread" (first and third terms on RHS) and the "meat" (second term on RHS) are scalars. For example, $I_i(\theta_j)$ is a scalar value. Incidentally, the "bread" in (11.8) is the inverse of the sum of information functions i over the item index $I_i(\theta_j) = a_i^2\mu_{ij}(\theta_j)\bar{\mu}_{ij}(\theta_j)$ in standard IRT. For the 2-PL model, the information function (Baker & Kim, 2004, p. 78; Lord, 1980), is given by $Var_{robust}(\hat{\theta}_j)$. The proposed IBCM sandwich estimate $Var_{robust}(\hat{\theta}_j)$ is distinct for each individual. The "bread" part of j in (11.8) involves only data from the specific individual. Accordingly, the piece of the sandwich in (11.8) carries no information whatsoever about the possible conditional residual dependency between item responses induced by the nuisance dimensions. Information concerning local dependency is drawn from the "meat" part of the sandwich in (11.8) through the responses from the entire sample of J individuals. Thus, to continue the culinary metaphor, Equation (11.8) represents a total of J different IBCM estimates, with R different kinds of breads and a common brand of meat (Ip & Chen, 2012).

Several types of common covariance structures have been proposed for the matrix θ (Fitzmaurice et al., 2004). The most commonly used covariance structures include exchangeable and unstructured. The former structure constrains all pairwise correlation to be uniform across item pairs; and the former allows any value within the range (–1,1) for any given pair of items. For IBCM, we respectively label the exchangeable and unstructured covariance IBCM(e) and IBCM(u). For SE estimate that is based on standard unidimensional IRT theory, we label it Conventional SE (CSE). Because the true value of θ is not known in general, we use the maximum *a posteriori* estimate for $\hat{\theta}$ in the place of θ for equations for SE estimates.

Simulation Experiments and Examples

Simulation Experiments for Assessing IBCM

We report the result of several simulation experiments for assessing RMSE and Type I coverage probability at the nominal level of 95 percent confidence for the proposed projective IRT procedure. The experiments were designed in such a way that response data θ_1 were all generated from the 2-D MIRT model in Equation (11.1) under a variety of conditions. By fixing the variances of both θ_2 and a_1 to 1.0 (and the means to 0.0), the strength of each dimension was controlled by the magnitude of the respective discrimination parameters, a_2 and θ_1. As indicated previously, the first dimension θ_2 is designated as the dominant trait, whereas the second dimension a_1 is assumed to be a nuisance factor. In the design, the strength of the first dimension, as indicated by the value of a_2 (assumed positive), was significantly higher—to various degrees—than that of the second, which is indicated by the value of I (also assumed positive).

A factorial design was used for generating Monte Carlo simulated data sets in the experiment. We list the factors and their respective levels as follows: (1) number of items J, four levels: 15, 25, 35, and 45 items; (2) number of individuals a_2, three levels: 500, 1,000, and 2,000 persons; (3) method of standard error estimation, three levels: CSE, IBCM(u), and IBCM(e); (4) relative strength of the minor dimension a_1 and distribution of the item parameters, three scenarios: (A) low minor dimension with diverse distribution on item parameters, (B) high minor dimension with diverse distribution, and (C) moderate minor dimension with non-diverse distribution, with *Unif* (1, 4) respectively sampled from *Unif* (1, 4), *Unif* (0.3, 1.2), and a_2 *Unif* (0.5, 1) respectively sampled from *Unif* (1, 2), *Unif* (0.1, 0.5), and *d*, and *Unif* (–5.0, 5.0), respectively sampled from *Unif* (–5.0, 5.0) *Unif* (–1.2, 1.2), and ρ; and (5) the correlation ρ between the two dimensions, five levels at $\rho = -0.6, -0.3, 0.0, 0.3$, and 0.6. For all of the specified conditions, we replicated the experiment 20 times using the same setting in order to obtain an estimate of the variability of the performance metrics. All in all, (4 × 3 × 3 × 3 × 5) = 10,800 data sets were generated and analyzed in the first experiment.

The metrics for assessing performance of an estimation procedure were the RMSE and the coverage probability of the 95 percent confidence intervals, which are respectively defined as follows:

$$RMSE = \sqrt{\frac{1}{J}\sum_{j=1}^{J}(\theta_j - \theta_j)^2}, \tag{11.9}$$

where θ is the estimate of ability, $\hat{\theta}$ is the true ability, and:

$$Coverage\ Probability = \frac{\#\text{ respondents whose } \theta \text{ fall within 95\% confidence limits}}{\#\text{ total respondents}}, \tag{11.10}$$

where the 95 percent confidence limits were centered at θ and were of length equal to 1.96 × standard error calculated from a specific in either direction. If the SE calculation is correct, then one expects the value θ to fall within the confidence limits with a probability approximately equal to the coverage probability.

Detailed results from the simulation experiments are reported in Ip and Chen (2012). Here, we only highlight some of the most important findings.

RMSE Assessment

Here, the 2-D MIRT SE estimate can be used as the benchmark reference because data were actually generated from the 2-D MIRT item response model.

Figure 11.4 shows the distribution of the RMSEs across different simulation conditions for scenario (B). The patterns seen in the other scenarios are rather similar and not shown here. In terms of RMSE, the projective IRT, regardless of the adjustment method used for SE, performs slightly better than the benchmark 2-D MIRT estimates for both scenarios (A) and (B). However, when the minor dimension is moderate and the distribution of item parameter distribution is tight (scenario C), the projected IRT does not enjoy an

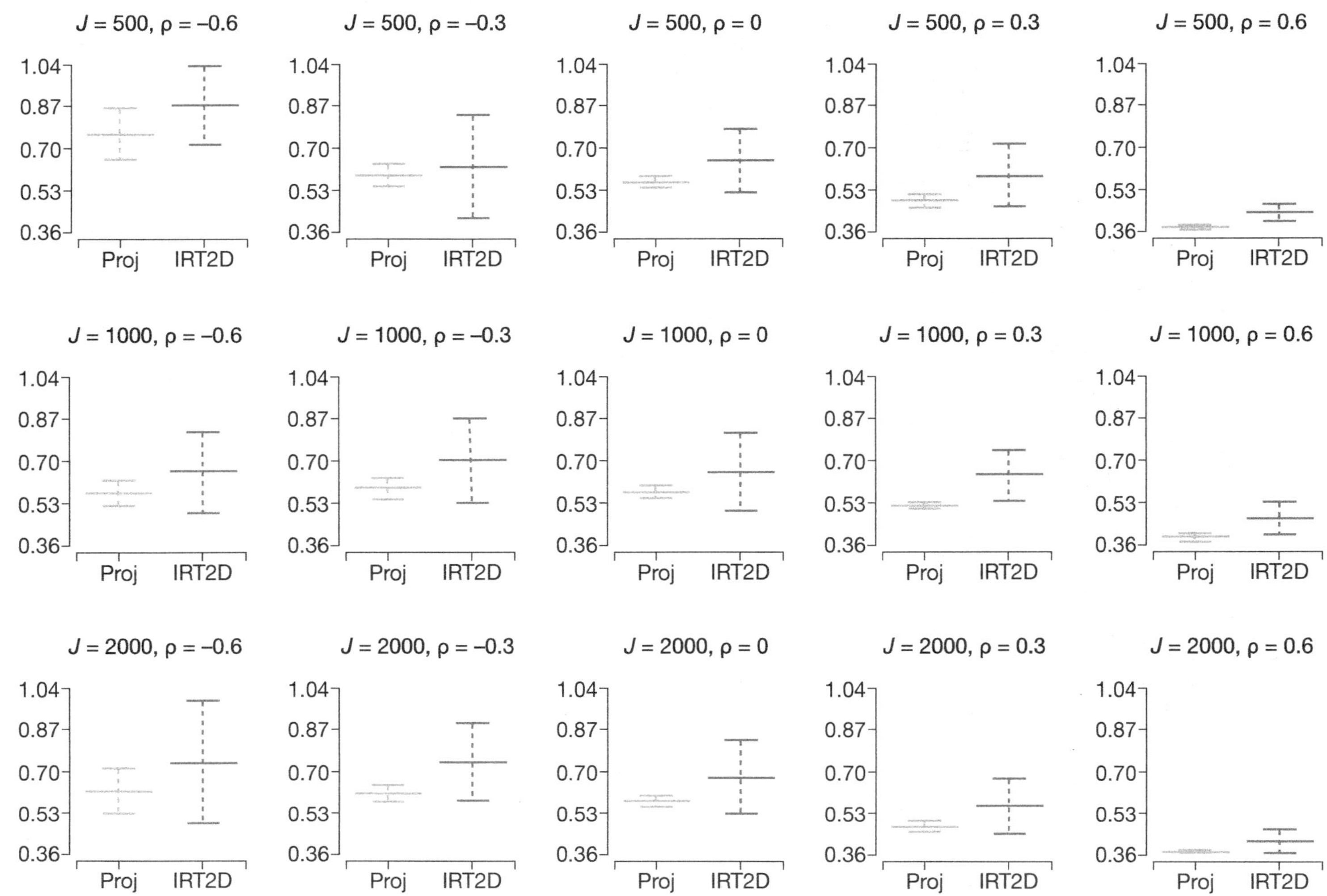

Figure 11.4 Distribution of RMSE for the projected IRT (Proj) and the 2-D MIRT (IRT2D) for the condition of strong minor dimension and diverse item parameter distribution with I = 45.

advantage in terms of smaller means and less variation any more, even though its performance is comparable to that of the benchmark 2-D MIRT.

95 Percent Coverage

The patterns and trends for 95 percent coverage probabilities for the projective IRT estimate show a high level of commonality among the first two scenarios: (A)—relatively weak minor dimension/high diversity of item parameters, and (B)—relatively strong minor dimension/high diversity of item parameters. The difference is in their magnitudes of coverage. Table 11.1 shows the 95 percent coverage probabilities for the projected IRT estimate using several estimates of SE of ability θ_1 for relatively strong minor dimension/high diversity of item parameters (scenario B). The reported numbers are the averaged percentages of correctly covered confidence intervals over 20 replications of the same experiment (same conditions and data-generating mechanism but different response data sets). In Table 11.1, the performances of four different SE estimates are compared: (1) CSE (i.e., as if no LD is present), (2) IBCM(e), (3) IBCM(u), and (4) 2-D MIRT SE estimate, for ability on the dominant dimension (I = 45). Of note, because of sampling error, the average could fluctuate around 95 percent even if the SE estimate is correct for the generative model.

Under scenario (B), both IBCM estimates seem to perform better than the CSE, with the IBCM(u) tracking higher coverage than those of the benchmark 2-D MIRT. This pattern is especially clear for a larger number of items (see ρ = 0, Table 11.1). When I = 45, and J = 500, the benchmark 2-D MIRT method only attains 69.9, 75.4, and 70.6 percent coverage respectively for θ, 1000, and 2000, whereas IBCM(u) achieves respective coverage of 81.0, 81.8, and 79.4. IBCM(e) tends to provide a little lower coverage than the benchmark. On the other hand, the coverage of the CSE method is quite poor; the method grossly underestimates SE, resulting in covering the true for θ only about half of the time for ρ = 0 and I = 45, which implies a Type I error rate of 50 percent.

For scenarios (A) and (C), the trends are rather different. For scenario (A), the coverage of CSE is generally better compared to scenario (B). For scenario (C), however, the CSE performs remarkably well. For example, when ρ = 0.6, for various values of I and J, the average coverage for the CSE, IBCM(e), and IBCM(u) are respectively 92.5, 93.6, and 82.6. When θ_1, the average coverage for the three methods are respectively 93.6, 95.1, and 89.3.

The results appear to suggest that IBCM(e) is useful when the minor dimensions are strong, and CSE surprisingly is a reasonably accurate measure for uncertainty when the minor dimensions are not strong and when distributions of item parameters are considered not diverse.

Application

Two data sets are used to illustrate the projective IRT approach: (1) clinical data collected from a study that measured the construct of older adults' desire for physical competency (Rejeski, Ip, Katula, & White, 2006); (2) clinical data collected from Wave 1 of a Patient Reported Outcomes Measurement Information System (PROMIS®) study on emotional distress. In the first example, we demonstrate how the projective model can be derived and further assess the robustness of the projective model, including its sensitivity to misspecification of the intermediate or "mother" MIRT using simulated data. The assessment of robustness used the following approach: first, we used parameters from real data to

Table 11.1 95% Coverage Probabilities for Scenario (B): Strong Minor Dimension, Diverse Item Parameters

		$\rho = -0.6$				$\rho = -0.3$				$\rho = 0$				$\rho = 0.3$				$\rho = 0.6$			
	J	*CSE*	*IBCM (e)*	*IBCM (u)*	*SE (2d)*	*CSE*	*IBCM (e)*	*IBCM (u)*	*SE (2d)*	*CSE*	*IBCM (e)*	*IBCM (u)*	*SE (2d)*	*CSE*	*IBCM (e)*	*IBCM (u)*	*SE (2d)*	*CSE*	*IBCM (e)*	*IBCM (u)*	*SE (2d)*
	500	75.9	69.9	70.7	74.1	69.3	76.3	77.3	70.0	75.3	69.2	82.8	78.7	78.2	83.8	89.9	83.2	82.4	84.8	91.4	86.0
$I = 15$	1000	80.5	71.2	78.4	76.1	76.4	68.1	77.0	76.4	76.1	73.6	82.6	81.5	76.6	79.3	85.8	82.7	83.6	91.7	94.1	89.8
	2000	77.7	84.5	81.2	78.9	73.1	72.5	74.9	75.8	76.3	70.9	77.4	76.3	82.7	78.5	85.6	88.9	83.6	76.4	91.4	87.7
	500	73.6	80.5	79.5	71.3	63.5	69.3	74.1	67.6	61.4	69.1	78.4	72.2	68.0	77.9	87.8	80.8	73.4	78.3	93.5	82.7
$I = 25$	1000	74.7	79.6	84.7	80.4	64.1	70.8	71.8	70.3	62.2	70.6	77.6	74.0	68.7	79.7	88.5	82.2	73.6	81.6	92.5	88.3
	2000	74.0	80.8	81.2	82.6	63.8	77.5	71.6	72.1	63.5	70.2	74.8	71.1	71.8	75.6	85.0	86.0	74.4	81.1	90.8	89.8
	500	62.0	71.7	77.7	69.6	60.1	66.2	79.5	70.6	57.3	66.4	85.6	73.6	58.5	74.2	86.7	75.1	64.8	84.0	92.4	81.6
$I = 35$	1000	64.2	70.3	79.4	72.6	57.3	66.3	75.0	67.4	56.7	70.9	77.9	71.9	61.9	67.7	82.7	79.4	66.0	75.1	87.8	82.8
	2000	63.3	67.8	73.0	67.4	56.1	68.7	71.0	66.4	56.6	65.9	81.0	80.7	63.9	76.7	85.8	85.7	69.3	76.7	92.6	86.6
	500	56.0	70.7	71.7	57.8	54.6	67.0	77.9	71.1	52.5	65.6	81.0	69.9	55.9	67.9	87.3	74.4	61.7	72.4	92.3	81.0
$I = 45$	1000	64.6	71.3	77.9	75.1	54.3	71.4	79.7	66.6	52.5	64.0	81.8	75.4	52.8	67.7	77.1	70.3	62.8	78.6	92.7	83.5
	2000	62.2	76.6	74.1	69.7	53.3	61.0	73.6	66.5	51.9	67.6	79.4	70.6	55.8	75.0	88.7	77.0	62.2	69.8	88.1	88.1

simulate multidimensional item responses, then based on the simulated data, we estimated provisional MIRT/bifactor models, including both correctly and incorrectly specified ones, and projected them onto a unidimensional IRT for analysis.

There are several reasons why we adopted this particular design. First, the projective IRT procedure directly operates on the MIRT parameters, not on the response data. Therefore, this design for assessing robustness does not entirely lose on the benefit of using real response data, but now it has the potential to provide more meaningful results as the underlying model becomes available. Second, the design allows a study of the sensitivity of projective IRT methods when the "mother" MIRT model is not correctly specified. In the first example, we fitted a (misspecified) 2-D MIRT model to a response data set generated from a 3-D bifactor model, which was based on parameters estimated from the real data. Then we compared the performance of the projected IRT from the misspecified model with the projected IRT from the correctly specified 3-D bifactor model. Specifically, we fitted to the response data a misspecified 2-D MIRT model with one dimension representing a general factor and another representing all of the other nuisance dimensions. Then we projected the 2-D model onto the general dimension (θ_1), which in our experiment was identified by matching the estimated factors to the general dimension in the 3-D bifactor model using a Euclidean distance metric.

The programs for generating simulated data, performing projection, and calculating ICBM were written in the statistical language R, whereas IRT/MIRT estimation was conducted using IRTPRO 2.1 (Scientific Software International, Inc., Lincolnwood, IL).

Example 1. Older Adults' Desire for Physical Competence

In the study of physical functioning in older adults, self-efficacy expectations are important in understanding falls and the decline of basic functional skills such as ambulation and transfer. The study for Desire for Physical Competence (DPC) was motivated by the need to understand the impact of self-efficacy expectations on behavior to the incentive value of behavior. This data set, collected under the auspices of the Pepper Older Americans Independence Center at Wake Forest University, contains response data from $J = 157$ older adults (mean age 73.3; SD = 8.0; n for men = 53; n for women = 140) to a 16-item measure that assesses a new construct termed DPC. The data resource and instrument design were described in detail by Rejeski and colleagues (2006).

Fourteen items were selected and the corresponding item responses had been dichotomized for this analysis. Table 11.2 shows several model statistics (–2 loglikelihood, AIC, BIC) for 2-D, 3-D, 4-D MIRTs. The 2-D model has the lowest AIC value while the 1-D model has the lowest BIC value. There was preliminary evidence that the items approximately separate into two groups (Rejeski et al., 2006): desire for basic physical tasks instrumental to daily living (e.g., having the ability to stand up from a low, soft couch or chair) and desire for more advanced but non-instrumental activities (e.g., having the ability to jog a short distance of 20–50 feet). An exploratory factor analysis revealed that the two groups were quite distinct. Under a two-factor model, for items identified as related to basic instrumental activities, the factor loadings were all higher than 0.74 (range 0.74–0.95) and below 0.13 (range 0.02–0.13) for the other factor. On the other hand, for items identified as related to non-instrumental activities, the factor loadings had a range of 0.64–0.89 on the dominant factor and a range of 0.05–0.12 on the other factor. We also fitted a bifactor model (one general plus two domain-specific dimensions that correspond to the factor analytic results), of which the model statistics are also given in Table 11.2.

To illustrate the projective procedure, we used the bifactor model as a starting point. Bifactor loadings of the DPC data and the results are presented in Table 11.3. In a

Table 11.2 Model Statistic for the Real Data Examples

Statistic	*1D*	*2D*	*3D*	*4D*	*Bifactor*
DPC data example					
−2xloglikelihood:	1690	1655	1638	1622	1657
Akaike Information Criterion (AIC)	1746	1737	1744	1762	1741
Bayesian Information Criterion (BIC)	1832	1862	1906	1976	1869
PROMIS® emotional stress example					
−2xloglikelihood:	52824	52353	52234	52180	52258
Akaike Information Criterion (AIC)	52916	52489	52412	52398	52396
Bayesian Information Criterion (BIC)	53268	53010	53094	53233	52925

Table 11.3 Estimated Factor Loading of DCP Data Using Bifactor Model Analysis and the Corresponding Item Parameters of the Projective Model

Item	*Estimated bifactor model*				*Projective model parameter*	
	a_1	a_2	a_3	d	a^*	d^*
1	2.18	1.61		1.38	1.58	1.00
2	1.99	1.32		−0.71	1.57	−0.56
3	5.77	4.35		0.78	2.10	0.28
4	2.16	1.04		1.32	1.84	1.13
5	3.5	0.42		−4.37	3.40	−4.25
6	5.79		1.12	−3.82	4.83	−3.19
7	6.17		2.64	−5.52	3.34	−2.99
8	2.79		1.13	−3.12	2.32	−2.60
9	4.23		1.13	−3.76	3.52	−3.13
10	3.37		−0.25	−3.15	3.33	−3.11
11	5.22	0.23		−4.05	5.18	−4.01
12	3.18	1.63		0.68	2.30	0.49
13	2.17	0.69		0.28	2.01	0.26
14	2.98	0.42		2.64	2.89	2.56

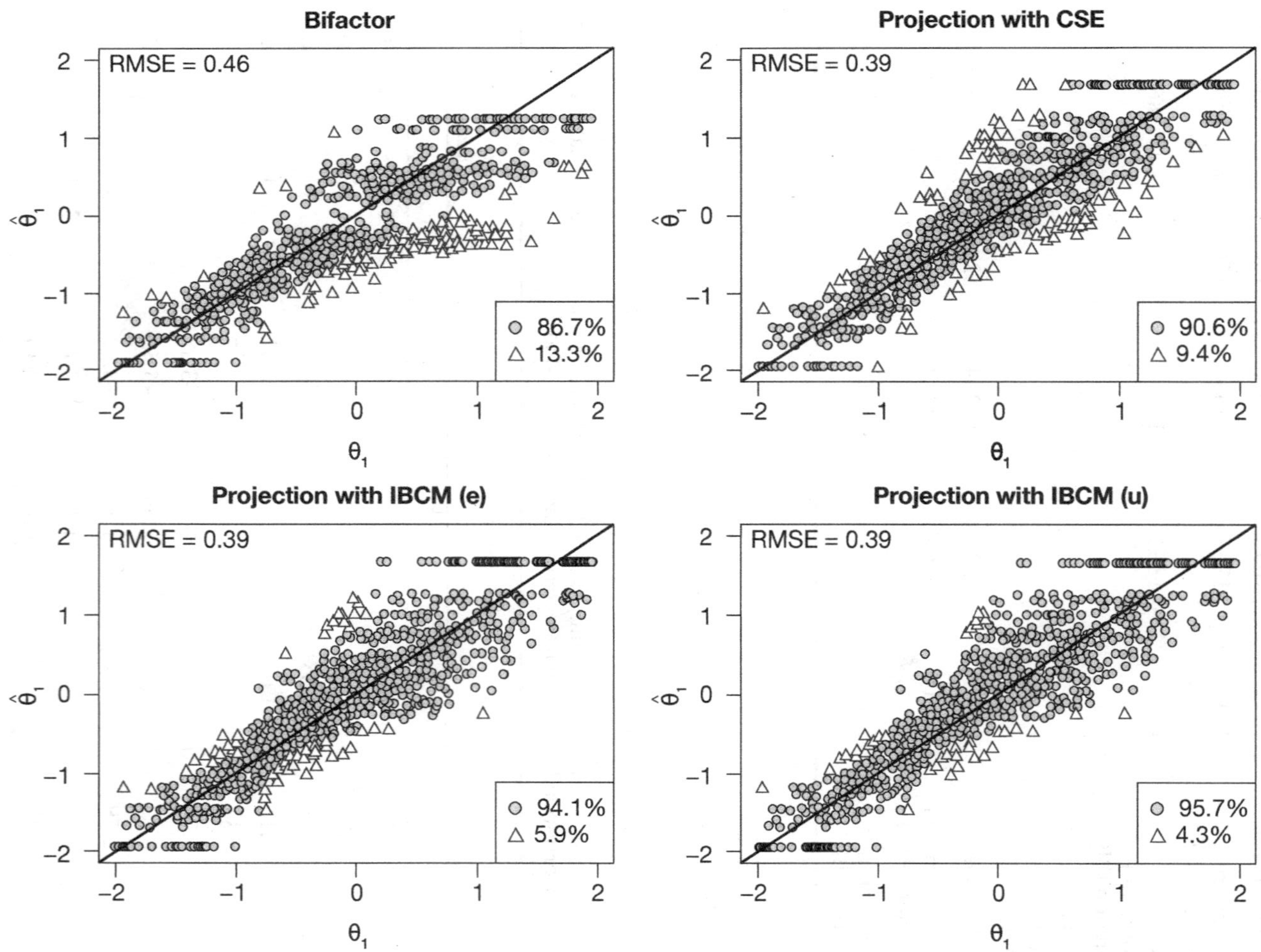

Figure 11.5 Scatterplots showing 95 percent confidence interval coverage for the true general trait $n = 15{,}707$ versus the estimated trait-2xloglikelihood. A dot indicates a case when the true general trait lies within the estimated 95 percent confidence interval (a "hit"), and a triangle indicates a case when the trait lies outside the interval (a "miss").

subsequent step, we projected the bifactor model onto a unidimensional model using Equations (11.1)–(11.3). For example, for item 1 Table 11.3), $\lambda_{logit} = \left[k^2 a_2^2 \left(1-\rho^2\right)\sigma_2^2 + 1\right]^{-1/2}$ $= \left[0.588^2 1.61 + 1\right]^{-1/2} = 0.726$, and $a^* = \lambda_{logit} a_1 = 0.726 \times 2.18 = 1.5$, given that $\rho = 0$, $\sigma_1 = \sigma_2 = 1$. Furthermore, we have $d^* = \lambda_{logit} d = 0.726 \times 1.38 = 1$.

It needs to be pointed out here that the bifactor model (Gibbons & Hedeker, 1992) assumes that all of the factors—general and domain specific—are independent. The simplifying assumption allows the projective IRT procedure described earlier in this chapter for 2-D MIRT to easily generalize to the higher-dimensional bifactor models: The projection of all blocks of items that have the same specific factor is treated as a separate 2-D MIRT projection problem.

In order to evaluate the sensitivity of the projected IRT model to misspecification of the "mother" MIRT, we followed the design described earlier with the following specification: item parameters from the 3-D bifactor model were used to generate responses from a random sample of 1,000 examinees drawn from the normal distribution $N(0, \Sigma)$ where Σ is a 3×3 identity matrix with $|\theta_k| < 2, k = 1,2,3$. We estimated the abilities and SE of the simulated data based on the item parameters listed in Table 11.2. Figure 11.5 shows the scatterplots and 95 percent confidence interval coverage for the true general trait $\hat{\theta}_1$ versus the estimated trait $\hat{\theta}_1$ with the corresponding SE for the following methods, respectively: (1) 3-D bifactor MIRT CSE, (2) projected $\hat{\theta}_1$ with SE estimated using CSE, (3) projected $\hat{\theta}_1$ with SE estimated using IBCM(e), and (4) projected $\hat{\theta}_1$ with SE estimated using IBCM(u). The covariance structures Cov_1 and Cov_2 respectively of IBCM(e) and IBCM(u) were specified as follows:

$$Cov_1(Y) = \begin{pmatrix} 1 & \phi & \cdots & \phi \\ \phi & 1 & \cdots & \phi \\ \vdots & & \ddots & \vdots \\ \phi & \phi & \cdots & 1 \end{pmatrix}; Cov_2(Y) = \begin{pmatrix} 1 & \phi_{21} & \cdots & \phi_{J1} \\ \phi_{21} & 1 & \cdots & \phi_{J2} \\ \vdots & & \ddots & \vdots \\ \phi_{J1} & \phi_{J2} & \cdots & 1 \end{pmatrix}. \tag{11.11}$$

The RMSE shows the projective IRT estimate of ability is both unbiased and accurate. The CSE estimate actually slightly under-covers, while both ICBM(e) and ICBM(u) provide reasonably accurate estimates. Note that the characteristics of item parameter values and their distributions for the bifactor model are somewhere between scenarios (A) and (B) in the simulation experiments described in Section 4. This explains the generally high performance of the ICBM in this example. The scatterplots for the correctly specified bifactor MIRT estimate and for the various SE methods are quite similar to the plot in Figure 11.4 and are not shown here. The RMSEs are 0.380 and 0.422 respectively for bifactor MIRT and projected IRT, which are of similar magnitudes to the RMSE in Figure 11.4. The coverage for the CSE (bifactor), CSE(projected), IBCM(u), and IBCM(e) are, respectively, 96.9, 92.7, 95.5, and 96.7, suggesting that both IBCM and CSE are performing quite well.

We further investigated the robustness of the projected IRT method by using a misspecified 2-D MIRT model and its corresponding projection. The RMSE of ability estimates of the projected IRT model from the misspecified 2-D MIRT model is 0.420, which is almost identical to that for the projected IRT for the 3-D bifactor model. The CSE (89.1%) performs reasonably well, whereas both IBCM(e) (95.9%) and IBCM(u) (94.8%) provide accurate coverage for the projective models from the incorrectly specified 2-D MIRT. This suggests that the projective model is quite robust to misspecification in the provisional MIRT model.

Table 11.4 Estimated Factor Loading of PROMIS® Data Using Bifactor Model Analysis and the Corresponding Item Parameters of the Projective Model

Estimated bifactor model	*Projective model*						
Item number	a_1	a_2	a_3	a_4	d	a^*	d^*
1	1.985	0.840			0.096	1.780	0.086
2	1.998	1.658			1.491	1.430	1.067
3	2.475	1.767			1.200	1.716	0.832
4	2.986	2.464			4.199	1.696	2.385
5	2.097	1.396			3.612	1.621	2.791
6	2.190	1.769			2.326	1.518	1.612
7	2.417	1.097			0.822	2.031	0.691
8	2.541	1.067			−0.075	2.153	−0.064
9	3.290		1.343		3.931	2.582	3.085
10	4.030		1.541		2.635	2.986	1.952
11	3.042		1.103		0.947	2.552	0.795
12	3.448		1.158		4.186	2.850	3.460
13	3.875		1.749		2.413	2.701	1.682
14	4.540		1.762		2.668	3.153	1.852
15	3.855		1.904		1.080	2.568	0.719
16	5.316			2.281	5.622	3.178	3.360
17	4.263			2.368	4.463	2.487	2.603
18	4.543			1.591	4.418	3.317	3.226
19	4.487			0.335	1.770	4.402	1.737
20	3.863			1.456	3.336	2.934	2.534
21	4.289			0.698	2.593	3.968	2.399
22	4.468			0.721	1.000	4.113	0.921
23	5.077			1.607	5.067	3.690	3.683

Example 2. Emotional Distress

The data set contained a subset of data collected from Wave 1 of the PROMIS® project, a large-scale National Institute of Health initiative to support research in PROs through the development of a range of measurements that cover physical, mental, and social health (Cella et al., 2010). The measurement tools can also be used across chronic conditions. The 23 items analyzed in this article covered three domains under emotional distress: Depression (8 items), Anxiety (7 items), and Anger (8 items), and data from a total of a^* participants were analyzed. Details about emotional distress measurement in PROMIS® is provided in Pilkonis and colleagues (2011).

We first fitted several different MIRT models including 2-D, 3-D, 4-D, and a bifactor model of one general and three domain-specific dimensions, to the data and then projected the data onto the dominant dimension. The bifactor model used the domains as specific dimensions and thus contained four dimensions. Table 11.2 shows the d^*, AIC, and BIC of the several fitted models, with the unidimensional (1-D) IRT also included as a reference. The bifactor model has the best fit in terms of both AIC and BIC and was used as a reference model for comparing with other fitted models. We fitted MIRT of different dimensions together with the bifactor model to the data and then derived the projected dimension for each "mother" MIRT. Our purpose is to compare projected values of the item parameters and, more important, the projected scores for emotional stress. Table 11.4 shows the estimated parameters for the bifactor model and the projected values of the discrimination and intercept parameters a^* and d^* (Equation (11.3)).

To summarize the comparison between the various projected scores, we used a scatterplot to show the estimated emotional distress score for the various projected models compared to that from the projected bifactor model in Figure 11.6. For readability, we only used the values from a random sample of 1,000 participants. We noted there were only 716 unique patterns (and thus IRT estimates) for the entire sample of n = 15,707. It can be seen from Figure 11.6 that the projected bifactor scores and the projected 2-D scores appear to be highly consistent, while the projected 4-D MIRT scores tend to deviate from the bifactor projected score. One possible explanation is that a high-dimensional MIRT model is often difficult to accurately calibrate. The uncertainties associated with the item parameters especially along the weaker dimensions are often large, leading to biases in the estimates for latent scores (emotional distress in this case). While there is no "true" underlying model for the data set, given the fact that the bifactor model has the best model fit statistic (both AIC and BIC), the result suggests that the bifactor model or the parsimonious 2-D MIRT could be a good starting "mother" MIRT for projective purpose.

Summary

The unidimensional item response model is a powerful tool for scaling multiple dichotomous and polytomous item responses. This class of parsimonious models has proved to be useful for handling multiple responses in many fields of study. As assessments become more complex, the undimensionality assumption for response data collected from health and medicine, education, and other social sciences becomes increasingly difficult to defend. However, it does not imply that unidimensional models are not helpful for measuring multidimensional response data. There are at least two directions for how unidimensional models can be used for measuring multidimensional response data: (1) First fit a multidimensional IRT model to the data and then somehow "project" the multidimensional model onto a unidimensional model, and (2) Directly fit a unidimensional IRT model to empirical data without going through the intermediate step of MIRT, and then assess the robustness of the model (e.g., Harrison, 1986; Junker & Stout, 1994; Kirisci, Hsu, & Yu, 2001; Reckase et al., 1986). If the fitted model is robust, then the unidimensional model could still serve the purpose of assessing some form of composite dimension. Which alternative is the preferred approach would depend on the purpose of the study. For example, if an overall single "representative dimension" or a functional dimension (Ip et al., 2013) is being sought for summarizing the multiple dimensions of the response data, then Direction (2) would be more appropriate.

The collection of methods described in this chapter—the projective IRT—is an approach along Direction (1), designed for researchers who are interested in using unidimensional models for measuring multidimensional data along a well-defined dominant dimension.

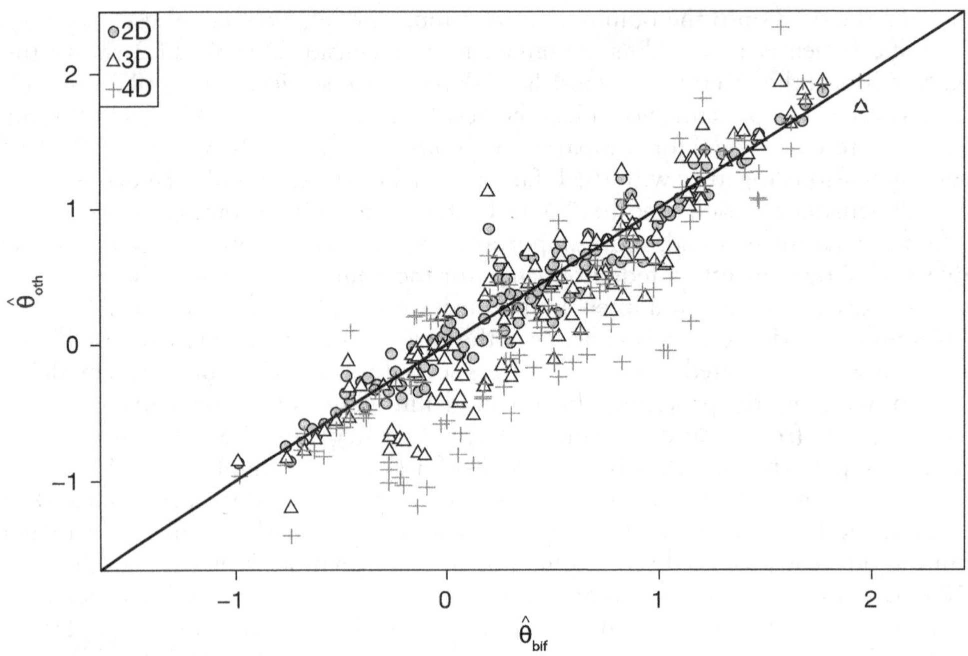

Figure 11.6 Scatterplot of projected person estimates from the bifactor model ($\hat{\theta}_{bif}$) and the projected person estimates from the other models ($\hat{\theta}_{oth}$) including 2-D, 3-D, and 4-D MIRT.

The technique, which we call "projection" here, is a marginalization or "integrating out" of the dimensions that are not of interest (see also footnote in Section 2b). Marginalization is a technique commonly used in the statistics literature; it is especially useful for comparing models that have different numbers of random effects (e.g., Heagerty & Zeger, 2000). The item parameters in the projected models represent unidimensional parameters averaged over other latent dimensions. As such, these parameters have been shown to be not sensitive to minor misspecification of the assumptions about the underlying multidimensional model. This alleviates concerns about the necessary accuracy of the provisional MIRT in the intermediate step of the projective model.

The findings from the Monte Carlo experiment and simulated data from realistic testing situations suggest that the uncertainty associated with score estimates in the projected IRT model can be approximated well by the conventional IRT SE estimates when the minor dimensions are not strong and when the item parameters are not extremely diverse. In cases when the minor dimensions are relatively strong (e.g., as suggested by high values of discrimination parameters in MIRT or bifactor analysis), then the IBCM(e) option for computing SE of the score should be considered.

In health and other sciences, the study of broad constructs such as depression is often hampered by the use of different measures across different studies, which makes cross-study comparison difficult. While efforts have been made to create common measures—an example of which is the PROMIS® initiative—it is unrealistic to expect a single definitive measure of depression will be agreed upon by everyone. More realistically, it is more likely that a number of scales will coexist, and that they all are more or less getting at the same construct, but are differentially contaminated by multidimensionality because of content differences and other substantive considerations. This is when the ability to extract accurate information along a defined dimension (signal) in the presence of a constellation of contaminating constructs (noise) of various mixes and various degrees could facilitate comparison across different data sets. The projective IRT is a tool for extracting information along a defined dimension.

The projective IRT framework described here should be of practical value to practitioners in the fields of education, psychology, and health sciences. For clinical researchers using PROs, they can now apply the method to enhance flexibility for designing questionnaires. For example, using the projective method, a question that apparently involves multiple features of interest but otherwise has strong face validity for a target construct could be retained. A cognitive scientist who wants to measure memory function of a subject could design ecologically valid tests that contain meaningful content and not worry that test items may involve memory and other cognitive domains such as spatial cognition and executive function. She could focus on designing the items. With these new tools, it is our hope that the psychometrician will wave a projective model "magic wand" and save her day.

Acknowledgments

This work is related to a follow-up study to a project originally supported by the NSF grant award SES-0719354 (PI: Edward Ip). One of the data sets used in this chapter was provided by PROMIS®. PROMIS® was funded with cooperative agreements from the National Institutes of Health (NIH) Common Fund Initiative (U54AR057951, U01AR052177, U54AR057943, U54AR057926, U01AR057948, U01AR052170, U01AR057954, U01AR052171, U01AR052181, U01AR057956, U01AR052158, U01AR057929, U01AR057936, U01AR052155, U01AR057971, U01AR057940, U01AR057967, U01AR052186). The contents of this chapter use data developed under PROMIS®. These contents do not necessarily represent an endorsement by the U.S. federal government or PROMIS®. See www.nihpromis.org for additional information on the PROMIS® initiative.

References

Ackerman, T.A., Gierl, M.J., & Walker, C.M. (2003). Using multidimensional item response theory to evaluate educational and psychological tests. *Educational Measurement: Issues and Practice, 22*, 37–51.

Adams, R.J., Wilson, M., & Wang, W.-C. (1997). The multidimensional random coefficient multinomial logit model. *Applied Psychological Measurement, 21*, 1–23.

Baker, F., & Kim, S. (2004). *Item response theory* (2nd ed.) New York: Marcel Dekker.

Bjorner, J.B., Wallenstein, G.V., Martin, M.C., Lin, P., Blaisdell-Gross, B., Piech, C.T., & Mody, S.H. (2007). Interpreting score differences in the SF-36 Vitality scale: Using clinical conditions and functional outcomes to define the minimally important difference. *Current Medical Research Opinion, 23*, 731–739.

Bradlow, E., Wainer, H., & Wang, X. (1999). A Bayesian random effects model for testlets. *Psychometrika, 64*, 153–168.

Braeken, J., Tuerlinckx, F., & De Boeck, P. (2007). Copulas for residual dependencies. *Psychometrika, 72*, 393–411.

Cella, D., Riley, W., Stone, A., Rothrock, N., Reeve, B., Yount, S., . . . the PROMIS Cooperative Group. (2010). Initial item banks and first wave testing of the Patient-Reported Outcomes Measurement Information System (PROMIS) network: 2005–2008. *Journal of Clinical Epidemiology, 63*, 1179–1194.

Embretson, S.E., & Reise, S.P. (2000). *Item response theory for psychologists*. Mahwah, NJ: Lawrence Erlbaum Associates.

Fitzmaurice, G.M., Laird, N.M., & Ware, J.H. (2004). *Applied longitudinal analysis*. New York: Wiley.

Forrest, C.B., Bevans, K.B., Tucker, C., Riley, A.W., Ravens-Sieberer, U., Gardner, W., & Pajer, K. (2012). Commentary: The Patient-Reported Outcome Measurement Information System (PROMIS) for children and youth: Application to pediatric psychology. *Journal of Pediatric Psychology, 37*, 614–621.

Gibbons, R.D., & Hedeker, D.R. (1992). Full-information item bifactor analysis. *Psychometrika, 57*, 423–436.

Gibbons, R.D., Immekus, J.C., & Bock, R.D. (2007). The added value of multidimensional IRT models. *Multidimensional and hierarchical modeling monograph 1*, Center for Health Statistics, University of Illinois at Chicago.

Hambleton, R. K., Swaminathan, H., & Rogers, H.J. (1991). *Fundamentals of item response theory*. Newbury Park, CA: Sage.

Harrison, D.A. (1986). Robustness of parameter estimation to violations to the unidimensionality assumption. *Journal of Educational Statistics, 11*, 91–115.

Heagerty, P.J., & Zeger, S.L. (2000). Marginalized multilevel models and likelihood inference. *Statistical Science, 15*, 1–26.

Holzinger, K.J., & Swineford, F. (1937). The bifactor method. *Psychometrika, 2*, 41–54.

Huber, P.J. (1964). Robust estimation of a location parameter. *Annals of Mathematical Statistics, 35*, 73–101.

Huber, P.J. (1981). *Robust statistics*. Hoboken, NJ: Wiley.

Hulin, C.L., Drasgow, F., & Parsons, C.K. (1983). *Item response theory: Application to psychological measurement*. Homewood, IL: Dow Jones-Irwin.

Humphreys, L.G. (1986). An analysis and evaluation of test and item bias in the predication context. *Journal of Applied Psychology, 71*, 327–333.

Ip, E.H. (2000). Adjusting for information inflation due to local dependency in moderately large item clusters. *Psychometrika, 65*, 73–91.

Ip, E.H. (2001). Testing for local dependency in dichotomous and polytomous item response models. *Psychometrika, 66*, 109–132.

Ip, E.H. (2002). Locally dependent latent trait model and the Dutch identity revisited. *Psychometrika, 67*, 367–386.

Ip, E.H. (2010). Empirically indistinguishable multidimensional IRT and locally dependent unidimensional item response models. *British Journal of Mathematical and Statistical Psychology, 63*, 395–415.

Ip, E.H., & Chen, S.-H. (2012). Projective item response model for test-independent measurement. *Applied Psychological Measurement, 36*, 581–601.

Ip, E.H., Molenberghs, G., Chen, S.-H., Goegebeur, Y., & De Boeck, P. (2013). Functionally unidimensional item response models. *Multivariate Behavioral Research, 48*, 534–562.

Ip, E.H., Wang, Y., De Boeck, P., & Meulders, M. (2004). Locally dependent latent trait model for polytomous responses with application to inventory of hostility. *Psychometrika, 69*, 191–216.

Junker, B.W., & Stout, W.F. (1994). Robustness of ability estimation when multiple traits are present with one trait dominant. In D. Laveault, B.D. Zumbo, M.E. Gessaroli, & M.W. Boss (Eds.), *Modern theories of measurement: Problems and issues* (pp. 31–61). Ottawa, Canada: University of Ottawa.

Kahraman, N., & Thompson, T. (2009, April). Relating unidimensional IRT parameters to a multidimensional response space: A comparison of two alternative dimensionality reduction approaches. Paper presented at the annual meeting of the National Council on Measurement in Education, San Diego, California.

Kelley, T.L. (1928). *Crossroads in the mind of man: A study of differentiable mental abilities*. Stanford, CA: Stanford University Press.

Kim, H. (1994). New techniques for the dimensionality assessment of standardized test data (Doctoral dissertation). Retrieved from Illinois Digital environment for Access to Learning and Scholarship (AAI9512427).

Kirisci, L., Hsu, T., & Yu, L. (2001). Robustness of item parameter estimation programs to assumptions of unidimensionality and normality. *Applied Psychological Measurement, 25*, 146–162.

Liang, K. Y., & Zeger, S. L. (1986). Longitudinal data analysis for discrete and continuous outcomes. *Biometrics, 42*, 121–130.

Lord, F. M. (1980). *Applications of item response theory to practical testing problems*. Mahwah, NJ: Lawrence Erlbaum Associates.

Luecht, R. M., & Miller, T. R. (1992). Unidimensional calibrations and interpretations of composite traits for multidimensional tests. *Applied Psychological Measurement, 16*, 279–293.

Muthén, B. O. (1989). Latent variable modeling in heterogeneous populations. *Psychometrika, 54*, 557–585.

Muthén, L. K., & Muthén, B. O. (2012). *Mplus user's guide* (7th ed.). Los Angeles, CA: Muthén & Muthén.

Ozer, D. (2001). Four principles of personality assessment. In L. A. Pervin & O. P. John (Eds.), *Handbook of personality: Theory and research* (2nd ed.) (pp. 671–688). New York: Guilford Press.

Pilkonis, P. A., Choi, S. W., Reise, S. P., Stover, A. M., Riley, W. T., & Cella, D. (2011). Item banks for measuring emotional distress from the Patient-Reported Outcomes Measurement Information System (PROMIS): Depression, anxiety, and anger. *Assessment, 18*, 263–283.

Reckase, M. D. (1997). A linear logistic multidimensional model for dichotomous item response data. In W. J. van der Linden & R. K. Hambleton (Eds.) *Handbook of item response theory* (pp. 271–286). New York: Springer.

Reckase, M. D., Carlson, J. E., Ackerman, T. A., & Spray, J. A. (1986). The interpretation of unidimensional IRT parameters when estimated from multidimensional data. Paper presented at the annual meeting of the Psychometric Society, Toronto.

Reise, S. P., Bonifay, W. E., & Haviland, M. G. (2013). Scoring and modeling psychological measures in the presence of multidimensionality. *Journal of Personal Assessment, 95*, 129–140.

Reise, S. P., Morizot, J., & Hays, R. D. (2007). The role of bifactor models in resolving dimensionality issues in health outcomes measures. *Quality of Life Research, 16*, 19–31.

Rejeski, J., Ip, E. H., Katula, J., & White, L. (2006). Older adults' desire for physical competence. *Medicine and Science in Sports and Exercise, 38*, 100–105.

Rijmen, F., & De Boeck, P. (2005). A relation between a between-item multidimensional IRT model and the mixture Rasch model. *Psychometrika, 70*, 481–496.

Spearman, C. (1933). The factor theory and its troubles: III. Misrepresentation of the theory. *Journal of Educational Psychology, 24*, 591–601.

Steinberg, L., & Thissen, D. (1996). Uses of item response theory and the testlet concept in the measurement of psychopathology. *Psychological Methods, 1*(1), 81.

Stout, W. (1987). A nonparametric approach for assessing latent trait unidimensionality, *Psychometrika, 52*, 586–617.

Stout, W., Froelich, A. G., & Gao, F. (2001). Using resampling methods to produce an improved DIMTEST procedure. In A. Boomsma, M. A. J. Duijn, & T. A. B. Snijders (Eds.), *Essays on item response theory* (pp. 357–376). New York: Springer-Verlag.

Thurstone, L. L. (1931). Measurement of social attitudes. *Journal of Abnormal and Social Psychology, 26*, 249–269.

van Abswoude, A. A. H., van der Ark, L. A., & Sijtsma, K. (2004). A comparative study of test data dimensionality assessment procedures under nonparametric IRT models. *Applied Psychological Measurement, 28*, 3–24.

Walker, C. M., Azen, R., & Schmitt, T. (2006). Statistical versus substantive dimensionality. *Educational and Psychological Measurement, 66*, 721–738.

White, H. (1980). A heteroskedasticity-consistent covariance matrix estimator and a direct test for heteroskedasticity. *Econometrica, 48*, 817–838.

Zeger, S. L., Liang, K. Y., & Albert, P. (1988). Models for longitudinal data: A generalized estimating equation approach. *Biometrics, 44*, 1049–1060.

Zhang, J. (2007). Conditional covariance theory and DETECT for polytomous items. *Psychometrika, 72*, 69–91.

12 Multidimensional Explanatory Item Response Modeling

Paul De Boeck and Mark Wilson

Introduction

In this chapter an item response modeling approach is discussed and illustrated that can be used for measurement and explanation at the same time. The main purpose of using item response models is the measurement of latent traits, to be considered as unobserved individual differences underlying human behavior and performances and also their test responses. In standard item response modeling, the items and the persons are represented by one or more parameters. The person parameter estimates provide us with a measurement of the latent trait(s). In an explanatory approach *properties* of the items and the persons are used to explain the responses. We will call this the "explanatory" approach (De Boeck & Wilson, 2004). The approach does not preclude measurement. Explanation and measurement can go hand in hand. The domain of application we will focus on is anger and aggression, but as will be explained in the Discussion section, the potential is much broader and includes other health-related variables.

Anger feelings and anger expression are psychologically important variables; they are similar, but also different, with different correlational patterns. Although anger feelings have been studied much more than their expression (Averill, 2001; Yousfi, Matthews, Amelang, & Schmidt-Rathjens, 2004), there is not only evidence for individual differences in anger feelings, but also for individual differences in the expression of anger (Deffenbacher, 1992; Spielberger, 1988), and these differences seem related to health and psychopathology. For example, anger-in expression (holding one's aggressive feelings) is correlated with blood pressure and cardiovascular problems (Jorgensen, Johnson, Kolodziej, & Schreer, 1996; Yousfi et al., 2004) and with depression (Brody, Haaga, Kirk, & Solomon, 1999), while anger-out expression (acting out one's anger feelings) is correlated with narcissism (Papps & O'Carroll, 1998) and impulsivity (Peños-Lledo, Fernandez, & Waller, 2004).

In a study by Smits and De Boeck (2007), three anger-related variables were investigated: anger feelings (A), verbally aggressive behavior tendency (T), and verbally aggressive behavior (B), all three with a situational self-report inventory. Based on a factor analysis and a rotation, three factors were found: anger feelings and two types of inhibition: T inhibition, the discrepancy between A and T, and B inhibition, the discrepancy between T and B. The idea underlying the interpretation of the two inhibition factors is that anger feelings lead to an aggressive behavior tendency and the behavior tendency in turn leads to aggressive behavior, while inhibition refers to new and negative input, when going from A to T (T inhibition), and from T to B (B inhibition).

The three factors were correlated with a rather broad array of variables. It was found that two of the three factors (B inhibition and A) had moderately strong relationships with other variables, while the correlations with T inhibition were much lower. B inhibition was positively correlated with Anger-in and Anger-out Control (controlling one's acting out) and negatively to Anger-out (acting out) as measured with the Self Expression and Control Scale (van Elderen, Maes, Komproe, & van der Kamp, 1997), an adaptation of Spielberger's (1996) Anger Expression Scale. Interestingly, B inhibition was also correlated with other variables: positively with the behavior inhibition system (BIS) and negatively with the behavior approach system (BAS) (Gray, 1990) as measured with the BIS/BAS inventory (Carver & White, 1994), positively with Agreeableness of the big five as measured with the NEO-FFI (Costa & McCrae, 1992), and negatively with verbal aggression as measured with the BPAQ (Buss & Perry, 1992). Compared with these correlations, the correlational pattern of T inhibition was very weak, while the correlational pattern of A was about equally strong but quite different. For example, anger feelings were positively correlated with Neuroticism and negatively with Agreeableness of the big five. Together, these findings suggest that individual differences with respect to anger expression are to be found mainly in B inhibition, and that individual differences in anger feelings are of a different nature than those with respect to B inhibition.

In the following we will concentrate on verbal aggression with situational items of the type used by Smits and De Boeck (2007), focusing on the verbally aggressive behavior tendency and on verbally aggressive behavior. We want to find out more about the functioning of verbal aggression, making use of *explanatory item response modeling* (EIRM; De Boeck & Wilson, 2004). As will be described, this implies that we will not start from the constructs and latent variables as such, but from the situational item responses, and that our motivation is to explain these responses. For example, T items and B items differ with respect to one important item feature. A T item is formulated as "Situation X. I would want to curse" (want mode), while a B item is formulated as "Situation X. I would curse" (do mode). B inhibition will be considered an interpretation of the varying effect induced by the want versus do mode of the items. In other words, the "latent trait" B inhibition corresponds to the varying effect of an item manipulation. Following the explanatory item modeling approach, the explanatory power is located in the item features, and the latent traits are varying effects of these features. At the same time, we will use a broader item design than just the contrast between the want and do modes, in order to study also other phenomena concerning verbal aggression, so that we can have a more global view on (self-reported) verbal aggressive responses. Before embarking on this endeavor, we will discuss item response modeling (IRT) and how it can be used in an explanatory way.

Research Methods

Item Response Models

Item response models (IRT) are a subclass of latent variable models. The common item response models are models with one latent variable, such as the unidimensional one-parameter, two-parameter, and three-parameter models (Embretson & Reise, 2000; van der Linden & Hambleton, 1997). Models with more than one latent variable are becoming more popular. A prominent example is the recently rediscovered bifactor model (Cai, Yang, & Hansen, 2011; Reise, 2012; Rijmen, 2010). The observations for an item response model are typically categorical item responses, either binary, ordered-category responses, or nominal responses. One can take different perspectives to latent variable models: a descriptive approach and three different approaches with explanatory purposes (outlined later). The third of these, called *explanatory item response modeling*, is the topic of the volume by De Boeck and Wilson (2004) and also of this chapter, and it will be employed to analyze verbal aggression data.

Measurement Perspectives

Descriptive Measurement Perspective

The first perspective is a *descriptive* measurement perspective. Following this perspective, the latent variables are given, as hypothetical constructs to be measured, such as Extraversion, Mathematical Ability, or Physical Well-being. Because the latent variables are unobserved one needs to rely on observed item responses. The selection of appropriate items and thus test construction is a crucial step in the process. The items are tools, the test is an instrument, while the latent traits are the ultimate aim of the exercise. The items are chosen to be descriptive indicators of constructs. Prominent examples of the perspective are Nunnally (1978), Jöreskog and Sörbom (1979), and Edwards and Bagozzi (2000). From a descriptive measurement approach, the items are an operational description or operational definition of the latent variable.

Reflective Measurement Perspective

The second perspective is *reflective measurement.* Following this perspective, the items and item responses are given and it is the role of the latent variables to "explain" the item responses (Bollen, 2002; Bollen & Lennox, 1991). The latent variables play the role of independent variables while the item response variables are the dependent variables. For example, the explanation for why a person gives mostly healthy responses in a health-related test is that he or she has a healthy lifestyle. The item responses reflect the underlying lifestyle latent variable (Figure 12.1 panel a). The latent variables are the explanatory tools or instruments for the item variables as the target. As an "explanation," the latent variables are internal to the responses because they are derived from these responses. A prominent indication of this reflective approach is the terminology of "effect indicators" for the observed variables (Bollen, 2002; Bollen & Lennox, 1991).

Formative Measurement Perspective

We will discuss this third perspective only briefly. Whereas in reflective measurement the latent variable has an explanatory role and the item responses are the effects of the latent trait, the roles are reversed in *formative measurement* (Figure 12.1 panel b). The items or indicators now have a causal role with respect to the latent variable and are called "causal indicators" (Bollen, 2002; Bollen & Lennox, 1991). The formative measurement

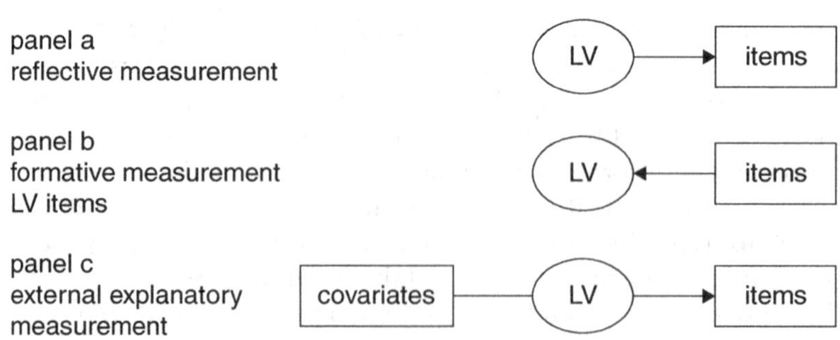

Figure 12.1 Three perspectives, with three different relationships between latent variables (LV) and items.

perspective has not been used in IRT thus far and will not be discussed further here because, for evident reasons, it does not provide an explanation of the item responses.

External Explanatory Perspective

The fourth perspective is based on external variables. It relates observables (covariates) to other observables (item responses). Unlike in the earlier two perspectives there are now three parties instead of just two (Figure 12.1 panel c). Note that there is only one arrow in panel c. It goes directly from the covariates, through the label "LV," to the item responses. The label LV indicates the strength of the effect that is represented by the one arrow. We focus in the following on the difference with reflective measurement (Figure 12.1 panel a). The explanation as provided by a reflective measurement perspective is limited, tautological, and arbitrary to some extent. It is limited because the focus is exclusively on the covariance of the item responses and not on their level (the means). It is tautological because the latent variables are supposed to explain something they will be inferred from. And the latent variables are arbitrary to some extent because of the property of rotational invariance.

A different kind of explanation relies on external variables of the items (item characteristics) and on external variables of the persons (person characteristics). These external variables are called *covariates* in the following. The latent variables are still part of the model, but they are redefined as varying effects of item covariates, as illustrated in panel c of Figure 12.1. Item covariates have an effect on item responses, more in particular on the level of the responses, the level of agreement, the level of certainty, and so forth, depending on the response scale. Latent variables can be seen as the individual variation in these effects, as will be explained later in this chapter. As a consequence, latent variables no longer have the role of being explanatory but rather the role of varying effect size, while the item covariates (i.e., the person and item characteristics) play the explanatory role instead. Within the domain of IRT, an early example is the linear logistic test model (LLTM, Fischer, 1973).

One way to see the difference between reflective measurement and explanatory measurement is the following. In the reflective case, we can think of the latent variable as the variable that stands in for all of the more complex variables we would use if we only knew what they were, and could measure them—that is, the latent variable acts "as if" it were genuinely causal, but the true causal model is most likely more complex. In the explanatory case, we now have advanced to the point where we believe that we do indeed have (at least some) potential causal variables identified and available—these are then the covariates in panel c of Figure 12.1.

Although it may not be immediately obvious, the construct modeling approach (Wilson, 2005, 2013) is also a version of this, where the external variables are the qualitatively ordered levels of mastery. The ordering of the item difficulties can be expected to be in line with the different levels in mastering a domain. The construct map shows the ordering based on the model estimation and the mastery levels to go through are the explanation for the difficulties.

Core Formula of Item Response Models

A Core Formula

Item response models for binary and ordered-category responses can all be formulated starting from a core formula, independent of the perspective (except for the third):

$$V_{pic} = \alpha_{i1}\theta_{p1} + .. + \alpha_{iD}\theta_{pD} - \beta_{ic} + \varepsilon_{pic}, \tag{12.1}$$

with V_{pic} as a latent response,[1] such that when $V_{pic} \geq 0$ a response category of the second set of compared categories is chosen, for person p ($p = 1, \ldots, P$) and item i ($i = 1, \ldots, I$), where c ($c = 1, \ldots, C$) as an index for the two sets of categories that are compared;

with θ_{pd} as the latent variable d ($d = 1, \ldots, D$);
with α_{id} as the weight of latent variable d;
with β_{ic} as an item category effect, depending on which categories are contrasted; and
and with ε_{pi} as a standard normal variable or a standard logistic variable, depending on whether a normal ogive or logistic model is used.

Note that {0} and {1} are the two sets of categories in the case of binary items (i.e., $C = 1$). For polytomous ordered-category items (i.e., $C > 1$) the sets of categories compared depend on whether the partial credit (Masters, 1982), the graded response (Samejima, 1969), or the sequential model (Tutz, 1990) is used. For example, suppose C = 3 and that the graded response model is being used, then there are three contrasted sets of categories: ({1} vs. {2,3,4}, {1,2} vs. {3,4}, and {1,2,3} vs. {4}). In that context, when $V_{pic} \geq 0$ for $c = 2$, then the second set ({3,4}) is chosen from the second contrast ({1,2} vs. {3,4}).

The Core Formula as a Regression Equation

The core formula can be read as a regression equation. V_{pic} is a latent item response and is explained by, regressed on, the D latent variables. The regression coefficients are α_{id} (slopes) and β_{ic} (intercept). Because of its bilinear character, the core formula can also be interpreted as V_{pic} being regressed on the following independent variables:

1. the α_{id}, with random slopes θ_{pd};
2. the binary item contrast indicators X_{pick} indicating to which latent response V_{pic} refers, with fixed effects β_{ic}.

The regression on X_{pick} can be clarified as follows:

$$\beta_{ic} = \sum_{k=1} \beta_k X_{pick},$$

where $X_{pick} = -1$ if $k = (i, c)$, $X_{pick} = 0$ otherwise, so that the regression on the binary indicators reduces to β_{ic}.

The two readings of Equation (12.1), either as a regression on latent variables (θ), or as a regression on item covariates (X) and item parameters (α), differ in the psychological meaning they have. The latent variables are either the independent variables (abilities, propensities, latent traits) attributed to the persons (first interpretation), or they are the varying effects of item variables, the α coefficients (second interpretation). Either α_{id} is the fixed effect of θ_{pd}, or θ_{pd} is the random effect of α_{id}.

1 In this context, the term "latent response" means that the response is not actually observed, but that it is a hypothetical continuous response that is used in the formulation of the statistical model. The term was used for the first time by Pearson (1901), and it is used later by several authors to formulate latent variable models for categorical responses and has become common terminology (e.g., Skrondal & Rabe-Hesketh, 2004). The more specific definition depends on the context and in this case is given in the equation. It is of course a construction, just as is θ.

Person and Item Covariates

In both interpretations, the independent variables, be they θ_{pd} (first interpretation) or α_{id} (second interpretation), have unknown values, which is of course unusual for independent variables. Suppose these values are observed indeed. Let us call the observed independent variables *covariates*: person covariates and item covariates, respectively, denoted as Z_{picj} (replacing θ_{pd}) for the person covariates, and X_{pick} (replacing α_{id}) for the item covariates, with *j* as an index for person covariates and *k* for an index of item covariates.

Replacing the α_{id} with *X* covariates means that V_{pic} is regressed on the *X* variables. These *X* variables can be:

(a) indicators of the pairs (*i*, *c*) as introduced before,
(b) characteristics of the items and the response categories, or
(c) both.

However, not all combinations are possible. For example, one can have item indicators with fixed effects that can be interpreted as thresholds, but one cannot also have item characteristics with fixed effects at the same time, because that would imply a deficient rank of the *X* variables. It is possible, however, to combine these two if the effects of the item characteristic type of covariates are random (varying) effects because they do not affect the rank for the fixed effect covariates.

In addition, person covariates *Z* can be added to the model, so that V_{pic} is regressed not only on *X* but also on *Z* variables, so that, for example, effects of gender, age, and so forth can be included. Because V_{pic} is the dependent variable, the two types of covariates, *Z* and *X*, also have subscripts *p*, *i*, and *c*, but the value of Z_{picj} does not vary with *i* because it is a person covariate, and the value of X_{pick} does not vary with *p* because it is an item covariate. Using covariates is crucial for an external explanatory approach, for the very reason that they are variables external to the item responses.

For a further analysis of verbal aggression, we plan to make use of *item covariates* in the first place, in an analysis based on an external explanatory perspective. In that way, three problems are solved associated with the reflective measurement perspective. First, item covariates with fixed and random effects offer an explanation for the covariance *and* for the level of the item responses. The fixed effects of the covariates explain the level and the varying effects explain the covariance. Second, the tautological explanatory role of latent variables is avoided. Instead the covariates take over the explanatory role. Third, the position of the latent variables in the multidimensional space is not arbitrary but fixed instead by the covariates. In fact, the latent variables are the individual differences in the effects of the item covariates.

Referring to the verbal aggression issue, this type of analysis allows us to establish the effect and individual differences therein of the kind of frustrating situation, of the specific type of verbally aggressive behavior, and of the difference between the do versus want mode. This analysis will also throw light on the B inhibition phenomenon and may lead to a better understanding of why it shows the correlational pattern as found by Smits and De Boeck (2007). Before describing the application, some model variants will be presented.

Three Model Types

In models with multiple response categories, it makes sense to have an item location, for example, the mean of the C thresholds, or the first threshold ($c = 1$) while the other parameters express the deviation of the (other) thresholds. Because for the application binary data will be used for reasons of simplification, there is only one threshold per item, which functions also as the location parameter. Therefore, the subscript c will be omitted from now on.

Using observed covariates, various transformations of Equation (12.1) are possible. Three possibilities are presented here:

1. with fixed item location parameters,
2. with fixed item covariate effects, and
3. with fixed item covariates and random item residuals.

Fixed Item Location Model (FI Model)

The FI model focuses on individual differences and leaves the differences between item locations unexplained. It has a fixed location parameter per item:

$$V_{pi} = \theta_{p1}X_{pi1} + .. + \theta_{pK}X_{piK} + \zeta_1 Z_{pi1} + .. + \zeta_J Z_{piJ} + \beta_i + \varepsilon_{pi}, \tag{12.2}$$

with $X_{pi1},..,X_{piK}$ as the item covariates from 1 to K;

$\theta_{p1},..,\theta_{pK}$ as the corresponding random person effects, $\theta_p \sim N(0,\Sigma_\theta)$;
$Z_{pi1},..,Z_{piJ}$ as the person covariates from 1 to J;
$\varsigma_1,..,\varsigma_J$ as the corresponding fixed person effects; and
β_i as the fixed location parameter for item i.

The model as defined in Equation (12.2) is a multidimensional model, with K dimensions, $\theta_{p1},..,\theta_{pK}$, and with J fixed person covariate effects, $\varsigma_1,..,\varsigma_J$. The K variables θ can be seen as the varying effects of the item covariates, while these X-values function as fixed discriminations. The J effects ς are the fixed effects of the J person covariates. In earlier work (Wilson & De Boeck, 2004), we have referred to this as a *person-explanative model*.

Fixed Item Covariate Effect Model (FIC Model)

In comparison with the FI model, the FIC model focuses in addition on an explanation of the item locations based on fixed item covariate effects:

$$V_{pi} = (\beta_1 + \theta_{p1})X_{pi1} + .. + (\beta_K + \theta_{pK})X_{piK} + \zeta_1 Z_{pi1} + .. + \zeta_J Z_{piJ} + \varepsilon_{pi}, \tag{12.3}$$

with β_k as the fixed effects of the K item covariates.

The individual item locations are now replaced with the sum $\beta_1 X_{pi1} + ... + \beta_K X_{piK}$. This model implies that the item locations are exhaustively determined by the item covariates and thus that a perfect explanation for the item location is provided by the item covariates. The well-known linear logistic test model (LLTM; Fischer, 1973) is an FIC model without person covariates. In earlier work (Wilson & De Boeck, 2004), we have referred to this as an *item-explanative model*. A perfect explanation of the item locations is perhaps too high an ambition, which is why the following model is useful. Note that the X covariates of Equation (12.3) do not need to be the same for fixed effects (β_k) and random effects (θ_{pk}), although in Equation (12.3) they are.

Fixed Item Covariate Effect Model Plus Item Residuals Model (FICIR Model)

In comparison with the FIC model, the FICIR model allows for a residual item location component, an unexplained part of the item location:

$$V_{pi} = (\beta_1 + \theta_{p1})X_{pi1} + .. + (\beta_K + \theta_{pK})X_{piK} + \zeta_1 Z_{pi1} + .. + \zeta_J Z_{piJ} + r_i + \varepsilon_{pi}, \tag{12.4}$$

with r_i as the item residual, $r_i \sim N(0, \sigma_r^2)$.

The FIC and FICIR models have a higher explanatory ambition than the FI model but they have also a reduced number of parameters. The item locations are reduced to the number of item covariates (FIC) plus one parameter for the residual variance (FICIR). The FIC model is the most ambitious explanatory model because it aims at a perfect explanation of the item locations, while the FICIR model can fill the commonly found explanation gap with a residual component. It is an item-explanative model with the flexibility that it allows for an unexplained part.

Multidimensionality

The FI, FIC, and FICIR as defined in Equations (12.2) to (12.4) are multidimensional models. They can be reduced to a *one-dimensional model* if an item covariate $X_{pi0} = 1$ (independent of p and i) with a random effect θ_{p0} replaces all other item covariates with random effects. Equation (12.2) then reduces to the simple one-parameter model with a regression on person covariates Z. Equation (12.3) reduces to the LLTM mentioned earlier with a similar regression component, and Equation (12.4) reduces to a latent regression version of the LLTM with error (Wilson & De Boeck, 2004).

In this chapter we are primarily interested in multidimensional models. Three forms of multidimensionality based on partition item covariates will be highlighted here: the correlated partition model, the correlated integrative processes model, and the bifactor model. The restriction to binary item covariates is not necessary, but it nicely leads to the three variants, each of them corresponding to known approaches from the literature.

The Correlated Partition Model for Multidimensionality

Suppose that the item set is partitioned, and that the partition is represented in a matrix **X**, such that for each item one and only one covariate k exists with $X_{ik} = 1$, see Table 12.1

Table 12.1 Item Partition Covariate Matrix, Integrative Processes Covariate Matrix, and Bifactor Covariate Matrix

	Partition			*Integrative Processes*			*Bifactor*			
i = 1	1	0	0	1	0	0	1	1	0	0
i = 2	1	0	0	1	0	0	1	1	0	0
i = 3	0	1	0	1	1	0	1	0	1	0
i = 4	0	1	0	1	1	0	1	0	1	0
i = 5	0	0	1	1	1	1	1	0	0	1
i = 6	0	0	1	1	1	1	1	0	0	1

(left part) for an example with six items, which would lead to $X_{pik} = 1$ for all values of p and the value of k in question. Without constraints on the corresponding covariance matrix, Σ_θ, this is the *correlated partition model.* It corresponds with a correlated group factor model, and has been referred to as a *between-item* model in earlier literature (Adams, Wilson, & Wang, 1997).

The Correlated Integrative Processes Model for Multidimensionality

The *correlated integrative processes model* can be used when the partition components are ordered, for example, because the same items are presented at different points in time (e.g., three, as in Table 12.1), or where the items integrate the dimensions successively. This can be expressed by assigning a one also to all items of a lower-ordered partition component, as illustrated in the central part of Table 12.1. It means that the random effects for an item belonging to subset k is the sum of random effects up to subset $k : \Sigma^{k}_{m=1}\theta_{pm}X_{pim}$. Without constraints on the covariance matrix, Σ_θ, this model is formally equivalent with the correlated partition model. It corresponds to Embretson's (1991) model for learning and change. This model as well as the following one, has been referred to as an example of a *within-item model* (Adams, Wilson, & Wang, 1997).

The Bifactor Model

The *bifactor model* can be used when the items belong to a common domain with subdomains. The commonality among the subdomains is expressed through an item covariate with a value of one for all items, from all subdomains, as in the right part of Table 12.1. The other item covariates indicate the subdomains. In order for this model to be identified, the covariance matrix, Σ_θ, needs to be diagonal (uncorrelated dimensions). The bifactor model is a constraint on the correlated partition model because it implies that:

1. all correlations between items stem from only two sources: the global domain and the specific subdomain, so that all correlations between the subdomains can be explained by one underlying dimension; and
2. the variance of the individual differences with respect to an item is the sum of two variances: the domain variance and the subdomain variance.

Although interesting in themselves, and certainly more explanative than a traditional unidimensional model, partitions have only a limited explanatory value, in two senses. First, the partition covariates do not provide an explanation for the item locations, unless one would be willing to make the strong assumption that the item locations are all equal within each subdomain. Second, the explanation for the correlations is that the correlations are equal within subdomains, which is perhaps too simplistic as an explanation. Partition covariates have by definition a limited meaning—they provide a categorization, but not anything more than that.

As will be explained in the application, it is also possible to use item covariates with a richer meaning than pure categorization. *Ordering* is an example. It is used in the integrative processes model. A stronger type of covariate, one that does imply ordering, is an interval scale covariate, such as when time since the first measurement functions as a covariate. Another organization principle is a *crossed design*, for example, a two-by-two design. The four cells define a partition, but, as a partition, they are not optimally informative. When the four cells (labeled in an intuitive way as A1B1, A1B2, A2B1, A2B2, respectively) are coded with four covariates (X1, X2, X3, and X4) as follows: (1,1,1,1),

(1,1,–1,–1), (1,–1,1,–1), and (1,–1,–1,1), then varying overall means (random effects of X1) can be separated from varying effects of A1 versus A2 (random effects of X2) and of B1 versus B2 (random effects of X3), taking into account whether the effects of one factor depend on the level of the other (random effects of X4). This kind of approach for individual differences and thus for dimensions clearly adds meaning if the contrasts A1 versus A2 and B1 versus B2 are meaningful contrasts. This latter approach will be used in the application and will be called a *general-plus-contrasts model.* It will be compared with the correlated partition model and the bifactor model for the same data.

Interaction Models

Thus far, the models are presented without interactions between item covariates and person covariates. It is rather easy to extend the equations with interactions. It suffices to add products of the X and Z covariates, terms we used earlier. For example, if it is hypothesized that there are gender differences with respect to the effect of X_k but not with respect to the effect of other item covariates, then one could add a term $\varsigma_{gender,k}X_{pik}Z_{pi,gender}$ to the global term $\varsigma_{gender}Z_{pi,gender}$. These interactions imply that the person covariates have a specific effect on the dimension that is induced by the item covariate *k*. For example, if $\varsigma_{gender,k}X_{pik}Z_{pi,gender} \neq 0$, then it implies that the individual differences induced by item covariate *k* are at least partly explained by the gender of the person. In the application, interaction effects will be included in the item response model analysis.

Application

Application Data

Items and Design

De Boeck and Wilson (2004) describe a data set from a personality scale inventory on verbal aggression. The same data set is used by De Boeck and colleagues (2011) and is available with the *lme4* package in R (Bates, Maechler, & Bolker, 2011). The measure has 24 items (in Dutch) and is based on a design with three item covariates. All items are defined on the basis of a situation and a behavior in the situation. Four frustrating situations are used, two of which where the source of frustration is another person and two of which where one is self to be blamed (other vs. self). For example, "I am waiting at a bus stop and the bus driver doesn't stop" is an other-situation, while "I arrived at the grocery store five minutes before closing time" is a self-situation. The corresponding item covariate is *Source of Frustration.* Three verbally aggressive behaviors were used as possible reactions in the situations: cursing, scolding, and shouting. Note that these have a somewhat more subtle usage in the original Dutch than in English, in that the first is cursing to oneself, the second is directed to another person, and the third is directed outwardly, to anyone in hearing. The corresponding covariate is *Behavior Type.* Given that there are two situations per source of frustration, this leads to 2 × 2 × 3 = 12 situation-behavior pairs. For each of these 12, two variants were formulated, one with a wanting mode (e.g., "Situation X. I would want to curse") and another with a doing mode (e.g., "Situation X. I would curse"). The corresponding item covariate is *Mode.* The wanting and doing modes refer to the Tendency concept and the Behavior concept from the introduction, respectively, and the discrepancy between the two modes refers to Behavior (B) inhibition. The 24 items are thus organized in a two (other vs. self) by two (want vs. do) by three (curse, scold, shout) design with two situations nested within self and also two situations nested within other.

Subjects and Response Scale

The subjects are 243 female and 73 male undergraduate students. The available person covariates are Gender and a Trait Anger score (Spielberger, 1988). The response scale for the inventory was a three-point scale: "yes," "perhaps," and "no." For the purpose of the application, the data are dichotomized such that "yes" and "perhaps" are one (agree, at least to some extent) and "no" is zero. The reason for this particular dichotomization is that verbal aggression is socially undesirable and a "perhaps" can therefore be understood as admitting verbal aggression. For a fine-grained analysis of this response scale based on the same data, see De Boeck and Wilson (in press), and for unidimensional models for the three-point data of this inventory, see Tuerlinckx and Wang (2004). Although the model formulations in Equations (12.2) to (12.4) are formulated for the more general case, we will focus here on binary data because the message is not related to the category parameters.

Application Models

Because of the complexity of the models we are considering here, we split up the presentation of the model(s) and the reporting of the results into four parts, in line with how the models are presented earlier in the chapter. The first is the multidimensionality part.

The Multidimensionality Part of the Model

Three multidimensional models will be estimated, two of which are the correlated partition model and the bifactor model. The third is a correlated general-plus-contrast model. The multidimensionality part of the model is explained in the following:

1. The *correlated partition model* has four dimensions: want&self, want&other, do&other, do&self, and thus this corresponds to a random effect for each cell of the 2 × 2 matrix arising from the crossing of want versus do with other versus self. More formally, the multidimensional part in Equation (12.1) is:

$$\theta_{p,wo}X_{pi,wo} + \theta_{p,ws}X_{pi,ws} + \theta_{p,do}X_{pi,do} + \theta_{p,ds}X_{pi,ds},$$

with $X_{pi,wo} = 1$ if the person p responds to a want-item (w) for a situation where another person is to be blamed (o), $X_{pi,wo} = 0$ otherwise, and similarly for the other three possibilities, with subscripts *ws*, *do*, and *ds*, for want and self, do and other, and do and self, respectively. The corresponding random effects $\theta_{p,wo}$, and so forth are random effects for the four combinations. The variance and covariance of the random effects are model parameters. The total number of parameters is $5 \times 4/2 = 10$.

2. The *bifactor model* with the same four dimensions plus a general dimension, but by the constraints of that model, they must all five be uncorrelated. More formally, the multidimensional part in Equation (12.1) is:

$$\theta_{p0}X_{pi0} + \theta_{p,wo}X_{pi,wo} + \theta_{p,ws}X_{pi,ws} + \theta_{p,do}X_{pi,do} + \theta_{p,ds}X_{pi,ds},$$

with $X_{pi0} = 1$ for all responses and θ_{p0} as the random intercept, while all other terms are the same as in the correlated partition model, except that the five random effects are uncorrelated, so that only their variances are model parameters. The total number of parameters is five. Given the constraint of uncorrelated dimensions, we do not expect that the bifactor model can recover the correlations between the four cells. We rather expect that a third and only three-dimensional model would have a better fit, as good or almost as good as the correlated partition model.

3. This three-dimensional *general plus contrast model* has the following dimensions:

- a general dimension, the random effect of item covariate 0 with $X_{pi0} = 1$ for all item responses;
- a Want vs. Do contrast dimension expressing individual differences in the discrepancy between wanting and doing (interpreted as B inhibition here), the random effect of the contrast covariate X_{w-d}, with $X_{pi,w-d} = 1$ for want-items and $X_{pi,w-d} = -1$ for do-items; and
- an Other vs. Self contrast dimension, which is the random effect of contrast covariate X_{o-s}, with $X_{pi,o-s} = 1$ for other-items and $X_{pi,o-s} = -1$ for self-items.

Taken together, the multidimensional part in Equation (12.1) is:

$$\theta_{p0}X_{pi0} + \theta_{p,w-d}X_{pi,w-d} + \theta_{p,o-s}X_{pi,o-s},$$

where the first term is the same as in the bifactor model, while the other two terms are different from the previous two models: $X_{pi,w-d} = 1$ for responses to want-items, and $X_{pi,w-d} = -1$ for responses to do-items; and $X_{pi,o-s} = 1$ for responses to other-items, and $X_{pi,o-s} = -1$ for responses to self-items. Because the whole variance-covariance matrix is estimated, the total number of parameters is $4 \times 3/2 = 6$. This model is a "main effects" model for the covariance between the four cells: an overall source of variance, and a source of variance per factor in the two-by-two design. In principle, an interaction random effect could be added (of the product $X_{pi,w-d}X_{pi,o-s}$), but it turned out that this is not needed. It means that B inhibition is not a different variable depending on whether self or other is the source of frustration.

Adding dimensions for the three behaviors crossed with the levels of Mode and Source of Frustration would lead to 12 dimensions in the correlated partition model and 13 in the bifactor model, which is too high for 24 items. Following the principles of the correlated general-plus-contrast model, only two more dimensions would be needed to account for the individual differences related to the three behaviors. We will check whether it pays off to include these two random effects in the model.

Also the following three parts of the model are explanatory extensions of the descriptive Equation (12.1): an item location explanatory part replacing β_i, a person explanatory part to explain the variation along the dimensions, and an interactive part of the model.

The Item Location Explanatory Part of the Model

This second part adds *explanatory terms for the item locations* to the multidimensionality part. We expect that the item locations can be roughly explained by the three item covariates: Mode, Source of Frustration, and Behavior Type, and that the residual terms will be small, which would show in a small residual variance σ_r^2. Effect coding will be used for the item covariates: want = 1, do = −1 ($X_{pi,w-d}$); other = 1, self = −1 ($X_{pi,o-s}$); curse = 1, scold = 0, shout = −1 ($X_{pi,c-sh}$); and curse = 0, scold = 1, shout = −1 ($X_{pi,sc-sh}$).

The corresponding model part is:

$$\beta_0 X_{pi0} + \beta_{w-d}X_{pi,w-d} + \beta_{o-s}X_{pi,o-s} + \beta_{curse}X_{pi,c-sh} + \beta_{scold}X_{pi,sc-sh} + \beta_{i0}X_{pi0}.$$

The first three item covariates are the same as in the correlated general-plus-contrast version of the multidimensionality part, while the next two, $X_{pi,c-sh}$ and $X_{pi,sc-sh}$, are not assumed to induce varying effects, but only fixed effects. Because all codings are effect codings, the fixed intercept, β_0, is the overall mean. The fixed effects other than β_0 are the main effects of the three inventory design factors. Finally, there is also a random item effect, β_{i0}, which is the residual item location, $\beta_{io} = r_i$ (see Equation (12.4)), unexplained by the main effects. Interactions of item covariates are not considered in this model because we know from earlier analyses that they are negligible (Wilson & De Boeck, 2004). The total number of parameters is 5 + 1, five fixed effects (main effects) and one residual variance. A successful explanation implies that the residual variance is very small.

The Person Explanatory Part of the Model

The third part adds *explanatory terms for the individual differences*. We expect that men are verbally more aggressive than women and also that respondents with a higher degree of trait anger are more verbally aggressive, in line with the study by Smits and De Boeck (2007), where anger was found to feed into the verbal aggression tendency and into verbally aggressive behavior. Gender will be contrast-coded such that the sum in the sample is zero, with a positive coding for women and negative for men. Trait Anger will be standardized before entering the analysis ($X_{pi,zTA}$). Overall individual differences that are not explained by the two person covariates are captured by the general dimension, which can be interpreted as the unexplained variation of the overall individual means.

The corresponding model part is:

$$\beta_G X_{piG} + \beta_{zTA} X_{pi,zTA},$$

with β_G and β_{zTA} as the fixed effects of the two person covariates. It is not expected that these two would explain a large share of the individual differences. The total number of parameters in this third part of the model is two.

The Interaction and Dimension-Specific Effects Part of the Model

The fourth part adds *person covariate by item covariate interactions* to the model, the effects of the products of the person covariates and item covariates. These interactions are of special interest in a multidimensional model, because they refer to specific types of individual differences. For example, an interaction between Gender and Mode means that men and women differ in how large the discrepancy is between wanting and doing, and thus in how much impact Gender has on the dimension induced by $X_{pi,w-d}$.

The corresponding model part is:

$$\beta_{G,w-d} X_{piG} X_{pi,w-d} + \beta_{G,o-s} X_{piG} X_{pi,o-s} + \beta_{zTA,w-d} X_{pi,zTA} X_{pi,w-d} + \beta_{zTA,o-s} X_{pi,zTA} X_{pi,o-s}.$$

These are four interaction effects, of Gender and Trait Anger with Mode and Source of Frustration. We expect that women express their verbally aggressive tendency less than men and thus have a higher degree of B inhibition, and that high trait anger leads to less B inhibition. Remember that B inhibition is an interpretation for the varying discrepancy between do and want. Unlike for Mode, we do not have expectations regarding the interactions with Source of Frustration.

If the interaction effects are significant, then the person covariates have specific effects on the dimensions, but, when they are negligible instead while the main effects are significant, then Gender and Trait Anger each have an overall effect and thus an effect on the general dimension. The total number of parameters in the fourth part of the model is four.

Model Estimation

The models are estimated with the *glmer* function from the *lme4* package in *R* (Bates, Maechler, & Bolker, 2011). The estimation method is not maximum likelihood but instead the Laplace approximation is used. How item response models can be estimated with this package and what the features are of the Laplace approximation is described by De Boeck and colleagues (2011).

Results

Multidimensionality

The multidimensional results are clear. The best of the three considered models is the correlated general-plus-contrast model. This is the model with one general dimension and two contrast dimensions (Want versus Do and Other versus Self). The first contrast dimension is the intended B inhibition dimension, while the second contrast dimension refers to how much easier verbal aggression is elicited when someone else is the source of frustration. The AIC and BIC values for this model are 7,988 and 8,113, respectively, which is slightly better than the correlated partition model (7,993 and 8,145) and the bifactor model (8,049 and 8,166). The correlated partition model is the model with a separate dimension for the two-by-two combinations of Want versus Do and Other versus Self. In the corresponding bifactor model, a general factor is added and all dimensions are orthogonal. The loglikelihood of the correlated general-plus-contrast model is –3,976 versus –3,974 and –4,007 for the correlated partition and bifactor models, respectively. The loglikelihood of the correlated general-plus-contrast model is only two units lower than that of the correlated partition model while the latter has four more parameters. In sum, the correlated general-plus-contrast method does slightly better, it requires only three dimensions and one of its dimensions is the intended B inhibition dimension. In this particular case, the result is rather clear although the differences are small. For a discussion of how to compare models with a different number of random effects (dimensions) in general, based on a likelihood ratio test, see De Boeck and colleagues (2011). The somewhat weaker performance of the bifactor model in this application is related to the matrix design of the inventory. For an inventory with a simple horizontal subscale structure, the bifactor model would likely have a better fit. The estimated multidimensional structure is presented in Table 12.2.

The general dimension is by far the strongest. The two contrast dimensions each contribute for only about 10 percent of the general dimension, and the Other versus Self dimension seems moderately correlated with the general dimension. The second and third dimensions can be understood as the random effect of item contrast covariates. The covariates induce varying discrepancies. This is a different interpretation of latent variables compared to the more common measurement context, where latent variables are preexisting variables that are measured through indicator variables. In addition, in an explanatory context, the interpretation of the dimensions borrows strength from the meaning of the item covariates. Regarding the investigation of B inhibition, the result for the Want versus Do dimension in Table 12.2 suggests that it is a rather independent source of individual differences.

Note on the Possibly Higher Dimensionality of the Data

When a model that added random effects of the two behavior type contrasts was estimated, this five-dimensional model turns out to have a better goodness of fit. The AIC and BIC values of the five-dimensional model are 7,704 and 7,891, which is better than those for the three-dimensional model. The fixed effects do not change much, but the result indicates the dimensionality is perhaps underestimated by the three-dimensional model reported earlier. An extension to a five-dimensional general-plus-contrast model may be needed, but, given that the ratio of five dimensions versus 24 items is rather high, we have not followed up here on this higher dimensionality.

Explanation of Item Locations

All main effects of the item covariates are statistically significant (at standard α settings); see Table 12.3. Subjects agree more with want-items than with do-items (0.281, $p < 0.01$), also more with other-items than with self-items (0.560, $p < 0.001$), and finally, depending on the behavior, more with curse-items than with scold-items and shout-items (1.152, $p < 0.001$). Because effect coding works with contrasts between 1 and –1, the effects are only half of the difference on the logit scale between want and do, and so forth. The means for want and do are –0.053 (intercept) + 0.281 = 0.228, and –0.053 – 0.281 = –0.334, corresponding to probabilities of 0.557 and 0.417 for wanting and doing, respectively (the B inhibition effect), when an average person is considered. The means for other and self are –0.053 + 0.560 = 0.507 and –0.053 – 0.560 = –0.613, corresponding to probabilities

Table 12.2 Estimated Variance-Covariance Matrix of the General-plus-Contrast Multidimensional Structure (the Off-diagonal Elements Are Correlations)

	General	*Want vs. Do*	*Other vs. Self*
General	2.217		
Want vs. Do	–0.115	0.240	
Other vs. Self	0.356	0.127	0.235

Table 12.3 Item Location Effects

	Fixed Effect	*Standard Error*	*p-value*
Intercept	–0.053	0.129	n.s.
Want vs. Do	0.281	0.089	<0.01
Other vs. Self	0.560	0.089	<0.0001
Curse vs. Shout	1.152	0.114	<0.0001
Scold vs. Shout	–0.001	0.113	n.s.

of 0.624 and 0.351 for other-situations and self-situations, respectively. The mean for curse is −0.053 + 1.152 = 1.099, the mean for scold is −0.053 − 0.001 = −0.054, and the mean of shout is −0.053 − 1.152 + 0.001 = −1.204. This means that the probabilities for cursing, scolding, and shouting are 0.750, 0.487, and 0.231, respectively. This ordering of estimated effects is consistent with the interpretation that more external expressions are harder to make than lesser ones.

Together, the item covariates explain most of the item location differences. The variance of the item location residual is only 0.135. The corresponding standard deviation of 0.367 is rather small in comparison with the range of the cumulated fixed effects, which runs from a minimum of −0.053 − 0.281 − 0.560 − 1.152 + 0.001 = −2.045 for items that combine do with self and shout to a maximum of −0.053 + 0.281 + 1.152 = 1.940 for items that combine want with other and curse. The corresponding probabilities of agreeing are 0.115 and 0.874, respectively. This range is more than 10 times larger than the standard deviation of the unexplained residual, so that one may conclude that the item locations are largely explained by the item covariates. Conditional on the validity of self-report, this means that we understand the variation in the average verbal aggressive responses. B inhibition is an important source of this variation, but other sources are the type of behavior and who is to blame. Based on the results from the previous subsection, the same item covariates are also sources of individual differences. This is not necessarily the case, but it happens to be so for our data. One further issue is how these individual differences be explained, individual differences in the overall level (the general dimension) and in the effect of the item covariates (the two contrast dimensions). These explanations are the subject of the next paragraphs.

Explanation of the Overall Individual Differences

First, do Trait Anger and Gender have an effect on the general dimension? The effect 1 sd of Trait Anger has on the general dimension (0.319) is smaller than 1 sd of that dimension (1.489). The effect range of +2 sd to −2 sd on the Trait Anger scale is 1.276 on the logit scale, which is still smaller than 1 sd of the general dimension (1.489). On the other hand, the effect of 1 sd on the Trait Anger scale (0.319) is larger than 1 sd on either of the two contrast dimensions, and, for an average person, for an increase of 1 sd on the Trait Anger scale, the probability of agreeing would increase from 0.487 to 0.566. The main effect of Gender is only marginally significant (−0.183, $p < 0.10$). Women are slightly less verbally aggressive.

The explanatory value of the two person covariates is much smaller than the explanatory value of the item covariates. The fixed effects are not only smaller, but the remaining unexplained variation is much larger, as one can infer from the diagonal values in Table 12.2 compared with the residual item location variance of 0.135.

Explanation of the Individual Differences in Covariate Effects

Second, do Trait Anger and Gender have an effect on the two contrast dimensions? Both of the interactions with Mode are significant: Mode by Gender (0.236, $p < 0.001$) and Mode by Trait Anger (−0.099, $p = 0.0156$). The discrepancy between wanting and doing is larger for women than for men, and the discrepancy decreases with Trait Anger. In terms of the dimensions it means that women tend to have a higher position (compared with men) on the first contrast dimension (want vs. do) and that the relative difference on the same dimension decreases with Trait Anger. In terms of B inhibition, it means that women have a higher level of B inhibition, and that higher anger levels are associated with lower levels of B inhibition. A third interaction is marginally significant, between Source of Frustration and Trait Anger (0.072, $p < 0.10$). With increasing Trait Anger, respondents are somewhat more verbally aggressive when someone else has caused the frustration than when they have caused the frustration themselves.

Although the person covariates do not have a large effect on the general dimension, they do have a relatively strong effect on the first contrast dimension. The individual differences in the discrepancy between wanting and doing (and thus B inhibition) are explained to a substantial degree by the Gender and the Trait Anger scores of the respondents.

Summary

We believe the application is helpful to better understand verbal aggression and B inhibition. Verbal aggression depends on the kind of behavior that is considered, on who is to blame, and on the mode of expression (wanting vs. doing). B inhibition has an overall effect and it shows at the same time individual differences, related to trait anger and gender. Individual differences in B inhibition are not different depending on who is to blame for the frustration (see correlated general-plus-contrast multidimensional structure) and they are independent of the individual differences in the effect the type of situation has (correlation of 0.127 in Table 12.2). Although a broader study would be needed, this suggests B inhibition is a general expression style, with interesting correlates, in line with its correlational pattern as found by Smits and De Boeck (2007).

More generally, the application illustrates how an explanatory item response modeling approach differs from other perspectives. The reported item response analysis is based in the first place on item covariates and their effects. The approach has provided an explanation for the responses the subjects gave, and, assuming that self-report is veridical to a reasonable extent, the analysis has revealed important phenomena with respect to verbal aggression. The explicit "latent traits" can be considered as individual variation in the overall mean (general dimension) or in the effect of item covariates (contrast dimensions).

The kind of explanation provided by an explanatory item response model is different from the explanation provided by a reflective measurement perspective. It is not the latent variables that have explanatory value, but the item covariates and the person covariates. In this view, latent traits are not preexisting ("real") variables that we cannot observe directly, but that merely require the discovery of indicator variables (i.e., manifest variable or items) in order to make them amenable to scientific investigation. Instead, they are thought of as the effect of the variation of factors in the design to study a phenomenon such as verbal aggression. Different factors in the design induce different effects and variations therein.

For example, one can think of a certainty versus uncertainty continuum of negative expectations. Some feelings express negative certainty (e.g., "hopeless" and "sad") and other feelings rather express negative uncertainty (e.g., "fearful" and "nervous"). An alternative but similar kind of continuum would be the degree of arousal (e.g., "hopeless" and "sad" do not imply arousal whereas "fearful" and "nervous" do). Instead of defining two latent variables, one for each type of negative feelings, one can make use of an item covariate (e.g., degree of uncertainty or arousal) and conduct a simple regression with random weights. The random intercept defines the general factor (e.g., negative affect) and the item covariate defines a bipolar factor (e.g., depression versus anxiety). We have tried this idea out in a pilot study for a depression and anxiety questionnaire and found that this redefinition of latent variables does indeed capture the covariance structure of the questionnaire. It was also possible to make the loadings of the bipolar factor a function of degree of arousal as an item covariate (Farouni, 2014). In other words, the latent variables can be understood as random regression coefficients.

However, it is perfectly possible to combine perspectives, and to measure the latent traits as viewed from a descriptive measurement perspective or from a reflective measurement perspective, supplemented with covariate effects—this would be a MIMIC model if the covariates are person covariates. The even more interesting case is where they are *item covariates*, as in the present application, because such covariates explain the nature of latent traits as individual differences in the effect the covariates have. This combination of measurement with explanation is called *explanatory measurement* by De Boeck and Wilson (2004). If one wants to estimate the person-specific effects of the item covariates, the classic approaches can still be used: maximum likelihood (ML), maximum *a posteriori* (MAP), expected *a posteriori* (EAP), and weighted maximum likelihood (WML) yielding Warm estimators. The traits that are measured in this way borrow meaning from both the item covariates and the person covariates.

Future Directions

The models we have used are not new models. They are members of the larger family of generalized linear mixed models (Breslow & Clayton, 1993; Fahrmeir & Tutz, 2001; McCulloch & Searle, 2001). They are logistic mixed models, and they are increasingly used for the analysis of experimental data in psychology (e.g., Baayen, Davidson, & Bates, 2008; Forster & Masson, 2008). This may eventually lead to a unification of data analysis methods in psychology. For example, for categorical data, an explanatory item response model can fulfill the role of an ANOVA model.

It is possible to extend this framework and to include degrees of discrimination, as in Equation (12.1). It is also possible to use item covariates to explain the degrees of discrimination, including a random residual for the non-explained part (e.g., Cho, De Boeck, Embretson, & Rabe-Hesketh, 2014; Klein-Entink, Kuhn, Hornke, & Fox, 2009). The degrees of discrimination and the loadings of factor analysis models are commonly interpreted on a mostly subjective basis, without objective explanation methods, whereas it is possible to use item covariates in explanatory models for discriminations and loadings.

Finally, an item multilevel structure can also be incorporated in the explanatory model. Suppose the set of items is divided into many non-overlapping subsets, each representing an aspect of a broader trait. For such a hierarchical trait structure covariates can be used for the first and second item level. The extensions needed for this kind of multilevel trait structure are described in Cho, De Boeck, Embretson, and Rabe-Hesketh (2014).

References

Adams, R.J., Wilson, M.R., & Wang, W.-C. (1997). The multidimensional random coefficients multinomal logit model. *Applied Psychological Measurement*, *21*, 1–23.

Averill, J.R. (2001). Studies on anger and aggression: Implications for theories of emotion. In W.G. Parrott (Ed.), *Emotions in social psychology: Essential readings* (pp. 337–352). Philadelphia, PA: Psychology Press/Taylor & Francis.

Baayen, R.H., Davidson, D.J., & Bates, D.M. (2008). Mixed effects modeling with crossed random effects for subjects and items. *Journal of Language and Memory*, *59*, 390–412.

Bates, D., Maechler, M., & Bolker, B. (2011). *lme4: linear mixed effects models using S4 classes*. R package version 0.999375–42, http://CRAN.R-project.org/package=lme4.

Bollen, K.A. (2002). Latent variables in psychology and the social sciences. *Annual Review of Psychology*, *53*, 605–634.

Bollen, K. A., & Lennox, R. (1991). Conventional wisdom on measurement: A structural equation perspective. *Psychological. Bulletin, 110*, 305–314.

Breslow, N. E., & Clayton, D. G. (1993). Approximate inference in generalized linear mixed models. *Journal of the American Statistical Association, 88*, 9–25.

Brody, C. L., Haaga, D. A. F., Kirk, L., & Solomon, A. (1999). Experiences of anger-in people who have recovered from depression and never-depressed people. *Journal of Nervous and Mental Disease, 187*, 400–405.

Buss, A. H., & Perry, M. (1992). The aggression questionnaire. *Journal Personality and Social Psychology, 63*, 452–459.

Cai, L., Yang, J. S., & Hansen, M. (2011). Generalized full-information item bifactor analysis. *Psychological Methods, 16*, 221–248.

Carver, C. S., & White, T. L. (1994). Behavioral inhibition, behavioral activation, and affective responses to impending reward and punishment: The BIS/BAS scales. *Journal of Personality and Social Psychology, 67*, 319–333.

Cho, S.-J., De Boeck, P., Embretson, S., & Rabe-Hesketh, S. (2014). Additive multilevel item structure models with random residuals: Item modeling for explanation and item generation. *Psychometrika, 79*, 84–104.

Costa, P. T., & McCrae, R. R. (1992). *Revised NEO personality inventory (NEO-PI-R) and the five factor inventory (NEO-FFI): Professional manual.* Odessa, FL: Psychological Assessment Resources.

De Boeck, P., Bakker, M., Zwitser, R., Nivard, M., Hofman, A., Tuerlinckx, F., & Partchev, I. (2011). The estimation of item response models with the lmer function from the lme4 package in R. *Journal of Statistical Software, 39*, 1–28.

De Boeck, P., & Wilson, M. (Eds.) (2004). *Explanatory item response models.* New York: Springer.

De Boeck, P., & Wilson, M. (in press). Explanatory item response models. In W. J. van der Linden & R. K. Hambleton (Eds.), *Handbook of item response theory, models, statistical tools, and applications.* Boca Raton, FL: Chapman & Hall/CRC Press.

Deffenbacher, J. (1992). Trait anger: theory, findings, and implications. In C. D. Spielberger & J. N. Butcher (Eds.), *Advances in personality assessment.* Vol. 9 (pp. 177–201). Hillsdale, NJ: Lawrence Erlbaum Associates.

Edwards, J. R., & Bagozzi, R. P. (2000). On the nature and direction of relationships between constructs and measures. *Psychologica Methods, 5*, 155–174.

Embretson, S. E. (1991). A multidimensional latent trait model for measuring learning and change. *Psychometrika, 56*, 495–516.

Embretson, S., & Reise, S. (2000). *Item response theory for psychologists.* Mahwah, NJ: Lawrence Erlbaum Associates.

Fahrmeir, L., & Tutz, G. (2001). *Multivariate statistical modeling based on generalized linear mixed models* (2nd ed.). New York: Springer-Verlag.

Farouni, T. (2014). *Theory-based constraints in a two-dimensional confirmatory item factor analysis model: An approach to disentangling the interference effects of latent variables.* Master's thesis, Ohio State University.

Fischer, G. (1973). The linear logistic test model as an instrument in educational research. *Acta Psychologica, 36*, 359–374.

Forster, K. I., & Masson, M. E. J. (2008). Special issue: Emerging data analysis. *Journal of Memory and Language, 59*, 387–556.

Gray, J. A. (1990). Brain systems that mediate both emotion and cognition. *Cognition and Emotion, 4*, 269–288.

Jöreskog, K. G., & Sörbom, D. (1979). *Advances in factor analysis and structural equation models.* Cambridge, MA: Abt Books.

Jorgensen, R. S., Johnson, B. T., Kolodziej, M. E., & Schreer, G. E. (1996). Elevated blood pressure and personality: A meta-analytic review. *Psychological Bulletin, 120*, 293–320.

Klein-Entink, R. H., Kuhn, J.-T., Hornke, L. F., & Fox, J.-P. (2009). Evaluating cognitive theory: A joint modeling approach using responses and response times. *Psychological Methods, 14*, 54–75.

Masters, G. N. (1982). A Rasch model for partial credit scoring. *Psychometrika, 47*, 149–174.

McCulloch, C.E., & Searle, S.R. (2001). *Generalized, linear, and mixed models.* New York: Wiley.
Nunnally, J.C. (1978). *Psychometric theory.* New York: McGraw-Hill.
Papps, B.P., & O'Carroll, R.E. (1998). Extremes of self-esteem and narcissism and the experience and expression of anger and aggression. *Aggressive Behavior, 24*, 421–438.
Pearson, K. (1901). Mathematical contributions to the theory of evolution VII. On the inheritance of characters not capable of exact quantitative measurement. *Philosophical Transactions of the Royal Society A, 195*, 79–150.
Peños-Lledo, E., Fernandez, J.D., & Waller, G. (2004). Association of anger with bulimic and other impulsive behaviours among non-clinical women and men. *European Eating Disorders Review, 12*, 392–397.
Reise, S.P. (2012). The rediscovery of bifactor measurement models. *Multivariate Behavioral Research, 47*, 667–696.
Rijmen, F. (2010). Formal relations and an empirical comparison among the bi-factor, the testlet, and a second-order multidimensional IRT model. *Journal of Educational Measurement, 47*, 361–372.
Samejima, F. (1969). Estimation of ability using a response pattern of graded scores. *Psychometrika* Monograph, No. 17.
Skrondal, A., & Rabe-Hesketh, S. (2004). *Generalized latent variable modeling. Multilevel, longitudinal, and structural equation models.* Boca Raton, FL: Chapman & Hall.
Smits, D., & De Boeck, P. (2007). From anger to verbal aggression: Inhibition at different levels. *Personality and Individual Differences, 43*, 47–57.
Spielberger, D. (1988). *State-Trait Anger Expression Inventory.* Professional manual. Odessa, FL: Psychological Assessment.
Spielberger, C.D. (1996). *State-Trait Anger Expression Inventory.* Professional manual. Odessa, FL: Psychological Assessment.
Tuerlinckx, F., & Wang, W.-C. (2004). Models for polytomous data. In P. De Boeck & M. Wilson (Eds.), *Explanatory item response modeling* (pp. 75–109). New York: Springer.
Tutz, G. (1990). Sequential item response models with an ordered response. *British Journal of Mathematical and Statistical Psychology, 43*, 39–55.
van der Linden, W.J., & Hambleton, R.K. (Eds.) (1997). *Handbook of modern item response theory.* New York: Springer.
Van Elderen, T., Maes, S., Komproe, I., & van der Kamp, L. (1997). The development of an anger expression and control scale. *British Journal of Health Psychology,* 2, 269–281.
Wilson, M. (2005). *Constructing measures: An item response modeling approach.* Mahwah, NJ: Lawrence Erlbaum Associates.
Wilson, M. (2013). *Challenges and opportunities of learning progressions for the psychometric community.* Paper presented at the annual meeting of the American Educational Research Association, San Francisco.
Wilson, M., & De Boeck, P. (2004). Descriptive and explanatory item response models. In P. De Boeck & M. Wilson (Eds.), *Explanatory item response modeling* (pp. 43–74). New York: Springer.
Yousfi, S., Matthews, G., Amelang, M., & Schmidt-Rathjens, C. (2004). Personality and disease: Correlations of multiple trait scores with various illnesses. *Journal of Health Psychology, 9*, 627–647.

13 Unipolar Item Response Models

Joseph F. Lucke

Introduction

Since its first application to the measurement of alcohol use disorder in 2003 (Kahler, Strong, Stuart, Moore, & Ramsey, 2003), item response theory (IRT; Embretson & Reise, 2000) has been applied with increasing frequency to addictions research. Dichotomous and polytomous IRT models have been applied to measures of alcohol use disorder (Keyes, Krueger, Grant, & Hasin, 2011, and references therein), nicotine use disorder (Liu, Hedeker, & Mermelstein, 2013, and references therein), illicit drug use disorders (Saha et al., 2012, and references therein), and gambling behavior disorder (Sharp et al., 2012, and references therein). The goal of these studies was to determine to what extent an addictive disorder could be adequately represented as a unidimensional continuum rather than the traditional categories of "use," "dependence," "abuse," and "addiction" (Orford, 2001).

IRT models, including all of the models referenced earlier, typically posit that the latent trait θ can take on any real value, that is, $-\infty < \theta < \infty$ an assumption I call the *bipolar trait* assumption. Bipolarity is appropriate for traits representing ability (e.g., music), achievement (e.g., mathematics), or attitude (e.g., gun control) for which everyone can be assigned a score, positive or negative, relative to the average score for that ability, achievement, or attitude.

The assumption of bipolarity, however, creates several problems for measuring levels of an addictive disorder. The first is that the assumption entrains trait scores that are not interpretable as a level of disorder. While it makes sense to assert that a person has a below-average ability in music or a right-of-center attitude toward gun control, it makes little or no sense to assert that a person has a below-average level of addiction to alcohol or an above-average level of addiction to gambling. The more meaningful assertion is that the person has a level of disorder relative to "no disorder." The anchor for the scale should therefore be "no disorder."

The second problem is the appropriate score θ_* for "no disorder." As there is no trait level less than that of "no disorder," the anchor should therefore be located at the least possible value for the trait. Under the assumption of bipolarity, we must have $\theta_* = -\infty$. If, in addition, the trait is assumed to be a random variable following a probability density on the entire real line, then the value θ_* must have probability density zero. The model thus formally assumes that there are no persons without a disorder. The empirical consequence is that any sample must include only those persons deemed at risk for the disorder because, from the model's perspective, persons without the disorder (e.g., one who never drinks alcohol cannot have an alcohol use disorder) do not exist.

This problem could be technically resolved by allowing positive probability density at $-\infty$, or, if the θ's are assumed fixed, by allowing $-\infty$ as a legitimate value. However, this solution induces an additional problem. Note that any person at risk for the disorder, even if endorsing no item, must have a trait score $\theta > \theta_*$. Under this scheme, the disorder score for any person at risk would be infinitely distant from persons without the disorder. Again, assuming an underlying bipolar trait effectively removes persons without the disorder from measurement.

The third and perhaps most important problem with bipolar traits is that they do not realistically represent an addictive disorder. Theories of addiction claim that "[an addictive disorder] can be usefully viewed as a behavioral manifestation of a chronic condition of the motivational system in which a reward-seeking behavior has become out of control" (West, 2006, p. 174). The excessive behavior is hypothesized to be caused by *cumulative ampliative effects* of an underlying reward system, itself arising from a nexus of personal dispositions and social influences, that are *inadequately damped* by eroded motivational constraints and ineffective social norms (Orford, 2001). Addiction is a *unipolar* disorder. Conceptualizing the level of addictive disorder as a latent trait and modeling the cumulative ampliative and dampening effects as infinitesimal multiplicative processes, Gibrat's "law of proportional effects" implies that the trait should asymptotically follow a lognormal density (Johnson, Kotz, & Balakrishnan, 1994). Population surveys of addictive behaviors (alcohol consumption, gambling activities, etc.) reveal unimodal, right-skewed empirical distributions, giving indirect support for an addictive disorder being a unipolar trait (Orford, 2001).

One of the advantages of IRT models is that they can be formulated to more realistically represent the underlying psychological processes that may explain an individual's response to items (De Boeck & Wilson, 2004). I recently proposed a class of IRT models, called *positive trait item response models*, that represents a person's response to items as a function of the unipolar latent trait presumed to underlie addictive disorders (Lucke, 2014). Here I update that class of models and rename it *unipolar item response models* (UIRMs).[1]

IRT models with unipolar traits are not new. The original Rasch (1966) model posited a unipolar trait for the subject's ability. Ramsay (1989) proposed a *quotient model*, similar to the Rasch model, that likewise employed a unipolar trait. Van der Maas, Molenaar, Maris, Kievit, and Borsboom (2011) proposed a *quotient-diffusion model* as a special case of *positive ability models*. Reise and Waller (2009) argued that clinical phenomena, such as depression, reflect unipolar *quasi-traits* that perhaps are being misidentified by standard (bipolar) IRT models. UIRMs attempt to appropriately measure unipolar traits with a flexible and interpretable model.

A New Research Method: The UIRM

A General UIRM

UIRMs are a psychometric implementation of Stevens's (1957) psychophysical power model (Thomas, 1983). According to his model, a psychological response $R > 0$ is related to a physical stimulus $S > 0$ by $R = \alpha S^\beta$, where $\alpha > 0$ and $\beta > 0$ are scale and shape parameters. Turning to the UIRM, let Y_{ik} be an observable Bernoulli random variable such that $Y_{ik} = 1$ if a person i endorses item k and $Y_{ik} = 0$ if i does not endorse the item. Let θ_i be a nonnegative latent variable denoting i-th person's level of addictive disorder such that $\theta_i = 0$ if i has no disorder and $\theta_i > 0$ if i has the disorder. Replace R with the expected response $E(Y_{ik})$ and S with θ_i. Next, reinterpret $\alpha_k = 0$ as the *easiness* parameter and $\beta_k = 0$ as the *discriminability*

1 I thank Steve Reise for suggesting the name.

parameter for item k. To ensure $0 \le \alpha_k \theta_i^{\beta_k} \le 1$, specify a link function F as an absolutely continuous distribution function with positive support. The general UIRM is thus:

$$\pi_k(\theta_i) = E(Y_{ik} \mid \theta_i, \alpha_k, \beta_k) = \Pr(Y_{ik} = 1 \mid \theta_i, \alpha_k, \beta_k) = F(\alpha_k \theta_i^{\beta_k}). \tag{13.1}$$

Two additional derivations are needed. The first is the derived parameter δ_k that represents the *severity* of the disorder as revealed by item k. The appropriate index of severity is the point on the θ axis such that:

$$\pi_k(\delta_k) = F(\alpha_k \delta_k^{\beta_k}) = \frac{1}{2}, \tag{13.2}$$

which yields:

$$\delta_k = \left[\frac{F^{-1}(0.5)}{\alpha_k}\right]^{1/\beta_k}. \tag{13.3}$$

The precision with which item k can estimate the underlying trait across varying values of θ is given by the *item information curve* (IIC). The general IIC for item k is:

$$\begin{aligned} I_k(\theta) &= E\left[\left(\frac{d\log\left\{\left[F(\alpha_k\theta^{\beta_k})\right]^{Y}\left[1-F(\alpha_k\theta^{\beta_k})\right]^{1-Y}\right\}}{d\theta}\right)^2\right] \\ &= \frac{\left[\alpha_k\beta_k\theta^{\beta_k-1}f(\alpha_k\theta^{\beta_k})\right]^2}{F(\alpha_k\theta^{\beta_k})[1-F(\alpha_k\theta^{\beta_k})]}, \end{aligned} \tag{13.4}$$

where f is the derivative of F. The precision with which a set of K items can estimate the underlying trait across varying values of θ and the corresponding asymptotic standard error of the estimate is given by the *total information function* (TIF):

$$I(\theta) = \sum_{k=1}^{K} I_k(\theta) \text{ and ase}(\theta) = I(\theta)^{-\frac{1}{2}}. \tag{13.5}$$

The choice of F specifies a UIRM, and here I consider two: the log-logistic and the Weibull. In what follows, the reader should note that I do not use notational elaborations to distinguish among the models. This approach reduces notational clutter, but requires the reader's careful attention to the context in which a model is presented.

The Log-Logistic UIRM

Because the logistic model is the canonical IRT model, I first present the UIRM analog, the *log-logistic* UIRM:

$$\pi_k(\theta_i) = \frac{\alpha_k \theta_i^{\beta_k}}{1 + \alpha_k \theta_i^{\beta_k}}. \tag{13.6}$$

As previously mentioned, Equation (13.6) with $\beta_k = 1$ for all k is Rasch's original item response model (Rasch, 1966, pp. 90–91).

From Equation (13.3), the item's severity is:

$$\delta_k = \left(\frac{1}{\alpha_k}\right)^{\frac{1}{\beta_k}}. \tag{13.7}$$

From Equation (13.4), the log-logistic IIC is:

$$I_k(\theta) = \left(\frac{\beta_k}{\theta}\right)^2 \frac{\alpha_k \theta^{\beta_k}}{\left(1+\alpha_k \theta^{\beta_k}\right)^2} = \left(\frac{\beta_k}{\theta}\right)^2 \pi_k(\theta)[1-\pi_k(\theta)]. \tag{13.8}$$

The Weibull UIRM

The second model is the *Weibull* UIRM:

$$\pi_k(\theta) = 1 - \exp\left(-\alpha_k \theta_i^{\beta_k}\right), \tag{13.9}$$

(Johnson et al., 1994, chapter 21). The Weibull model with $\theta > 0$ is a canonical model in bio-statistics for survival analysis and in engineering for failure analysis. Its application here is, I believe, new. For $\beta_k = 1$, the Weibull reduces to the exponential distribution.

From Equation (13.3), the item's severity is:

$$\delta_k = \left(\frac{\log_2}{\alpha_k}\right)^{\frac{1}{\beta_k}}. \tag{13.10}$$

Compare Equation (13.10) to Equation (13.7). From Equation (13.4), the Weibull IIC is:

$$I_k(\theta) = \left[\alpha_k \beta_k \theta^{\beta_k - 1}\right]^2 \frac{\exp(-\alpha_k \theta^{\beta_k})}{1-\exp(-\alpha_k \theta^{\beta_k})} = \left[\alpha_k \beta_k \theta^{\beta_k - 1}\right]^2 \frac{1-\pi_k(\theta)}{\pi_k(\theta)}. \tag{13.11}$$

Comparing Equation (13.8) to Equation (13.11), note that the log-logistic IIC is a function of the variance of the item whereas the Weibull IIC is a function of the odds of not endorsing the item.

Bayesian Inference

Bayesian inference was used to obtain posterior densities of the parameters. The analysis yields posterior density of a parameter, thereby allowing one to compute any statistic regarding the parameter. Furthermore, the Bayesian approach uses the responses of all respondents, including those who endorsed no items and those who endorsed all items.

Let N be the number of persons and K be the number of items. Adopt the standard IRT assumptions of (1) unidimensionality of the trait, (2) independence among subjects, (3) local independence among items, along with (4) no missing data and (5) prior independence among the parameters. From Bayes's Theorem, the joint posterior density of the $2K + N$ model parameters for the general UIRM given the data is:

$$\begin{aligned}
&p(\alpha_i,\ldots,\alpha_K;\beta_i,\ldots,\beta_K;\theta_1,\ldots,\theta_I \mid y_{11},\ldots,y_{IK}) \\
&\propto p(y_{11},\ldots,y_{IK} \mid \alpha_i,\ldots,\alpha_K;\beta_i,\ldots,\beta_K;\theta_1,\ldots,\theta_I)p(\alpha_i,\ldots,\alpha_K;\beta_i,\ldots,\beta_K;\theta_1,\ldots,\theta_I) \\
&= \prod_{i=1}^{N}\prod_{k=1}^{K} p(y_{ik} \mid \alpha_K,\beta_K,\theta_i)p(\alpha_K)p(\beta_K)p(\theta_i) \\
&= \prod_{i=1}^{N}\prod_{k=1}^{K} \pi_k(\theta_i)^{y_{ik}}[1-\pi_k(\theta_i)]^{1-y_{ik}}\, p(\alpha_K)p(\beta_K)p(\theta_i),
\end{aligned} \tag{13.12}$$

where $p(\alpha_K)$, $p(\beta_K)$, and $p(\theta_i)$ are the prior densities. The product over 1, ..., N is justified by independence over persons, the product over 1, ..., K is justified by local independence, and the product among the prior densities of the parameters follows from the assumed independence of parameters.

For the log-logistic model, substitution of Equation (13.6) for (13.1) into (13.12) yields:

$$\pi_k(\theta_i)^{y_{ik}}[1-\pi_k(\theta_i)]^{1-y_{ik}} = \frac{(\alpha_k\theta_i^{\beta_k})^{y_{ik}}}{1+\alpha_k\theta_i^{\beta_k}}.$$

For the Weibull model, substitution of Equation (13.9) for (13.1) into (13.12) yields:

$$\pi_k(\theta)^{y_{ik}}[1-\pi_k(\theta_i)]^{1-y_{ik}} = [\exp(\alpha_k\theta^{\beta_k})-1]^{y_{ik}}\exp(-\alpha_k\theta^{\beta_k}).$$

Following the reasoning given in Section 13, the prior densities for the N traits θ_i were assumed to be log-normal(0, 1) for all i. The K parameters α_k were given low-information log-normal priors with location 0 and scale 10, so that $\Pr(0 < \alpha_k < 181.5) = 0.95$. The K parameters β_k were given the moderate-information gamma priors with scale 0.1 and shape 0.1, so that $\Pr(0 < \beta_k < 5.8) = 0.95$. All priors were assumed to be mutually independent.

The $2K + N$ posterior parameter densities were obtained by Markov chain Monte Carlo (MCMC) simulation using Metropolis-Hastings-within-Gibbs sampling (Fox, 2010). Equation (13.12) was coded into the MCMC program *JAGS* (Plummer, 2003, 2011). All data management, analyses, and graphical displays were conducted in *R* (R Core Team, 2014) using *Rstudio* (RStudio, Inc, 2013). The interface between *R* and *JAGS* was managed by the *r2jags* package (Su & Yajima, 2012). Graphics were produced with the *lattice* (Sarkar, 2008) and *directlabels* (Hocking, 2014) packages.

Application

Data Set

The data set to demonstrate these models comprised a nationwide (United States, 50 states + DC) random sample of 2,432 adult (18+ years of age) respondents to a 12-item survey over 14 months on the prevalence of gambling pathology (Welte, Barnes, Wieczorek, Tidwell, & Parker, 2001). The 12 items consisted of the Diagnostic Interview Schedule (DIS) (Robins, Marcus, Reich, Cunningham, & Gallagher, 1996) for the DSM-IV (American Psychiatric Association, 1994). A condensed description of the items is given in Table 13.1. There was no DIS08 as the item was a filler item and was not analyzed.

Table 13.1 Condensed Description of the 12 DIS Items

Name	*Item: In your lifetime have you ever . . .*
DIS01	Spent a lot of time thinking about ways to get money so you could gamble?
DIS02	Sometimes kept thinking repeatedly about the times you won?
DIS03	Spent a lot of time planning your bets when you could be doing other things?
DIS04	Used gambling as a way to relieve a bad mood?
DIS05	Increased the amount you gamble over time to keep up the excitement?
DIS06	Gone back to try to recover the money you lost?
DIS07	Tried to quit or reduce your gambling?
DIS09	Kept family & friends from knowing how much you gambled?
DIS10	Raised money for gambling by writing bad checks or other illegal ways?
DIS11	Gambled so much as to require borrowing money?
DIS12	Risked loss of your job because of your gambling?
DIS13	Ever caused trouble with spouse/partner because of your gambling?

Results

Simulations and Convergence Diagnostics

Both the log-logistic and Wiebull models were analyzed in two runs. The first run consisted of 1,000 simulations with three chains. The second run used the terminal densities of the first run to obtain 10,000 simulations, thinned by 10, again for three chains. The final densities were based on the final 3,000 (1,000 simulations × 3 chains) simulations. All MCMC convergence diagnostics were satisfactory. In particular, the potential scale reduction factor $\hat{R}$(Brooks & Gelman, 1997) was less than the recommended 1.05 for all parameters, the maximum being $\hat{R} \leq 1.008$ for both log-logistic and Weibull models. The effective sample size exceeded the recommended 100 for all parameters, the minima being 270 for the log-logistic and 250 Weibull models. For both models, autocorrelations were effectively zero for all positive lags.

Parameter Estimates

The model contains $2K + N = 2 \times 12 + 2342 = 2456$ parameters. Of the $4096 = 2^{12}$ possible response patterns, 124 were observed. Of the 12 possible sum scores, 1,934 were zero. Thus 498 respondents (20.5%) endorsed at least one item. Of these, 251 (50.4%) endorsed exactly one item. No one endorsed all 12 items, but three endorsed 11 items and five endorsed 10 items.

Table 13.2 displays for each item its count of endorsement, the posterior mean easiness α and its standard deviation, the posterior mean discriminability β and its standard deviation, and the posterior median δ. The models yielded remarkably similar posterior estimates. The severity represented by an item (δ) was likewise similar for both models, with the exception of the two extreme items DIS10 and DIS12. The Weibull model found these items less severe than the log-logistic model. Both models ordered the items identically in terms of severity. Table 13.2 also displays the deviance information criterion (DIC), a Bayesian measure of model fit (Spiegelhalter, Best, Carlin, & Linde, 2002). According to the DIC, the log-logistic model gives better fit to the data than does the Weibull.

Table 13.2 The counts of each item's endorsement, posterior means (standard deviations) for each item's easiness ($\alpha \times 10^3$), discriminability (β), and posterior median severity (δ) parameters for the log-logistic and Weibull UIRMs. The last row presents each model's goodness of fit by the deviance information criterion (DIC).

Item	*Count*	*Log-Logistic*			*Weibull*		
		$\alpha \times 10^3$	β	δ	$\alpha \times 10^3$	β	δ
DIS01	46	1.4 (0.7)	2.7 (0.3)	12.6	1.3 (0.7)	2.6 (0.3)	11.4
DIS02	201	8.3 (2.9)	3.0 (0.3)	5.0	12.9 (3.2)	2.4 (0.2)	5.3
DIS03	80	2.4 (1.1)	2.8 (0.3)	8.9	2.9 (1.2)	2.6 (0.3)	8.8
DIS04	134	8.1 (2.5)	2.5 (0.2)	7.1	10.4 (2.7)	2.1 (0.2)	7.4
DIS05	92	4.6 (1.6)	2.5 (0.2)	8.9	5.5 (1.8)	2.2 (0.2)	8.9
DIS06	242	21.3 (5.0)	2.5 (0.2)	4.8	28.1 (5.0)	2.0 (0.1)	5.2
DIS07	186	14.7 (3.7)	2.4 (0.2)	5.9	16.7 (3.7)	2.1 (0.2)	6.0
DIS09	77	1.1 (0.6)	3.3 (0.4)	8.2	1.5 (0.8)	3.0 (0.3)	8.3
DIS10	5	0.5 (0.4)	1.9 (0.5)	63.7	0.5 (0.5)	1.9 (0.5)	55.4
DIS11	19	0.0 (0.1)	4.0 (0.6)	14.7	0.0 (0.1)	4.0 (0.6)	13.2
DIS12	4	0.1 (0.2)	2.7 (0.6)	39.9	0.1 (0.2)	2.8 (0.6)	29.9
DIS13	40	1.2 (0.7)	2.6 (0.3)	13.7	1.3 (0.7)	2.5 (0.3)	12.5
	DIC		6312			6362	

Item Analyses

Figure 13.1 displays the item characteristic curves (ICCs) for each model. Both models yielded three "bundles" of items, which are more apparent in the log-logistic than the Weibull model. The extreme bundle comprises items DIS10 and DIS12. The less extreme bundle consists of items DIS01, DIS11, and DIS13. The bundle comprising items DIS02 through DIS09 represents the least severity of use disorder.

Figure 13.2 displays the item information curves (IICs) for each model. In contrast to the ICCs, the IICs are quite different between models, with the Weibull IICs being more diffuse than the log-logistic IICs. Recall the log-logistic ICC is a function of the variance of the item, Equation (13.8), whereas the Weibull ICC is a function of the odds of non-endorsement, Equation (13.11).

An overall assessment of the DIS as a whole is given by the estimated TIF and the corresponding estimated standard error of the trait, both as a function of the trait level. Figure 13.3 displays from Equation (13.5) the TIFs and the standard error for each model. To obtain comparable vertical scaling, each TIF has been multiplied by 20; this rescaling has no effect on its interpretation. As with individual items, the TIF for the Weibull is more diffuse than that for the log-logistic. For both models, the standard error in the estimated trait becomes increasingly large beyond the trait level of 15.

Person Scores

Perhaps the most important aspect of IRT is the ability to estimate each person's trait, in this case gambling use disorder, given a vector of item responses. The posterior density of person scores, the θ s, is an automatic result of the Bayesian analysis. Figure 13.4 displays the posterior mean gambling disorder scores against themselves for both the log-logistic

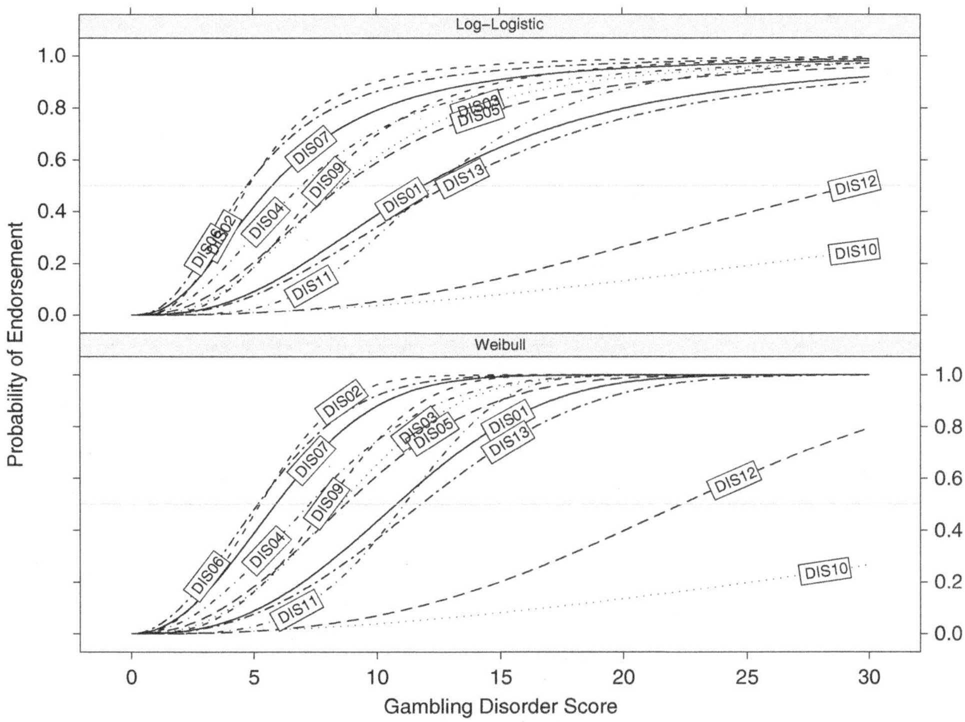

Figure 13.1 Item characteristic curves for the 12 DIS items under the log-logistic and Weibull unipolar models.

and Weibull models. The straight line connects the mean scores and the 50 percent (darker lines) and 95 percent (lighter lines) probability intervals for each mean score. The scaling is intrinsic to each model, and the scales can be compared between models only in terms of ordering. Consonant with the item analyses earlier in this chapter, the log-logistic person scores are relatively precise for scores less than 10 with the precision decreasing as scores increase, and the Weibull person scores are relatively precise for scores less than 15 with the precision decreasing as scores increase.

Of particular use is the *predicted* expected posterior score for a given set of item responses. Let $a_k = E(\alpha_k \mid y_{1k}, \ldots, y_{Nk})$ and $b_k = E(\beta_k \mid y_{1k}, \ldots, y_{Nk})$ for each k. Further, let

$$\tilde{\pi}_k(\theta) = pr(Y_{ik} = 1 \mid \alpha_k = a_k, \beta_k = b_k, \theta),$$

where π is given by Equations (13.6) or (13.9). The predicted posterior person score can be approximated by:

$$\tilde{\theta}_i = E(\theta \mid a_k, b_k, y_{i1}, \ldots, y_{iK}) = \frac{\int_0^\infty \prod_{k=1}^{K} \theta[\tilde{\pi}_k(\theta)]^{y_{ik}}[1 - \tilde{\pi}_k(\theta)]^{1-y_{ik}}\, p(\theta) d(\theta)}{\int_0^\infty \prod_{k=1}^{K} [\tilde{\pi}_k(\theta)]^{y_{ik}}[1 - \tilde{\pi}_k(\theta)]^{1-y_{ik}}\, p(\theta) d(\theta)}.$$

Figure 13.4 also displays $\tilde{\theta}_i$ as filled points for all persons. The predicted scores from the log-logistic model appear to adequately approximate the expected scores, with the predicted scores falling within the corresponding 50 percent probability intervals. However,

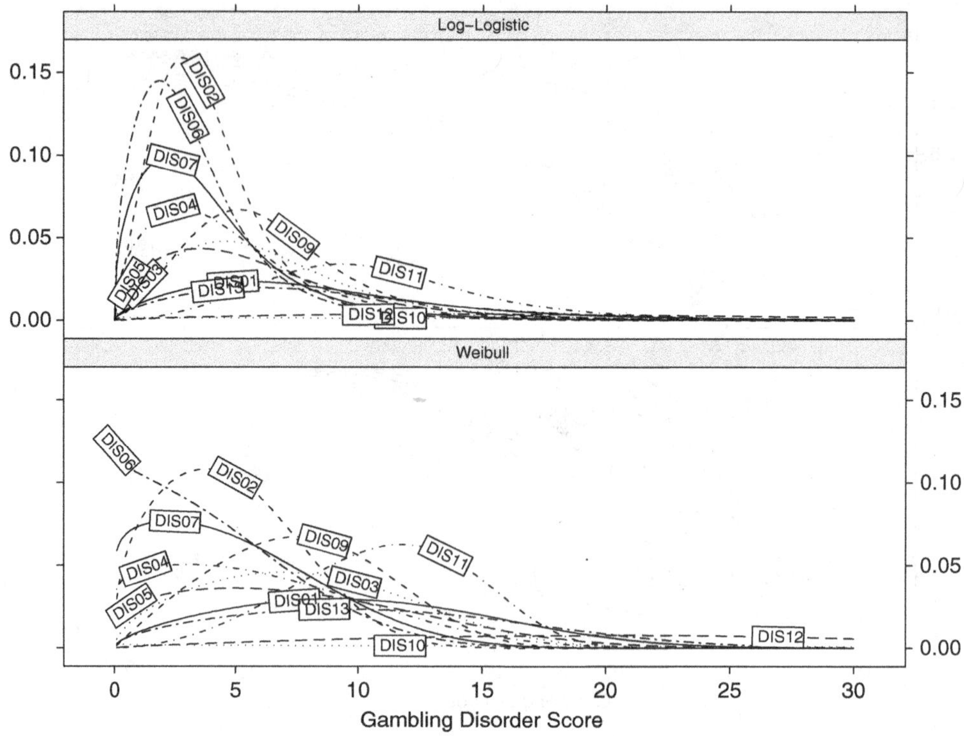

Figure 13.2 Item information curves for the 12 DIS items under the log-logistic and Weibull unipolar models.

the predicted scores from the Weibull model are less satisfactory approximations as some of them fall outside the corresponding 50 percent probability interval. The source of this lack of fit remains unknown and is under investigation.

Summary

The purpose here was to introduce a class of unipolar item response models (UIRMs) that could more realistically represent traits such as addictive disorders (Lucke, 2014). This new class of models was proposed on theoretical rather than empirical grounds. Theories of addictive disorders emphasize the increasingly ampliative effects worsening the disorder over a baseline of no disorder. This theoretical premise is not consistent with the standard IRT assumption that the trait can lie anywhere along the real line. The UIRM assumes the trait representing an addictive disorder to be positive with the baseline of no disorder fixed at zero.

UIRMs are a psychometric implementation of Stevens's (1957) psychophysical power law. The general UIRM and two specific UIRM models were introduced—the log-logistic and the Weibull—along with subsidiary derivations of item severity and item information functions. These models were here applied to a data set surveying gambling use disorder. A previous study applied these models to alcohol use disorder (Lucke, 2014).

Bayesian inference via Markov chain Monte Carlo methods provided a satisfactory method for obtaining posterior distributions for item parameters and the person traits. The estimates of the item parameters were quite similar between the two models. The item severity parameters ranked in the items in the same order for both models. The

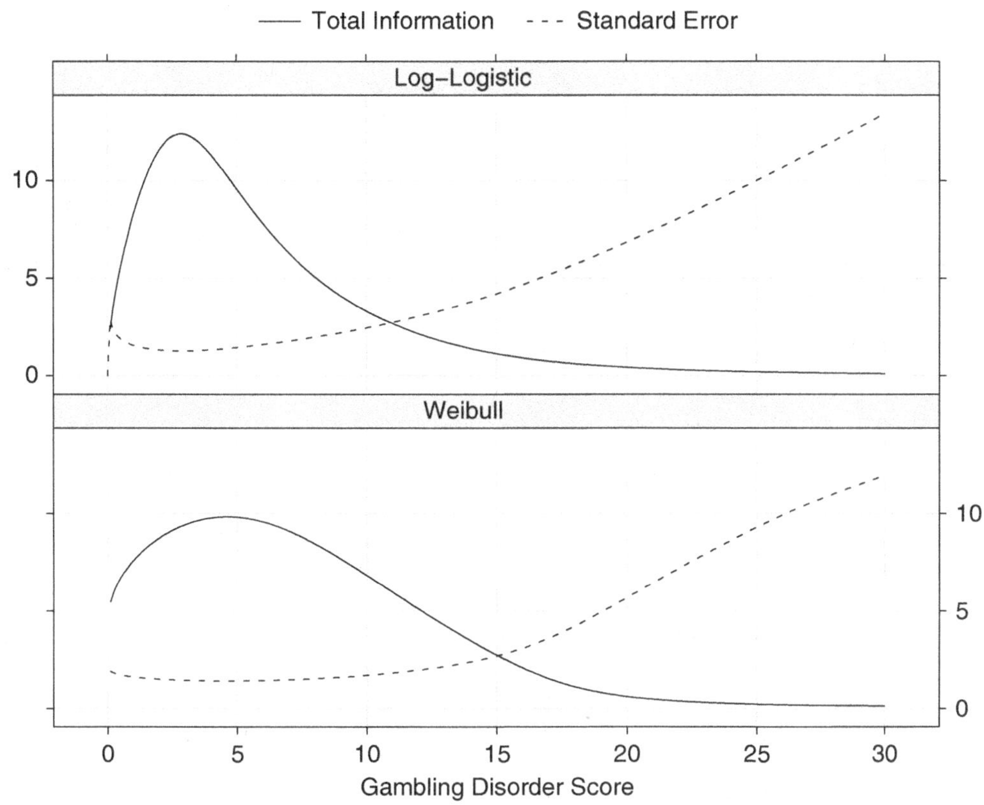

Figure 13.3 Total Information Curve (solid line) and Trait Standard Error Curve (dashed line) for the log-linear and Weibull unipolar models.

two UIRMs yielded slightly differently shaped item characteristic curves that nonetheless retained the same ordering of items across models. However, the two UIRMS yielded quite distinct item information curves. The item total information was also different between the two models because of differences in the link function. The Bayesian approach also allows model comparisons using the DIC. For example, the two-parameter UIRMs could be compared to a one-parameter model or, based on the three "bundles" of items discovered earlier, a two-parameter model with constraints.

Reise and Waller noted "striking contrasts between the IRT modeling of clinical and cognitive tests," finding that several standard, bipolar IRT studies have shown the maximum item information to be in the pathological range of the trait with little precision in the non-pathological range (Reise & Waller, 2009, pp. 29–32). The typical conclusion is that the items were poorly chosen for the non-pathological region and new items need to be created to address this range. Reise and Waller, however, suggest that the problem may not lie with the items but with the IRT model itself—using a bipolar IRT model where a unipolar model would be more appropriate.

The results here show that the UIRMs, in contrast, may not possess this problem. The two models here show maximum information at the lower end of the trait scale with diminishing precision as the trait level increases. Furthermore, the person trait scores are meaningful under the UIRM. UIRMs thus provide a viable alternative to the standard IRT models for phenomena such as addictive disorders.

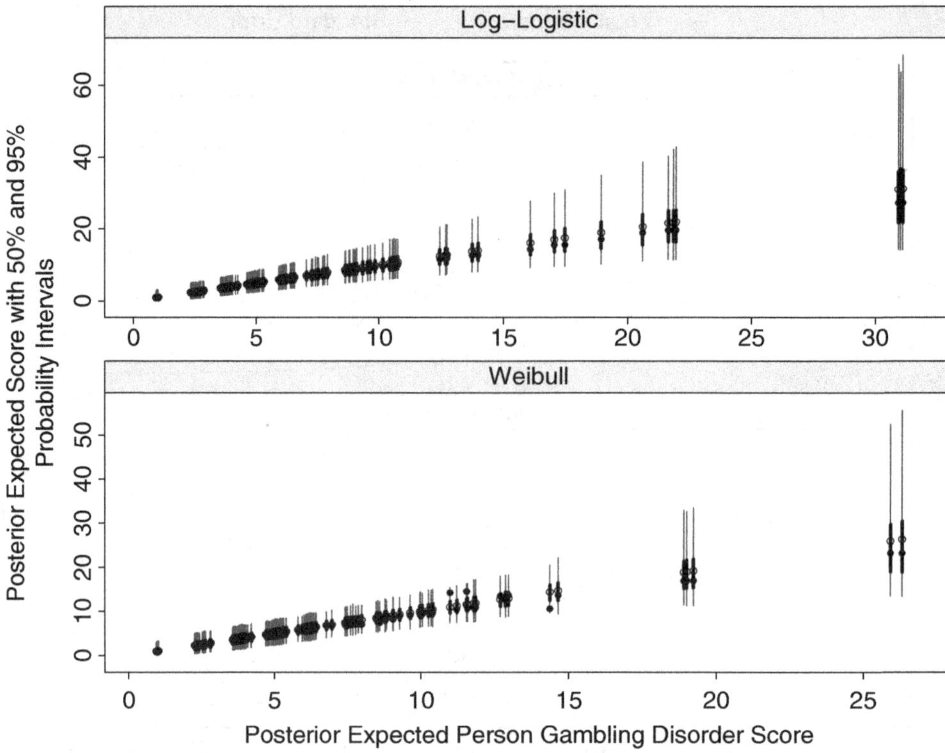

Figure 13.4 Posterior Expected Person Scores (circles) their 50 percent (dark line) and 95 percent (light line) probability intervals supplemented with the Estimated Expected Scores (points) for the log-logistic and Weibull unipolar models.

Future Directions

UIRMs have the potential for several extensions. The first extension lies in the choice of link functions. Here we considered only two, the log-logistic and the Weibull, but any non-negatively supported distribution function, such as the log-normal or log-Cauchy, could be used. Justification of the link function on substantive grounds would be essential.

Setting the prior density for the latent trait as lognormal was based on the presumed infinitesimal multiplicative process underlying an addictive disorder. A second extension would be the use of other priors based on other psychological processes. A related issue is whether the trait value of zero can be estimated from the test instrument itself or must be determined by procedures external to the test, for example, never drinks or never gambles.

The UIRMs proposed here assumed that the probability of item endorsement was zero for those persons with a trait level at zero. Although this makes sense for measures of addictive disorders, it need not be the case for measures of other unipolar traits such as depression, chronic pain, or mobility assessment. The third extension would include an item parameter for the probability of an item's endorsement when the trait level is zero.

A fourth extension would be an integrated Bayesian differential item functioning (DIF) model for UIRMs similar to the model proposed for bipolar IRT (Soares, Gonçalves, & Gamerman, 2009). A fourth extension would include item and person covariates as in explanatory item response models (De Boeck & Wilson, 2004). These extensions are currently being explored.

Acknowledgments

I thank John Welte and Grace Barnes for providing the data set. I also thank Samara Rice for reviewing a previous version of this chapter.

References

American Psychiatric Association. (1994). *Diagnostic and statistical manual of mental disorders* (4th ed.). Washington, DC: American Psychiatric Publications.

Brooks, S.P., & Gelman, A. (1997). General methods for monitoring convergence of iterative simulations. *Journal of Computational and Graphical Statistics*, *7*, 434–455.

De Boeck, P., & Wilson, M. (2004). *Explanatory item response models: A generalized linear and nonlinear approach*. New York: Springer.

Embretson, S.E., & Reise, S.P. (2000). *Item response theory for psychologists*. Mahwah, NJ: Lawrence Erlbaum Associates.

Fox, J.-P. (2010). *Bayesian item response modeling: Theory and applications*. New York: Springer.

Hocking, T.D. (2014). *Direct labels for multicolor plots in lattice or ggplot2*. (Available at http://directlabels.r-forge.r-project.org/).

Johnson, N.L., Kotz, S., & Balakrishnan, N. (1994). *Continuous univariate distributions* (2nd ed., vol. 1). New York: Wiley.

Kahler, C.W., Strong, D.R., Stuart, G.L., Moore, T.M., & Ramsey, S.E. (2003). Item functioning of the alcohol dependence scale in a high-risk sample. *Drug and Alcohol Dependence*, *72*(2), 183–192.

Keyes, K.M., Krueger, R.F., Grant, B.F., & Hasin, D.S. (2011). Alcohol craving and the dimensionality of alcohol disorders. *Psychological Medicine*, *41*(03), 629–640.

Liu, L.C., Hedeker, D., & Mermelstein, R.J. (2013). Modeling nicotine dependence: An application of a longitudinal IRT model for the analysis of Adolescent Nicotine Dependence Syndrome Scale. *Nicotine & Tobacco Research*, *15*(2), 326–333.

Lucke, J.F. (2014). Positive trait item response models. In R.E. Millsap, L.A. van der Ark, D.M. Bolt, & C.M. Woods (Eds.), *New developments in quantitative psychology: Presentations from the 77th annual psychometric society meeting*. New York: Springer.

Orford, J. (2001). *Excessive appetites: A psychological view of addictions* (2nd ed.). Chichester, UK: Wiley.

Plummer, M. (2003). JAGS: A program for analysis of Bayesian graphical models using Gibbs sampling. In K. Hornik, F. Leisch, & A. Zeileis (Eds.), *Proceedings of the 3rd international workshop on distributed statistical computing*. Vienna, Austria: Technische Universität Wien. (Available at http://sourceforge.net/projects/mcmc-jags/.)

Plummer, M. (2011). *JAGS version 3.1.0 user manual*. (Available at http://sourceforge.net/projects/mcmc-jags/files/Manuals/3.x/jags user manual.pdf/download.)

R Core Team. (2014). *R: A language and environment for statistical computing*. Vienna, Austria. (Available at http://cran.us.r-project.org/.)

Ramsay, J.O. (1989). A comparison of three simple test theory models. *Psychometrika*, *54*(3), 487–499.

Rasch, G. (1966). An individualistic approach to item analysis. In P.F. Lazarsfeld & N.W. Henry (Eds.), *Readings in mathematical social science* (pp. 89–108). Chicago, IL: Chicago Science Research Associates.

Reise, S.P., & Waller, N.G. (2009). Item response theory and clinical measurement. *Annual Review of Clinical Psychology*, *5*(1), 27–48 (PMID: 18976138).

Robins, L., Marcus, L., Reich, W., Cunningham, R., & Gallagher, T. (1996). *NIMH Diagnostic Interview Schedule: Version IV (DIS-IV)*. St Louis, MO.

RStudio, Inc. (2013). *Rstudio*. Boston, MA. (Available at www.rstudio.com/.)

Saha, T.D., Compton, W.M., Chou, S.P., Smith, S., Ruan, W.J., Huang, B., et al. (2012). Analyses related to the development of DSM-5 criteria for substance use related disorders: 1. Toward amphetamine, cocaine and prescription drug use disorder continua using item response theory. *Drug and Alcohol Dependence*, *122*(1–2), 38–46.

Sarkar, D. (2008). *Lattice: Multivariate data visualization with R*. New York: Springer. (Available at http://lattice.r-forge.r-project.org/.)

Sharp, C., Steinberg, L., Yaroslavsky, I., Hofmeyr, A., Dellis, A., Ross, D., et al. (2012). An item response theory analysis of the Problem Gambling Severity Index. *Assessment*, *19*(2), 167–175.

Soares, T. M., Gonçalves, F. B., & Gamerman, D. (2009). An integrated Bayesian model for DIF analysis. *Journal of Educational and Behavioral Statistics*, *34*(3), 348–377.

Spiegelhalter, D. J., Best, N. G., Carlin, B. P., & Linde, A. van der. (2002). Bayesian measures of model complexity and fit. *Journal of the Royal Statistical Society: Series B (Statistical Methodology)*, *64*(4), 583–639.

Stevens, S. S. (1957). On the psychophysical law. *Psychological Review*, *64*(3), 153–181.

Su, Y.-S., & Yajima, M. (2012). *R2jags: A package for running JAGS from R*. (Available at http://cran.r-project.org/web/packages/R2jags/R2jags.pdf.)

Thomas, H. (1983). Parameter estimation in simple psychophysical models. *Psychological Bulletin*, *93*(2), 396–403.

van der Maas, H. L. J., Molenaar, D., Maris, G., Kievit, R. A., & Borsboom, D. (2011). Cognitive psychology meets psychometric theory: On the relation between process models for decision making and latent variable models for individual differences. *Psychological Review*, *118*(2), 339–356.

Welte, J., Barnes, G., Wieczorek, W., Tidwell, M.-C., & Parker, J. (2001). Alcohol and gambling pathology among U.S. adults: Prevalence, demographic patterns and comorbidity. *Journal of Studies on Alcohol and Drugs*, *62*(5), 706–712.

West, R. (2006). *Theory of addiction*. Oxford, UK: Blackwell.

14 Selecting Among Polytomous IRT Models

Remo Ostini, Matthew Finkelman, and Michael Nering

Introduction

Polytomous item response theory (IRT) has proven fertile ground for psychological measurement model development. While unidimensional dichotomous IRT models primarily come in three basic choices, the measurement practitioner has many more potential models from which to choose when working with polytomous response data, even within the subset of unidimensional models. Ostini and Nering (2006) provide a consideration of some of the ways polytomous IRT models differ as a class from dichotomous models. Nering and Ostini (2010) provide a deeper investigation of the historical and conceptual origins of the most influential models in a collection of chapters written by the researchers most closely associated with the development of the models.

The larger range of models from which to choose results in part from attempts to address the larger number of item formats that polytomous items can take. It also reflects an increased number of possibilities for representing the relationships among category responses within an item—when there are more than two categories into which a respondent can be categorized. However, having a larger number of models from which to choose potentially complicates the question of how to select a model for a particular application, particularly if the concern is with choosing the "correct" model.

This chapter will outline some of the more commonly applied polytomous IRT models, including some of their more salient differences. This chapter will then consider a strategy for choosing among polytomous IRT models, presenting some research that has a bearing on how the strategy may play out in practice.

What Are the Choices?

Influential polytomous IRT models include a model for response data from items with categories that do not have a pre-specified order—the Nominal Response model (NRM; Bock, 1972, 1997) (see also Chapter 18). Multiple-choice items, where there is no explicit order of "correctness" to the distractor items, are often considered potential candidates for the application of the NRM. This provides an opportunity to make use of the distractor items, rather than treating the multiple-choice item as dichotomously scored items (where all distractor responses are marked as incorrect). The model is not, however, limited to multiple-choice items, as Chapter 18 shows. The mathematical form of the NRM is shown in Equation (14.1).

$$P_{jk}\left(u=k\middle|\theta;\mathbf{a},\mathbf{c}\right)=P_{jk}\left(\theta\right)=\frac{\exp\left(a_k\theta+c_k\right)}{\sum_{l=1}^{m}\exp\left(a_l\theta+c_l\right)}, \tag{14.1}$$

where $P_{jk}(\theta)$ is the probability that a response u to item j is in category k $(l = 1, 2, \ldots, k, \ldots, m)$, as a function of the ability or trait continuum θ, with a category slope parameter a_k and category intercept parameter c_k and with $(a_k\theta + c_k) \equiv Z_k$. The form of Equation (14.1), where the denominator is the sum of all possible numerators, is described as a divide-by-total model by Thissen and Steinberg (1986). This model is unusual in that it involves directly estimating a category response function ($P_{jk}(\theta)$) for each item response option.

One of the earliest polytomous IRT models for items with ordered response categories is the Logistic Graded Response model (L-GRM; Samejima, 1969, 1997b). This model is from a family of graded models developed by Samejima for application to polytomous items where there is a clear order to the amount of a trait required to answer each item category. Likert-type items are a clear example of such an item, but the model can be equally applied to constructed response items, which are scored into better and worse responses to a test question or item. The mathematical form of the L-GRM is shown in Equation (14.2).

$$P_{jk}(\theta) = \frac{\exp\left[a_j\left(\theta - b_{jk}\right)\right]}{1 + \exp\left[a_j\left(\theta - b_{jk}\right)\right]} - \frac{\exp\left[a_j\left(\theta - b_{j(k+1)}\right)\right]}{1 + \exp\left[a_j\left(\theta - b_{j(k+1)}\right)\right]}, \tag{14.2}$$

which can be summarized as $P_{jk} = P^*_{jk} - P^*_{j(k+1)}$, where* $P_{jk}(\theta)$ is the probability of responding in category k $(k = 0, 1, \ldots, m)$ of item j, P^*_{jk} represents the category boundary (threshold) function for category k of item j, a_j is the item discrimination parameter and b_{jk} is the difficulty (location) parameter for category boundary (threshold) parameter k of item j. The form of Equation (14.2), which involves subtracting an element ($*_{j(k+1)}$) from a preceding element ($*_{jk}$), is described as a difference model by Thissen and Steinberg (1986). The difference model approach to modeling response probabilities is required when polytomous category boundaries—the P* elements in the summary equation—are modeled as cumulative probabilities. This process is described in Ostini and Nering (2006) where this form of polytomous model is characterized as a cumulative boundary (CUM) model.

The Rating Scale model (RSM; Andrich, 1978a, 1978b) is another early IRT model for ordered polytomous items and like the L-GRM (Samejima, 2010) represents a specific instance of a broader approach to modeling polytomous items (Andrich, 2010). The RSM was specifically developed for measurement situations using rating scales (such as Likert scales), which were assumed or expected to operate in the same way across all items in a test, survey, or questionnaire. The model is shown in Equation (14.3).

$$P_{jk}(\theta) = \frac{\exp\sum_{v=1}^{k}\left(\theta - \left(\delta_j + \tau_v\right)\right)}{\sum_{c=1}^{m_j}\exp\sum_{v=1}^{c}\left(\theta - \left(\delta_j + \tau_v\right)\right)}, \tag{14.3}$$

where $P_{jk}(\theta)$ is the probability of responding in category k $(k = 1, 2, \ldots, m)$ of item j, δ_i is the item difficulty (location) parameter, and τ_k is the common category boundary (threshold) parameter for all the items using a particular rating scale. The τ_k define how far from any given item location a particular threshold for the scale is located. The form of Equation (14.3) is another example of a divide-by-total model in Thissen and Stenberg's (1986) terminology. In the case of ordered polytomous IRT models, the divide-by-total model is constructed on the basis of category boundaries that are defined by the probability of responding in either response category adjacent to (either side of) the category boundary. Models of this type are therefore referred to as adjacent category models (ACM) by Ostini and Nering (2006) in contrast to the approach taken in CUM models such as the L-GRM. Other ACM models include the Partial Credit [14.4] and [14.5]).Generalized Partial Credit model described later in this chapter (Equations (14.4) and (14.5)).

As can be seen in Equation (14.3), the RSM approach to modeling polytomous item responses involves a distinct method for representing model item parameters with reference to a central item location. Figure 14.1 provides a graphical representation of this approach for two items b_1 and b_2, at different locations on the trait scale. The three tau at the end of the arrows for each item represent the common distance from the item location to the boundary locations for two four-category rating scale items.

This approach is quite flexible in its capacity to model item complexity while keeping the number of estimated parameters low. Examples of this approach incorporating a dispersion parameter (Dispersion Location model, DLM; Andrich, 1982), a skew parameter (Dispersion, Skew Location model, DSLM; Andrich, 1985), and a combination of rating scale and dispersion parameters that reflects Thurstone's (Edwards & Thurstone, 1952) method of successive intervals (Successive Intervals model, SIM; Rost, 1988) are described and compared in Ostini (2002). Figure 14.2 shows how these different models can be represented using the general approach shown for the RSM in Figure 14.1. Vertical lines in the figure represent category boundary locations for two different items (Item *i* and Item *j*) on equivalent θ scales. In Figure 14.1, these locations are represented by the end points of the arrows for each item category. In the mathematical representation of these models, the boundary locations are at the inflection point of the category boundary functions.

The Partial Credit model (PCM; Masters, 1982) provides a more general parameterization for ordered polytomous items than the RSM. In the PCM each category boundary is modeled separately, allowing for items within a scale to vary in the number of categories that they contain. Equation (14.4) shows the PCM.

$$P_{jk}(\theta) = \frac{\exp\sum_{v=1}^{k}(\theta - \delta_{jv})}{\sum_{c=1}^{m_j}\exp\sum_{v=1}^{c}(\theta - \delta_{jv})}, \tag{14.4}$$

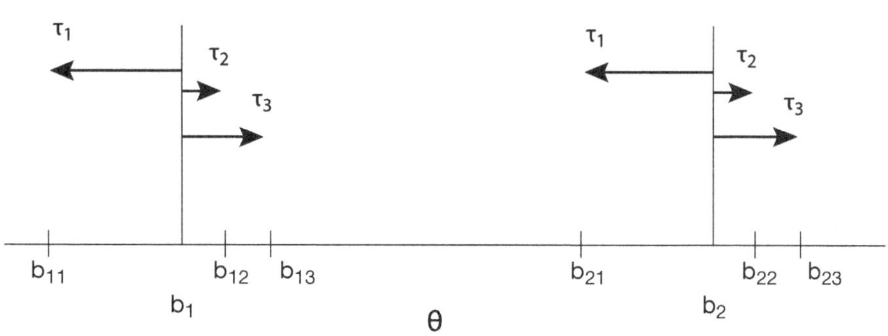

Figure 14.1 Graphical representation of the RSM approach to modeling category boundaries.

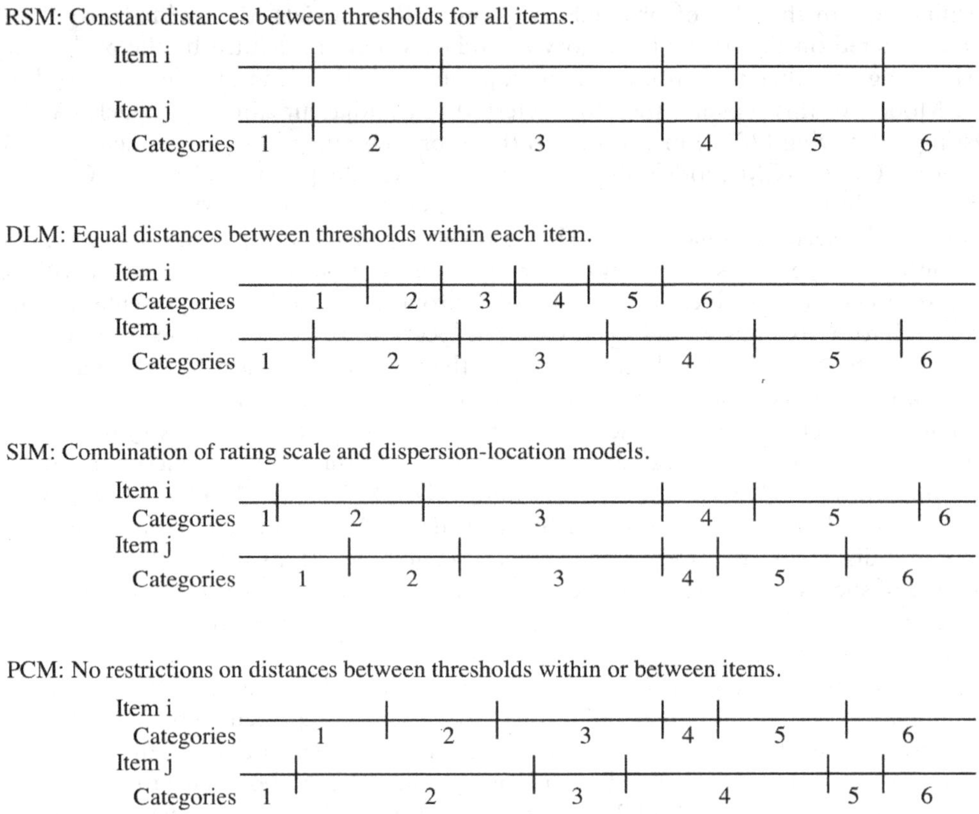

Figure 14.2 Graphical representation of different ways to simplify models by constraining the relationship between category boundaries using the RSM modeling approach.

where $P_{jk}(\theta)$ is the probability of responding in category *k* ($k = 1, 2, \ldots, m$) of item *j*, δ_{jv} is the difficulty (location) parameter for category boundary (threshold) parameter *v* of item *j*. The RSM and the PCM are both Rasch-type polytomous IRT models.

The Generalized Partial Credit model (GPCM; Muraki, 1992) extends the PCM by modeling a separate discrimination parameter for each item. In this respect, the GPCM is equivalent to the L-GRM although it becomes so by extending the PCM, and is therefore an adjacent category model whereas the L-GRM is a cumulative model. The GPCM also uses the central item location parameterization approach used in the RSM and other Andrich models, as is shown in Equation (14.5).

$$P_{jk}(\theta) = \frac{\exp \sum_{v=1}^{k} 1.7a_j(\theta - b_j + d_v)}{\sum_{c=1}^{m_j} \exp \sum_{v=1}^{c} 1.7a_j(\theta - b_j + d_v)}, \tag{14.5}$$

where $P_{jk}(\theta)$ is the probability of responding in category *k* ($k = 1, 2, \ldots, m$) of item *j*, a_j is the item discrimination parameter, b_j is the item difficulty (location) parameter, and d_v is the category boundary (threshold) parameter for an item. The d_v define how far from an item location a threshold is located. Adding a discrimination parameter results in the GPCM no longer adhering to the tenets of Rasch measurement—for example, specific objectivity.

Other more recently developed, distinctive polytomous IRT models include the Sequential model (Tutz, 1990, 1997) and the Acceleration model (Samejima, 1995). The Sequential model is a hybrid model incorporating elements of adjacent category and cumulative boundary modeling to represent boundaries as discrete sequential steps in responding to an item (Ostini & Nering, 2006). The Acceleration model is a rare example of a model in Samejima's heterogeneous class of graded models that was developed to provide a way to model complex cognitive tasks in detail (Ostini & Nering, 2006). It is an exponential model that treats test items as cognitive tasks made up of a number of problem-solving steps.

Distinctions Among Models

Differences among polytomous IRT models might be considered important when deciding which model to use in a specific measurement context. As with dichotomous IRT, polytomous IRT models can be distinguished in terms of whether or not a guessing parameter is employed, and whether or not item discrimination is modeled as a separate parameter. Polytomous IRT models also differ with respect to whether or not they were developed within the Rasch measurement approach. The distinction between polytomous Rasch and non-Rasch models is not as clear or philosophically rigorous as it is in the dichotomous case and largely revolves around the question of whether or not sufficient statistics are available for model parameter estimation.

A major distinction that applies only to polytomous IRT models pertains to the way that category boundaries within an item are modeled. Boundary locations can either be modeled across an item, in terms of cumulative category responses (GRM-type models), or locally, with respect to adjacent category responses only (Rasch-type models). They can also be modeled in a combination of adjacent and cumulative boundaries as in sequential models. The statistical basis of this distinction is described in Agresti's (1997) work on the classification of response process and in Mellenberg's (1995) conceptual treatment of polytomous IRT models.

Table 14.1 shows how the category boundary function locations differ between a cumulative category model (L-GRM) and an adjacent category model (GPCM) for an item from a scale measuring moral conceptualization (Ostini, 2010). While these parameters were estimated using the same software program and a common set of data, the type of boundary categorization used by each model is still only one of the factors affecting these parameter estimates. Boundary location values are also influenced by differing discrimination parameter estimates and differences in parameter estimation routines across IRT

Table 14.1 Item Category Parameter Comparison for an Item Modeled by a Cumulative Model (L-GRM) and an Equivalent Adjacent Category Model (GPCM)

Model	*Category Boundary*			
	1	*2*	*3*	*4*
L-GRM	–2.502	–0.766	0.848	2.419
GPCM	–2.415	–0.688	0.992	2.111

models—even within a single software program. The differences in boundary location estimates shown in the table are therefore only indicative of the effects of the two ways of modeling category boundaries.

Polytomous models can also be constrained in pre-specified ways. The most common example of this is where polytomous items elicit responses using a rating scale. Rating scale versions of both cumulative (RS-GRM; Muraki, 1990) and adjacent category (RSM) models exist. Conversely, polytomous models can be generalized to become able to operate with data where the ordering of response categories is unknown or not specified (NRM) or where the data to be modeled are essentially continuous (Samejima, 1973).

A factor that might be considered important in selecting among the variety of polytomous IRT models available for use is the question of how they differ in terms of measurement outcomes. In a comparison of eight different polytomous IRT models with model parameters estimated using seven different software programs (for 26 different model x software conditions) applied to two common data sets, Ostini (2002) investigated measurement outcomes in terms of variation in item and respondent trait level parameter estimates. The results of that research inform some of our consideration of model selection issues later in this chapter.

A Selection Strategy

In the remainder of this chapter we will outline a strategy for making an informed decision about which polytomous IRT model to use in a specific context. Cella and colleagues (2007) provide a good outline addressing the more fundamental question of why IRT would be used in preference to classical test theory. These ideas are explained in more detail in the work of Lord (1980; Lord & Novick, 1968) and Hambleton and Swaminathan (1985).

Background Considerations

A number of preliminary issues must be considered before IRT model selection takes place. These include the assumptions that underpin IRT, the question of measurement philosophy, and the possible processes that give rise to polytomous item responses.

IRT Assumptions

IRT is known as a strong measurement theory because it makes strong assumptions about the condition of the data to which the model is being fit. To begin with, item data must be of known dimensionality. In practice, especially for polytomous models, this usually comes down to data being unidimensional—that is, only one latent trait is needed to account for test item responses. A second assumption is that test items produce data that are locally independent. This assumption is clearly described in a number of places (Hambleton & Swaminathan, 1985; Lord & Novick, 1968; Weiss & Yoes, 1991). For a test measuring just one trait, the assumption of unidimensionality is equivalent to the assumption of local independence, although this is not the case for multidimensional tests (Crocker & Algina, 1986)—making model assumption testing much more difficult for multidimensional tests. A third key assumption is that the latent variable is monotonically related to item response probability. That is, people with greater levels of a trait have higher probabilities of responding in the item category that indicates the presence (or greater presence for polytomous items) of the trait (Lord, 1980). In the simplest case, for a test of ability consisting of dichotomous items, a response indicating "greater presence" of the trait typically refers to a correct response.

A further issue that arises for polytomous IRT models is the question of whether each response category for an item is, for some range of the trait continuum, the most probable response category. The contention is that an item is not working as intended or expected if it has modeled response categories that are never the most probable response category. In essence, the argument is that an item category that is never the most probable category is not required. Having such a category suggests that an item has too many categories for use in making meaningful measurement distinctions. This is seen as an important diagnostic tool (Andrich, 1995) with implications for combining data across response categories (joining assumption) and for category boundary parameterization. For polytomous models, such as Rasch models and the GPCM, which use ACM boundaries, the presence of unordered boundary locations (boundary reversals) is a clear indicator of an item category that is never most probable. For models built on CUM boundaries, category response functions need to be explicitly plotted for such categories to be identified. In the CUM case, a category response function that never rises in probability above the height of all other category functions at some point on the trait scale is a category that is never the most probable category.

Testing of IRT and model assumptions is sometimes seen as something to be done prior to model fitting; however, assumption testing usually requires fitting IRT models as part of the testing process. This was the approach explicitly used in the development of PROMIS® item banks, where, for example, items selected for the Emotional Distress domain were calibrated using the GRM and the response categories for each item were inspected to determine whether they were "most probably" categories at any point on the trait continuum (Cella et al., 2007). Our research suggests that substantive differences among polytomous IRT models are more pronounced to the extent that data do not meet IRT model assumptions (Ostini, 2002). That is, where data meet IRT model assumptions, substantive differences in the measurement outcomes of different polytomous IRT models tend to be small. Examples of how this can occur are described over the following sections of this chapter.

Measurement Philosophy

While the practical difference between Rasch and non-Rasch models is less distinct for polytomous IRT, the difference in underlying measurement philosophy remains. If measurement practitioners are convinced that specific objectivity is an important feature of their measurement enterprise, they will need to use a Rasch model. Specific objectivity can be thought of as the capacity to provide invariant comparisons among people and among items. At the model parameter level, this requires that comparisons among item parameter values be independent of person parameter values and vice versa. In practice this means expecting, or being willing to treat items as if they are equally discriminating across an item set. IRT models that include a separately modeled discrimination parameter are not therefore Rasch models.

An important element of measurement philosophy is the question of whether tests should be designed so that responses fit measurement theory or whether the goal is to find a model that reflects how people actually respond to tests. The argument from a Rasch perspective is that meaningful measurement only occurs if specific objectivity holds, which requires data that fit a Rasch model. In practice, items typically vary in their discriminating power but this cannot be modeled in a separate discrimination parameter (with the potential decrease in model fit) for specific objectivity to hold. Considering the response processes that have been proposed for different polytomous IRT models helps clarify the distinction between selecting a model based on data and selecting data to fit a model.

Response Processes

The logistic ogive is the mathematical function at the heart of IRT. It represents the probability of a person responding to an item with a specific response in terms of the standing of that person on the trait that the item is measuring. Figure 14.3 shows the shape of a logistic ogive modeling a hypothetical response to a health outcome item. In Figure 14.3, Person H has more of the trait in question (the health outcome) and therefore has a higher probability of endorsing this item.

This function was adopted for this purpose early in the development of IRT, in part because it was found to closely resemble the item response behavior that people exhibit (see, e.g., Lord, 1980). There are a number of further assumptions implicit in the different types of polytomous IRT models about the way responses are generated when a respondent is faced with a test item. Different polytomous models make different assumptions about the psychological processes that might lead to a particular person responding in a

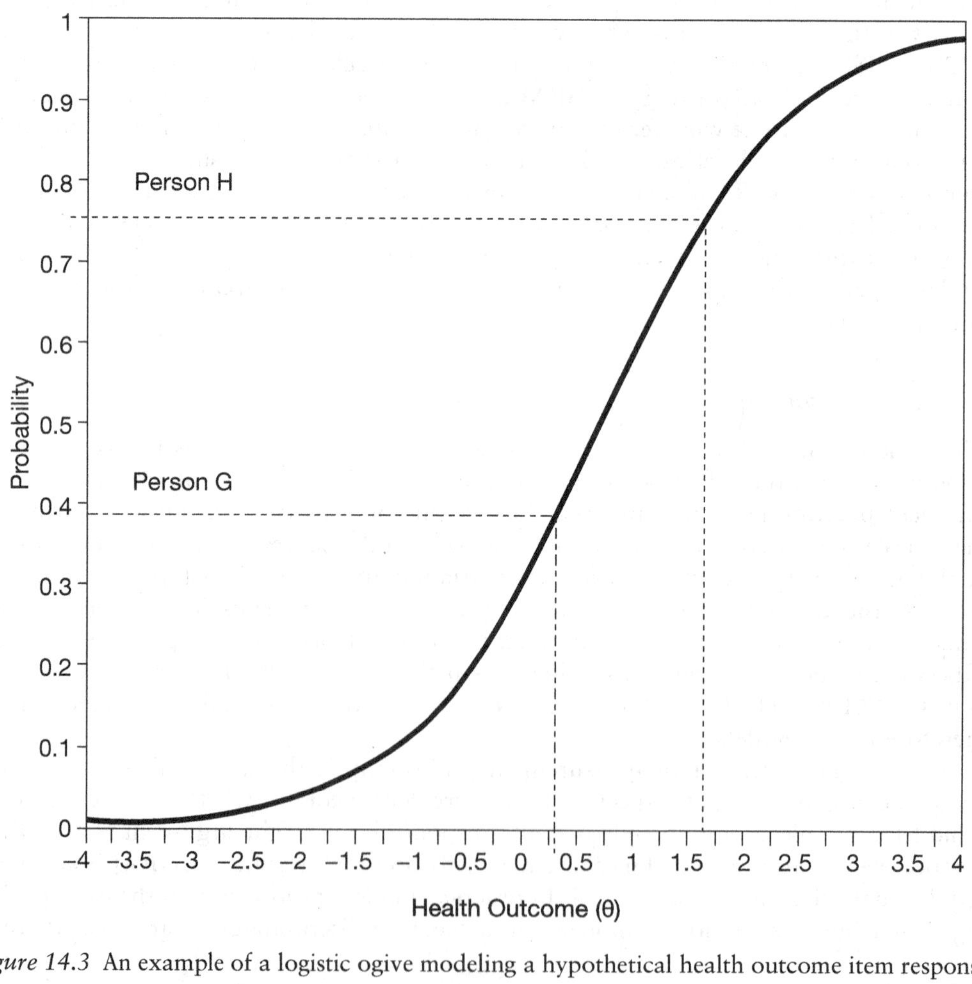

Figure 14.3 An example of a logistic ogive modeling a hypothetical health outcome item response.

particular category of a polytomous item. Curiously, and unfortunately, research into the response processes that people actually employ when faced with different types of testing situations is very rare. There is therefore little empirical data to suggest which models might be more appropriate for a given testing situation.

Cognitive interviewing can provide a method for assessing the response processes that people use when responding to polytomous items (see, e.g., Castillo-Díaz & Padilla, 2013). It could conceivably be used to test the hypothesized response processes for polytomous IRT models. For example, Samejima (1972) proposed a response process for cumulative models in her Graded Response framework whereby a respondent who has been attracted by a response category ($g - 1$) to item i is subsequently further attracted by the next category (g). This hypothesized response process is the building block of her cumulative polytomous IRT model—and could conceivably be tested, through a process such as cognitive interviewing.

RATING SCALE

The fact that the RSM models item category boundaries in terms of adjacent categories implies a response process that treats each category boundary as a separate dichotomous item (Masters, 1982; Masters & Wright, 1984; Wright & Masters, 1982). This suggests that a person giving a response in the third category of an ordered polytomous item has effectively responded positively to two successive dichotomous items (the boundary between the first and second item categories, and then again at the boundary between the second and third categories).

Rather than focusing on how people respond to polytomous items, in more recent work, Andrich (2010) begins with the theoretical measurement requirement of invariant comparisons among people and among items (i.e., specific objectivity) and shows how this is accomplished in a general polytomous Rasch model. Applying different parameter restrictions then results in specific models, such as the PCM and the RSM. The parameterization of the RSM and the PCM specifically were described earlier.

Andrich (2010) then focuses on two properties of the RSM and polytomous Rasch models that can seem counterintuitive. The first is that, with polytomous Rasch models, it is not possible to combine responses from two adjacent categories into a single response category without changing how an item is measuring the trait in question or changing the model-data fit for the item—that is, these models violate the "joining assumption" (Jansen & Roskam, 1986). The second property that he addresses is how the trait level ordering of Rasch model category boundary locations need not be the same as the intended order of the item categories (i.e., boundary reversals). Rather than treating these properties as problems with polytomous Rasch models, Andrich (2010) argues that a strength of polytomous Rasch models is that they provide a way to test whether ordered, categorical items are operating in the manner intended. For example, finding boundary reversals shows that an ordered categorical item is not functioning as intended.

Our empirical comparison of item parameters and boundary functions across different polytomous IRT models suggested that the rating scale parameterization of the RSM was more plausible than the within-item dispersion parameterization of the DLM but produced greater modeled discrepancies in comparisons with more general polytomous models such as the DSLM, PCM, and SIM (Ostini, 2002). In trait parameter comparisons, RSM trait estimates correlated perfectly with almost all other Rasch models in an IRT assumption-fitting data set. However, specific, estimated individual trait locations differed more for people modeled with the RSM than other Rasch models. This set of results suggests that the rating scale assumption may be overly restrictive—even with data collected using a rating scale format (Ostini, 2002). That is, while trait estimate rank ordering was very similar for RSM and more general models, trait estimates across test respondents showed larger differences for RSM modeled estimates compared to more general models than among the different general models themselves. This suggests that keeping category "widths" constant in a test using an ostensibly common rating scale (such as a Likert scale) may not be empirically supported.

PARTIAL CREDIT MODEL (AND GENERALIZED PCM)

The idea that polytomous Rasch models (and adjacent category models generally) model successive dichotomous choices at each category boundary was initially proposed in the context of the development of the PCM (Masters, 1982; Masters & Wright, 1984; Wright & Masters, 1982). In early descriptions of this response process, each category boundary decision was described as an independent step. However, Tutz (1990), Molenaar (1983), and Verhelst and Verstralen (1997) showed clearly that adjacent category boundaries for an item are not modeled independently of each other—and Masters (1988) ultimately conceded that this was the case.

In his more recent exposition of the development of the PCM, Masters (2010) focuses on the importance of specific objectivity—describing it in terms of the independent estimation of different people's abilities that allows "objective" comparisons. As with Andrich (2010) as described in the previous section, the argument essentially becomes a justification of the adjacent category response process (whatever it may represent) because it allows specific objectivity.

This essentially leaves the GPCM without a clear underlying response process because the estimation of a discrimination parameter renders the model unable to meet the requirements of specific objectivity; and the critique of the step notion of a response process applies equally to the GPCM as to polytomous Rasch models.

GRADED RESPONSE MODEL FRAMEWORK

Samejima (1972) describes a response process for her class of models (including the L-GRM), which is based on a function that denotes the probability that someone who has been attracted by an item response category will be further attracted by the next category. The probability of being attracted to a specific response category is the serial product of this function for all preceding categories. The probability of responding in a particular response category is then the probability of being attracted to that category minus the probability of being attracted to the next response category. This cumulative response process applies specifically to polytomous items with ordered response categories.

More recently, Samejima (1996, 2010) has proposed a set of five criteria with which to evaluate polytomous IRT models. The first criterion explicitly states that models and their accompanying assumptions must fit with the psychological processes that gave rise to the data. The remaining four criteria are mathematical criteria that define requirements for meeting the joining assumption; that describe the general shape of category response functions; and that define the ordered nature of response categories.

Samejima appears to allow for the possibility that different psychological response processes will operate in different testing contexts. This has led her to introduce a number of new polytomous models within her graded response model framework, which operate quite differently from the L-GRM for which she is best known. These include a logistic positive exponent family of models (Samejima, 2008) and the acceleration model (Samejima, 1995). The details of the psychological processes that these models are intended to capture are described in the relevant publications, but the driving assumption behind

Samejima's work is that IRT models should be selected on the basis of their conformity to the nature of the response data. This insistence has most recently taken Samejima into the realm of nonparametric estimation methods (Samejima, 2010).

Parameter Estimation

Fitting a polytomous IRT model to a set of data effectively comes down to estimating a set of model parameters—for both item characteristics and person trait levels. Modeling multiple categories for each item adds a level of complexity to polytomous IRT modeling beyond that entailed in dichotomous IRT, particularly for models that allow for different numbers of categories for different items in a test. Simultaneously estimating invariant item and person parameters on the same measurement scale is computationally complex and intensive. It also requires data to provide information about each item parameter, in sufficient quantity to estimate the parameters with precision.

Amount of Data

Another related consideration is the amount of data being collected. As a general rule, the more item parameters being estimated, the more data that will be required to accurately estimate those parameters. Another consideration here is that more complex data collection processes can result in more missing data (planned or unplanned). Data need to be collected in a way that ensures that there are enough responses in each response category of every item to allow category boundaries to be estimated with some degree of precision.

In general terms, this requires that enough information is available in the data (item responses) to estimate a parameter with some precision. This typically requires a larger sample for more complex models, such as those that require estimation of a discrimination parameter. However, a number of factors come into play when considering sample size requirements, and no simple, generally applicable sample size guidance is possible. Data sets should be checked to identify response categories that are rarely or never selected prior to attempting to fit an IRT model. Their presence will cause estimation difficulties and indicate that more data is required—or that responses across categories must be collapsed into a combined (post hoc) category. The standard error of parameter estimates can also be checked after model fitting to identify possible estimation problems—one cause of which may be insufficient response data.

For example, the distribution of the trait in a sample, relative to the trait location of an item, is a complicating factor. The problem can be seen in an item that is not difficult to endorse fully (or answer correctly in an ability test), which may fail to elicit responses in response categories that indicate less of a trait (e.g., the "disagree" categories in a rating scale) in a sample of respondents with moderate or high levels of the trait. This can result in difficulty in accurately estimating category boundaries between the categories that are infrequently selected simply because little information is available to inform the parameter estimation.

The PROMIS® Block item collection procedure is a good example of ensuring sufficient data is collected to allow accurate parameter estimation. In the first wave of data collection, responses were obtained from a sample of 21,133 people, 7,005 of whom completed the full item bank, with 14,128 completing overlapping blocks of items (Cella et al., 2007; Hays, Morales, & Reise, 2000).

In previous research we found parameter estimation convergence to be a problem for some estimation programs, when small numbers of items were being modeled—even when there was data from a large number of respondents, with data present in every response category of every item (Ostini, 2002). This problem can sometimes be avoided by changing the default estimation procedures in a program. An example of this that we experienced with the now superseded Multilog program (Thissen, 1991) required changing person parameter estimation from maximum likelihood to maximum *a posteriori*.

Type of Parameter

Beyond the question of amount of data, however, is the question of the type of parameter being modeled. Modeling a discrimination parameter for each item will require a broad range of responses to each item in a measurement scale. Modeling a "guessing" parameter, as, for example, in the three-parameter logistic model for dichotomous data, will require a substantial amount of data at low trait levels for the parameter to be estimated with any precision.

In a health outcome context, "guessing" types of responding could occur with any self-report measure that provides an exhaustive list of response options from which respondents can choose (such as multiple-choice, True/False, or rating scale formats). This situation allows respondents to select a trait-indicating response (e.g., health status) that is not a true indication of their health status. Such responding can occur in situations where people are disinterested in responding to a test, fatigued, or distracted, where the response becomes essentially random. Responding that is not a true reflection of a person's trait can also arise in measures of typical performance, such as self-reported health outcomes, when respondents deliberately choose a response that suggests that their health is worse than it really is. For example, a respondent may select 1 = Very Poor on a five-point scale (from Very Poor to Very Good) in order to increase their chance of obtaining a desired health care outcome. The converse is also possible with, for example, a question regarding health risk behavior, where a respondent may select a more socially desirable response indicating low-risk behavior when their true behavior is in fact more risky. While the latter two examples differ from the more random forms of responding typically associated with a guessing parameter, they contribute to potential estimation difficulties when they represent responding at low trait levels.

Aside from the "guessing" parameter, the discrimination parameter is the most difficult to estimate. This was certainly found to be the case in our model comparison research where parameter estimation problems only arose for models that required the estimation of a discrimination parameter (Ostini, 2002). Such parameter estimation problems had flow-on effects on respondent trait estimates. That is, when an estimation routine was unable to converge on a parameter estimate, the parameter (discrimination in this case) had to be artificially constrained and this process influenced the person parameter estimates that were subsequently calculated.

This issue was also more pronounced for data that demonstrated worse fit to IRT model assumptions—particularly the unidimensionality assumption. While different parameter estimation methods could overcome this problem, this in turn also differentially affected modeled trait estimate outcomes (Ostini, 2002). Indeed, it was disconcerting to find that a software program's default estimation method setting could have a greater influence on trait distribution characteristics than choice of polytomous model appeared to have (Ostini, 2002).

Another finding from our model comparison research was that discrimination parameter estimates were strongly related across models and estimation software—except for the RS-GRM. This suggests that the rating scale approach of constraining boundary parameters to be equivalent across items substantially influences the estimation of the discrimination parameter for an item (Ostini, 2002). This is perhaps unsurprising when it is recalled that discrimination in the polytomous IRT case is composed of a combination of an item discrimination component and the widths of item categories. Constraining category boundaries across items will then necessarily require the item discrimination parameter to be entirely responsible for modeled differences in discrimination across items.

In the context of the computationally intensive parameter estimation demands of polytomous IRT models, the availability of sufficient statistics for Rasch model parameter estimation can be an advantage. The availability of sufficient statistics can improve the robustness of the parameter estimation process, irrespective of any measurement philosophy considerations. On the other hand, this robustness may also mask instances of poor model-data fit (Ostini, 2002), indicating an interaction between model type, parameter estimation, and model data fit.

In previous research we found evidence of interaction between polytomous IRT models and estimation software due to the different estimation routines used; for example, maximum likelihood versus Bayesian methods (Ostini, 2002). A general finding from our previous model comparison research was that parameter estimation effects tended to be more pronounced for the data set that more poorly met IRT assumptions (Ostini, 2002).

Model Fit

Model fit is an important tool in the test construction process but also has a potential role in model selection (see Chapter 6). Ideally, model fit testing will provide an indication of whether the response process underlying the model being fitted to a set of response data accurately represents the way the response data was produced or generated. In practice, it is not clear that either the response specification for most polytomous IRT models or the available tests of model fit, are adequate for this task.

An outline of some of the different mathematical approaches to assessing model-data fit are listed in Ostini and Nering (2006) together with a discussion of the problems associated with the fit statistics available for polytomous IRT model testing. That book also provides a worked example comparing the different results produced by two fit statistics (x^2, and Q_i) when they are applied to a five-category item modeled by four different polytomous IRT models (RSM, PCM, GPCM, and L-GRM).

The discussion in Ostini and Nering (2006) focuses on model-data fit and this is the most obvious level at which to assess fit as part of the model selection process. In IRT, however, fit can also be evaluated at the individual item or the specific person level. While this level of fit assessment is often part of the test construction process, it can also be implicated in model misfit during the model selection process. In part this is because item selection decisions made during test construction have model selection implications. More generally, the processes of test construction and model selection are rarely completely separate.

Broadening the idea of statistical model selection beyond model specific fit statistics raises the notion of a simultaneous consideration of the goodness of fit of a model and the number of parameters required to achieve that fit. This typically involves a penalty term that increases with the number of parameters in the fitted models, allowing the comparison of models with different numbers of parameters. The Akaike information criterion (AIC; Akaike, 1977) and various modifications of the AIC implement an approach to model selection along these lines.

A recent comprehensive evaluation of six model selection methods (Whittaker, Chang, & Dodd, 2012), including the likelihood ratio test and five information criteria methods, found that all of the methods were able to accurately select models from data generated by simple IRT models. However, these methods for assessing overall model-data fit were unable to correctly assess model fit for models involving discrimination or "guessing" parameters.

Glas (2010) provided an innovative framework for evaluating polytomous IRT model fit. The framework allows for the assessment of item and person fit, as well as evaluation of the form of the item response function, local stochastic independence, and subpopulation invariance, the latter of which is also known as differential item functioning (DIF). This potentially allows a more integrated approach to assessing model-data fit and testing fundamental IRT assumptions together. While this framework has not been implemented in IRT modeling software, Glas provides examples of methods that can be used to apply this framework.

Two methods for assessing fit were described by Glas (2010) in the context of two common IRT parameter estimation methods: marginal maximum likelihood (MML) and Bayesian estimation. Modification indices based on Lagrange multiplier statistics were developed for the MML estimation context, and demonstrated for three polytomous IRT models (GPCM, Sequential model, and L-GRM) and for person fit. Glas (2010) also developed the application of posterior predictive checks for the evaluation of model fit in a Bayesian parameter estimation context. It is not yet clear whether this promising approach can become a practical tool in the model selection toolkit or whether it will primarily remain a research tool.

In our earlier model comparison research, identification of misfitting items was not consistent even within the same model as fit by different software programs. Furthermore, more general models did not show better item-model fit than more restrictive models beyond the very restrictive rating scale models (Ostini, 2002). This could be a reflection of model fit; an example of the deficiencies among available model fit statistics; an example of Samejima's contention that estimation procedures unduly affect fit results (Samejima, 1997a); or some combination of these three factors.

Item-model fit analysis was the area that showed the largest potential to substantively affect measurement outcomes in our model comparison research (Ostini, 2002). This was due to the fact that applying the fit results from the different model and parameter estimation software conditions would have led to the retention of different items in the tests being modeled. However, the major substantive differences that would have resulted from this process did not appear to be based on sound fit test criteria (Ostini, 2002).

The process of ascertaining whether a chosen polytomous IRT model is the best model for a set of response data involves a number of interacting factors. The fundamental question is whether the modeled response process corresponds to the process evident in the response data—whether that process is pragmatically conceived (per Samejima) or driven by measurement theory (per Rasch). Any test of this proposition, however, is influenced by the presence of items that are not operating as intended; people who are not responding as expected; software that is imperfectly estimating model parameters; and fit statistics that are unable to provide an unbiased test of the data's deviation from model expected responses. Given this interwoven complexity and the need for substantial amounts of data for parameter estimation purposes, the p-value of any given fit test is unlikely to be the best way to select a polytomous IRT model for any given testing situation. For some model comparison procedures, in certain model comparison situations, however (e.g., with nested models), the comparative magnitude of the fit test statistic may be a pragmatic factor in selecting among models.

Reporting and Interpretation of Results

It is generally easier to report and explain results from simpler models. For example, modeling discrimination may result in respondents' latent trait ranking among a testing cohort being different from their summed ("number correct") score ranking. This can be difficult to explain and justify to those who commissioned a testing program or who took a particular test, for whom "number correct" may make intuitive sense. Because Rasch trait scores are based on number correct scores given their reliance on sufficient statistics for their estimation, this can make them easier for people to understand.

In terms of specific models, Smits, Cuijpers, and van Straten (2011) selected the L-GRM over the GPCM for their modeling project because of the ease with which L-GRM item parameters can be interpreted for items generated by a Likert rating scale and because of the authors' perception that a model with cumulative category boundaries is simpler to explain to test users.

Interpreting the meaning of score categories is assisted by the capacity to equate IRT outcomes across different groups of test takers. Unlike CTT, this means score categories and IRT test results generally can be meaningfully interpreted across testing settings—temporally and across groups of test takers.

Equating is more complicated when a discrimination parameter is involved, and this may be a consideration for model selection. Equating processes are also more readily accomplished within some parameter estimation programs than others—and the polytomous IRT models for which those programs can estimate parameters may then influence model selection decision making.

Available Model Estimation Software

The availability and associated features of model estimation software can be a pragmatic factor that influences model selection decision. Early RSM software availability helped the RSM to become a model of choice (Hambleton, van der Linden, & Wells, 2010). This is not always the case, however, as in the example of WinMira software (von Davier, 1998), which had one of the earlier and more useable graphical user interfaces. The availability of this feature nevertheless did not make the Successive Integers Model or the Q fit statistic that WinMira estimated more widely adopted. Graphical user interfaces are now much more common but sometimes still require knowledge of Fortran data specification code, simply to read data in to an estimation routine.

Different parameter estimation software often provides different fit statistics, making it difficult to obtain consistent conclusions on model fit, even for a single specific polytomous IRT model when fit by different software. Furthermore, program documentation rarely gives clear guidance on how to use the fit indicators provided (Ostini, 2002). This contributes to the effect described earlier where different programs, using different methods to test fit, identify different items as misfitting—even when fitting the same polytomous model. The process of identifying and removing "misfitting" items in this way has more influence on modeled outcome than model type.

Other diagnostic features, particularly graphic displays of results such as plots of parameter estimates, are very helpful in understanding how a model is operating with a particular set of data. Most programs provide these in some form; for example, even a generic statistical program like R (R Development Core Team, 2011) has libraries such as MIRT (Chalmers, Pritikin, & Zoltak, 2014) and SIRT (Robitzsch, 2014) that provide histograms and graphs of item and person parameter results. The reliance of IRT modeling on specific forms of response functions makes graphical representations of modeled outcomes particularly useful for seeing what is actually happening in a modeling situation.

Measurement Differences

To the extent that substantive measurement differences are the result of selecting test items based on item-data fit, the fact that different model-estimation program combinations provide highly inconsistent guidance on items to retain (Ostini, 2002) is a matter of significant concern.

In terms of the distinction between CUM and ACM models, our model comparison research suggests that differences in modeled probabilities of test-taker responses in a given item category between CUM and ACM models are smaller than the difference found among different ACM models. For example, L-GRM and GPCM results were more similar than PCM and GPCM modeled probabilities, even though the latter two are both ACM models. The presence of an estimated discrimination parameter has more effect on modeled outcomes than does the CUM—ACM distinction (Ostini, 2002). This becomes an important consideration in model choice for polytomous models, both because discrimination parameter estimation can be more difficult to achieve without imposing external constraints, and because polytomous item discrimination is modeled through a combination of a slope parameter and the width between item-category boundaries (Muraki, 1992; Muraki & Bock, 1999).

In the data set that better met IRT assumptions, the most general model (GPCM) was the only model that produced trait distribution estimates that differed markedly from those produced by other models—largely as a result of trait estimate convergence problems resulting from a small number of cases with extreme parameter estimates (Ostini, 2002). Those estimates were themselves evidently the product of discrimination parameter estimation difficulties. Aside from these GPCM results, substantive measurement differences across the 25 remaining model conditions were not reflected in large differences in trait estimate distributions (Ostini, 2002).

More generally, when a data set meets fundamental IRT assumptions, and to the extent that substantive measurement differences are thought of in terms of respondent trait estimates—especially the rank ordering of those estimates—different polytomous IRT models produce very similar results (Ostini, 2002). Therefore, while concerns remain about the utility of available item-model fit procedures, once a set of items has been selected, the many different polytomous IRT models produce remarkably similar respondent measurement. This indicates that the most important factor when using polytomous IRT models is to invest care and effort in the initial item analysis and IRT assumption testing stages. Selection of the particular polytomous IRT model that is applied to a given set of data appears to be a far less important issue (Ostini, 2002).

Results from our model comparison work (Ostini, 2002) suggest that models can be too restrictive (e.g., RSM, DLM, RS-GRM). However, the most general models investigated (L-GRM & GPCM) did not produce substantially different results from less general models such as the PCM, SIM, and DLSM. This result reaffirms a perception among polytomous IRT practitioners. For example, when considering whether to use the PCM or the L-GRM in a measurement project, Smits and colleagues (2011) noted that the choice between the two models made little difference in terms of the resulting person parameters.

Strategy Simplified

In summary, selecting from among the polytomous IRT models available for a given measurement task can be thought of as requiring an answer to three basic questions, following which, two important tests of data condition are required. These steps are outlined next.

(1) *Why are you measuring?*

- is there an implied response process?
- have you ascribed to a particular philosophy of measurement?

- how are you going to use the results (decision making; explain to respondents or test commissioning body)?

(2) *What data are (will be) available?*

- less data may require fitting a simpler model (which is likely to fit the data less well)
- fewer parameters to estimate; or—if responses are relatively evenly distributed across item response categories for all items—perhaps choose a Rasch model because then you have sufficient statistics on which to base parameter estimation.

(3) *What software is available?*

- Understanding the parameter estimation methods used by specific software and the way outlying estimates are constrained may be important for parameters that are difficult to estimate

Test IRT assumptions—including assumption of uniform discrimination if you do not want to estimate a discrimination parameter.

Test model fit—both item-model fit and person-model fit, as well as overall model-data fit. This is primarily to get to know your particular set of data better, rather than for the purpose of item or model selection.

Summary

Our research suggests that the most important factor when thinking about applying a polytomous IRT model is to test model assumptions carefully and thoroughly, with special consideration of the unidimensionality assumption. Deviation from the unidimensionality assumption has undue, differential effects on parameter estimation across different polytomous models and different software. One consequence is that, even though polytomous Rasch model estimation procedures are more robust in the face of violation of the unidimensionality condition, the resulting item and person parameters are nevertheless affected by the assumption's violation.

It is also important to consider whether the availability of sufficient statistics in the parameter estimation procedure would be advantageous—if, for example, there is a limited amount of data available. This would suggest using a Rasch model. However, this would also mean that respondent trait order would be the same irrespective of which Rasch model is used. And, as mentioned in the previous paragraph, special care will need to be taken to ensure that IRT assumptions are met before modeling takes place.

Awareness of the default settings of the parameter estimation software being used to model data is also important, as they can have undue effects on the values of the parameters that are estimated. This can occur when estimation routines fail to constrain parameter estimates; or conversely, when estimation routines unduly restrict parameter estimates, thereby artificially restricting parameter variability across items or respondents.

Finally, and to repeat the first point, it is crucial that IRT model assumptions are carefully tested and item selection results should be based on assumption testing outcomes, rather than IRT item-model fit statistics, as fit results may not be reliable and have a disproportionate effect on modeled outcomes based on the inconsistent guidance that they give across different models.

References

Agresti, A. (1997). Connections between loglinear models and generalized Rasch models for ordinal responses. In J. Rost & R. Langeheine (Eds.), *Applications of latent trait and latent class models in the social sciences* (pp. 209–218). Münster: Waxmann.

Akaike, H. (1977). On entropy maximization principle. In P.R. Krishnaiah (Ed.), *Applications of statistics* (pp. 27–41). Amsterdam: North Holland.

Andrich, D. (1978a). Application of a psychometric rating model to ordered categories which are scored with successive integers. *Applied Psychological Measurement, 2*, 581–594.

Andrich, D. (1978b). A rating formulation for ordered response categories. *Psychometrika, 43*(4), 561–573.

Andrich, D. (1982). An extension of the Rasch model for ratings providing both location and dispertion parameters. *Psychometrika, 47*(1), 105–113.

Andrich, D. (1985). An elaboration of Guttman scaling with Rasch models for measurement. In N.B. Tuma (Ed.), *Social methodology* (1st ed., pp. 33–80). San Francisco, CA: Jossey-Bass.

Andrich, D. (1995). Models for measurement, precision, and the nondichotomization of graded responses. *Psychometrika, 60*(1), 7–26.

Andrich, D. (2010). Understanding the response structure and process in the polytomous Rasch model. In M. Nering & R. Ostini (Eds.), *Handbook of polytomous item response theory* (pp. 123–152). New York: Taylor & Francis.

Bock, R.D. (1972). Estimating item parameters and latent ability when responses are scored in two or more nominal categories. *Psychometrika, 37*(1), 29–51.

Bock, R.D. (1997). The nominal categories model. In W.J. van der Linden & R.K. Hambleton (Eds.), *Handbook of modern item response theory* (pp. 33–49). New York: Springer.

Castillo-Díaz, M., & Padilla, J.-L. (2013). How cognitive interviewing can provide validity evidence of the response processes to scale items. *Social Indicators Research, 114*(3), 963–975.

Cella, D., Yount, S., Rothrock, N., Gershon, R., Cook, K., Reeve, B., . . . Rose, M. (2007). The Patient-Reported Outcomes Measurement Information System (PROMIS): Progress of an NIH Roadmap cooperative group during its first two years. *Medical Care, 45*(5 Suppl 1), S3–S11.

Chalmers, P., Pritikin, J., & Zoltak, M. (2014). Multidimentsional item response theory, 1.3. York: Authors.

Crocker, L., & Algina, J. (1986). *Introduction to classical and modern test theory*. Fort Worth, TX: Harcourt Brace Jovanovich.

Edwards, A.L., & Thurstone, L.L. (1952). An internal consistency check for scale values determined by the method of successive intervals. *Psychometrika, 17*(2), 169–180.

Glas, C.A.W. (2010). Testing fit to IRT models for polytomously scored items. In M. Nering & R. Ostini (Eds.), *Handbook of polytomous item response theory* (pp. 185–208). New York: Taylor & Francis.

Hambleton, R.K., & Swaminathan, H. (1985). *Item response theory: Principles and applications*. Boston, MA: Kluwer Nijhoff.

Hambleton, R.K., van der Linden, W.J., & Wells, C.S. (2010). IRT models for the analysis of polytomously scored data: Brief and selected history of model building advances. In M. Nering & R. Ostini (Eds.), *Handbook of polytomous item response theory* (pp. 21–42). New York: Taylor & Francis.

Hays, R.D., Morales, L.S., & Reise, S.P. (2000). Item response theory and health outcomes measurement in the 21st century. *Med Care, 38*(9 Suppl), II28–42.

Jansen, P.G.W., & Roskam, E.E. (1986). Latent trait models and dichotomization of graded responses. *Psychometrika, 51*(1), 69–91.

Lord, F.M. (1980). *Applications of item response theory to practical testing problems*. Hillsdale, NJ: Lawrence Erlbaum Associates.

Lord, F.M., & Novick, M.R. (1968). *Statistical theories of mental test scores*. Reading, MA: Addison-Wesley.

Masters, G.N. (1982). A Rasch model for partial credit scoring. *Psychometrika, 47*(2), 149–174.

Masters, G.N. (1988). Measurement models for ordered response categories. In R. Langeheine & J. Rost (Eds.), *Latent traits and latent class models* (pp. 11–29). New York: Plenum Press.

Masters, G.N. (2010). The partial credit model. In M. Nering & R. Ostini (Eds.), *Handbook of polytomous item response theory* (pp. 109–122). New York: Taylor & Francis.

Masters, G.N., & Wright, B.D. (1984). The essential process in a family of measurement models. *Psychometrika, 49*(4), 529–544.

Mellenbergh, G.J. (1995). Conceptual notes on models for discrete polytomous item responses. *Applied Psychological Measurement, 19*(1), 91–100.

Molenaar, I.W. (1983). Item Steps: Heymans Bulletins Psychological Institute, University of Groningen.

Muraki, E. (1990). Fitting a polytomous item response model to Likert-type data. *Applied Psychological Measurement, 14*(1), 59–71.

Muraki, E. (1992). A generalized partial credit model: Application of an EM algorithm. *Applied Psychological Measurement, 16*(2), 159–176.

Muraki, E., & Bock, R.D. (1999). PARSCALE: IRT item analysis and test scoring for rating-scale data. (Version 3.5). Chicago: Scientific Software International.

Nering, M., & Ostini, R. (Eds.). (2010). *Handbook of polytomous item response theory*. New York: Taylor & Francis.

Ostini, R. (2002). *Identifying substantive measurement differences among a variety of polytomous IRT models*. PhD dissertation, University of Minnesota, Minneapolis. PsycINFO database.

Ostini, R. (2010). Measuring conceptualisations of morality: Or how to invent a construct and measure it too. In G. Walford, M. Viswanathan, & E. Tucker (Eds.), *The SAGE handbook of measurement* (pp. 337–352). Los Angeles, CA: Sage.

Ostini, R., & Nering, M. (2006). *Polytomous item response theory models*. Thousand Oaks, CA: Sage.

R Development Core Team. (2011). R: A language and environment for statistical computing. (Version 2.13.1). Vienna: R Foundation for Statistical Computing. Retrieved from www.R-project.org/.

Robitzsch, A. (2014). Supplementary item response theory models, 0.45–23. Salzburg: Author.

Rost, J. (1988). Measuring attitudes with a threshold model drawing on a traditional scaling concept. *Applied Psychological Measurement, 12*, 397–409.

Samejima, F. (1969). Estimation of latent ability using a response pattern of graded scores. *Psychometrika, Monograph Supplement No. 17*.

Samejima, F. (1972). A general model for free response data. *Psychometrika, Monograph Supplement No 18*.

Samejima, F. (1973). Homogeneous case of the continuous response model. *Psychometrika, 38*(2), 203–219.

Samejima, F. (1995). Acceleration model in the heterogeneous case of the general graded response model. *Psychometrika, 60*(4), 549–572.

Samejima, F. (1996). Evaluation of mathematical models for ordered polychotomous responses. *Behaviormetrika, 23*(1), 17–35.

Samejima, F. (1997a). Departure from normal assumptions: A promise for future psychometrics with substantive mathematical modeling. *Psychometrika, 62*(4), 471–493.

Samejima, F. (1997b). Graded response model. In W.J. van der Linden & R.K. Hambleton (Eds.), *Handbook of modern item response theory* (pp. 85–100). New York: Springer.

Samejima, F. (2008). Graded response model based on the logistic positive exponent family of models for dichotomous responses. *Psychometrika, 51*, 567–577.

Samejima, F. (2010). The general graded response model. In M. Nering & R. Ostini (Eds.), *Handbook of polytomous item response theory* (pp. 77–107). New York: Taylor & Francis.

Smits, N., Cuijpers, P., & van Straten, A. (2011). Applying computerized adaptive testing to the CES-D scale: a simulation study. *Psychiatry Research, 188*(1), 147–155.

Thissen, D. (1991). Multilog, 6.0. Chicago: Scientific Software International.

Thissen, D., & Steinberg, L. (1986). A taxonomy of item response models. *Psychometrika, 51*(4), 567–577.

Tutz, G. (1990). Sequential item response models with an ordered response. *British Journal of Mathematical and Statistical Psychology, 43*, 39–55.
Tutz, G. (1997). Sequential models for ordered responses. In W. J. van der Linden & R. K. Hambleton (Eds.), *Handbook of modern item response theory* (pp. 139–152). New York: Springer.
Verhelst, N. D., & Verstralen, H. H. F. M. (1997). Modeling sums of binary responses by the partial credit model. Cito, Arnhem, The Netherlands.
von Davier, M. (1998). WINMIRA 32—Online users manual. (Version Windows 95). Kiel: Institute for Science Education (IPN).
Weiss, D. J., & Yoes, M. E. (1991). Item response theory. In R. K. Hambleton & J. Zaal (Eds.), *Advances in educational and psychological testing* (pp. 69–95). Boston, MA: Kluwer.
Whittaker, T. A., Chang, W., & Dodd, B. G. (2012). The performance of IRT model selection methods with mixed-format tests. *Applied Psychological Measurement, 36*(3), 159–180.
Wright, B. D., & Masters, G. N. (1982). *Rating scale analysis*. Chicago, IL: MESA.

Part III

Using IRT Models in Applied Problems

15 Scoring and Estimating Score Precision Using Multidimensional IRT Models

Anna Brown and Tim J. Croudace

Introduction

The ultimate goal of measurement is to produce a score by which individuals can be assessed and differentiated. Item response theory (IRT) modeling views responses to test items as indicators of a respondent's standing on some underlying psychological attributes (van der Linden & Hambleton, 1997)—we often call them latent traits—and devises special algorithms for estimating this standing. This chapter gives an overview of methods for estimating person attribute scores using one-dimensional and multidimensional IRT models, focusing on those that are particularly useful with patient-reported outcome (PRO) measures.

To be useful in applications, a test score has to approximate the latent trait well, and importantly, the precision level must be known in order to produce information for decision-making purposes. Unlike classical test theory (CTT), which assumes the precision with which a test measures the same for all trait levels, IRT methods assess the precision with which a test measures at different trait levels. In the context of PRO measurement, this enables assessment of the measurement precision for an individual patient. Knowing error bands around the patient's score is important for informing clinical judgments, such as deciding upon significance of any change, for instance in response to treatment. (Reise & Haviland, 2005). At the same time, summary indices are often needed to characterize the overall precision of measurement in a research sample, population group, or in the population as a whole. Much of this chapter is devoted to methods for estimating measurement precision, including the score-dependent standard error of measurement and appropriate sample-level or population-level marginal reliability coefficients.

Patient-reported outcome measures often capture several related constructs, the feature that may make the use of multidimensional IRT models appropriate and beneficial (Gibbons, Immekus, & Bock, 2007). Several such models are described, including a model with multiple correlated constructs, a model where multiple constructs are underlain by a general common factor (second-order model), and a model where each item is influenced by one general and one group factor (bifactor model). To make the use of these models more easily accessible for applied researchers, we provide specialized formulae for computing test information, standard errors, and reliability. We show how to translate a multitude of numbers and graphs conditioned on several dimensions into easy-to-use indices that can be understood by applied researchers and test users alike. All described methods and techniques are illustrated with a single data analysis example involving a popular PRO measure, the 28-item version of the General Health Questionnaire (GHQ28; Goldberg & Williams, 1988), completed in mid-life by a large community sample as a part of a major UK cohort study.

Common Factor Model and Item Responses

Psychometric tools measuring PROs or health-related quality of life (HRQoL) often necessitate the capture of several related constructs (Fayers & Machin, 2007). For example, the Quality of Life Interview for the Chronically Mentally Ill differentiates seven subdomains (Gibbons et al., 2007), each a distinct area of functioning. Hence, we will use multidimensional models as the basis (Gibbons, Immekus, & Bock, 2007), and consider a one-dimensional model as the simplest special case.

Let $\theta = (\theta_1, \theta_2, ..., \theta_T)'$ be a set of *T* psychological attributes (traits). We assume that the latent traits are normally distributed random variables; they have the mean of zero, unit variance, and are freely correlated (their covariance matrix is Σ). In a test with *m* items, each item is designed to elicit an internal response (denoted u_i^*), which depends on one or more attributes, as described by a common factor model:

$$u_i^* = \mu_i + \lambda_{1i}\theta_1 + \lambda_{2i}\theta_2 + ... + \lambda_{Ti}\theta_T + \varepsilon_i . \qquad (15.1)$$

In this expression, μ_i is the mean utility for the population of respondents; $\lambda_{1i}, \lambda_{2i}, ..., \lambda_{Ti}$ are factor loadings of item *i* on each of the attributes; and ε_i is the unique part (or error). The error terms are normally distributed random variables with the mean zero and are uncorrelated with the common factors and among themselves, so that their covariance matrix Ψ^2 is diagonal.

The internal response u_i^* can represent, for example, the degree of agreement with the item or the value the respondent attaches to the item (item *utility*); however, this *response tendency* is not observed directly. The actual observed item response u_i will typically constitute an option that the respondent chose from available options, either dichotomous ("yes"–"no", "agree"–"disagree") or polytomous ("never"–"sometimes"–"often"–"always"; or "strongly disagree"–"disagree"–"neutral"–"agree"–"strongly agree" etc.). In IRT models, the observed response u_i is related to the latent response tendency u_i^* through a threshold process. For instance, it is assumed that the response is positive when the response tendency is over a threshold value τ_i, and the response is negative otherwise:

$$u_i = \begin{cases} 1 & \text{if } u_i^* \geq \tau_i \\ 0 & \text{if } u_i^* < \tau_i \end{cases}. \qquad (15.2)$$

In what follows we give formulae for the dichotomous case, mentioning how to extend them to polytomous cases in passing. All response models can be extended to the polytomous case by considering, for example, a graded response approach (Samejima, 1969), or from the Rasch modeling perspective, a partial credit model (Masters & Wright, 1997).

Given the item-factors relationship (15.1) and the threshold relationship (15.2), the item response function for item *i* in a *threshold / loading* form is given by:

$$P(u_i) = \Pr(u_i = 1|\theta) = \Phi\left(\frac{-\tau_i + \lambda_{1i}\theta_1 + ... + \lambda_{Ti}\theta_T}{\sqrt{\psi_i^2}}\right), \qquad (15.3)$$

where $\Phi(x)$ denotes the cumulative standard normal distribution function evaluated at *x*, and ψ_i^2 is the residual variance for item *i*. Without loss of generality, we use the normal-ogive link here. Alternatively, the logistic link function $L(x) = 1/(1+e^{-x})$ can be used (Reckase, 2009).

Because the continuous response tendency u_i^* is unobserved (only its dichotomization u_i is observed), the variance ψ_i^2 cannot be identified in typical single-group models. It is customary to parameterize IRT models (e.g., McDonald, 1999) by letting:

$$\alpha_i = \frac{-\tau_i}{\sqrt{\psi_i^2}} \text{ and } \beta_{ij} = \frac{\lambda_{ij}}{\sqrt{\psi_i^2}}. \tag{15.4}$$

With this, the item response function (IRF) can be written in an *intercept / slope* form as:

$$P_i = \mathrm{P}(u_i|\theta) = \Phi(\alpha_i + \beta_{1i}\theta_1 + \ldots + \beta_{Ti}\theta_T). \tag{15.5}$$

The multidimensional response model is flexible in terms of how many attributes can influence a particular item. For instance, every item in a multi-trait test might measure one trait only and therefore will have only one nonzero slope (we say that items "possess an independent-clusters basis"; McDonald, 1999, p. 179). When this is the case, the IRF is a familiar s-shaped item characteristic curve. The IRF becomes a surface when the item depends on two attributes. In these two cases of low dimensionality, the IRF can be easily plotted.

Latent Trait Estimation

Latent trait scores can be estimated by treating the model parameters (item intercepts and slopes, trait covariances, etc.) as if they were known. This is reasonable if model parameters have been accurately estimated. When the model parameters are fixed to their estimated values, the probability of every item response depends only on the latent traits, and the fundamental approach to estimating the trait scores is to search for values that maximize the joint likelihood of each response pattern $\mathbf{u} = (u_1, u_2, \ldots u_m)$. The maximum likelihood (ML) approach assumes local independence, that is, the item responses are independent after conditioning on the latent traits. The ML scores are found iteratively by maximizing the mode of the likelihood function:

$$l(\mathbf{u}|\theta) = \prod_{i=1}^{m} P_i(\theta)^{u_i}(1 - P_i(\theta))^{1-u_i}. \tag{15.6}$$

Maximum likelihood estimation uses information from the item responses only and is philosophically uncontroversial (McDonald, 2011). The score, however, is undefined for some response patterns, notably for "perfect" patterns (for instance by answering "yes" to all items or selecting the top rating category such as "strongly agree"). The likelihood of such a pattern increases infinitely when the latent trait score increases. The score is also undefined when non-keyed responses are given to all items (for instance by answering "no" or selecting the bottom rating category such as "strongly disagree"). Such extreme patterns can be quite common in PRO measures, for example in screening tests.

An alternative approach is to use prior information about the trait distribution in addition to the actual item responses. With this Bayesian approach, the likelihood of a score given the observed response pattern (posterior distribution) is computed from known density of the score in the population (prior distribution, usually standard normal), and the likelihood of the observed response pattern given the score (joint likelihood value used in ML estimation). Two alternative methods using this approach are *expected a posteriori* (EAP) estimation, which computes the mean of the posterior distribution; and *maximum a posteriori* (MAP) estimation, which maximizes the mode of the posterior distribution (Embretson & Reise, 2000). By adding information from the prior distribution, the problem of undefined trait scores for "perfect" patterns is overcome, that is, a score is always defined when the posterior approach is used.

The EAP estimation is most often used when only one trait θ is measured. The EAP score is computed as the ratio between the integral of the posterior function weighted by the latent trait θ, and the unweighted integral of the posterior function. The EAP scores are approximated using numerical integration:

$$\mathrm{EAP}(\mathbf{u}|\theta) \approx \frac{\sum_q \theta_q \left[\prod_{i=1}^{m} P_i(u_i)\right] \phi(\theta_q) d\theta_q}{\sum_q \left[\prod_{i=1}^{m} P_i(u_i)\right] \phi(\theta_q) d\theta_q}, \tag{15.7}$$

where q are quadrature points selected along the latent trait continuum. For a discussion regarding the number of points necessary for precise estimation, see Thissen and Orlando (2001). It is evident that an EAP score is non-iterative and easy to compute when only one or two dimensions are involved. The EAP estimation, however, becomes computationally demanding when the number of traits increases, as the number of points on the multidimensional grid used for integration increases exponentially.

The MAP scores are found iteratively by maximizing the mode of the posterior distribution:

$$l_P(\mathbf{u}|\theta) = \phi(\theta) \prod_{i=1}^{m} \left[P_i(\theta)^{u_i} (1 - P_i(\theta))^{1-u_i} \right]. \tag{15.8}$$

Finding the best set of scores optimizing the multidimensional function requires iterative procedures using gradients. For one-dimensional models this seems a complication compared to the non-iterative EAP; however, in multidimensional models this estimation method is much more efficient because it searches for the optimal set of theta values for all traits simultaneously and the number of iterations is unaffected by the number of traits.

The posterior EAP and MAP approaches have been shown to achieve precise estimates with fewer items than the ML method; however, they are known to shrink the latent trait distribution toward the population mean. The amount of shrinkage depends on several factors, including the test length, and can be quite substantial in short tests (Thissen & Orlando, 2001).

Standard Error of Measurement and Information

Score estimates are only our best guess at estimating the true score, and inevitably, all estimation methods are associated with a certain degree of error. The likelihood of a response pattern **u**, or the posterior likelihood, is a function that is typically Gaussian in appearance and has a single peak. The mode (or the mean) provides a limited summary of the likelihood function. The width or the spread of the likelihood, on the other hand, indicates the degree of uncertainty around the estimated score—the narrower the spread, the more confident we can be that the true theta value is close to the estimated value. The spread of the likelihood for approximately Gaussian distributions is meaningfully described by its standard deviation. The standard deviation of the likelihood of a response pattern, therefore, is a measure of the **standard error** of estimation in IRT.

For the EAP estimator, it is natural to compute the standard deviation from the mean (which is the estimated EAP score) directly, by taking values of the likelihood function at the quadrature points:

$$\mathrm{SE}_{EAP}\left(\hat{\theta}\right) \approx \sqrt{\frac{\sum_q \left(\theta_q - \mathrm{EAP}[\theta]\right)^2 \left[\prod_{i=1}^{m} P_i\left(u_i\right)\right] \phi\left(\theta_q\right) d\theta_q}{\sum_q \left[\prod_{i=1}^{m} P_i\left(u_i\right)\right] \phi\left(\theta_q\right) d\theta_q}}. \tag{15.9}$$

For the methods maximizing the mode of the likelihood function (ML and MAP), the variance of the score estimate is obtained as the inverse of the expected value of the second derivative of $l\left(\mathbf{u}|\theta\right)$ or $l_P\left(\mathbf{u}|\theta\right)$ with respect to $\boldsymbol{\theta}$ (Fisher, 1921). The expected value of the second derivative of likelihood function is called the *Fisher information*:

$$\mathcal{I}\left(\theta\right) = -E\left(\frac{\partial^2 l\left(|\theta\right)}{\partial \theta^2}\right), \tag{15.10}$$

and the variance of the likelihood function (the squared standard error of the score) is the reciprocal of the Fisher information:

$$SE^2\left(\theta\right) = \frac{1}{\mathcal{I}\left(\theta\right)}. \tag{15.11}$$

The Fisher information is inversely related to the error variance and therefore provides a measure of the test precision. Applying the general formula (15.11) to the ML estimator, we obtain for the *one-dimensional case* $SE_{ML}\left(\hat{\theta}\right) = 1/\sqrt{\mathcal{I}\left(\hat{\theta}\right)}$. The standard error of the MAP estimator involves the information of the posterior likelihood function instead:

$$SE_{MAP}\left(\hat{\theta}\right) = \frac{1}{\sqrt{\mathcal{I}_P\left(\hat{\theta}\right)}}. \tag{15.12}$$

For the *multidimensional case*, the standard error of the MAP-estimated score for the latent trait θ_a involves the directional posterior information evaluated at the point-estimates of the trait scores $\hat{\boldsymbol{\theta}} = (\hat{\theta}_1, \hat{\theta}_2, \ldots, \hat{\theta}_T)$:

$$SE^a\left(\hat{\boldsymbol{\theta}}\right) = \frac{1}{\sqrt{\mathcal{I}_P^a\left(\hat{\boldsymbol{\theta}}\right)}}. \tag{15.13}$$

The following section shows how to compute the Fisher information in both one-dimensional and multidimensional cases.

Item Information Function (IIF)

When responses to test items depend on *one latent trait*, the maximum likelihood Item Information Function (IIF) for item *i* is given by:

$$\mathcal{I}_i\left(\theta\right) = \frac{\left[P_i'\left(\theta\right)\right]^2}{P_i\left(\theta\right)\left[1 - P_i\left(\theta\right)\right]}, \tag{15.14}$$

where $P_i'(\theta)$ denotes the first derivative of the item response function (McDonald, 1999). For items with graded response categories, the item information can be derived from category response functions as follows (Dodd, De Ayala, & Koch, 1995; Samejima, 1969):

$$\mathcal{I}_i(\theta) = \sum_{x=0}^{k} \frac{\left[P_{ix}'(\theta)\right]^2}{P_{ix}(\theta)}. \tag{15.15}$$

A challenging feature of many PRO measures is their potentially multidimensional structure, whereby item responses may depend on *two or more latent traits*. When this is the case, the *direction* of information must also be considered (Ackerman, 2005; Reckase, 2009). The definition of item information is generalized to accommodate the change in slope with direction $\boldsymbol{\alpha}$ taken from a point in the latent trait space:

$$\mathcal{I}_i^{\alpha}(\theta) = \frac{\left[\nabla_{\alpha} P_i(\theta)\right]^2}{P_i(\theta)\left[1 - P_i(\theta)\right]}, \tag{15.16}$$

where $P_i(u_i = 1|\theta)$. Let $\boldsymbol{\alpha}$ be a vector of angles to all T axes that defines the direction from a point $\boldsymbol{\theta}$, and $\nabla_{\alpha} P_i(\theta)$ be the gradient in direction $\boldsymbol{\alpha}$, which is given by (Reckase, 2009):

$$\nabla_{\alpha} P_i(\theta) = \frac{\partial P_i(\theta)}{\partial \theta_1}\cos(\alpha_1) + \frac{\partial P_i(\theta)}{\partial \theta_2}\cos(\alpha_2) + \ldots + \frac{\partial P_i(\theta)}{\partial \theta_T}\cos(\alpha_T). \tag{15.17}$$

For each item, we might consider one or more directions of information. Often, these would correspond to the direction(s) of the trait(s) in which we are interested. When computing the information along the axis θ_a, the angle to θ_a is 0° and therefore $\cos(\alpha_a) = 1$, whereas the angle to any other axis, say θ_b, is determined by the correlation between θ_a and θ_b so that $\cos(\alpha_b) = \text{corr}(\theta_a, \theta_b)$ (Bock, 1975). It follows that the information in direction of the trait θ_a is given by:

$$\nabla_{a} P_i(\theta) = \frac{\partial P_i(\theta)}{\partial \theta_1}\text{corr}(\theta_1, \theta_a) + \ldots + \frac{\partial P_i(\theta)}{\partial \theta_a} + \ldots + \frac{\partial P_i(\theta)}{\partial \theta_T}\text{corr}(\theta_T, \theta_a). \tag{15.18}$$

In the applications sections of this chapter we will provide specific information functions for models commonly used to score responses to PRO measures.

Test Information Function (TIF)

When local independence holds, the Test Information Function (TIF) is simply the sum of the item information functions. In one-dimensional cases, the TIF is $\mathcal{I}(\theta) = \sum_{i=1}^{m} \mathcal{I}_i(\theta)$. In multidimensional cases, the total information in direction $\boldsymbol{\alpha}$ is the sum of all item information functions (15.16). Thus, the test information about trait θ_a is:

$$\mathcal{I}^{a}(\theta) = \sum_{i=1}^{m} \mathcal{I}_i^{a}(\theta). \tag{15.19}$$

So far, we have taken into account information provided by the item responses, that is, the maximum likelihood (ML) information. When Bayesian estimators are used, information given by the prior distribution will also contribute to the latent trait estimation. The so-called *posterior test information* function, $\mathcal{I}_P(\theta)$, reflects contributions provided by the item responses and the prior distribution. For a *single latent trait*, the standard normal prior distribution adds unity to the information across the latent trait continuum (Du Toit, 2003):

$$\mathcal{I}_P(\theta) = \mathcal{I}(\theta) + 1. \tag{15.20}$$

For *multiple latent traits*, the multivariate standard normal prior with correlation matrix Σ adds to the ML test information function as follows:

$$\mathcal{I}_P^a(\theta) = \mathcal{I}^a(\theta) + \left[\Sigma^{-1}\right]_a, \tag{15.21}$$

where $\left[\Sigma^{-1}\right]_a$ is the ath diagonal element of the inverted latent trait correlation matrix (for proof, see Appendix B in Brown & Maydeu-Olivares, 2011). When all traits are uncorrelated, the term added to the ML test information in Equation (15.21) equals unity. When the traits are correlated positively, the term is greater than unity (and therefore the prior distribution contributes more information for the trait estimation).

Reliability

While the standard error functions (15.12) to (15.13) characterize the precision of measurement provided by an instrument completely, it may be convenient in applications to offer a single index of precision. Such a single index is more likely to appeal to, and be understood by, the test user, and it enables a quick evaluation of a PRO measure's overall measurement quality by third parties, such as regulatory authorities. Provision of simple indices is particularly beneficial for multi-trait measures, where the main challenge is to present and summarize the information functions in a comprehensible fashion. Contour plots and "clam shell" plots (see Ackerman, 2005; Reckase, 2009) are already complicated when just two dimensions are involved, but with more dimensions, they become quite impractical.

One such index, *marginal reliability*, was suggested by Green and colleagues (1984):

$$\rho = \frac{\sigma^2 - \bar{\sigma}^2_{error}}{\sigma^2} = 1 - \frac{\bar{\sigma}^2_{error}}{\sigma^2}. \tag{15.22}$$

This coefficient follows the fundamental definition of reliability as the proportion of variance in the observed score due to true score (equal to observed minus error variance). Provided the standard error function is relatively uniform, the marginal reliability estimate will be representative of the test's overall reliability, and may be used for comparison with classical reliability statistics. In addition, the reliability is an important quantity because it describes how closely the estimated trait resembles the latent (true) trait score:

$$\text{corr}(\theta, \hat{\theta}) = \sqrt{\rho}. \tag{15.23}$$

There are two ways to compute the marginal reliability coefficient. One way, referred to as *theoretical reliability* (du Toit, 2003), involves averaging the squared standard error for all trait values **in the theoretical distribution** to obtain the error variance in (15.22):

$$\bar{\sigma}^2_{error} = \int_{-\infty}^{\infty} SE^2(\theta)\phi(\theta)\,d\theta. \tag{15.24}$$

Once the error variance has been estimated (usually by approximating the integral (15.24)), the marginal reliability is computed by assuming the latent trait score variance in (15.22) $\sigma^2 = 1$, giving:

$$\rho = 1 - \bar{\sigma}^2_{error}. \tag{15.25}$$

With multiple traits, the theoretical reliability procedure becomes unattractive because it involves multidimensional integration. An alternative approach, *empirical reliability*, involves averaging the squared standard errors of estimated trait scores **in a sample** to obtain the error variance in (15.22). That is, the observed and the error variance are computed from the estimated trait scores $\hat{\theta}$ and their standard errors in a sample of N respondents:

$$\hat{\sigma}^2 = \frac{1}{N}\sum_{j=1}^{N}\left(\hat{\theta}_j - \bar{\hat{\theta}}\right)^2, \qquad \bar{\hat{\sigma}}^2_{error} = \frac{1}{N}\sum_{j=1}^{N} SE^2\left(\hat{\theta}_j\right). \tag{15.26}$$

The standard error is computed as appropriate for the estimator, using the standard deviation of the posterior likelihood (15.9) for the EAP estimator, the inverse of the Fisher information for the ML estimator, and the inverse of the posterior information (15.12) for the MAP estimator. Conveniently, some software packages such as TESTFACT (Bock et al., 2003) or *Mplus* (Muthén & Muthén, 1998–2010) compute the standard error of a score as part of the score estimation process.[1]

The empirical reliability is very easy to compute for a single trait, but its computational simplicity becomes especially advantageous when dealing with multi-trait measures. The sample-based empirical reliability approach essentially uses the estimated scores $\hat{\theta}_j = (\hat{\theta}_{1j}, \hat{\theta}_{2j}, \ldots, \hat{\theta}_{Tj})$ for every respondent j as a sample of points on the multidimensional grid.

Typically, single reliability indices provide good summaries of measurement precision for instruments with relatively uniform test information functions. For instruments with peaked information functions, summary indices are unlikely to be representative indicators of precision for any ranges of the latent trait. In addition, Bayesian estimators tend to shrink the scores toward the population mean, particularly when the number of items is small. When this is the case, the observed variance $\hat{\sigma}^2$ computed using (15.26) may be low, and the empirical index might underestimate the actual reliability.

RESEARCH METHODS

Scoring and Estimating Measurement Precision in Applications

Application

In the following sections, we show how test scores and their standard errors are estimated for a range of item response models popular in patient-reported outcomes applications. Four models—the unidimensional model, the correlated traits model, the second-order model, and the bifactor model—are included in the discussion. We illustrate all points made with the same data analysis example.

1 *Mplus* 7 provides standard errors for the estimated scores only when the EAP estimator is used.

Data Example: The 28-Item "Scaled" General Health Questionnaire (GHQ-28) in a General Population Birth Cohort Sample (the NSHD)

The 28-item version of Goldberg's General Health Questionnaire (GHQ-28; Goldberg, 1972; Goldberg & Hillier, 1979; Goldberg & Williams, 1988) is a popular instrument that was initially developed as a screening questionnaire for detecting psychiatric disorders in community settings and nonpsychiatric clinical settings, such as primary care or general practice (Croudace et al., 2003; Goldberg et al., 1997). A vast literature of clinical and general population studies has indicated that the 28-item version of the GHQ[2] performs well as a screening instrument for minor psychiatric disturbance and as an indicator of psychiatric morbidity. Although the GHQ-28 was developed to detect potential psychiatric cases by measuring the level of nonspecific psychiatric morbidity by probing for signs and symptoms, it is often considered as a potentially multidimensional measure. It can be used as a population-wide measure of psychological distress, for example in the first stage of a two-stage epidemiological study of mental health. It is also a candidate outcome measure for clinical trials, as a primary or secondary measure of emotional distress.

Respondents completing the GHQ questionnaire are asked to think about their health in general and any medical complaints they have had over **the past few weeks**. The version used here consists of 28 items designed to measure four **a priory** facets of mental health variation (four subscales): Somatic Symptoms, Social Dysfunction, Anxiety / Insomnia, and Severe Depression / Hopelessness. Each facet is measured with seven questions (for item content see Table 15.1), and responses are given by selecting one of four categories. These are indicated by a set of "verbal anchors." On the copyrighted forms, no numbered scoring is displayed for each anchor and there is subtle variation in their wording, which varies according to the phrasing of the questions. The response categories refer to either absence of the symptom ("*not at all*"), or presence of the symptom in relation to the "usual" amount—that is, "*no more than usual*," "*rather more than usual*," "*much more than usual*," for instance:

> "Have you recently lost much sleep over worry?"
> *(Not at all—No more than usual—Rather more than usual—Much more than usual)*

For some questions, response categories are unique but still follow the same pattern of comparison with the "usual" state of things, for instance:

> "Have you recently felt capable of making decisions about things?"
> *(More so than usual—Same as usual—Less so than usual—Much less capable)*

The GHQ-28 has 20 items that are worded in terms of "psychological problems / distress" (i.e., negatively worded) as the former example question, and eight items that are worded in terms of "psychological health" (i.e., positively worded) as the latter question. Regardless of whether the question is worded positively or negatively, the response categories are always presented in the order of increasing problems or symptomatic distress. Thus, the last category represents the most severe symptoms or the greatest *psychological / emotional distress* for all items.

2 Copyrighted instrument distributed by GL Assessment, see FAQ at www.gl-assessment.co.uk/health_and_psychology/resources/general_health_questionnaire/faqs.asp?css=1.

Our data set comprises responses from the ongoing Medical Research Council National Survey of Health and Development (NSHD), also known as the British 1946 birth cohort. We refer to the wave of interviewing undertaken in 1999 when the participants were aged 53 (Wadsworth et al., 2003). At that time, 2,901 respondents (1,422 men and 1,479 women, about 99 percent of the total number of study participants) provided answers on all items of the GHQ-28, and this is the full-response-set sample we consider here.

As would be expected, in this predominantly healthy mid-life community sample, most respondents selected either the first or the second response categories for most questions (corresponding to an absence or only a small amount of symptoms or distress). All item responses were positively skewed, particularly for the rather extreme items of the Severe Depression facet. Despite the large size of the data set, the last response category yielded only single frequency figures for some items, and to avoid instability of parameter estimates we *collapsed the two top response categories prior to any analyses*, effectively resulting in the item coding **0–1–2–2**.

We start by exploring the factor structure of these data in *Mplus*[3] (Muthén & Muthén, 1998–2010) using diagonally weighted least squares (DWLS) estimation (the software default) based on the matrix of polychoric correlations (Muthén, du Toit, & Spisic, 1997). Considering that the instrument was designed to measure four facets of psychological distress, we expect to find that four moderately correlated factors underlie the data. However, there is also a clear possibility of one general "psychological distress" construct underpinning the associations between these four related facets.

An exploratory analysis yielded five eigenvalues greater than one (12.9, 2.6, 2.2, 1.5, and 1.1). As the ratio of the first to the second eigenvalue is very large, a strong general factor is evident, together with three or four further factors. Goodness of fit of this exploratory solution is $\chi^2 = 3917$, $df = 272$, $p < 0.001$, RMSEA = 0.068, CFI = 0.959.

A target rotation of the four-factor solution to a hypothesized structure (where items designed to measure a facet have zero loadings on all other facets) yielded what we consider a well-behaved solution. Items designed to measure a facet had large loadings on the corresponding factor and mostly near-zero loadings on the other three factors (see Table 15.1). As expected, these four factors were moderately correlated (their intercorrelations ranged from 0.33 to 0.56).

Based on theoretical considerations governing the design of the GHQ-28 and the exploratory solution, any psychometric model for this data should reflect the interrelated nature of the measured facets. These relationships could be modeled through a factor capturing variation between individuals on the primary psychological adjustment / distress continuum, and possibly further factors, that may exist over and above the general factor. In what follows, we consider four alternative models for the GHQ-28 data.

The first model is a **unidimensional** model, in which one common factor explains all variation in the data (Figure 15.1a). This is the most basic IRT model and we use it here for illustration of the basic scoring principles.

The second model is a **correlated traits** model, in which four freely correlated facets are indicated by their respective items (Figure 15.1b). This model is useful if the focus of measurement is on the four facets.

The third model is a **second-order** model, in which a second-order factor explains common variance in the four facets (see Figure 15.1c). This model is useful when scores on the general factor as well as scores on its facets are of interest.

3 Analyses can also be performed using the freeware FACTOR program, available on http://psico.fcep.urv.es/utilitats/factor/index.html.

Table 15.1 Standardized Factor Loadings in the Oblique Four-Factor Solution for GHQ-28

Item	*Wording*	*Factor 1 Somatic Symptoms*	*Factor 2 Anxiety*	*Factor 3 Social Dysfunction*	*Factor 4 Depression*
S1	good health	0.53		0.39	
S2	need good tonic	0.62	0.36		
S3	run down	0.72	0.32		
S4	felt ill	0.69			
S5	pains in head	0.97			
S6	pressure in head	0.97			
S7	hot and cold spells	0.39			
A1	lost sleep over worry		0.79		
A2	difficulty staying asleep		0.67		
A3	constant strain		0.73		
A4	edgy		0.58		
A5	panicky/scared		0.49		0.33
A6	everything on top of you		0.69		
A7	nervous		0.59		0.36
SD1	manage to keep busy			0.52	
SD2	take longer time			0.55	
SD3	doing things well			0.95	
SD4	satisfied with tasks			0.86	
SD5	play a useful part			0.76	
SD6	making decisions			0.61	
SD7	enjoy daily activities		0.35	0.41	
D1	worthless				0.61
D2	hopeless				0.72
D3	not worth living				0.79
D4	thoughts of suicide				0.95
D5	nerves too bad				0.53
D6	wishing dead				0.86
D7	suicidal ideas				0.92

Note: Loadings below 0.3 in magnitude are omitted. S = Somatic Symptoms, A = Anxiety / Insomnia, SD = Social Dysfunction, D = Depression.

The fourth and the last model is a **bifactor** model, in which every item is influenced by two factors—the general factor and a group factor (Figure 15.1d). The general factor accounts for the common variance shared by all items. Group factors are "residual" dimensions, which account for any remaining common variance specific to the items forming the facets. The bifactor model is a useful representation of data where the general factor is of particular, but not sole interest.

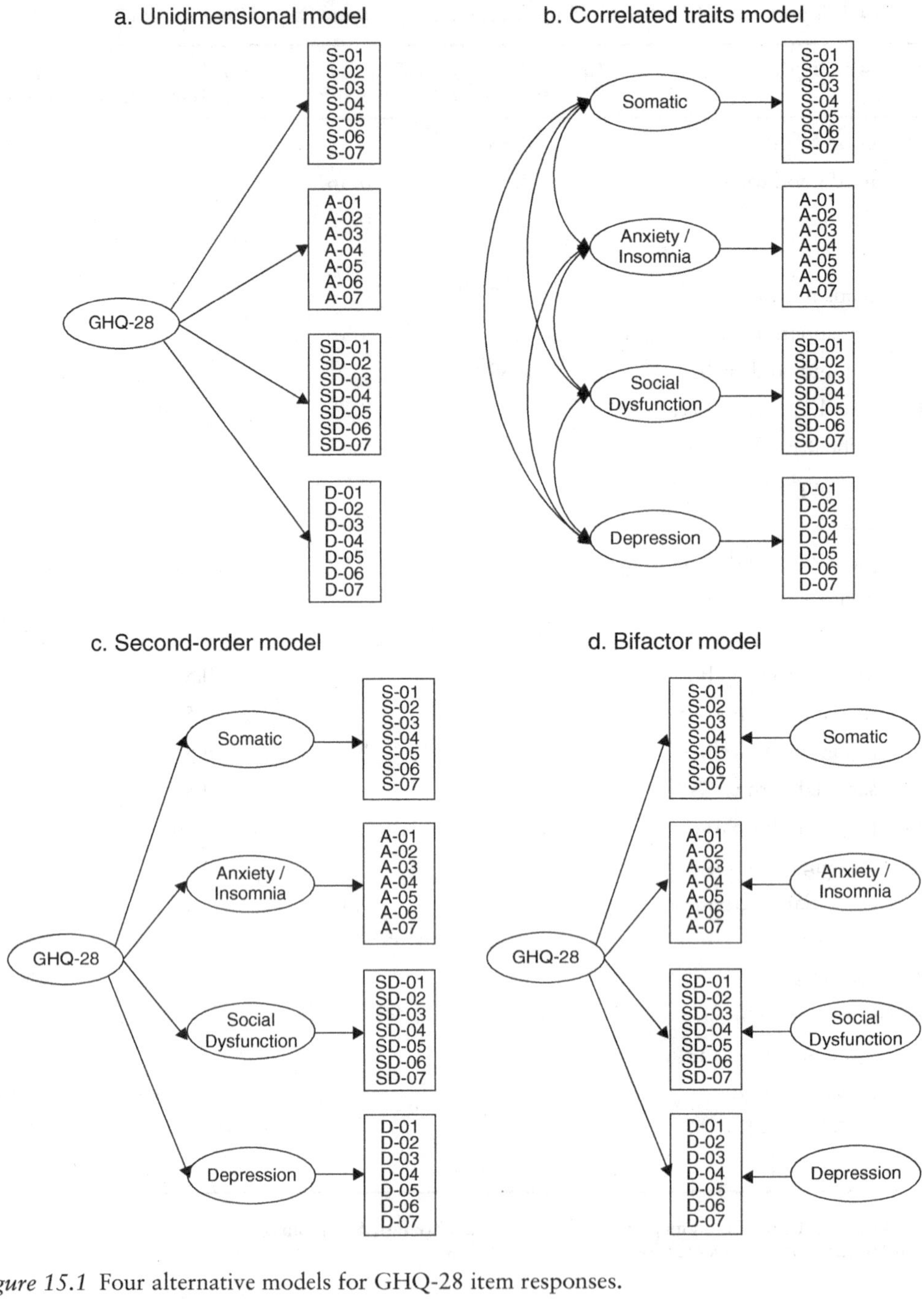

Figure 15.1 Four alternative models for GHQ-28 item responses.

Scoring Under the Unidimensional IRT Model

When the instrument items depend on one latent trait, the ML item information function (15.14) is calculated from the normal ogive item response function $P_i(\theta) = \Phi(\alpha_i + \beta_i\theta)$ as follows (McDonald, 1999, p. 284):

$$\mathcal{I}_i(\theta) = \frac{\beta_i^2 \left[\phi(\alpha_i + \beta_i\theta)\right]^2}{\Phi(\alpha_i + \beta_i\theta)\left[1 - \Phi(\alpha_i + \beta_i\theta)\right]}. \tag{15.27}$$

Here, $\phi(x)$ denotes a standard normal density function evaluated at x. Having computed the item information functions for all items, the ML test information is computed by adding all item contributions, and the posterior information is computed using (15.20).

When the logistic link $P_i(\theta) = \mathrm{L}(\mathrm{D}\alpha_i + \mathrm{D}\beta_i\theta)$ is used,[4] the item information function (15.14) amounts to:

$$\mathcal{I}_i(\theta) = (\mathrm{D}\beta_i)^2 \mathrm{L}(\mathrm{D}\alpha_i + \mathrm{D}\beta_i\theta)\left[1 - \mathrm{L}(\mathrm{D}\alpha_i + \mathrm{D}\beta_i\theta)\right]. \tag{15.28}$$

All formulae for item information involving the normal-ogive link function given further in this chapter can be adopted for the logistic link by using the general expression given earlier.

Illustration: GHQ-28 General Factor Scored Under the Unidimensional Model

It is important to note that these formulae for unidimensional IRT models cannot be applied if the key assumption of local independence does not hold in the data. In particular, when local independence does not hold the test information cannot be decomposed into the sum of item information functions. We know that dependencies exist between items within the four facets of GHQ-28; however, for purposes of illustration we proceed as if the GHQ-28 really did measure only one underlying trait, "psychological distress." This analysis, using the simplifying assumption of local independence, will be later compared with analyses using other models, and we shall investigate the extent to which the simplification affects the results.

Item parameters were estimated according to the single factor model depicted in Figure 15.1a, using the DWLS estimator in *Mplus* software. We report the chi-square and other fit indices for this and subsequent models in Table 15.2. As expected, the model fitted the data poorly, with RMSEA and CFI/TLI indicating unsatisfactory fit. Specifically, this model failed to reproduce correlations between the items within the four facets.

The individual trait scores were estimated using two Bayesian methods—the EAP and the MAP. The EAP scores ranged from –2.96 to 3.52 (mean 0.03 and standard deviation 0.90). The MAP scores ranged from –2.87 to 3.42 (mean 0.03 and standard deviation 0.89).The two sets of scores correlate almost perfectly, with the correlation being different from one in the fifth decimal place, and in the rest of this chapter we therefore use the EAP score only.

The standard errors of the EAP score estimates were computed according to Equation (15.9). Figure 15.2 shows the EAP standard errors plotted against the estimated trait scores for all individuals in the NSHD sample. For comparison, we also plot the standard errors computed from the Fisher information of the posterior likelihood function using

Table 15.2 Goodness of Fit for Alternative GHQ-28 Models

Model	*Chi-square*	*df*	*RMSEA*	*CFI*	*TLI*
Unidimensional	15314	350	.121	.831	.818
Second-order	5920	346	.075	.937	.931
Correlated traits	5870	344	.074	.938	.932
Bifactor	4142	323	.064	.957	.950

4 D = 1.7 is the scaling constant used with the intercept and slope parameters from the normal ogive metric.

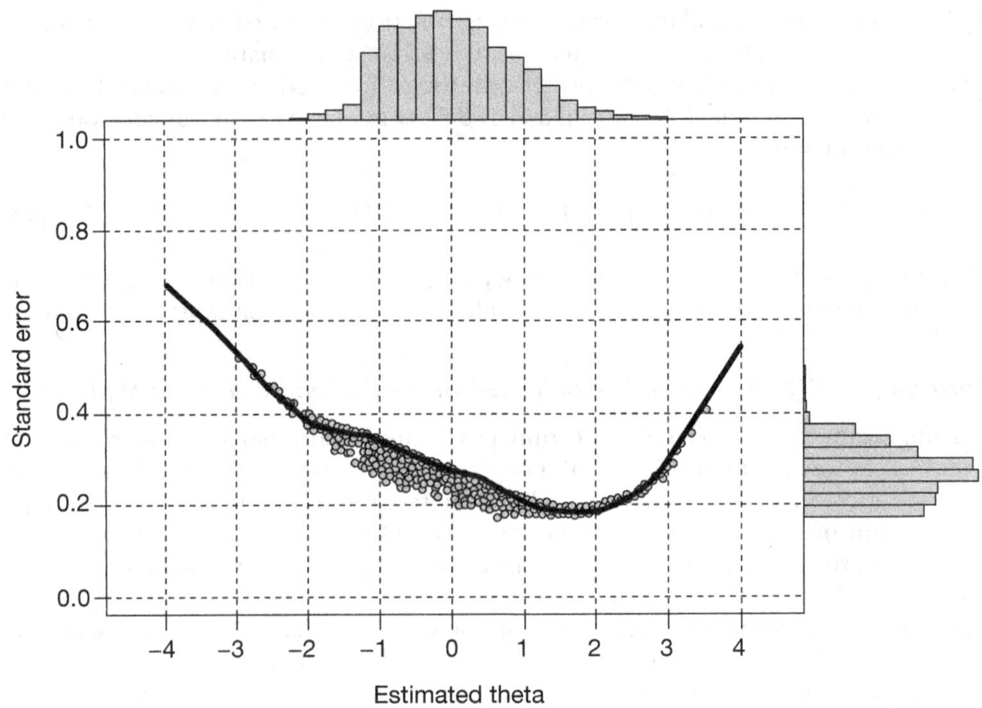

Figure 15.2 Standard errors for the general psychological distress factor under the unidimensional model, with distributions of estimated scores and standard errors.

Note: Points represent standard errors of individual EAP scores; solid line is the standard error function derived from the Fisher posterior information.

Equation (15.20). It can be seen that the standard error function based on the Fisher information traces the errors of the EAP scores almost perfectly. Figure 15.2 shows that for the most of the latent score range (between –3 and 3) the precision of measurement is good, with the standard errors below 0.5.

The empirical reliability of the MAP sample scores (computed from Fisher information) is 0.899, and empirical reliability of EAP sample scores computed from the squared EAP standard errors is 0.908. In this case, the two empirical estimators give similar results. We, however, suspect that these high reliability values are an overestimation, due to ignoring the local dependencies between items measuring the same facets in this simple model.

Scoring Under the Correlated Traits IRT Model

In measures where each item indicates only one of T correlated facets f_1, f_2, ..., f_T (the items possess an independent-clusters basis), such as our hypothesized structure for the GHQ-28 depicted in Figure 15.1b, the one-dimensional theory applies when it comes to computing the ML item information and test information functions. Because each item response is conditional on a single trait, there is no difference between estimating trait scores by using a model with multiple correlated traits and by using separate unidimensional models, provided that the item parameters in both models are identical.

There is, however, a difference between estimating the trait scores in univariate and multivariate fashion when Bayesian estimators are used. In a model with correlated traits, the latent trait correlations will be taken to account as a feature of the multivariate prior distribution. When the traits are associated, the population-based likelihood of having a certain score on one trait will vary depending on the levels of other traits. For example, in the GHQ-28 with its positively correlated facets, a combination of four scores that are all one standard deviation below the population mean is more likely than a combination of scores where two facet scores are one standard deviation above and two facet scores are one standard deviation below the population mean. When the appropriate prior population density is used in Bayesian estimation, it increases the estimation precision by "borrowing" information from related trait scores. To quantify how much information is added by related scores, we refer to Equation (15.21).

Illustration: GHQ-28 Facets Scored Under the Correlated Traits Model

The correlated traits model (see Figure 15.1b) was estimated using the DWLS estimator. Goodness-of-fit indices are reported in Table 15.2. As expected, the model fitted much better than the unidimensional model. After the model parameters were estimated, the individual responses were scored using the MAP estimator (because the EAP estimator is very computationally heavy with as many as four dimensions). Model-based correlations between the latent traits are given in Table 15.3. These correlations are used to assess the contributions from the prior multivariate normal distribution to estimation of each subscale score. Because the four facets are positively correlated, the prior information provided by each facet in (15.21) is greater than one. For instance, the prior distribution adds an impressive 3.33 to the information function for the Anxiety / Insomnia subscale.

The standard errors of the facet scores estimated in the multivariate fashion as described earlier are given in Figure 15.3(a–d). Corresponding standard errors of the univariate score estimation (if the scores were MAP-estimated without the knowledge of the related facets) are shown for comparison. It can be seen that the multivariate scoring yields higher accuracy than the scale-by-scale univariate scoring when traits are correlated.

Marginal reliabilities computed for each estimated facet are given in Table 15.4. It can be seen that the Severe Depression score shows particularly high shrinkage toward the population mode, producing low observed score variance (0.64). The empirical reliabilities for Somatic Symptoms and Anxiety subscales are above 0.8, but fall short of 0.7 for Social Dysfunction and Severe Depression.

Scoring Under the Bifactor IRT Model

In this section, we use the general formulation for response functions and multidimensional information given earlier in this chapter to provide formulae necessary to compute the item and test information for bifactor models. Let g be a *general factor* measured by

Table 15.3 Estimated Latent Trait Correlations Under the Correlated Traits Model

	S	*A*	*SD*	*D*
(S) Somatic Symptoms	1			
(A) Anxiety / Insomnia	.70 (.01)	1		
(SD) Social Dysfunction	.59 (.01)	.60 (.01)	1	
(D) Severe Depression	.54 (.02)	.76 (.01)	.57 (.02)	1

Note: Standard errors are in parentheses. S = Somatic Symptoms, A = Anxiety / Insomnia, SD = Social Dysfunction, D = Severe Depression.

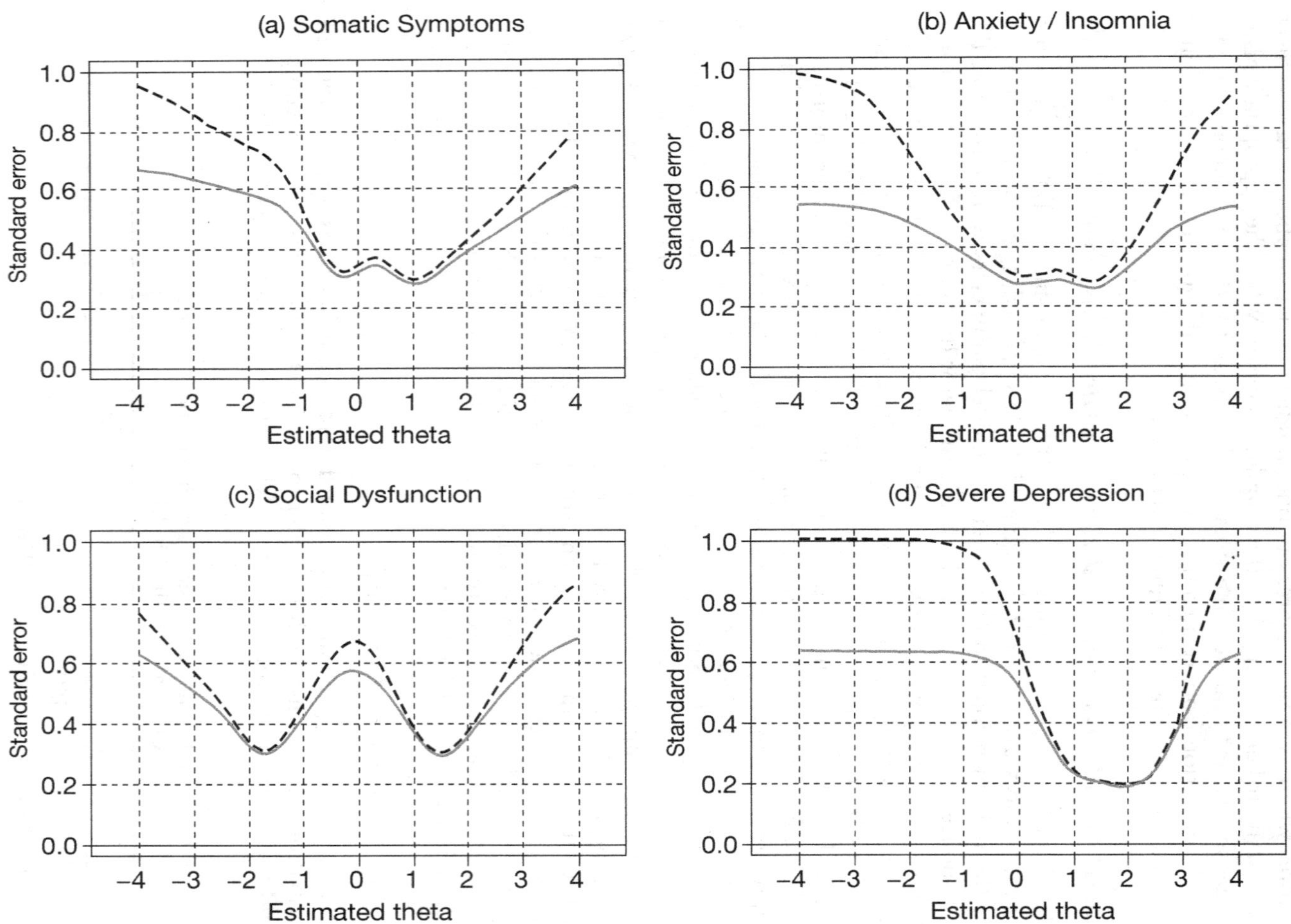

Figure 15.3 Standard error functions for the four subscales in the GHQ-28 data example; univariate versus multivariate scoring using the MAP estimator.

Note: Solid line is the standard error function for the multivariate estimation; dashed line is the standard error function for the univariate (scale-by-scale) estimation.

the instrument, and $s_1, s_2, \ldots, s_T$ be T *group factors* (for instance, related to facets). The set of factors underlying item responses is therefore $\mathbf{g}^* = (g, s_1, s_2, \ldots, s_T)'$. At this point, it is important to emphasize the difference in conceptual meaning between subscales / facets and "group factors." In bifactor models, group factors do **not** have the same interpretation as facets in correlated traits models. Statistically, they are residuals left after accounting for the general factor, and therefore represent unique features common to groups of items that are not explained by the general factor. The group factors, therefore, cannot be thought of as "Anxiety" or "Depression" or whatever meaning we associate with facets—instead, they represent common features of "Anxiety" or "Depression" items that are not captured by "Psychological Distress."

The general factor and the group factors are assumed mutually uncorrelated, have zero means and unit variances so that their distribution is multivariate standard normal $\mathbf{g}^* \sim N_{T+1}(0, \mathbf{I})$, where $\mathbf{I}$ denotes the identity covariance matrix. In the bifactor model, the item response tendency is influenced by two factors—the general factor g and one group factor, say s_a.

$$u_i^* = \alpha_i + \beta_{0i} g + \beta_{ai}\, s_a + \varepsilon_i. \tag{15.29}$$

In this expression, α_i is the intercept, β_{0i} is the slope parameter for the general factor g, β_{ai} is the slope for the group factor s_a, and ε_i is the error. Assuming the error is distributed normally with the mean 0 and unit variance, the item response function given in the intercept / slope parameterization is, therefore, the two-dimensional normal ogive:

$$P_i\left(\mathbf{g}^*\right) = P\left(u_i = 1 \middle| \mathbf{g}^*\right) = \Phi\left(\alpha_i + \beta_{0i} g + \beta_{ai} s_a\right). \tag{15.30}$$

Because all the factors in this model are uncorrelated, the gradient in direction of the general factor g in Equation (15.17) becomes

$$\nabla_g P_i\left(\mathbf{g}^*\right) = \frac{\partial P_i\left(\mathbf{g}^*\right)}{\partial g} = \beta_{0i}\phi\left(\alpha_i + \beta_{0i} g + \beta_{ai} s_a\right), \tag{15.31}$$

where $\phi(x)$ is the normal density function evaluated at x. Thus, the IIF in direction of the general factor g for the bifactor model is:

$$\mathcal{I}_i^g\left(\mathbf{g}^*\right) = \frac{\left(\beta_{0i}\right)^2 \left[\phi\left(\alpha_i + \beta_{0i} g + \beta_{ai} s_a\right)\right]^2}{\Phi\left(\alpha_i + \beta_{0i} g + \beta_{ai} s_a\right)\left[1 - \Phi\left(\alpha_i + \beta_{0i} g + \beta_{ai} s_a\right)\right]}. \tag{15.32}$$

Because the item information function is conditioned on both the general and the group factor, local independence holds and the IIFs are additive. The test information about the general factor g is the sum of all IIFs in the direction of g. This summation, however, will make the test information function for the general factor **conditional on all group factors**, although each item information function is only conditional on **one** group factor (in addition to the general factor).

When prior knowledge about the population distribution is used for score estimation, the prior information must be added to the ML test information to compute the posterior test information. In the bifactor model, the latent covariance matrix is $\Sigma = \mathbf{I}$ and the information added in (15.21) is simply 1:

$$\mathcal{I}_P^g\left(\mathbf{g}^*\right) = \mathcal{I}^g\left(\mathbf{g}^*\right) + \left[\mathrm{I}^{-1}\right]_g = \sum_i \mathcal{I}_i^g\left(\mathbf{g}^*\right) + 1. \tag{15.33}$$

Illustration: GHQ-28 General and Group Factors Scored Under the Bifactor Model

The bifactor model illustrated in Figure 15.1d, with the latent factor variances set to one and the item uniqueness set to one, involved estimating 28 slope parameters β_{0i} related to the general factor, and 28 slope parameters $\beta_{Si}, \beta_{Ai}, \beta_{SDi}, \beta_{Di}$ related to the four group factors s_S, s_A, s_{SD}, s_D. In addition, 56 = 28*2 category thresholds were estimated (two thresholds for each three-category item). Goodness-of-fit indices for this model are reported in Table 15.2. The model shows acceptable CFI/TLI, and it is an improvement compared to the correlated traits model. The person parameters (general and group scores) for the GHQ-28 were estimated using the MAP estimator.

The properly conditioned and therefore additive **item** information functions (IIFs) for this model depend on two factors only (one general and one group factor) and can be plotted as surfaces. However, the **test** information function (TIF) in the direction of the general factor depends on five factors (the general factor as well as four group factors), and therefore cannot be presented easily.

We use estimated scores for each person j $\left(\hat{g}_j, \hat{s}_{Sj}, \hat{s}_{Aj}, \hat{s}_{SDj}, \hat{s}_{Dj}\right)$ as sampled points on the multidimensional grid to summarize high-dimensional information functions, in the following manner. For each sampled point, item information functions will yield scalar values; the TIF for the general factor can be easily computed by summing the scalar IIF values. Finally, the standard errors can be computed and plotted against estimated values of the general factor for all individuals in the sample. Figure 15.4 illustrates such a scatter for the GHQ-28 data. It can be seen that the standard errors for most participants were below 0.4, and only two participants out of 2,901 had

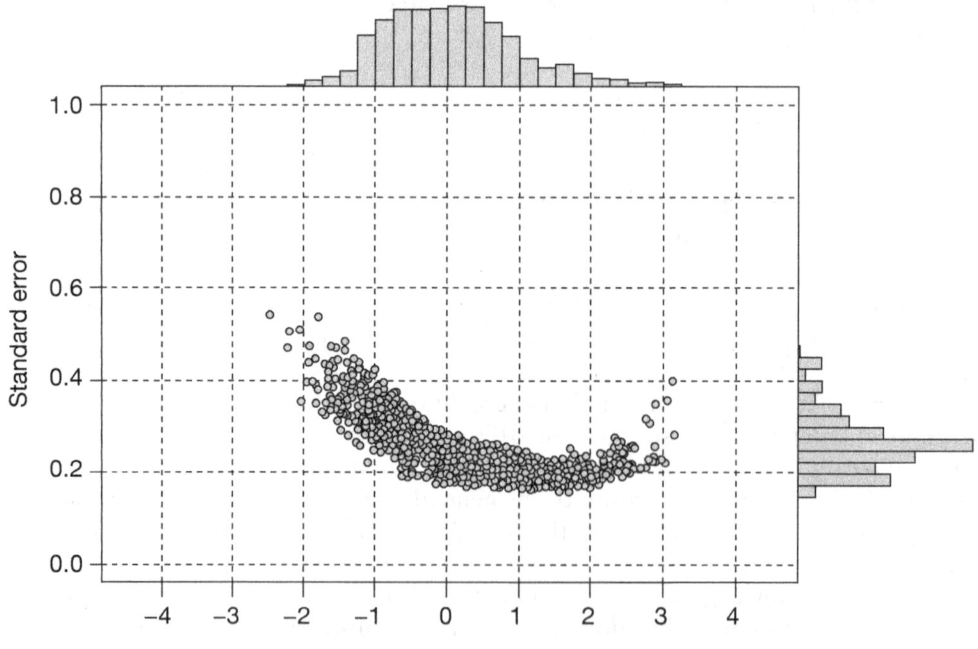

Figure 15.4 Standard errors of MAP general factor scores under the bifactor model in the GHQ-28 data example; fully conditioned on all latent factors.

the standard errors above 0.5. These larger standard errors were associated with low scores on the general factor ($\theta = -1.78$ and $\theta = -2.48$). The empirical reliability of MAP scores calculated from these standard errors is 0.901, very close to the estimate given by the unidimensional model.

Scoring Under the Second-Order IRT Model

In measures with a second-order factorial structure (such as the model depicted in Figure 15.1c), common variance in T facets $f_1, f_2, \ldots, f_T$ is explained by one general factor g, and every item response tendency depends on one first-order factor (facet), say f_a:

$$u_i^* = \alpha_i + \beta_{ai} f_a + \varepsilon_i. \tag{15.34}$$

Here, α_i is the item intercept, β_{ai} is the slope for the facet f_a, and ε_i is the error distributed with the mean 0 and unit variance (thus we keep the standard IRT intercept/slope parameterization for the measurement part of the model).

Each facet factor, in turn, is an indicator of the general factor, g:

$$f_a = \lambda_a g + d_a, \tag{15.35}$$

where d_a is a residual term, also called "disturbance" in structural equation modeling (SEM) literature. The residual terms are uncorrelated with the general factor and with each other. The structural part of the model in Equation (15.35) is parameterized so that the general factor g and the facet factors $f_1, f_2, \ldots, f_T$ have unit variances, that is, the factor loadings λ_a are standardized. It is convenient to work with standardized facet scores, and use the established formulae for the standard normal ogive. In order for the facet scores to be standardized, the disturbance terms must have variances $var(d_a) = 1 - \lambda_a^2$.

It follows that the set of latent factors in the measurement model (15.34) $\mathbf{f} = (f_1, f_2, \ldots, f_T)'$ is distributed $\mathbf{f} \sim N_T(0, \Sigma)$, where Σ is the covariance matrix:

$$\Sigma = \begin{pmatrix} 1 & \lambda_1\lambda_2 & \cdots & \lambda_1\lambda_T \\ \lambda_2\lambda_1 & 1 & \cdots & \lambda_2\lambda_T \\ \vdots & \vdots & \ddots & \vdots \\ \lambda_T\lambda_1 & \lambda_T\lambda_2 & \cdots & 1 \end{pmatrix}. \tag{15.36}$$

The item response function can be written as the standard normal ogive:

$$P_i(\mathbf{f}) = P(u_i = 1 | \mathbf{f}) = \Phi(\alpha_i + \beta_{ai} f_a). \tag{15.37}$$

Because the item response tendency u_i^* depends on one facet f_a only, and does not depend on the general factor, the partial derivatives with respect to the general factor and irrelevant facets are zero, and the gradient in direction of the general factor g in Equation (15.17) becomes:

$$\nabla_g P_i(\mathbf{f}) = \frac{\partial P_i(\mathbf{f})}{\partial g} \text{corr}(g, g) + \sum_{k=1}^{T} \left(\frac{\partial P_i(\mathbf{f})}{\partial f_k} \text{corr}(f_k, g) \right) = \frac{\partial P_i(\mathbf{f})}{\partial f_a} \text{corr}(f_a, g). \tag{15.38}$$

The partial derivative with respect to f_a in (15.38) is:

$$\frac{\partial P_i(\mathbf{f})}{\partial f_a} = \beta_{ai}\phi(\alpha_i + \beta_{ai} f_a), \tag{15.39}$$

where $\phi(x)$ is the normal density function evaluated at x. It follows from (15.35) that the correlation between the general factor g and the facet factor f_a is $\mathrm{corr}(f_a, g) = \lambda_a$, and the gradient is:

$$\nabla_g P_i(\mathbf{f}) = \beta_{ai}\lambda_a\,\phi(\alpha_i + \beta_{ai} f_a). \tag{15.40}$$

Finally, the IIF **in the direction of the general factor *g*** for an item measuring the facet factor f_a in the second-order model, parameterized as described earlier, is:

$$\mathcal{I}_i^g(\mathbf{f}) = \frac{(\beta_{ai}\lambda_a)^2\left[\phi(\alpha_i + \beta_{ai} f_a)\right]^2}{\Phi(\alpha_i + \beta_{ai} f_a)\left[1 - \Phi(\alpha_i + \beta_{ai} f_a)\right]}. \tag{15.41}$$

In the second-order model, local independence holds and the item information functions are additive. The TIF about the general factor g is the sum of all IIFs in the direction of g. This summation, just as it was the case with the bifactor model, makes the test information function for the general factor **conditional on all facet factors**, although each item information function is only conditional on one facet factor.

When Bayesian methods are used for score estimation, the prior information must be added to the ML test information to compute the posterior test information. In the second-order model, the general factor is estimated from continuous facet indicators, and the amount of information added by the univariate normal prior is one:

$$\mathcal{I}_P^g(\mathbf{f}) = \mathcal{I}^g(\mathbf{f}) + 1. \tag{15.42}$$

An added advantage of the second-order model is that along with the scores for the general factor, scores for the facets can also be estimated. It follows from Equation (15.37) that the ML item information **in direction of the facet factor f_a** is:

$$\mathcal{I}_i^a(\mathbf{f}) = \frac{\beta_{ai}^2\left[\phi(\alpha_i + \beta_{ai} f_a)\right]^2}{\Phi(\alpha_i + \beta_{ai} f_a)\left[1 - \Phi(\alpha_i + \beta_{ai} f_a)\right]}. \tag{15.43}$$

The TIF about the facet factor f_a is the sum of all IIFs in the direction of f_a. Just like in the model with correlated traits, relationships between the facet factors described by (15.36) will be taken to form the covariance matrix for the multivariate normal distribution used as a prior. To quantify how much information is added by related scores, we refer to Equation (15.21).

The Second-Order Model as a Special Case of the Bifactor Model

If we substitute the expression for the facet factor (15.35) into the expression for the item response tendency (15.34), we obtain an expression of the response tendency as a direct function of the general factor and the residual (disturbance) term:

$$u_i^* = \alpha_i + \beta_{ai}\lambda_a g + \beta_{ai} d_a + \varepsilon_i. \tag{15.44}$$

The only difference between this expression and the bifactor Equation (15.29) is the naming convention for the residual / disturbance term, and choice of regression parameters (slopes). We keep notation for the disturbance terms d_a in the second-order model distinct from the group terms s_a in the bifactor model only to emphasize that they have different variances in our chosen parameterization. Recall that while variances of the group terms in the bifactor model are set to one, variances of the disturbance terms in the second-order factor model are set to one minus squared factor loading on the general factor ($1-\lambda_a^2$). Otherwise, these entities have equivalent roles in the models and equivalent meaning.

It follows that any second-order model can be equivalently parameterized as a bifactor model with some restrictions on slope parameters (Rindskopf & Rose, 1988). That is, the slope on the general factor in a bifactor representation of the second-order model is proportionate to the respective slope on the group factor, with one common proportion coefficient λ_a for all items related to the same group factor s_a:

$$\beta_{0i} = \beta_{ai}\lambda_a. \tag{15.45}$$

Consequently, the bifactor model estimates twice as many slope parameters as there are items, while the second-order model estimates as many slopes on the group factors as there are items plus as many common facet coefficients as there are facets. Put simply, the second-order model is nested within the bifactor model.

It is now clear that the expression for the IIF in the direction of the general factor for the second-order model (15.41) is identical to the expression for the bifactor model (15.32), when the two models are parameterized as described. That is, in the bifactor model we set variances for the general, group, and unique factors equal one. In the second-order model, we set variances for the general, facet, and unique factors equal one (this means that variances for the facet residuals/disturbances are constrained to one minus squared factor loading on the general factor). This parameterization ensures a familiar *z*-score metric interpretation, and scale, for all model-estimated factors.

Illustration: GHQ-28 General Factor and Facets Scored Under the Second-Order Model

The second-order model for the GHQ-28 illustrated in Figure 15.1c, with the general and facet factors' variances set to one (and recall that item unique variances are set to one), estimates four facet loadings on the general factor, and 28 item slope parameters relating to the four facet factors f_S, f_A, f_{SD}, and f_D. There are also 56 = 28*2 category threshold parameters (two thresholds for each three-category item). Goodness-of-fit indices for this model are reported in Table 15.2. This model fitted much better than the unidimensional model and almost as well as the correlated traits model. The scores on the general factor and the facets were estimated using the MAP estimator.

The resulting TIF in direction of the general factor depends on all four facets, although information functions for each item depend on one facet only. This means that the properly conditioned and therefore additive **item** information functions can be plotted as curves; however, the four-dimensional **test** information function cannot be plotted. Again, we use the sample-based approach to working with information functions here, as follows.

Once the factor scores $\hat{\mathbf{f}}_j = \left(\hat{f}_{Sj}, \hat{f}_{Aj}, \hat{f}_{SDj}, \hat{f}_{Dj}\right)$ have been estimated for each individual j, they are used as sampled points. For each point, the item information functions yield scalar values, and the TIF for the general factor is easily computed by summing the IIFs. The prior contribution is then added as described by Equation (15.42). Finally, the standard errors can be computed and plotted against the estimated values of the general factor

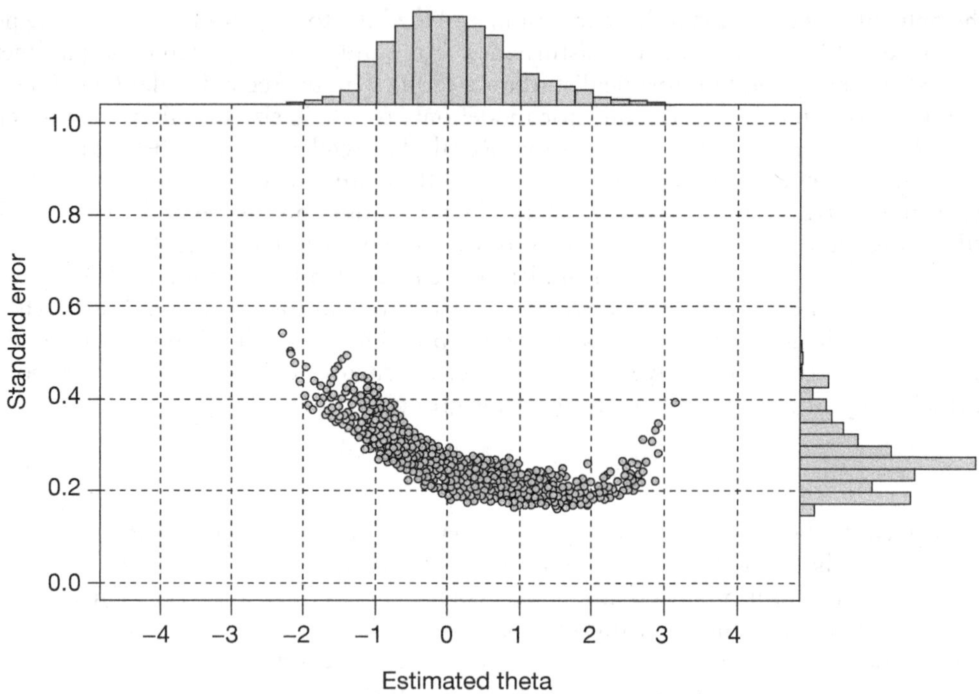

Figure 15.5 Standard errors of MAP general factor scores under the second-order factor model in the GHQ-28 data example; fully conditioned on all latent factors.

for all individuals in the sample. Figure 15.5 illustrates this scatter for our GHQ-28 data example. It can be seen that the standard errors for most participants were below 0.4, and only one participant out of 2,901 had the standard error above 0.5. This larger standard error (SE = 0.54) was associated with a low score on the general factor ($\theta = -2.32$). The empirical reliability of MAP scores calculated from these standard errors is **0.891**, lower than the estimate for the unidimensional model, and the bifactor model.

The standard errors of the facet scores were computed using the information function (15.43). The resulting standard error functions were very similar to the respective functions estimated under the correlated traits model. The empirical reliabilities for each facet are given in Table 15.4. It can be seen that they are very similar to the respective reliability coefficients for the correlated traits model.

Evaluation of the Alternative Scoring Methods for GHQ-28 Data Example

A range of scoring options for a typical, ordinal-response patient-reported outcome measure with a general-group structure was discussed and illustrated with the GHQ-28 data set. The unidimensional model, violating the assumption of local independence, showed poor fit to the data (see Table 15.2). The other models, which accommodated the multidimensional faceted structure of the GHQ-28, fitted the data nearly acceptably, and the bifactor model showed the best fit.

Table 15.5 reports correlations between the **general psychological distress** scores estimated with the alternative scoring models. It can be seen that all methods yielded highly similar scores (the correlations ranged from 0.960 to 0.987). The lowest correlation was observed between our worst-fitting model—the unidimensional model—and our best fitting model—the bifactor model. Figure 15.6 presents scatterplots for the general factor scores estimated under different models. It can be seen that there was a slight departure from linearity in the relationship between the unidimensional scores and the bifactor scores, and the unidimensional scores and the second-order scores. The second-order model yielded general factor scores that were very close to the bifactor scores, and the relationship between these two sets of scores was linear.

Reliability estimates obtained using the marginal (empirical) coefficients, which were fully conditioned on all latent traits in the multidimensional models, reached around 0.9 for all models. These estimates, however, are likely to be overly optimistic for the unidimensional model, which ignored local dependencies between the items within facets and therefore likely overestimated the test information and underestimated the standard errors.

We expect the bifactor reliability estimates to be an accurate reflection of the real measurement precision provided by this well-fitting scoring model. To examine how accurate the estimated scores really were for all models, we conducted a simulation study, where the bifactor model was the generating model for item responses. The estimated item parameters from the GHQ-28 bifactor model were used to generate true scores and categorical item responses for $N = 2{,}901$ cases in 100 replications. The simulated item responses were scored using the same methods we applied to the real GHQ-28 data set. The correlation between the true and the estimated scores on the general factor was computed. Recall that, according to (15.23), the squared correlation between the true and the estimated score is a measure of test reliability.

Results of this simple simulation study are reported in the last column of Table 15.4. The highest squared correlation between the true and the estimated score (the test reliability) is for the bifactor model (0.869) and the lowest for the unidimensional model (0.824). Comparing these figures with the reliability estimates in the same table, we can

Table 15.4 Marginal (Empirical) Reliabilities Under Alternative GHQ-28 Scoring Models.

Model	*Estimator*	*S*	*A*	*SD*	*D*	General	$[\text{corr}(\theta,\hat{\theta})]^2$
Unidimensional	MAP					**.899**	.824
	EAP					**.908**	
Correlated traits	MAP	.817	.871	.666	.639	-	-
Second-order	MAP	.813	.867	.665	.607	**.891**	.852
Bifactor	MAP	-	-	-	-	**.902**	.869

Note: S = Somatic Symptoms, A = Anxiety / Insomnia, SD = Social Dysfunction, D = Depression.

Table 15.5 Correlations Between GHQ-28 General Distress Scores Estimated Using Alternative Scoring Models.

	Second-order	*Bifactor*
Unidimensional	.987	.960
Second-order		.982

Note: Both EAP and MAP scoring for the unidimensional model yield identical correlations with the other models.

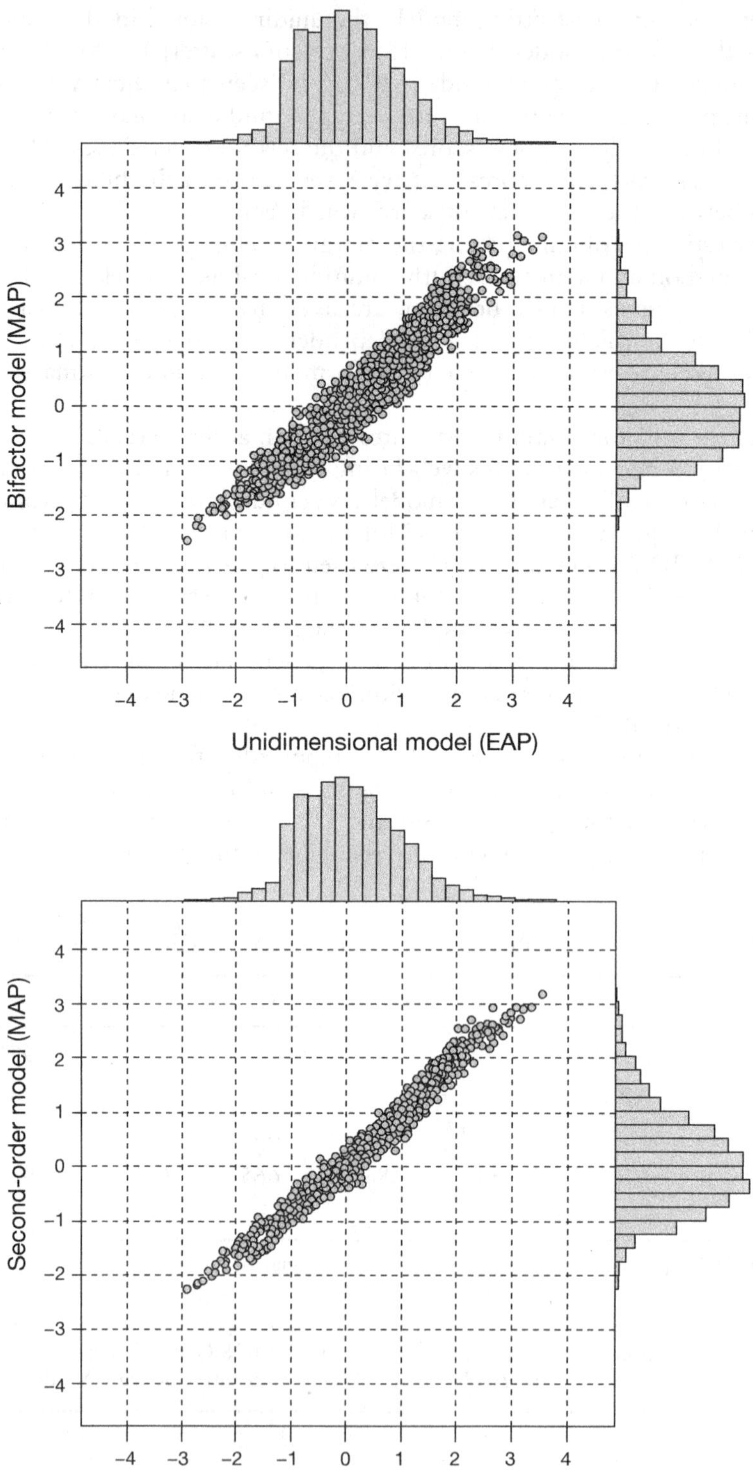

Figure 15.6 Comparison of the GHQ-28 general factor score estimates under different scoring models.

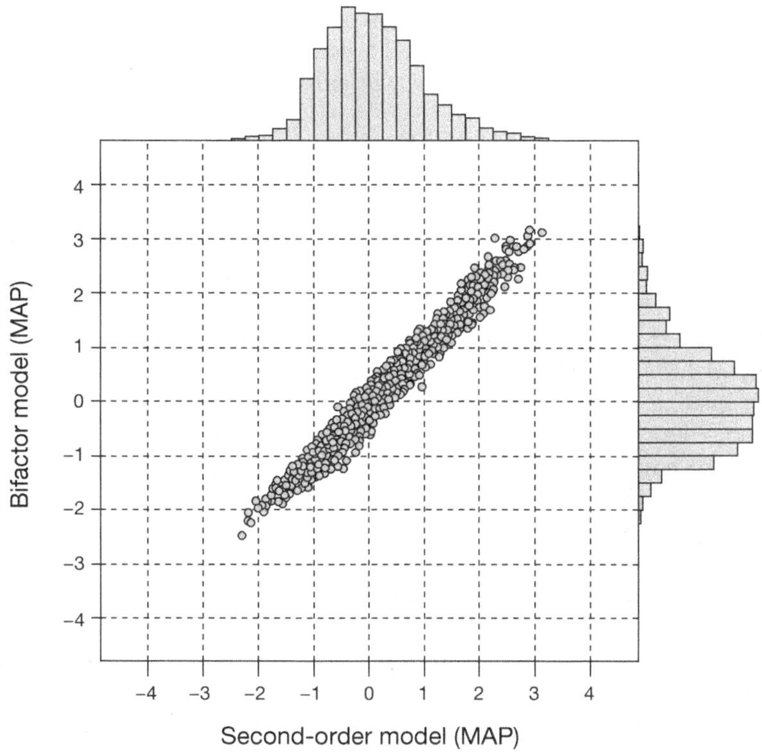

Figure 15.6 (*Continued*)

see that the test information methods overestimated the reliability slightly for the bifactor and the second-order models (by 3.8% and 4.6% respectively), and more substantially for the unidimensional model (by 9.1%). The slight overestimation with the well-fitting bifactor model is likely due to remaining local dependencies between items within the Somatic Symptoms subscale.

Overall, we conclude that the bifactor model is the most suitable for these data, and that it produces scores with good measurement precision that can be reasonably accurately estimated using the described sample-based methodology involving multidimensional information. When assessment on the general factor is desired, the second-order model is the second best from the fit and the measurement precision point of view; and it may be preferred to the bifactor model in situations when scoring on the subscales is also required.

Summary

Which model is the most suitable for a particular measurement instrument should be a decision based largely on conceptual grounds, not merely model fit. Furthermore, particular measurement focus (e.g., whether the general factor or the facet factors are of interest) imposes practical requirements on the scoring model. Approaching the model choice from the theoretical perspective governing the instrument's design, the GHQ-28 used as an example patient-reported outcome measure was developed to measure four conceptually distinct constructs that were expected to show moderate to strong associations in most samples (clinical or general population). The correlated traits model is clearly suitable from this point of view. However, this model fails to capture any common variance existing among the subscales, and therefore is only suitable for measuring the facets but not the overall psychological distress.

The second-order model, on the other hand, captures not only the facets but also the general factor underlying them. The researcher may consider the four health facets to be manifestations of the common construct (psychological distress), which represent specific features that go beyond this common view/summary. For example, the individual facets may have differential prognostic significance. In such a framework, it certainly makes sense to estimate and report individual scores on the four "subscales," and the second-order model is well suited to this purpose.

In the bifactor model, no familiar "subscale" scores are estimated in addition to the general factor. Instead, group factors are estimated, which capture residual variance after the general factor has been accounted for. Although not commonly used, these residual scores can be also considered in applied research. We expect to see them exploited in longitudinal studies with repeated PRO measures, in parallel with examining a process of change in general score values.

The second-order model would be the model of choice for understanding the GHQ-28 from the perspective that gave rise to its four-subscale structure and the perspective of its classical scoring. If, however, the researcher believes that all individual variation is caused by the general psychological distress continuum, and common content shared by the items within each subscale is in fact a "method" factor related to specific manifestation of distress symptoms, the bifactor model is more suitable. It might also be the case that only *some* of the group factors are interpretable as method factors.[5]

REFERENCES

Ackerman, T.A. (2005). Multidimensional item response theory modeling. In A. Maydeu-Olivares & J.J. McArdle (Eds.), *Contemporary psychometrics* (pp. 3–26). Mahwah, NJ: Lawrence Erlbaum Associates.

Bock, R.D. (1975). *Multivariate statistical methods in behavioral research.* New York: McGraw-Hill.

Bock, R.D., Gibbons, R., Schilling, S.G., Muraki, E., Wilson, D.T., & Wood, R. (2003). *TESTFACT 4.0 user's guide.* Chicago, IL: Scientific Software International.

Brown, A., & Maydeu-Olivares, A. (2011). Item response modeling of forced-choice questionnaires. *Educational and Psychological Measurement, 71*(3), 460–502.

Croudace, T.J., Evans, J., Harrison, G., Sharp, D.J., Wilkinson, E., McCann, G., Spence, M., Crilly, C., & Brindle, L. (2003). Impact of the ICD-10 Primary Health Care (PHC) diagnostic and management guidelines for mental disorders on detection and outcome in primary care: Cluster randomised controlled trial. *British Journal of Psychiatry, 182*, 20–30.

Dodd, B.G., De Ayala, R.J., & Koch, W.R. (1995). Computerized adaptive testing with polytomous items. *Applied Psychological Methods, 19*, 5–22.

Du Toit, M. (Ed.). (2003). *IRT from SSI.* Chicago, IL: Scientific Software International.

Embretson, S.E., & Reise, S. (2000). *Item response theory for psychologists.* Mahwah, NJ: Lawrence Erlbaum Associates.

Fayers, P.M., & Machin, D. (2007). *Quality of Life: The assessment, analysis and interpretation of patient-reported outcomes. Second edition.* John Wiley & Sons.

5 Acknowledgments: The authors are grateful to Marcus Richards of the MRC Unit for Lifelong Health and Ageing for allowing us to use the GHQ-28 data for the numerical example. Work on this chapter was supported by a grant from the Isaac Newton Trust (grant number RG63087) awarded to the first author, and by a grant from the Wellcome Trust (grant number 088869/Z/09/Z) awarded to the second author.

Fisher, R.A. (1921). On the mathematical foundations of theoretical statistics. *Philosophical Transactions A, 222*, 309–368.
Gibbons, R.D., Bock, R.D., Hedeker, D., Weiss, D.J., Segawa, E., Bhaumik, D.K., Kupfer, D.J., Frank, E., Grochocinski, V.J., & Stover, A. (2007). Full-information item bifactor analysis of graded response data. *Applied Psychological Measurement, 31*, 4–19.
Gibbons, R.D., Immekus, J.C., & Bock, R.D. (2007). The added value of multidimensional IRT models. Didactic workbook. Retrieved on June 1, 2011 from http://outcomes.cancer.gov/areas/measurement/multidimensional_irt_models.pdf.
Goldberg, D.P. (1972). *The detection of psychiatric illness by questionnaire*. London: Oxford University Press.
Goldberg, D.P., Gater, R., Sartorius, N., Ustun, T.B., Piccinelli, M., Gureje, O., & Rutter, C. (1997). The validity of two versions of the GHQ in the WHO study of mental illness in general health care. *Psychological Medicine, 27*, 191–197.
Goldberg, D.P., & Hillier, V.F. (1979). A scaled version of the General Health Questionnaire. *Psychological Medicine, 9*, 139–145.
Goldberg, D.P., & Williams, P. (1988). *A user's guide to the general health questionnaire*. NFER Nelson: Windsor.
Green, B.F., Bock, R., Humphreys, L.G., Linn, R.L., & Reckase, M.D. (1984). Technical guidelines for assessing computerized adaptive tests. *Journal of Educational Measurement, 21*, 347–360.
Masters, G.N., & Wright, B.D. (1997). The partial credit model. In W.J. van der Linden & R. Hambleton (Eds.), *Handbook of modern item response theory*. New York: Springer-Verlag.
McDonald, R.P. (1999). *Test theory: A unified approach*. Mahwah, NJ: Lawrence Erlbaum Associates.
McDonald, R.P. (2011). Measuring latent quantities. *Psychometrika, 76*(4), 511–536.
Muthén, B., du Toit, S.H.C., & Spisic, D. (1997). *Robust inference using weighted least squares and quadratic estimating equations in latent variable modeling with categorical and continuous outcomes*. Unpublished manuscript, College of Education, UCLA. Los Angeles, CA.
Muthén, L.K., & Muthén, B.O. (1998–2010). *Mplus user's guide. Sixth edition*. Los Angeles, CA: Muthén & Muthén.
Reckase, M. (2009). *Multidimensional item response theory*. New York: Springer.
Reise, S., & Haviland, M. (2005). Item response theory and the measurement of clinical change. *Journal of Personality Assessment, 84*(3), 228–238.
Rindskopf, D., & Rose, T. (1988). Some theory and applications of confirmatory second-order factor analysis. *Multivariate Behavioral Research, 23*, 51–67.
Samejima, F. (1969). *Estimation of latent ability using a response pattern of graded scores* (Psychometric Monograph No. 17). Richmond, VA: Psychometric Society. Retrieved from www.psychometrika.org/journal/online/MN17.pdf.
Thissen, D., & Orlando, M. (2001). Item response theory for items scored in two categories. In D. Thissen & H. Wainer (Eds.), *Test scoring*. Mahwah, NJ: Lawrence Erlbaum Associates.
Van der Linden, W.J., & Hambleton, R. (1997). Item response theory: Brief history, common models and extensions. In W.J. van der Linden & R. Hambleton (Eds.), *Handbook of modern item response theory*. New York: Springer-Verlag.
Wadsworth, M.E., Butterworth, S.L., Hardy, R.J., Kuh, D.J., Richards, M., Langenberg, C., Hilder, W.S., & Connor, M. (2003). The life course prospective design: An example of benefits and problems associated with the study of longevity. *Social Science and Medicine, 57*, 2193–2205.

16 Developing Item Banks for Patient-Reported Health Outcomes

Dennis A. Revicki, Wen-Hung Chen, and Carole Tucker

Introduction

Over the past 30 years, health outcome assessments have been increasingly used in clinical trials and clinical practice settings. Health outcomes assessment is now commonly incorporated into clinical practice and patient health care. In clinical trials and comparative effectiveness research studies, health outcomes assessments are used to demonstrate treatment effectiveness (Ahmed et al., 2012). Health outcomes are also playing a larger role in health system performance assessments by providing critical information on health care quality from the consumer perspective (National Quality Forum, 2013). However, for years, the development of health outcomes assessments was not systematic or consistent, and multiple assessments for different purposes and of varying quality have been developed. Many instruments were developed to meet the immediate needs of a specific clinical study or clinical development program, and often multiple instruments covering the same health domains were simultaneously developed by competing health outcomes researchers. The development of item banks using item response theory (IRT) methods for different health domains provides a way to standardize the health outcomes assessment by drawing from a pool of items that are systematically and consistently developed and that have scores on a standardized metric (Cella et al., 2007; Cella et al., 2010). In addition, a tailored health outcomes assessment can be developed using a subset of items from an item bank so that the assessment is more efficient and less burdensome to patients yet retains adequate precision.

This chapter discusses the necessary components to develop and evaluate the measurement qualities of an item bank. The chapter includes examples from completed research and development activities from the Patient Reported Outcomes Measurement Information System (PROMIS®) network, sponsored by the National Institutes of Health. First, a clear and well-defined health concept needs to be developed because this conceptual framework (content map) provides the fundamental structure for the item bank. Second, factor analyses and item response theory analyses are applied to determine an optimal set of items for the item bank. This chapter summarizes the systematic process used to develop the conceptual framework through qualitative methods, and to describe the item bank construction and calibration phases through quantitative evaluation.

Conceptual Framework

As with the development of any measure that includes a patient-reported outcome (PRO), the initial step in development is identifying the conceptual framework for the item bank. This conceptual framework, or item map, provides a representation of the content of the item bank. The conceptual framework needs to capture the range of experience intended

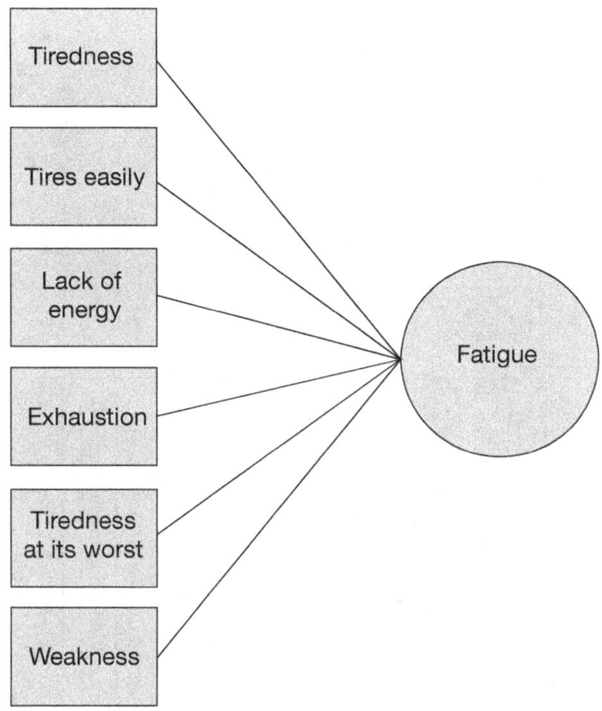

Figure 16.1 Conceptual framework for Anemia Impact Measure Fatigue Scale.

to be reflected in the item bank. The conceptual framework for an item bank is generated based on information from the health-related literature and clinician and patient input (see later in this chapter). An example of the conceptual framework underlying the Anemia Impact Measure (AIM) fatigue experience scale is shown in Figure 16.1 (Kleinman et al., 2012). As can be seen, the tiredness, weakness, lack of energy, and other items fit into the concept of fatigue from the patients' perspective.

The complete PROMIS® domain framework includes physical, mental, and social health (Cella et al., 2010; Riley et al., 2010). This tripartite framework is consistent with the health framework defined by the World Health Organization (World Health Organization, 1958). The PROMIS® domain framework is depicted in Figure 16.2. For example, in the PROMIS® project, emotional distress was conceptualized as including depression, anxiety, and anger domains (Pilkonis, 2011), and the physical function item bank included lower and upper extremity and central neck and back subdomains (Fries, Krishnan, Rose, Lingala, & Bruce, 2011). The conceptual framework for the PROMIS® health domains was originally established based on review of the health outcomes and medical literature, patient qualitative research, and interviews with clinicians and health outcomes researchers. The conceptual framework and item bank content was subsequently rigorously reviewed, and revisions were made to the conceptual framework (Cella et al., 2010; Riley et al., 2010), with more recent revisions made in 2012 (www.nihpromis.org).

Research Methods

Qualitative Item Bank Development

Qualitative development needs to be carefully and systematically conducted to assure and provide evidence of the content validity of a new item bank (Brod, Tesler, & Christensen,

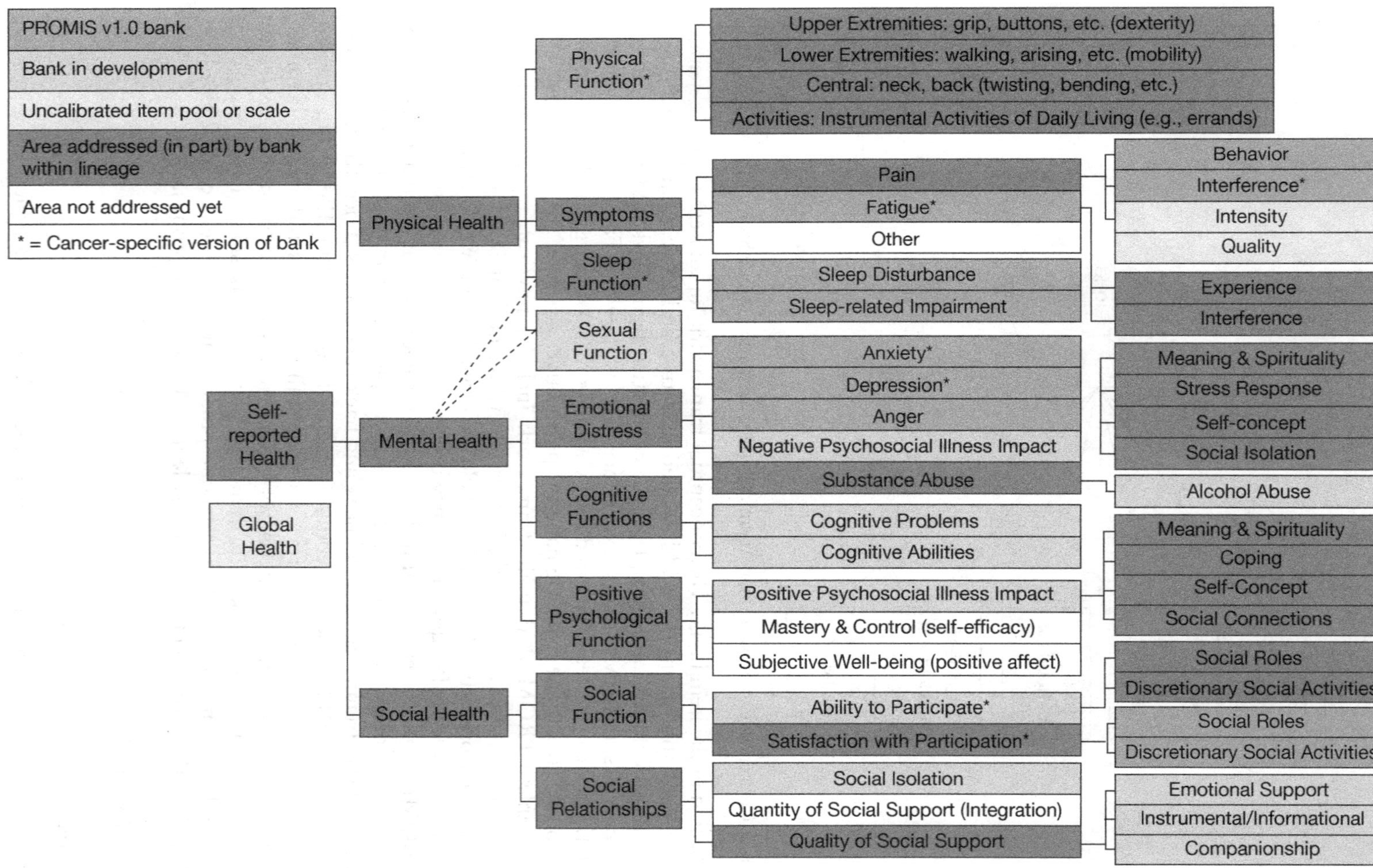

Figure 16.2 PROMIS® conceptual framework.

2009; Lasch et al., 2010; Magasi et al., 2012). Focus groups and cognitive interview study methods are described and examples are provided based on the development research conducted as part of PROMIS® and other projects. This section summarizes the steps in using the qualitative data, combined with information from existing health outcomes instruments, to develop and populate the pool of potential questions for the item bank. Attention to response scales and recall period, depending on the health domain, are also discussed.

The initial stage of item bank development begins with populating the conceptual framework with possible item content. The main sources of potential items are previously developed and published items in the same domain or content area and qualitative interviews. A systematic literature search should be conducted to identify and select possible items for the new item bank. In the PROMIS® project, investigators reviewed the health outcomes, psychological, and medical literature to identify instruments that assessed the target domain (e.g., fatigue, physical function, pain interference, etc.). Given that thousands of items may be initially identified, a system for organizing and evaluating the items is needed. Therefore, the identified items were pooled and a systematic process of "binning and winnowing" was completed followed by item revision, focus group exploration of domain coverage, cognitive interviews on individual items, and final revision before field testing (DeWalt, Rothrock, Yount, Stone, & P.C. Group, 2007).

Binning

Binning refers to a systematic process for grouping items according to content and the specific latent construct (DeWalt et al., 2007). By grouping items systematically, the item bank developer can identify redundancy among different content-relevant items and identify the best potential items based on qualitative characteristics. In the PROMIS® project, the binning of items was accomplished by the domain work groups and the bins were based on previous factor analyses of domain items and theory-based studies of the domain structure. Items that did not fit an existing bin were set aside and reviewed, and new bins were subsequently defined based on emergent groups of these items. Single items that did not fit within a bin were reviewed by content experts, placed within an existing bin, or recorded for possible inclusion later in the conceptual framework. The final set of items in each of the bins was then reviewed to ensure content coverage.

Winnowing

Winnowing refers to the process used to reduce the large item pool to a smaller representative set of items that are consistent with each domain definition and to reduce item redundancy in each domain. Each item was systematically reviewed by two to three team members based on a set of criteria. The specific criteria were:

1. Item content was inconsistent with domain definition.
2. Item was semantically redundant with another item.
3. Item content was too narrow to be universally applicable.
4. Stem of the item was disease specific, reducing general applicability.
5. Item content was confusing.

In the PROMIS® project, across all health domains, about 30 percent of items were removed because of redundancy and about 45 percent of the items were removed because they did not fit within the domain definitions and structure (DeWalt et al., 2007). During the winnowing process, multiple researchers within the domain workgroup reviewed the items and the decisions about eliminating or including specific items within each domain. For example, in the fatigue item bank the question "How much have you gotten fatigued easily?" was determined to be redundant with other items and was removed, because these other items covered the same concept using simpler language. The item "Do you feel much too much tiredness with normal or soft efforts?" was reviewed and deleted because the content of the item was considered confusing. This process of binning and winnowing resulted in a smaller set of items that was more representative of the structure and definition of each health domain.

Focus Groups

As for any PRO, participant qualitative research is needed to ensure that the individual's experiences with the targeted health domain are covered adequately in the item bank (Brod et al., 2009; Lasch et al., 2010; Magasi et al., 2012; Strauss & Corbin, 1998). Focus group sessions assist the item bank developer to understand and determine the vocabulary and experiences of the targeted group to help inform the development of the domain item bank. The information from focus groups and individual concept elicitation interviews can confirm the domain definitions, identify common language for describing concepts, and identify important gaps in coverage of the targeted domains and concepts. Finally, it is important to cover the patient experience with each domain to ensure that the patient perspective is included in the content of the item banks. Although the PROMIS® project used focus groups for concept elicitation, individual interviews can also be used to identify relevant item bank content for the targeted domain.

A key challenge in developing item banks that will be applied across demographic groups and diseases relates to selecting participants for the focus groups. To adequately cover the experience of all individuals across different demographic and disease groups would likely require thousands of participants, which is not practical. Therefore, some sort of targeting needs to be applied to make sure that age, gender, and racial/ethnic diversity is achieved and that a range of chronic illnesses is covered.

For the PROMIS® project, where multiple item banks were developed to assess multiple domains, three to five focus groups were organized for each domain, except for emotional distress, which held 13 focus groups given the number of domains (i.e., depression, anxiety, anger, alcohol abuse) (DeWalt et al., 2007). Participants were recruited from general medical clinics, outpatient psychiatry clinics, arthritis registries, rehabilitation centers, and schools for the pediatric domains. An attempt was made to achieve diversity in gender, age, and racial/ethnic group diversity (see Table 16.1). Semi-structured interviews were also used to develop concepts within some of the pediatric PROMIS® projects as an alternative approach to focus groups. For these interviews, a script was developed and interviewers were trained to maximally elicit the range of the child's experience within the domains (Forrest et al., 2012).

PROMIS® investigators moderated the focus groups and the participants discussed the range of their experience with the targeted domain (e.g., fatigue, pain, physical function, etc.). After the completion of the focus groups or the interviews, content analysis was performed on the transcripts, investigator notes, and recall of the discussions. The content analysis identified key words and phrases, emergent themes for each domain, and areas incompletely addressed in the domains. This information was then used to enrich and expand the item pools and to revise items to better cover the content from the patient's perspective.

Table 16.1 PROMIS® Network Focus Group Participant Characteristics for Five Health Domains

	Domains				
	Emotional Distress	*Fatigue*	*Social Function*	*Physical Function*	*Pain*
Number groups	13	3	5	3	4
Total participants	104	17	31	15	24
Female, %	50%	65%	65%	80%	79%
Race, %					
White	57%	94%	65%	94%	88%
African American	38%	6%	29%	0%	8%
Other	6%	0%	6%	7%	4%
Hispanic, %	2%	0%	0%	7%	0%
Age, Mean (range)	50 (23–88)	48 (26–65)	53 (23–83)	56 (31–86)	61 (26–76)
Education, %					
<11th grade	5%	6%	3%	7%	0%
High school	18%	18%	19%	13%	25%
Some college	33%	29%	45%	13%	46%
College degree	28%	24%	13%	40%	13%
Advanced degree	16%	24%	19%	27%	17%

Source: DeWalt et al. (2007).

Item Revision, Response Options, and Recall Periods

After the binning and winnowing process and the focus groups, the domain workgroups each had a set of items covering the domain content. However, the set of items included a variety of phrases, recall time frames, response options, and literacy demands (DeWalt et al., 2007). This variation in item content and style would make it difficult to administer as a coherent measure or computerized adaptive test (CAT). The domain item set was then revised to provide a uniform format, make the item content understandable to a range of literacy levels, and minimize ambiguity and cognitive difficulty. A sixth-grade reading level was targeted for all item content in the adult banks, and a third-grade reading level in most pediatric banks. Item stems were revised to be single-barreled (one concept being queried) and grammatically simple. Consideration was also given to consistency in both tense and person within a given item bank.

Next, it is necessary to determine the response options for the items in the domain item bank. For health outcome domains, the variety of different response options can be classified into categories of frequency, duration, intensity, and capability. For any domain item bank, the response scale needs to fit the construct being assessed and make cognitive sense to the respondent. For an item bank, it is important that there is a consistent set of response options and number of response levels within the bank. For item banks, four-to six-level response scales allow for a range of responses and work well for IRT analyses (Bode, Lai, Cella, & Heinemann, 2003). However, more research is needed on response scales and number of response scale levels (Preston, Reise, Cai, & Hays, 2011).

In the PROMIS® project, after review of different response options and psychometric considerations, a small set of different response options were specified (DeWalt et al., 2007) (Table 16.2), which has been further expanded as the number of item banks has grown (www.nihpromis.org). The set of different possible recall periods allowed for flexibility and uniformity among the PROMIS® item banks. The uniformity across different PROMIS® item banks has been key to ensure consistent response options for the profile instruments that use items from several different banks. Most of the PROMIS® item banks used one or more of these response options. The pain behavior item bank used frequency response options, and added, based on cognitive interviews, the response option "*had no pain*" (response scale: 1 (*had no pain*) to 6 (*always*)) (Revicki, Chen, Harnam, et al., 2009).

Finally, the recall period needs to be specified. A variety of recall periods can be used from the past 24 hours, past seven days, past two weeks, or past four weeks. Most important, the recall period needs to fit the health domain. The decision about recall period is complex and there is not much guidance on the best way to select a recall period. For example, there is research evidence that identifies problems associated with respondent recall of health and other concepts related to memory and cognitive heuristics for recalling experiences (Bradburn, Rips, & Shevell, 1987; Erskine, Morley, & Pearce, 1990; Gorin & Stone, 2001; Menon & Yorkston, 2000; Redelmeier & Kahneman, 1996; Robinson & Clore, 2002; Schwartz & Sudman, 1994). Recall accuracy may be improved if a single-day interval is used, but this result may lack generalizability if that particular day was different than most days. Longer recall periods provide a broader report of the behavior, symptom, or experience of interest, but often tend to more heavily weight the most recent days and "estimate" the previous days. This can add to the respondent's cognitive burden by requiring more thought to estimate and recall.

For example, during the development of the AIM, a 24-hour recall period was determined for the anemia-related symptoms (i.e., fatigue, feeling lightheaded, etc.) as symptom experience may vary considerably day to day, while for the daily activities, social activities, cognitive function, and emotions subscales, a seven-day recall period was specified (Kleinman et al., 2012).

For most of the PROMIS® domains, a seven-day recall period was selected. This recall period was selected because it is short enough to minimize biases due to memory and long

Table 16.2 Response Option Examples for PROMIS® Item Banks

Category	*Response Options*	
Intensity	None	Not at all
	Mild	A little bit
	Moderate	Somewhat
	Severe	Quite a bit
	Very severe	Very much
Frequency	Never	Never
	Rarely	Once a week or less
	Sometimes	Once every few days
	Often	Once a day
	Always	Every few hours

Source: DeWalt et al. (2007).

enough to have ecological validity. The main focus was to minimize the patient recall biases, but to have a recall period sufficient to capture experiences that were clinically relevant for health outcomes research. However, not all the PROMIS® domains use a seven-day recall period. For example, the sexual dysfunction domain uses a 30-day recall period, as this longer time period allows for the respondent to experience several sexual events and activities in order to be able to complete the questions (Flynn et al., 2013). The adult physical function domain items do not include any recall period, as the developers considered that function was assessed by self-reported capability rather than self-reported performance (Fries et al., 2011).

Cognitive Interviews

After final revisions to the item content, response scales, and recall period, a cognitive interview study is needed to make certain that respondents understand the meaning of the questions and how to make a response. Cognitive interviewing can be conducted using a variety of techniques, although most studies incorporate a retrospective verbal probing method (Willis, 2005). In retrospective verbal probing, participants are asked to read and complete the item, and then an interviewer asks the participant questions about their understanding of the item content and response scale.

Cognitive interviewing is an integral part of the PRO instrument development process and is essential for ensuring the content validity of the resulting instrument or item bank. Cognitive interviewing examines whether the respondent understands the instrument's instructions, item content, and response scales. Cognitive interviewing focuses on the respondent's comprehension of the item stem and content, the process the respondent uses to retrieve relevant information from memory, decision processes (e.g., social desirability, motivation), and response processes.

The usual process for cognitive interviewing starts with the respondent completing the items or instrument. Next, trained interviewers use a script to query the respondent for other specific information relevant for each item, that is, they probe systematically into the basis for each response (Willis, 2005). Cognitive debriefing studies often include small samples (N = 10–30) depending on the number of items and the complexity of the PRO measure. Often, an iterative approach is taken where each item of the draft instrument is reviewed by 5 to 10 participants, and then revisions, if necessary, are made to the instrument and additional cognitive interviews are completed. The process continues until no further changes are required for the item bank or instrument. The qualitative data from the cognitive interviews are content analyzed to identify misunderstandings, absence of comprehension, and other problems with the item stems and response scales.

For example, in the development of the Anemia Impact Measure (Kleinman et al., 2012), based on the cognitive interviews, the instructions were changed. "Please complete the daily diary every evening after you have eaten dinner" was revised to "Please complete the daily diary every evening at approximately the same time." This was done because patients with chemotherapy-induced anemia reported eating dinner at different times or not eating dinner at all on some days. Also, based on the interviews, the stem of all symptom impact items was changed to read "To what extent during the past 7 days" to improve comprehension of the participants. Several items were also modified based on the cognitive interviews; for example, "Did you need to rest during the day?" was changed to "Did you need to rest more during the day?" The results of cognitive interviewing provide guidance to the item bank developers as to necessary revisions that will ensure comprehension and understanding of the item bank instructions, item content, and response scales.

In the PROMIS® project, sets of 30 items were developed and each item was evaluated by five respondents using cognitive interviewing methods (DeWalt et al., 2007). Trained interviewers used the retrospective verbal probing method for this cognitive debriefing. The small sample size was selected for practical reasons, and each item was reviewed by at least two participants with one of the following: a) education less than high school, b) reading level less than ninth grade, or c) cognitive impairment diagnosis. Interviews were conducted in the South, Northeast, Midwest, and Western regions of the United States. Table 16.3 provides a summary of the demographic characteristics of the PROMIS® adult cognitive interviewing participants by domain. Final revisions to the questions were made, as needed, based on the results of the cognitive interviews. The resulting item banks for the various domains were then ready for field testing and psychometric analyses.

Quantitative Evaluation

Once a draft item bank is developed and available for field testing, it is necessary to collect data to enable psychometric evaluation. Ideally, the data collected for psychometric evaluation will be from the general population to allow for normative scoring and interpretation. A sufficiently large sample is necessary at this stage for evaluating dimensionality, item parameters, model fit, differential item functioning, reliability, validity, and responsiveness.

The recommended sample size for psychometric testing depends on the complexity of domain structure and number of items in an item bank. For most item banks, a sample size of 500 is probably reasonable, and a rule of thumb of 10 participants per item makes

Table 16.3 PROMIS® Network Cognitive Interview Study Participant Characteristics for Five Health Domains

	Domains				
	Emotional Distress	*Fatigue*	*Social Function*	*Physical Function*	*Pain*
Total participants	33	22	21	18	44
Female, %	64%	55%	40%	67%	59%
Race, %					
White	76%	50%	71%	67%	82%
African American	38%	6%	29%	0%	8%
Other	2%	0%	0%	7%	0%
Hispanic, %	2%	0%	0%	7%	0%
Age, Mean (range)	50 (23–88)	48 (26–65)	53 (23–83)	56 (31–86)	61 (26–76)
Education, %					
<11th grade	5%	6%	3%	7%	0%
High school	18%	18%	19%	13%	25%
Some college	33%	29%	45%	13%	46%
College degree	28%	24%	13%	40%	13%
Advanced degree	16%	24%	19%	27%	17%

Source: DeWalt et al. (2007).

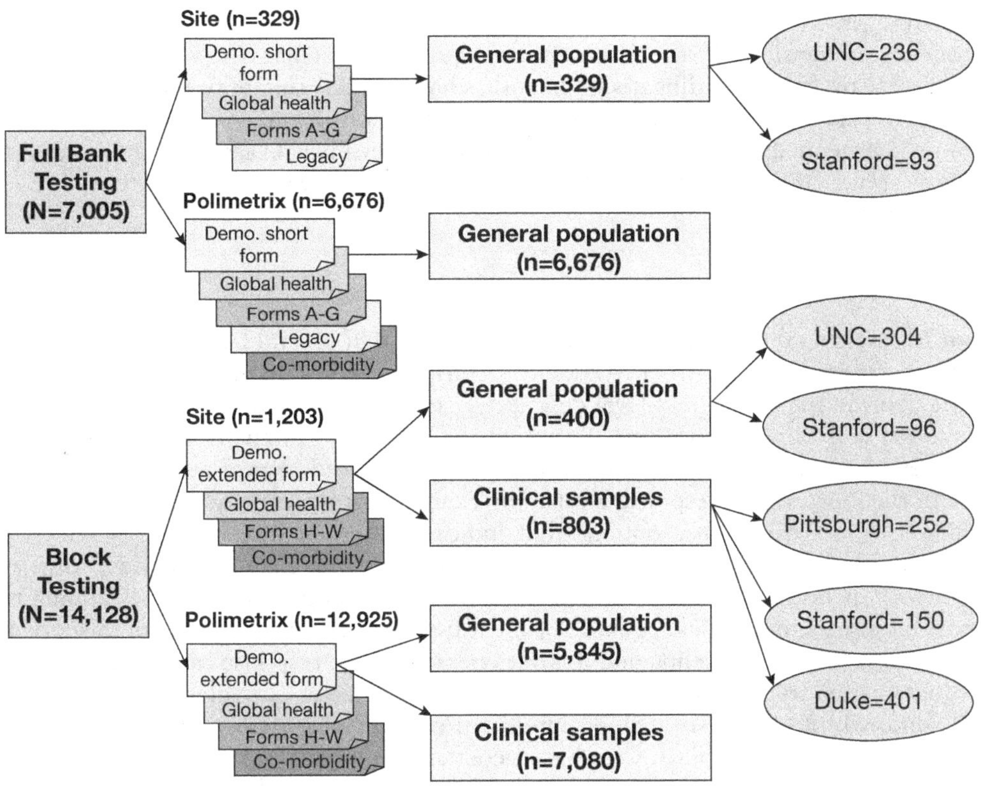

Figure 16.3 PROMIS® Wave 1 samples

psychometric sense. For the multi-domain PROMIS® I project, a sample size of more than 21,000 was recruited because of the large number of domains (14) and items within each domain, to minimize respondent burden, and for the planned psychometric analyses. Because of the number of item banks tested in PROMIS®, a complex data collection strategy was employed (see Figure 16.3). This strategy included two arms and a total sample size of 21,133. A total of 19,601 individuals were recruited by Polimetrix, with the remaining 1,532 recruited from selected PROMIS® primary research sites. Similarly, in the PROMIS® pediatric work, 12,488 children and 5,037 parents were recruited to assess the psychometric properties of the 10 new item banks. An additional 5,000 children and 7,500 parents were recruited for prospective norming of the pediatric item banks.

Unidimensionality

One critical assumption of IRT models relates to the unidimensionality of the set of items, that is, whether the items represent a single underlying construct. No set of items will ever perfectly meet strictly defined unidimensionality assumptions (McDonald, 1981; Reise et al., this volume). All health outcome data contain some multidimensionality. The objective is to assess whether scales are "essentially" or "sufficiently" unidimensional (McDonald, 1999; see also Chapter 2) to allow unbiased scaling of individuals on a common latent trait or construct. One important criterion is the robustness of item parameter estimates, which can be examined by removing items that may represent a significant secondary dimension. If the item parameters (in particular the item discrimination parameters or factor loadings) significantly change, then this may indicate insufficient unidimensionality (Drasgow & Parsons, 1983; Harrison, 1986). A number of researchers have recommended methods and considerations for evaluating essential unidimensionality (Lai et al., 2006; McDonald, 1981, 1999; Roussos & Stout, 1996; Stout, 1987; see also Chapter 2).

Classical Test Theory Methods to Assess Unidimensionality

Prior to assessing dimensionality, it is recommended that several basic classical test theory statistics are estimated in order to provide descriptive information about the performance of the items in the bank. Item-level descriptive statistics are useful for identifying patterns of skewed and missing responses. Based on the PROMIS® Network experience with the pain behavior item bank, it is essential to identify skewed response patterns and sparse data in the more severe response levels. For example, in the general population, few participants endorsed response options that indicated more frequent pain behaviors. Two distributions of responses were observed, one involving no pain and at least some pain, which was dichotomous, and then a more normal distribution of responses among those reporting some pain (Revicki et al., 2009). Clearly, response distributions of this type have implications for IRT modeling and analyses because some response categories may not be adequately used to provide robust and stable item parameter estimates (see Chapter 13).

Additional analyses may include inter-item correlations, item-scale correlations, and internal consistency reliability. Cronbach's coefficient alpha (Cronbach, 1951) can be used to examine internal consistency with 0.70 to 0.80 as an accepted minimum for group-level measurement and 0.90 to 0.95 as an accepted minimum for individual-level measurement (Hays & Revicki, 2005). Cronbach's alpha provides a measure of the reliability of the composite, which is influenced by all sources of common variance. With large item banks (i.e., > 20 items) of small to moderately correlated items, the coefficients are often very large even when subsequent factor analyses reveals significant multidimensionality. Based on PROMIS® and other experience (Cortina, 1993), coefficient alpha is not a very useful indicator of unidimensionality in health domain item banks.

Factor Analytic Methods to Assess Unidimensionality

Confirmatory factor analysis (CFA) is recommended to evaluate the extent that the item pool measures a dominant dimension that is consistent with the content experts' definition of the domain (Reeve et al., 2007). Exploratory factor analysis (EFA) is recommended and is often used as the first step to explore dimensionality. In very specific situations, CFA can be selected as the first step when the pool of items are carefully developed to represent a dominant construct based on an exhaustive literature review and qualitative research. However, in most cases it is advisable to start with EFA to understand potential multidimensionality in the item bank data. Because of the ordinal nature of the patient-reported outcome data, appropriate software (e.g., MPLUS (Muthén & Muthén, 1998) or LISREL (Jöreskog, Sörbom, & Du Toit, 2003)) should evaluate polychoric correlations using an appropriate estimator. Polychoric correlations are used because of the ordinal nature of the data. Recommendations from PROMIS® include weighted least squares with adjustments for the mean and variance estimator in MPLUS or diagonally weighted least squares estimator in LISREL for the confirmatory factor analysis.

The CFA model fit needs to be assessed by examining multiple indices. Given that statistical criteria like the chi-square statistic are sensitive to sample size, a range of practical fit indices needs to be examined such as the comparative fit index (CFI > 0.95 for good fit), root mean square error of approximation (RMSEA < 0.06 for good fit), Tucker-Lewis Index (TLI > 0.95 for good fit), standardized root mean residuals (SRMR < 0.08 for good fit), and average absolute residual correlations (< 0.10 for good fit) (Bentler, 1990; Browne & Cudeck, 1993; Hu & Bentler, 1999; Kline, 2010; McDonald, 1999; Reeve et al., 2007). However, these CFA fit indices do not always provide useful information on unidimensionality when alternative multidimensional structures may underlay the data (Reise et al., 2012).

EFA needs to be conducted to explore unidimensionality and to determine the multidimensional structure of the data. The magnitude of eigenvalues for the larger factors (at least 20 percent of the variability on the first factor is especially desirable), differences in the magnitude of eigenvalues between factors, scree test, parallel analysis, correlations among factors, and factor loadings may be inspected to determine the underlying structural patterns. The concept of simple structure needs to be considered in interpreting the derived factor structure. Simple structure is present when items load primarily on only one factor, with minimum loadings on other factors in an EFA.

An alternate method to determine whether the items are "sufficiently" unidimensional is the bifactor item factor analysis model (Gibbons, Hedeker, & Bock, 1992; McDonald, 1999). The bifactor approach to assessing unidimensionality is to assign each item to a specific subdomain based on theoretical considerations. A model is then fit with each item loading on a common factor and on a specific subdomain ("group" factor). The common factor is defined by all the items, while each subdomain is defined by subsets of items in the bank. The factors are constrained to be mutually uncorrelated so that all covariance is partitioned either into loadings on the common factor or onto the subdomain factors. If the standardized loadings on the common factor are all salient (i.e., greater than 0.30) and substantially larger than loadings on the group factors, the item bank is considered to be "sufficiently homogeneous" (McDonald, 1999). In addition, the researcher can compare individual scores under a bifactor and unidimensional model. If scores are highly correlated (e.g., $r > 0.90$), this provides further evidence that the effects of multidimensionality are ignorable (Reise & Haviland, 2005).

For example, a single factor CFA was fit to the PROMIS® pain interference and pain behavior item banks (Amtmann et al., 2010; Revicki et al., 2009). Table 16.4 summarizes the fit statistics for the two item banks. Clearly, there is evidence supporting essential unidimensionality for both item banks. In addition, the first extracted factor in an exploratory

Table 16.4 Confirmatory Factor Analysis Goodness of Fit Statistics for PROMIS® Pain Interference and Pain Behavior Item Banks

	Pain Interference	*Pain Behavior*
Number of items	41	52
CFI	0.97	0.90
TLI	0.99	0.99
RMSEA	0.175	0.156
SRMRR	0.033	0.035

Source: Revicki et al. (2009); Amtmann et al. (2010).

factor analysis accounted for 86 percent and 90 percent of the variance for pain interference and pain behavior, respectively. The RMSEA values exceed recommended criteria; however, this finding is not surprising given that Cook, Kallen and Amtmann (2009) found that RMSEA values tend to be elevated when there are larger numbers of items, and that this statistic may not be appropriate for evaluating dimensionality of large item banks.

Caution should be exercised when interpreting fit based on the usual CFA fit indices (i.e., CFI, RMSEA, etc.), as they may indicate relatively good fit, when more multidimensional models may more likely fit the data. For example, Reise and colleagues (2012) demonstrated that the usual structural equation modeling fit indices such as CFI or SRMR routinely reject unidimensional measurement models even in contexts in which the structural coefficient bias is low. If there is any indication of multidimensionality, Reise and colleagues (2012) recommend examining factor strength indices (e.g., explained common variance, OmegaH) and applying bifactor models to determine if the data is sufficiently unidimensional for IRT analyses.

Local Independence

Local independence assumes that once the dominant factor influencing an individual's response to an item is controlled, there should be no significant association among item responses (Steinberg & Thissen, 1996; Wainer & Thissen, 1996; Yen, 1993). The presence of local dependence influences IRT parameter estimates and represents a problem for scale construction and computerized adaptive test (CAT) applications. Uncontrolled local dependence among items in a CAT assessment may result in a score unrelated to the PRO construct being assessed. Scoring respondents based on mis-specified models will result in inaccurate estimates of their level on the underlying trait (specifically, the standard errors will be too small). This problem occurs frequently in health outcomes measurement because of narrowly defined constructs and similar repeated items. For example, two items on current pain (i.e., How intense is your pain right now? What is your level of pain right now?) showed evidence of local dependency.

Identification of local dependence among polytomous response items includes examining the residual correlation matrix produced by the single factor CFA. High residual correlations (greater than 0.2) are flagged and considered for possible local dependence. In addition, IRT-based tests of local dependence can be utilized including Yen's (1984) Q3 statistic and Chen and Thissen's (1997) local dependence indices. These statistics are based on a process that involves fitting a unidimensional IRT model to the data, and then examining the residual covariation between pairs of items, which should be zero or near zero if the unidimensional model fits.

The modification indices (MIs) of structural equation modeling (SEM) software may also be used as statistics to detect local independence. When inter-item polychoric correlations are fitted with a one-factor model, the result is a limited information parameter estimation scheme for the graded normal ogive model. The MIs for such a model are one degree of freedom chi-square scaled statistics that suggest unmodeled excess covariation between items, which, in the context of item factor analysis, is indicative of local independence.

Items flagged as locally dependent are then examined to evaluate their potential effect on IRT parameter estimates. One test is to remove one of the locally dependent items, and to examine changes in IRT model parameter estimates and in factor loadings for all the other items.

To handle local dependence on item and person parameter estimates, one of the items can be removed from the item bank. If this is not feasible because both items provide a substantial amount of contextual information, then locally dependent items can be marked as "enemies," preventing them from being administered in a single assessment to any individual. Local dependence needs to be controlled in the calibration step to remove the influence of these highly correlated items. In all cases, the locally dependent items should be evaluated to understand the source and resultant impact of this dependency.

Monotonicity

In the context of health outcomes research, the assumption of monotonicity means that the probability of endorsing or selecting an item response indicative of better health status should increase as the underlying level of health increases. This is a basic requirement for IRT models of items with ordered response categories. Approaches for evaluating monotonicity include examining graphs of item mean scores conditional on "rest-scores" (i.e., total raw scale score minus the item score) using the MOKKEN package in R, or fitting a nonparametric IRT model (Ramsay, 1997) to the data that yields initial IRT probability curve estimates. A nonparametric IRT model fits trace lines for each response to an item without any a priori specification of the order of the responses. The data analyst then examines the fitted trace lines to determine which response alternatives are associated with lower levels of the domain and which are associated with higher levels. The shapes of the trace lines may also indicate other departures from monotonicity, such as bimodality. While nonparametric IRT may not be the most efficient way to produce the final item analysis and scores for a scale, this type of analysis can be very informative about the tenability of the assumptions of parametric IRT.

Item Calibration and Item Response Theory Model

Once the assumptions have been confirmed, IRT models are fit to the data for item and scale analysis as well as for item calibration. IRT refers to a family of models that describe, in probabilistic terms, the relationship between a person's response to a question and his or her level on the PRO latent construct (e.g., physical function, fatigue, etc.) that the scale measures (Embretson & Reise, 2000; Hambleton, Swaminathan, & Rogers, 1991). For every item in the item bank, item parameters are estimated. The item slope or discrimination parameter describes how well the item performs in the scale in terms of the strength of the relationship between the item and the underlying scale. The item difficulty or threshold parameters identify the location along the construct's latent continuum where the item best discriminates among individuals.

The PROMIS® network evaluated both a general IRT model—the graded response model (GRM; Samejima, 1969, 1997)—and two models based on the Rasch model framework—the partial credit model (Masters, 1982) and the rating scale model (Andrich, 1978; Wright & Masters, 1982). Based on these analyses, PROMIS® network recommended using the GRM in item bank development work. The GRM is a very flexible model of the parametric, unidimensional, polytomous-response IRT family of models. Because it allows discrimination to vary item by item, it typically fits response data better than a one-parameter model (Embretson & Reise, 2000; Thissen & Orlando, 2001). Compared to alternative models such as the generalized partial credit model, the GRM is relatively easy to understand and illustrate and retains its functional form when response categories are merged. The GRM offers a flexible framework for modeling the participant responses to examine item and scale properties, to calibrate the items of the item bank, and to score individual response patterns in the health outcomes assessment. In PROMIS®, other IRT models were fit as needed. For example, in the analysis of the pain behavior item bank, nominal and hybrid nominal and partial credit IRT models were examined (Revicki et al., 2009). The GRM was the primary IRT method used in PROMIS® (Cella et al., 2010).

The unidimensional GRM is a generalization of the IRT two-parameter logistic model for dichotomous response data. The GRM is based on the logistic function that describes, given the level of the trait being measured, the probability that an item response will be observed in *category k or higher*. For ordered responses $X = k$, $k = 1,2,3, \ldots, m_i$, where response m reflects the highest theta (latent ability) value, this probability is defined (Samejima, 1969, 1997; Thissen, 2001) as:

$$P(X_i = k|\theta, b_i, a_i) = \frac{1}{1+\exp\left[-a_i(\theta - b_{i,k-1})\right]} - \frac{1}{1+\exp\left[-a_i(\theta - b_{i,k})\right]}.$$

This function models the probability of observing each category as a function of the underlying construct. The subscript on m indicates that the number of response categories does not need to be equal across items. The discrimination (slope) parameter a_i varies by item i in a scale. The threshold parameters b_{ik} varies within an item with the constraint $b_{k-1} < b_k < b_{k+1}$, and represents the point on the theta axis where the probability passes 50 percent that the response is in category k or higher.

IRT model fit is assessed using a number of indices. Residuals between observed and expected response frequencies by item response category are compared, and the fit for different models is based on analyses of the relative magnitudes of the differences (residuals). IRTFIT (Bjorner et al., 2006) is used to assess model fit for each item and computes the extension of S-X^2 and S-G^2 for items with more than two responses (Orlando & Thissen, 2000, 2003). These statistics estimate the fit of the item responses to the IRT model, that is, whether the responses follow the pattern predicted by the model. Statistically significant differences indicate poor fit. The S-X^2 (a Pearson X^2 statistic) and S-G^2 (a likelihood ratio G^2 statistic) are fit statistics that use the sum score of all items and compare the predicted and observed response frequencies for each level of the scale sum score. The ultimate goal is to determine the extent to which misfit affects model performance in terms of the valid scaling of individual differences (Hambleton & Han, 2005).

For example, the IRT parameters and fit statistics for selected pain behavior items are summarized in Table 16.5 for participants who reported more than mild pain (Revicki et al., 2009). The item on "isolating myself from others" had a slope (a) of 2.71 and assessed a broad range of the construct of pain behavior. Although the item on "moving slowly" had a similar slope (2.67), a narrower range of the pain behavior construct was assessed.

Once the fit of the IRT model to the response data is considered satisfactory, attention is shifted to analyzing the item and scale properties of the PROMIS® domains. The psychometric properties of the items will be examined by review of their item parameter estimates, CRCs, and item information curves (Reeve, 2003; Reeve & Fayers, 2005). Information curves indicate the range of theta where an item best discriminates among individuals. Higher information indicates greater precision for measuring a person's domain level. The height of the curves (denoting more information) is a function of the discrimination power (*a* parameter) of the item. The location of the information curves is determined by the threshold (*b*) parameter(s) of the item. Information curves indicate which items are most useful for measuring different levels of the measured construct. The information curves for selected items from the PROMIS® pain behavior item bank are depicted in Figure 16.4.

Table 16.5 IRT Item Parameters and Fit Statistics for PROMIS® Pain Behavior Items, Excluding Subjects With 0 or 1 Global Pain Responses: Pooled WAVE-1 and ACPA Data (N = 9,589)

ID	*Item*	*Slope*[1]	*Category Threshold*[1]					*Item Fit Statistics*[2]				*df*
		A	*b1*	*b2*	*b3*	*b4*	*b5*	*S-G2*	*Prob_G2*	*S-X2*	*Prob_X2*	
PAINBE2	When I was in pain I became irritable	2.90	–2.16	–0.82	–0.07	0.81	1.64	55.97	0.2936	52.29	0.4236	51
PAINBE3	When I was in pain I grimaced	2.55	–2.24	–0.86	–0.03	1.02	2.03	46.83	0.6770	47.95	0.6338	52
PAINBE8	When I was in pain I moved extremely slowly	2.67	–2.22	–0.93	–0.18	0.68	1.49	59.31	0.2266	57.11	0.2911	52
PAINBE24	When I was in pain I moved stiffly	2.15	–2.37	–1.11	–0.42	0.57	1.48	73.67	0.0317	67.45	0.0875	53
PAINBE25	When I was in pain I called out for someone to help me	2.51	–2.01	0.58	1.25	2.07	2.83	35.09	0.8792	35.73	0.8625	46
PAINBE31	I limped because of pain	1.81	–2.41	–0.47	0.06	0.93	1.71	55.35	0.3859	55.70	0.3735	53
PAINBE37	When I was in pain I isolated myself from others	2.71	–2.26	–0.24	0.26	0.92	1.85	76.82	0.0039	64.82	0.0433	47

[1] Using IRT software MULTILOG (Thissen et al., 2002).
[2] Using SAS macros IRTFIT (Bjorner et al., 2006).
*Two highest response categories are collapsed for Items 40 and 41.

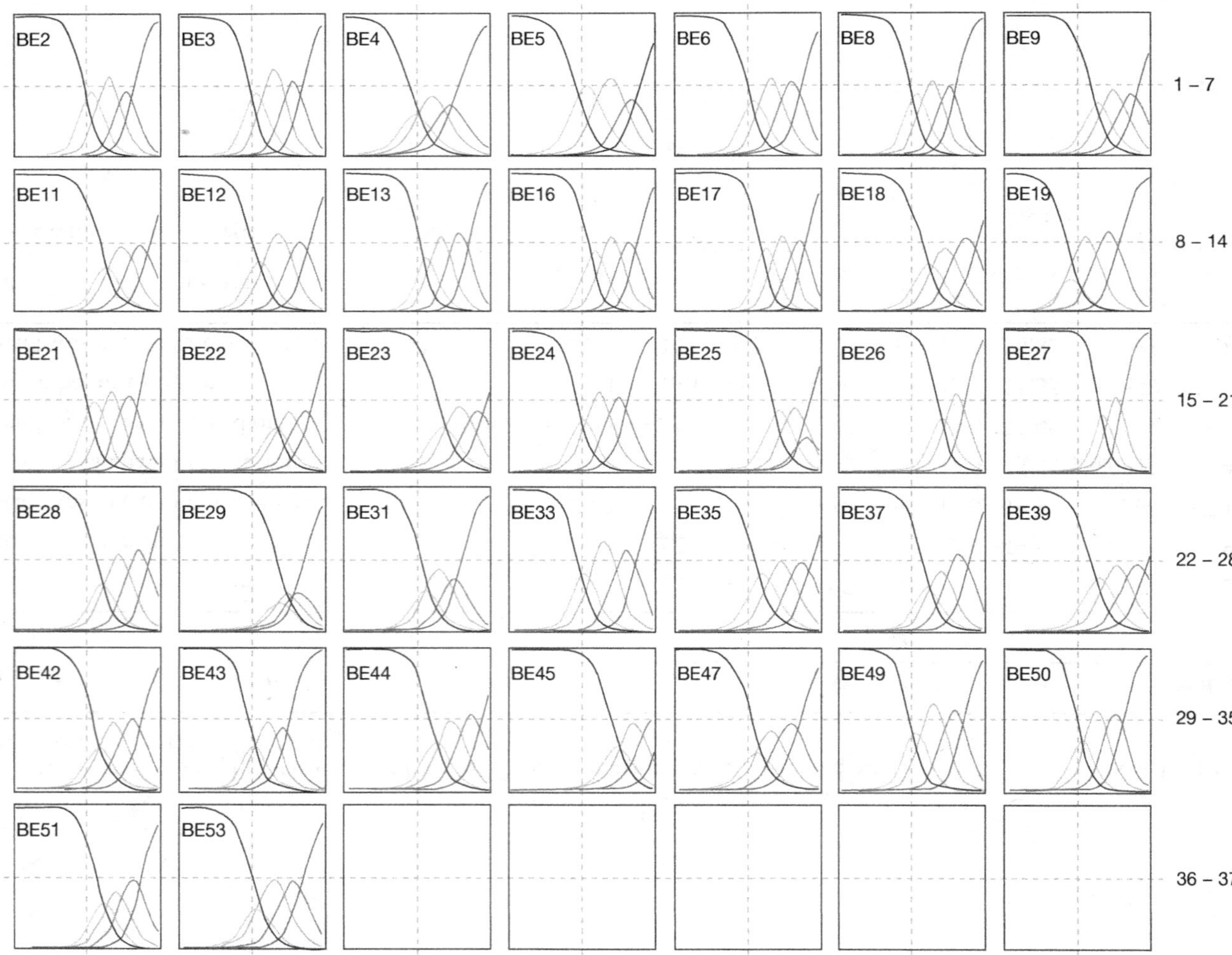

Figure 16.4 Category response curves for pain behavior items.

Poorly performing items are reviewed by content experts before the item bank is established. Misfitting items may be retained or revised when they are identified as clinically relevant and when alternative, better-fitting items are not available. Low discriminating items in the tails of the theta distribution (at low or at high levels of the construct being measured) may be retained or revised to add information for extreme scores though they would not have been retained in regions of the continuum better populated by items.

Differential Item Functioning

Differential item functioning (DIF) refers to the situation where members from different groups (i.e., age, gender, race, education, culture) on the same level of the latent trait have a different probability of giving a certain response to a particular item. DIF is a threat to the validity of any health outcome instrument. DIF occurs when subjects on the same level of the latent trait, such as disease severity, answer the same item differently depending on their group membership (Chang, 2005; Holland & Thayer, 1988). The concept of uniform and nonuniform DIF was first introduced by Mellenbergh (Mellenbergh, 1982). Uniform DIF occurs when the discrepancy between groups is constant across the range of the latent construct. Whereas, with nonuniform DIF, the discrepancy between groups differs depending on the level of the latent construct. The validity of the PRO measure may be compromised because the response to the item with DIF may be due to some external factor other than the intended construct. For example, crying spells is one of the symptoms of patients with depression, but this concept is endorsed more often by women than men with the same level of depression severity (Teresi et al., 2009). Therefore, the crying item is said to exhibit DIF due to gender for assessing depression.

DIF is a discrepancy between two groups of subjects in the conditional probability of a response to an item conditioned on the level of the latent construct. Because IRT consists of mathematical models already expressed as the conditional probability of a certain item response given the latent trait, its application to DIF detection is straightforward. Two methods commonly used for DIF detection for polytomous response items are the IRT log-likelihood ratio (IRTLR) (Cohen, Kim, & Wollack, 1996; Kim & Cohen, 1998; Thissen et al., 1986; Thissen et al., 1993) and ordinal logistic regression (Zumbo, 1999). The IRTLR is based on a multidimensional model of DIF that formally defines a second latent trait that contributes to the DIF. The ordinal logistic regression method of detecting DIF is a straightforward application of logistic regression modeling. Because an interaction term of latent trait by groups can be included in the model, the logistic regression method can be used to detect the nonuniform DIF directly. A method based on complex multiple indicators, multiple causes (MIMIC) confirmatory factor analysis model can also be used for DIF detection (Finch, 2005).

In the PROMIS® project, most of the domain item bank investigators used either ordinal logistic regression or IRTLR modeling; however, the investigators primarily used logistic regression and ordinal logistic regression using an observed conditioning score. A modification, IRTOLR (Crane, van Belle, & Larson, 2004; Crane, Gibbons, Jolley, & van Belle, 2006), was used in some analyses. Estimates from a latent variable IRT model, rather than the traditional observed score, are used as the conditioning variable; this method incorporates effect sizes into the uniform DIF detection procedure. This allows for DIF criteria specification, that is, statistical tests of uniform and nonuniform (Swaminathan & Rogers, 1992), or an effect size modification based on changes in the pseudo-R^2 in nested model (Zumbo, 1999).

An alternative method involving IRTLR likelihood ratio tests (Cohen et al., 1996; Kim & Cohen, 1998; Thissen et al., 1986; Thissen et al., 1993) in IRTLRDIF, MULTILOG (Thissen & Orlando, 2001; Thissen et al., 2002), and IRTPRO (Cai et al., 2011), can be used for DIF detection, accompanied by magnitude measures (Teresi, Kleinman, & Ocepek-Welikson, 2000), such as the non-compensatory DIF index (Flowers, Oshima, & Raju, 1999; Raju, Van Der Linden, & Fleer, 1995). Scale-level impact can be assessed using expected scale scores, expressed as group differences in the total test (scale) response functions, that show the extent to which DIF cancels at the scale level.

Given that numerous factors can impact DIF assessment, it is difficult to recommend a single, best method for evaluating DIF. However, generally, IRT-based methods are recommended. The best recommendation is to have a primary method and secondary method used for sensitivity analyses. Moreover, the magnitude of DIF should be assessed together with both scale and individual impact.

Multiple factors may impact DIF and the assessment of PROs. In many cases, differences in item responses are expected for members of different groups. An item may cover very important content for assessing a health outcome despite different groups of participants responding to it differently. In this case, the item should be retained in the item bank, but each individual's response should be compared within his or her reference group. This requires the item to be treated differently according to group membership, for example, different item scores between male and female. An ideal assessment of health outcomes involves tailoring the items to the unique characteristics of the individual for maximum information. This is possible by using CAT with a large item bank. In this case, items with DIF are no longer a threat to the validity of the test and become assets of the instrument.

Evaluating Psychometric Characteristics

The calibrated item bank can be used to develop dynamic (CAT) or fixed length static forms for application in clinical trials and other studies. As with any PRO measure, the measurement properties of the CAT or static forms need to be evaluated. The most relevant psychometric characteristics that need to be evaluated include test-retest reliability, construct validity, and responsiveness. While a comprehensive review of these measurement properties is beyond the scope of this chapter, we will briefly summarize each approach. More comprehensive reviews are available (De Vet, Terwee, Mokkink, & Knol, 2011; Fayers & Machin, 2007; Hays & Revicki, 2005; Nunnally & Bernstein, 1994).

Reliability

In classical test theory, the concept of reliability is at the scale score level. For IRT, the concept of reliability is conceptualized as "information" and examines measurement precision that can differ across the levels of a construct. The relationship between information and standard error (SE) is defined by the formula $SE(\theta) = 1/\sqrt{I(\theta)}$, where θ is the estimated trait level, SE is the standard error of θ, and I is information. As the formula indicates, increased scale information is associated with smaller SEs and, therefore, greater precision.

Figure 16.5 summarizes the standard errors over the range of pain behavior scores for the total item bank, a seven-item short form, and a seven-item computerized adaptive test (Revicki et al., 2009). For the full item bank, reliability is 0.90 or greater across most of the score distribution, and the short form and CAT have reliabilities exceeding 0.80 across the majority of the score distribution. In comparison, Cronbach's alpha for the full pain behavior item bank was 0.98.

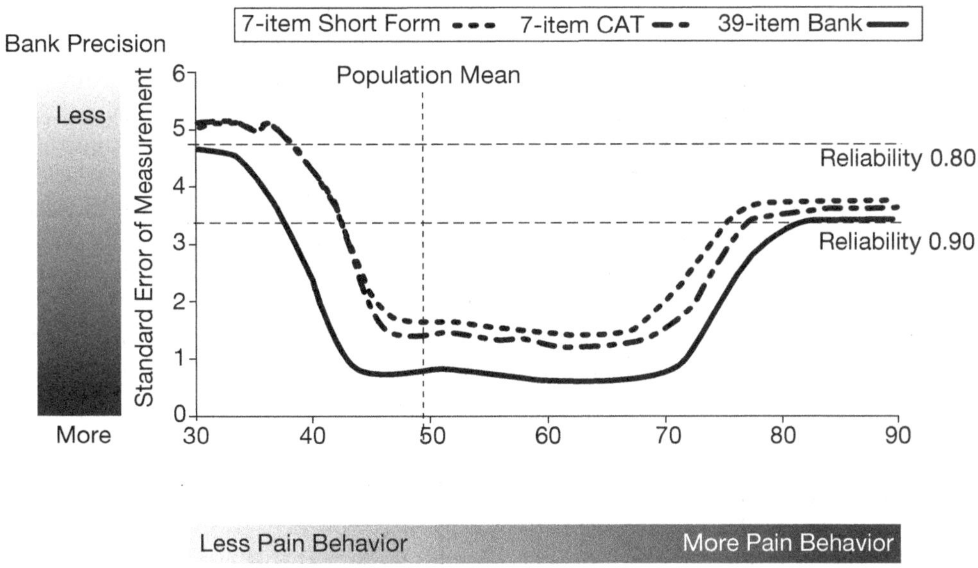

Figure 16.5 SEM for pain behavior item bank, short-form and CAT.

Test-Retest Reliability

Test-retest reliability, or reproducibility, is the relationship between scores obtained by the same individual on two or more separate occasions (Hays & Revicki, 2005). Most often test-retest reliability is tested over short periods of time (i.e., one to two weeks) in individuals who are not expected to change. Intraclass correlation coefficients (ICCs), based on one-way, two-way fixed, or two-way random analysis of variance models depending on data structure, are normally used to assess test-retest reliability (Hays & Revicki, 2005). For PROMIS® CAT and static scores, test-retest reliability is evaluated in a number of clinical samples. For example, the pain behavior domain scores are evaluated in patients with low back pain, osteoarthritis, and multiple sclerosis.

Currently, there is some evidence supporting the stability of the short form and CAT scales based on the PROMIS® item banks. Pilkonis and colleagues (2011) examined the test-retest reliability of the emotional distress and sleep function scales. Based on a seven- to 14-day period, test-retest reliability (ICCs) was 0.79 to 0.89 for anger, 0.85 to 0.86 for anxiety, 0.76 to 0.90 for depression, 0.89 to 0.93 for sleep disturbance, and 0.83 to 0.95 for sleep impairment. In a recent study, Bajaj and colleagues (2011) evaluated the psychometric characteristics of multiple PROMIS® CATs (i.e., anger, anxiety, depression, fatigue, physical function, pain interference, pain behavior, social activities, social roles, sleep disturbance, sleep impairment) in 200 patients diagnosed with cirrhosis. These investigators found that test-retest reliability (ICCs) ranged from 0.76 to 0.99 for the CAT scores over a 14-day interval.

Construct Validity

Validity represents the extent to which a PRO measure reflects what it is intended to measure rather than something else (Hays & Revicki, 2005; Nunnally & Bernstein, 1994). The process of evaluating the validity of PRO measures involves accumulating evidence that reflects the degree to which the measures denote what they were intended to represent. To evaluate construct validity, a series of hypotheses are generated as to how measures should "behave" and then observed data are used to test these hypotheses (Cronbach & Meehl, 1955). Hypotheses are stated regarding the direction (and sometimes the strength) of relationships that might be expected, and validity is supported when the associations are consistent with hypotheses. The evaluation of construct validity is iterative by its nature with empirical results accumulating to provide further support and increasing confidence in the validity of the PRO measure. The main types of validity assessed for PRO measures include concurrent, predictive, and known-groups validity.

Both concurrent and known-groups validity are being used to evaluate the measurement properties of the CAT and static form scores from the PROMIS® item banks (Cella et al., 2010; Rothrock et al., 2010). Concurrent validity, for most of the item banks, is evaluated by correlations with legacy instruments that assess comparable health outcome domains (Cella et al., 2010). Table 16.6 provides a summary of the concurrent validity findings for several of the PROMIS® domains. The PROMIS® pain interference scores were correlated with Brief Pain Inventory interference scores (Amtmann et al., 2010). The PROMIS® pain interference score was correlated 0.90 with the BPI pain interference scale, 0.48 with pain intensity, –0.84 with the SF-36 bodily pain scale, and 0.55 with PROMIS® physical function scores.

Known-groups validity, that is, whether the PRO score varies significantly by levels on a criterion variable (i.e., clinical severity) or some other characteristic, has been evaluated for many of the PROMIS® item bank scores (Cella et al., 2010). For example, pain interference and behavior scores have been compared by levels of pain intensity (Amtmann

Table 16.6 Concurrent Validity of Selected PROMIS® Domains

PROMIS® Domain		*Legacy Measure*
Physical Function		
–0.88		Health Assessment Questionnaire
0.88		SF-36 Physical Function Scale
Fatigue		
0.95		FACIT-Fatigue Scale
0.88		SF-36 Vitality Scale
Anxiety	**Depression**	
0.75	0.83	Center for Epidemiologic Studies-Depression Scale
0.80	0.72	Mood and Anxiety Symptom Questionnaire
Pain Interference		
0.81		Brief Pain Inventory-Severity Scale
0.85		Brief Pain Inventory—Interference Scale
–0.83		SF-36 Bodily Pain Scale
Sleep Disturbance		
0.85		Pittsburgh Sleep Quality index
0.70		Epworth Sleepiness Scale

et al., 2010; Revicki et al., 2009). PROMIS® pain behavior scores varied significantly by ratings of pain intensity with higher pain behavior scores in those with greater pain intensity numerical rating scale (NRS) (see Figure 16.6). Mean pain interference scores varied significantly by levels of general health status (see Figure 16.7). Rothrock and colleagues (2010) compared various PROMIS® domain scores by chronic disease groups and those without reported chronic diseases to evaluate the validity of the PROMIS® scores. The results indicated that across the different PROMIS® domains, the presence of chronic conditions was associated with more impaired scores compared with those without chronic medical conditions.

Responsiveness

Responsiveness is critical for clinical trial applications, and refers to the ability of a PRO measure to detect changes in health status in those individuals who are changing in clinical status (Hays & Revicki, 2005; Revicki et al., 2008). Responsiveness of health outcome assessments is evaluated by using anchor-based or distribution-based methods. However, the anchor-based methods provide the most insight into responsiveness with the distribution-based methods providing additional supportive information on the magnitude of effects. In the anchor-based approach, multiple relevant anchors are identified and changes in health outcome scores are evaluated by these anchors.

The selected anchors can be clinical measures (i.e., hemoglobin levels, clinician severity ratings, signs and symptoms, etc.) or other patient-reported measures (i.e., patient ratings of disease severity, other measures with known response scales and interpretation). Often, clinicians and patients are asked to rate the change in the patient's health

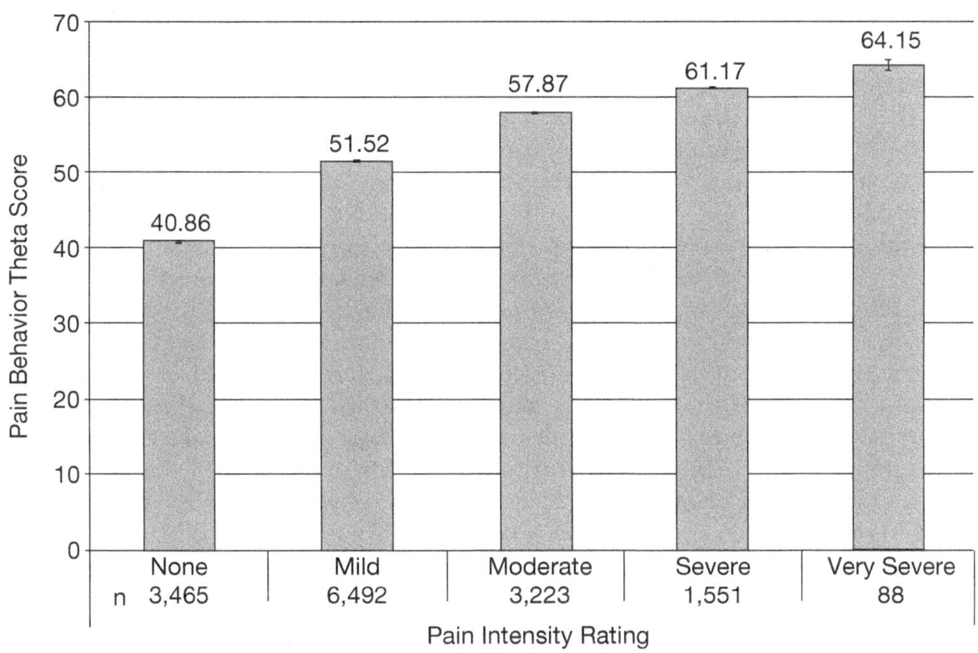

Figure 16.6 Mean pain behavior T-scores by pain intensity.

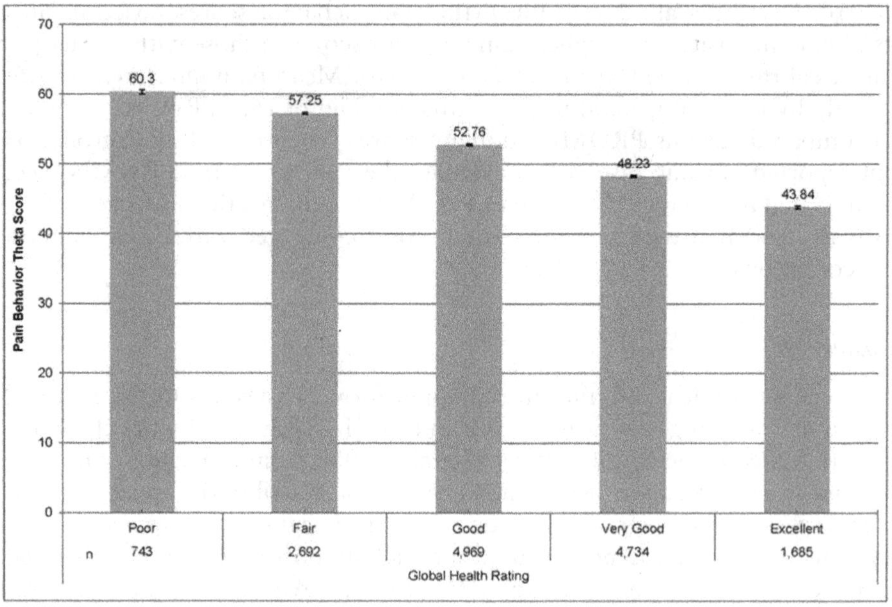

Figure 16.7 Mean pain interference T-scores by general health status.

status from baseline in a longitudinal study. However, limitations in recall for baseline health status may limit the usefulness of patient global ratings of change, and variations in clinician understanding of facets of the patient's health status may also limit the clinician ratings. Anchors should be correlated at least moderately (> 0.35) with the targeted health domain. Ideally, multiple anchors are available and responsiveness can be estimated across the anchors to get a sense of the responsiveness of the item bank derived CAT or short-form scale.

A number of studies have been completed or are under way to document the responsiveness of the PROMIS® measures in patients with low back pain, osteoarthritis, depression, COPD, heart transplantation, and various cancer diagnoses. The PROMIS® depression scores have been demonstrated to be responsive to antidepressant treatment in patients with major depressive disorder (Pilkonis et al., 2011), across multiple domains after heart transplantation (Weinfurt, 2011), in rheumatoid arthritis patients (Fries et al., 2011), and for pain interference after treatment for low back pain (Revicki & Cook, 2011). In fact, the PROMIS® 20-item physical function scale outperformed the Health Assessment Questionnaire in sensitivity to changes in clinical status among rheumatoid arthritis patients (Fries et al., 2011). For low back pain in those patients who achieved a 50 percent improvement in pain intensity NRS, the PROMIS® pain interference scale demonstrated a 1.72 effect size compared with a 0.97 effect size for the Brief Pain Inventory interference scale (Revicki & Cook, 2011).

Yost, Eton, Garcia and Cella (2011) recruited 101 cancer patients and administered the PROMIS® fatigue, pain interference, physical function, anxiety, and depression short form scales at baseline and after 6 to 12 weeks to evaluate responsiveness and to determine minimum important differences. All the PROMIS® scales were responsive to changes in clinical status, and minimal important differences ranged from 2.5 to 6.0 points on the T-score metric for different domain scale scores.

Further Development and Evolution of Existing Item Banks

Item banks may need to be updated and revised over time when there are changes in the context of measurement and in the population. Some of the questions in the item bank may reference everyday activities or items that change over time. For example, some older items may reference technologies that become outdated, such as rotary landline telephones changing to cellular telephones and smartphones. Health domain item banks should be reviewed on a regular basis to ensure that the items include culturally relevant content. Item shift may occur over time; thus, developers need to review their item banks to make sure they are relevant for respondents. There need to be iterations between qualitative development and quantitative evaluation, and continued focus on the evolution of health domain item banks.

Challenges and Future Development of Item Banks

Challenges for Item Bank Development

There are several obstacles and challenges associated with developing health domain item banks, especially for item banks that will be used to assess outcomes in both the general population and chronic disease populations. First, the content of the item bank needs to be relevant across the continuum of the targeted health domain. Therefore, the initial development of the item bank needs to focus on the health experience of the diverse representatives of the general population and selected chronic disease samples that represent the range of impairments in the targeted domain. The main challenge is in identifying these representative patient groups and engaging them in qualitative research.

Second, some health domains are fairly narrow in definition and in some cases only a limited number of unique items can be generated. Health domains with narrow bands are challenging such as depression, anxiety, and anger, and may result in small sets of items that cover the range of the trait continuum. These nearly redundant, narrow item sets may result in problems of local dependence. These narrower constructs also challenge the need for other IRT applications, such as computerized adaptive testing.

Third, there are limitations in the number of DIF analyses that may be feasible given the size of typical psychometric evaluation studies. At a minimum, DIF should be assessed for gender, age groups, race/ethnicity, education level, and language groups. However, a number of other evaluations of DIF might also be relevant to understand the performance and bias in item banks, including comparing different chronic disease groups and other demographic characteristics. Additional DIF analyses can be planned once there are sufficient sample sizes in demographically varied populations. DIF analyses should always be conducted to compare different language translations as they are developed. However, for DIF to be meaningful, it is important to fully understand the dimensionality of an item bank.

Fourth, existing item banks may need to be extended to cover a broader range of the health domain continuum depending on the planned applications for short form scales and CATs based on the item banks. Many of the existing item banks cover unidirectional concepts (i.e., pain behavior, depression, anxiety, fatigue, etc.), and it is difficult to extend these banks further into the "healthy" end of the continuum of the latent construct. For example, the existing PROMIS® item banks are beginning to be administered to military personnel who may have physical functioning and other domain levels at the highest end of the health domain. Additional items may need to be developed and calibrated to enable discrimination of functioning at these higher levels of functioning. There may be cases where it is necessary to extend the item banks to better cover the most impaired part of the health domain. As with better functioning, additional items may need to be developed and calibrated to cover the more impaired part of the health domain continuum. As research is completed with different chronic disease groups, additional items may need to be added to existing item banks. For example, research with individuals with spinal cord injury and HIV disease may result in the identification of additional concepts in a depression domain that may require new items. As further research is conducted with different chronic disease groups, more items may need to be included in existing item banks to extend relevant domain coverage. These items will then need to be calibrated and included in the item banks.

Finally, as additional items are included in existing item banks, item calibration will need to be conducted and updated. Methods will need to be applied to ensure that the revised item calibrations continue to maintain the original domain item bank metrics. This is important for maintaining continuity with the initial item banks, short form scales, and CAT forms. The score metric is important for linking the domain scores over the years and for continued interpretation of these scores across studies and across time.

Summary

Item banks and computerized adaptive testing based on these item banks represent the future of health outcomes assessment. The flexibility and added measurement precision of item banks and short form scales and CAT forms allows for more efficient assessment of health outcomes. Central to PROMIS® are multiple item banks that include a comprehensive set of questions assessing each health domain. Items can be selected from the PROMIS® item banks to create targeted static short forms for specific patient populations. Such static short forms are not adaptive, and consist of the same items, such as an eight-item depression-specific or pain interference measure. Profile measures, covering multiple health domains, can also be developed from selected static short forms. As an alternative, researchers can use the PROMIS® measures to assess a patient's health status using computerized adaptive testing. CAT tailors the items administered to any specific patient to the actual health status of the patient and potentially represents a more efficient assessment method, often with improved precision.

Given the increase in access to computers and other electronic technologies, health assessments based on item banks may be more feasible in the future. The increasing development of the infrastructure for electronic health records may enable the accommodation of health outcome data from multiple domain item banks. Such clinical applications for measures based on item banks may be useful for monitoring the health status of patients in clinical practice and for improving clinicians' understanding of the effectiveness of health care interventions. These health outcome measures may also be used to examine the quality of the delivery of health care services. The increased emphasis on comparative effectiveness research requires access to large data sets that include information on treatments, clinical outcomes, and patient-reported outcomes (Ahmed et al., 2012). The availability of efficient and standardized multi-domain health assessments as part of the medical record may assist in developing a relevant database for conducting comparative effectiveness research.

The value of health assessments based on item banks will be demonstrated with the increased application of short form scales and CAT forms based on multi-domain item banks. Clearly, these health outcomes assessments can be used to increase the precision and efficiency of patient-reported outcomes in clinical trials, epidemiologic studies, and clinical practice. The availability of comprehensive item banks covering multiple health domains, as with the PROMIS® project, provides for flexible and efficient assessment of health-related outcomes.

References

Ahmed, S., Berzon, R.A., Revicki, D.A., Lenderking, W.R., Moinpour, C.M., Basch, E., . . . International Society for Quality of Life (2012). The use of patient-reported outcomes (PRO) within comparative effectiveness research: Implications for clinical practice and health care policy. *Medical Care, 50*, 1060–1070.

Amtmann, D., Cook, K.F., Jensen, M.P., Chen, W-H, Choi, S., Revicki, D., . . . Lai, J.S. (2010). Development of a PROMIS item bank to measure pain interference. *Pain, 150*, 173–182.

Andrich, D. (1978). A rating formulation for ordered response categories. *Psychometrika, 43*, 561–573.

Bajaj, J.S., Thacker, L.R., Wade, J.B., Sanyal, A.J., Heuman, D.M., Sterling, R.K., . . . Revicki, D.A. (2011). PROMIS computerized adaptive tests are dynamic instruments to measure health-related quality of life in patients with cirrhosis. *Alimentary Pharmacology & Therapeutics, 34*, 1123–1132.

Bentler, P.M. (1990). Comparative fit indexes in structural models. *Psychololological Bulletin, 107*, 238–246.

Bjorner, J.B., Smith, K.J., Orlando, M., Stone, C., Thissen, D., & Sun, X. (2006). *IRTFIT: A macro for item fit and local dependence tests under IRT models*. Lincoln, RI, QualityMetric Incorporated.

Bode, R.K., Lai, J.S., Cella, D., & Heinemann, A.W. (2003). Issues in the development of an item bank. *Archives of Physical Medicine & Rehabilatation, 84*(4 Suppl 2), S52–60.

Bradburn, N.M., Rips, L.J., & Shevell, S.K. (1987). Answering autobiographical questions: The impact of memory and inference on surveys. *Science, 236*, 157–161.

Brod, M., Tesler, L.E., & Christensen, T.L. (2009). Qualitative research and content validity: Developing best practices based on science and experience. *Quality of Life Research, 18*, 1263–1278.

Browne, M.W., & Cudeck, R. (1993). Alternative ways of assessing model fit. In K.A. Bollen & J.S. Long (Eds.), *Testing structural equation models* (pp. 136–162). Newbury Park, CA: Sage.

Cai, L., Thissen, D., & du Toit, S.H.C. (2011). *IRTPRO for windows*. Lincolnwood, IL: Scientific Software International.

Cella, D., Yount, S., Rothrock, N., Gershon, R., Cook, K., Reeve, B., . . . P.C. Group. (2007). The Patient-Reported Outcomes Measurement Information System (PROMIS): Progress of an NIH roadmap cooperative group during its first two years. *Medical Care, 45*(5 Suppl 1), S3–S11.

Cella, D., Riley, W., Stone, A., Rothrock, N., Reeve, B., Yount, S., . . . P.C. Group. (2010). The Patient-Reported Outcomes Measurement Information System (PROMIS) developed and tested its first wave of adult self-reported health outcome item banks: 2005–2008. *Journal of Clinical Epidemiology, 63*, 1179–1194.

Chang, C.H. (2005). Item response theory and beyond: Advanced in patient-reported outcomes measurement. In W.R. Lenderking & D.A. Revicki (Eds.), *Advancing health outcomes research methods and clinical applications* (pp. 37–55). McLean, VA: International Society for Quality of Life Research.

Chen, W.H., & Thissen, D. (1997). Local dependence indexes for item pairs using item response theory. *Educational and Behavioral Statistics, 22*, 264–289.

Cohen, A.S., Kim, S.H., & Wollack, J.A. (1996). An investigation of the likelihood ratio test for detection of differential item functioning. *Applied Psycholological Measurement, 20*, 15–26.

Cook, K.F., Kallen, M.A., & Amtmann, D. (2009). Having a fit: Impact of number of items and distribution of data on traditional criteria for assessing IRT's unidimensionality assumption. *Quality of Life Research, 18*, 447–460.

Cortina, J.M. (1993). What is coefficient alpha? An examination of theory and applications. *Journal of Applied Psychology, 78*, 98–104.

Crane, P.K., Gibbons, L.E., Jolley, L., & van Belle, G. (2006). Differential item functioning analysis with ordinal logistic regression techniques. DIFdetect and difwithpar. *Medical Care, 44*(11 Suppl 3), S115–123.

Crane, P.K., van Belle, G., & Larson, E.B. (2004). Test bias in a cognitive test: Differential item functioning in the CASI. *Statistics in Medicine, 23*, 241–256.

Cronbach, L.J. (1951). Coefficient alpha and the internal structure of tests. *Psychometrika, 16*, 297–334.

Cronbach, L.J., & Meehl, P.E. (1955). Construct validity in psychological tests. *Psychological Bulletin, 52*, 281–302.

De Vet, H.C.W., Terwee, C.B., Mokkink, L.B., & Knol, D.L. (2011). *Measurement in medicine: A practical guide*. Cambridge, UK: Cambridge University Press.

DeWalt, D.A., Rothrock, N., Yount, S., Stone, A.A., & P.C. Group. (2007). Evaluation of item candidates: The PROMIS qualitative item review. *Medical Care, 45*(5 Suppl 1), S12–21.

Drasgow, F., & Parsons, C.K. (1983). Application of unidimensional item response theory models to multidimensional data. *Applied Psycholological Measurement, 7*, 189–199.

Embretson, S.E., & Reise, S.P. (2000). *Item response theory for psychologists*. New York: Psychology Press.

Erskine, A., Morley, S., & Pearce, S. (1990). Memory for pain: A review. *Pain, 41*, 255–265.

Fayers, P.M., & Machin, D. (2007). *Quality of life: Assessment, analysis, and interpretation*. Chichester, UK: Wiley.

Finch, H. (2005). The MIMIC model as a method for detecting DIF: Comparison with Mantel-Haenszel, SIBTEST, and the IRT likelihood ratio. *Applied Psychological Measurement, 28*, 278–295.

Flowers, C.P., Oshima, T.C., & Raju, N.S. (1999). A description and demonstration of the polytomous DFIT framework. *Applied Psychological Measurement, 23*, 309–332.

Flynn, K.E., Lin, L., Cyranowski, J.M., Reeve, B.B., Reese, J.B., Jeffery, D.D., . . . Weinfurt, K.P. (2013). Development of the NIH PROMIS (R) sexual function and satisfaction measures in patients with cancer. *Journal of Sexual Medicine, 10*(Suppl 1), 43–52.

Forrest, C.B., Bevans, K.B., Tucker, C., Riley, A.W., Ravens-Sieberer, U., Gardner, W., & Pajer, K. (2012). Commentary: The patient-reported outcome measurement information system (PROMIS(R)) for children and youth: Application to pediatric psychology. *Journal of Pediatric Psychology, 37*, 614–621.

Fries, J.F., Krishnan, E., Rose, M., Lingala, B., & Bruce, B. (2011). Improved responsiveness and reduced sample size requirements of PROMIS physical function scales with item response theory. *Arthritis Research & Therapeutics, 13*, R147.

Gibbons, R.D., Hedeker, D., & Bock, R.D. (1992). Full-information item bi-factor analysis. *Psychometrika, 57*, 423–436.

Gorin, A., & Stone, A.A. (2001). Recall biases and cognitive errors in retrospective self-reports: A call for momentary assessments. In A. Baum, T.A. Revenson, & J.E. Singer (Eds.), *Handbook of health psychology* (pp. 405–413). Mahwah, NJ: Lawrence Erlbaum Associates.

Hambleton, R.K., & Han, N. (2005). Assessing the fit of IRT models to educational and psychological test data: A five step plan and several graphical displays. In W.R. Lenderking & D.A. Revicki (Eds.), *Advances in health outcomes research methods and clinical applications* (pp. 57–78). McLean, VA: International Society for Quality of Life Research.

Hambleton, R.K., Swaminathan, H., & Rogers, H. (1991). *Fundamentals of item response theory*. Newbury Park, CA: Sage.

Harrison, D.A. (1986). Robustness of IRT parameter estimation to violations of the unidimensionality assumption. *Journal of Educational Statistics, 11*, 91–115.

Hays, R.D., & Revicki, D.A. (2005). Reliability and validity, including responsiveness. In P. Fayers & R.D. Hays (Eds.), *Assessing quality of life in clinical trials* (pp. 25–39). New York: Oxford University Press.

Holland, P.W., & Thayer, D.T. (1988). Differential item performance and the Mantel-Haenszel procedure. In H. Wainer & H.I. Braun (Eds.), *Test validity* (pp. 129–145). Hillsdale, NJ: Lawrence Erlbaum Associates.

Hu, L.T., & Bentler, P. (1999). Cutoff criteria for fit indices in covariance structure analysis: Conventional criteria versus new alternatives. *Structural Equation Modeling, 6*, 1–55.

Jöreskog, K.G., Sörbom, D., & Du Toit, S. (2003). *LISREL 8: New statistical features*. Lincolnwood, IL: Scientific Software International.

Kim, S.H., & Cohen, A.S. (1998). Detection of differential item functioning under the graded response model with the likelihood ratio test. *Applied Psychological Measurement, 22*, 345–355.

Kleinman, L., Benjamin, K., Viswanathan, H., Mattera, M.S., Bosserman, L., Blayney, D.W., & Revicki, D.A. (2012). The anemia impact measure (AIM): Development and content validation of a patient-reported outcome measure of anemia symptoms and symptom impacts in cancer patients receiving chemotherapy. *Quality of Life Research, 21*, 1255–1266.

Kline, R.B. (2010). *Principles and practice of structural equation modeling*. New York: Guilford Press.

Lai, J.S., Crane, P.K., & Cella, D. (2006). Factor analysis techniques for assessing sufficient unidimensionality of cancer related fatigue. *Quality of Life Research, 15*, 1179–1190.

Lasch, K.E., Marquis, P., Vigneux, M., Abetz, L., Arnould, B., Bayliss, M., . . . Rosa, K. (2010). PRO development: Rigorous qualitative research as the crucial foundation. *Quality of Life Research, 19*, 1087–1096.

Magasi, S., Ryan, G., Revicki, D., Lenderking, W., Hays, R.D., Brod, M., . . . Cella, D. (2012). Content validity of patient-reported outcome measures: Perspectives from a PROMIS meeting. *Quality of Life Research, 21*, 739–746.

Masters, G.N. (1982). A Rasch model for partial credit scoring. *Psychometrika, 47*, 149–174.

McDonald, R.P. (1981). The dimensionality of test and items. *British Journal of Mathematical Statistical Psychology, 34*, 100–117.

McDonald, R.P. (1999). *Test theory: A unified treatment*. Mahwah, NJ: Lawrence Erlbaum Associates.

Mellenbergh, G.J. (1982). Contingency table models for assessing item bias. *Journal of Educational Statistics, 7*, 105–118.

Menon, G., & Yorkston, E. (2000). The use of memory and contextual cues in the formation of behavioral frequency judgments. In A. Stone, J. Turkkan, & C. Bachrach (Eds.), *The science of self-report: Implications for research and practice* (pp. 63–79). Mahwah, NJ: Lawrence Erlbaum Associates.

Muthén, L.K., & Muthén, B.O. (1998). *Mplus user's guide*. Los Angeles, CA: Muthén & Muthén.

National Quality Forum (2013). *Patient-reported outcomes in performance measurement*. Washington, DC: National Quality Forum.

Nunnally, J.C., & Bernstein, I.H. (1994). *Psychometric theory*. New York: McGraw-Hill.

Orlando, M., & Thissen, D. (2000). Likelihood-based item-fit indices for dichotomous item response theory models. *Applied Psychological Measurement, 24*, 50–64.

Orlando, M., & Thissen, D. (2003). Further investigation of the performance of S-X2: An item fit index for use with dichotomous item response theory models. *Applied Psychological Measurement, 27*, 289–298.

Pilkonis, P. (2011, April). *Pittsburgh PROMIS wave II protocols*. PROMIS Steering Committee Meeting, Bethesda, MD.

Pilkonis, P., Choi, S.W., Reise, S.P., Stover, A.M., Riley, A.W., & Cella, D. (2011). Item banks for measuring emotional distress from the Patient-Reported Outcome Measurement Information System (PROMIS): Depression, anxiety, and anger. *Assessment, 18*, 263–283.

Preston, K.S.J., Reise, S.P., Cai, L., & Hays, R. (2011). Using the nominal response model to evaluate response category discrimination in the PROMIS emotional distress item pools. *Educational & Psychological Measurement, 71*, 523–550.

Raju, N.S., Van Der Linden, W.J., & Fleer, P.F. (1995). IRT-based internal measures of differential functioning of items and tests. *Applied Psychological Measurement, 19*, 353–368.

Ramsay, J.O. (1997). A functional approach to modeling test data. In W.J. van der Linden & R.K. Hambleton (Eds.), *Handbook of modern item response theory* (pp. 381–394). New York: Springer.

Redelmeier, D.A., & Kahneman, D. (1996). Patients' memories of painful medical treatments: Real-time and retrospective evaluations of two minimally invasive procedures. *Pain, 66*, 3–8.

Reeve, B. B. (2003). Item response theory modeling in health outcomes measurement. *Expert Review Pharmacoeconomics & Outcomes Resesearch, 3*(2), 131–145.

Reeve, B. B., & Fayers, P. (2005). Applying item response theory modeling for evaluating questionnaire item and scale properties. In P. Fayers & R. D. Hays (Eds.), *Assessing quality of life in clinical trials* (pp. 131–145). New York: Oxford University Press.

Reeve, B. B., Hays, R. D., Bjorner, J. B., Cook, K. F., Crane, P. K., Teresi, J. A., . . . Cella, D. (2007). Psychometric evaluation and calibration of health-related quality of life items banks: Plans for the patient-reported outcome measurement information system (PROMIS). *Med Care, 45*(5 Suppl 1): S22–S31.

Reise, S. P., & Haviland, M. G. (2005). Item response theory and the measurement of clinical change. *Journal of Personality Assessment, 84*, 228–238.

Reise, S. P., Scheines, R., Widaman, K. F., & Haviland, M. G. (2012). Multidimensionality and structural coefficient bias in structural equation modeling: A bifactor perspective. *Educational & Psychological Measurement, 73*, 5–26.

Revicki, D. A., Chen, W. H., Harnam, N., Cook, K. F., Amtmann, D., Callahan. L. F., . . . Keefe, F. J. (2009). Development and psychometric analysis of the PROMIS pain behavior item bank. *Pain, 146*, 158–169.

Revicki, D. A., & Cook, K. F. (2011, May). *Development and psychometric evaluation of the PROMIS pain interference item bank.* Presentation at the 30th Annal Scientific Meeting of the American Pain Society. Austin, TX.

Revicki, D. A., Hays, R. D., Cella, D., & Sloan, J. (2008). Recommended methods for determining responsiveness and minimally important differences for patient-reported outcomes. *Journal of Clinical Epidemioliology, 61*, 102–109.

Riley, W. T., Rothrock, N., Bruce, B., Christodolou, C., Cook, K., Hahn, E. A., & Cella, D. (2010). Patient-reported outcomes measurement information system (PROMIS) domain names and definitions revisions: Further evaluation of content validity in IRT-derived item banks. *Quality of Life Research, 19*, 1311–1321.

Robinson, M. D., & Clore, G. L. (2002). Belief and feeling: Evidence for an accessibility model of emotional self-report. *Psychological Bulletin, 128*, 934–960.

Rothrock, N. E., Hays, R. D., Spritzer, K., Yount, S. E., Riley, W., & Cella, D. (2010). Relative to the general US population, chronic diseases are associated with poorer health-related quality of life as measured by the Patient-Reported Outcomes Measurement Information System (PROMIS). *Journal of Clinical Epidemioliology, 63*, 1195–1204.

Roussos, L., & Stout, W. (1996). A multidimensionality-based DIF analysis paradigm. *Applied Psychological Measurement, 20*, 355–371.

Samejima, F. (1969). Estimation of latent ability using a response pattern of graded scores. *Psychometrika Monograph* 17.

Samejima, F. (1997). Graded response model. In W. J. van der Linden & R. K. Hambleton (Eds.), *Handbook of modern item response theory* (pp. 85–100). New York: Springer.

Schwartz, N., & Sudman, S. (1994). *Autobiographical memory and the validity of retrospective reports.* New York: Springer-Verlag.

Steinberg, L., & Thissen, D. (1996). Uses of item response theory and the testlet concept in the measurement of psychopathology. *Psychological Methods, 1*, 81–97.

Stout, W. (1987). A nonparametric approach for assessing latent trait unidimensionality. *Psychometrika, 52, 589–617.*

Strauss, A., & Corbin, J. M. (1998). *Basics of qualitative research: Techniques and procedures for developing grounded theory.* Thousand Oaks, CA: Sage.

Swaminathan, H., & Rogers, H. J. (1992). Detecting differential item functioning using logistic regression procedures. *Journal of Educational Measurement, 27*, 361–370.

Teresi, J. A., Kleinman, M., & Ocepek-Welikson, K. (2000). Modern psychometric methods for detection of differential item functioning: Application to cognitive assessment measures. *Statistics in Medicine, 19*, 1651–1683.

Teresi, J. A., Ocepek-Welikson, K., Kleinman, M., Eimicke, J. P., Crane, P. K., Jones, R. N., . . . Cella, D. (2009). Analysis of differential item functioning in the depression item bank from the

Patient Reported Outcome Measurement Information System (PROMIS): An item response theory approach. *Psychological Science Quarterly, 51*, 148–180.

Thissen, D. (2001). *IRTLRDIF v2.0b: Software for the computation of the statistics involved in item response theory likelihood-ratio tests for differential item functioning.*

Thissen, D., Chen, W.H., & Bock, D. (2002). *MULTILOG*. Lincolnwood, IL, Scientific Software International.

Thissen, D., & Orlando, M. (2001). Item response theory for items scored in two categories. In D. Thissen & H. Wainer (Eds.), *Test scoring* (pp. 73–140). Mahwah, NJ: Lawrence Erlbaum Associates.

Thissen, D., Steinberg, L., & Gerard, M. (1986). Beyond group-mean differences: The concept of item bias. *Psychological Bulletin, 99*, 118–128.

Thissen, D., Steinberg, L., & Wainer, H. (1993). Detection of differential item functioning using the parameters of item response models. In P.W. Holland & H. Wainer (Eds.), *Differential item functioning* (pp. 123–135). Hillsdale, NJ: Lawrence Erlbaum Associates.

Wainer, H., & Thissen, D. (1996). How is reliability related to the quality of test scores? What is the effect of local dependence on reliability? *Educational Measurement, 15*, 22–29.

Weinfurt, K. (2011, October). *Validity of PROMIS measures in patients undergoing heart transplantation for congestive heart failure.* PROMIS Steering Committee Meeting, Bethesda, MD.

Willis, G. (2005). *Cognitive interviewing.* Thousand Oaks, CA: Sage.

World Health Organization (1958). *The first ten years of the World Health Organization.* Geneva, Switzerland: World Health Organization.

Wright, B.D., & Masters, G.N. (1982). *Rating scale analysis.* Chicago, IL: MESA Press.

Yen, W.M. (1984). Effect of local item dependence on the fit and equating performance of the three-parameter logistic model. *Applied Psychological Measurement, 8*, 125–145.

Yen, W.M. (1993). Scaling performance assessments: Strategies for managing local item dependence. *Journal of Educational Measurement, 30*, 187–213.

Yost, K.J., Eton, D.T., Garcia, S.F., & Cella, D. (2011). Minimally important differences were estimated for six Patient-Reported Outcomes Measurement Information System-Cancer scales in advanced-stage cancer patients. *Journal of Clinical Epidemioliology, 64*, 507–516.

Zumbo, W.M. (1999). *Logistic regression modeling as a unitary framework for binary and likert-type (ordinal) item scores.* Ottawa, ON: Directorate of Human Resources Research and Evaluation, Department of National Defense.

Using Item Response Theory to Evaluate Measurement Invariance in Health-Related Measures

Roger E. Millsap, Heather Gunn, Howard T. Everson, and Alex Zautra

Introduction

For more than a decade, the National Institutes of Health (NIH) has supported the development of the Patient Reported Outcomes Information System (PROMIS®) Roadmap initiative (www.nihpromis.org). This effort reflects the growing importance of and interest in the use of measures of patients' self-reported health status in medical and health care research, as well as in clinical practice. The goal of the NIH initiative is to support the development of a large bank of items for measuring patient-reported outcomes (PROs), which, ultimately, could be assembled into measurement scales for use in both clinical and research settings. With NIH support the PROMIS® development initiative has been able to make both the items and the scales available to clinicians and researchers (Cella et al., 2007).

Our main goal in this chapter is to present researchers and others working with PROMIS® and other scales with a model-based psychometric perspective about how best to identify items that may function differently for different patient groups, and thereby contribute to the challenge of maintaining validity in these health-related measurement scales. In the psychometric literature these model-based methods are described more formally under the general headings of differential item functioning (DIF) or measurement invariance (Millsap, 2011; Osterlind & Everson, 2009; Widaman & Reise, 1997). With this context in mind, we begin with a review of the definition of measurement invariance and how violations of invariance are distinguished from simple group differences in scores. Also, we demonstrate how contemporary methods based on *item response theory* are applied to the challenge of empirically investigating measurement invariance. We illustrate these methods using a running example based on responses from a community sample of a widely used health survey measure, the *SF-36* scale.

Measurement Invariance

The idea of measurement invariance originated through attempts to model formally how item responses and test scores vary as a function of the respondent's status on the latent (unobserved) variable to be measured. A test or questionnaire item may have been designed to measure a particular psychological attribute, for example, a depression scale item asking about the presence of a symptom of depression. From a psychometric measurement model perspective, we can express the probabilities of possible responses to this item as a function of the respondent's location on a hypothesized latent scale of depression. We say the depression item is *measurement invariant* to the extent that, after accounting for the respondent's status on the latent depression scale, no other systematic influence on the response probabilities exists. Another way of expressing this idea is to say that if two different people have the same score on the latent depression scale, their response probabilities will be identical, regardless of their differences on other variables such as gender, race, age, or general health status. Measurement models can take different forms; in this chapter we focus on models in item response theory (IRT).

We can express the idea of measurement invariance formally. Let X_{ij} be the score for the ith person on the jth questionnaire item, and let θ_i represent the latent variable score (e.g., depression score) for the ith person. We assume here that there is only one relevant latent variable. Let V_i represent any other measured characteristic for the ith person, such as gender or age. Then we say that X is measurement invariant in relation to θ and V if:

$$P(X_{ij} = x \mid \theta_i, V_i) = P(X_{ij} = x \mid \theta_i), \tag{17.1}$$

(Mellenbergh, 1989; Meredith & Millsap, 1992). Once θ is taken into account, no other characteristic V is important in determining the item response probabilities.

Measurement invariance is a useful property, particularly if we wish to describe group differences on variables defined by V. For example, if V represents gender, and we wish to study gender differences in depression as measured by X, we need to assume that the gender differences are due to θ, rather than artifactual influences. For example, if men and women vary systematically in their willingness to report depression symptoms, this variation will violate measurement invariance for X. A man and a woman who are identical on θ will then *not* have the same probabilities of response to X. When measurement invariance is violated, we say further that *measurement bias* is present for X, or that X shows *differential item functioning* (DIF) (Holland & Thayer, 1988; Osterlind & Everson, 2009).

Although measurement invariance may hold for X, there may still be large group differences in scores on X. A depression item that is measurement invariant in relation to gender may still be endorsed more often by women than men, if women have higher scores on average for θ, the latent depression variable. Group differences in item scores that simply reflect differences on the latent variable measured by the item denote *impact* (Dorans & Holland, 1993; Holland & Thayer, 1988), rather than measurement bias or DIF. The key distinction between impact and bias is that impact is driven by actual differences on the targeted latent variable, while bias is produced by other, construct-irrelevant influences. These other influences may be only partially understood in practice.

Statistical methods for testing measurement invariance are now widely available; for recent general reviews, see Millsap (2011) and Osterlind and Everson (2009). The central notion underlying all of these methods is the *matching principle* (Angoff, 1993): individuals should be matched on θ before groups are compared on X. Once individuals are properly matched, if X is indeed measurement invariant, there should be no group differences on X beyond random influences such as sampling error or unreliability. The difficulty here is that θ is latent, so no explicit match on θ is possible. This problem is addressed in two different ways by available statistical methods. One approach matches individuals on a measured proxy variable Z that serves as a substitute for θ. In practice, the usual choice for Z is the total score on the scale in which X is embedded. These methods then condition on Z when examining group differences on X.

The second approach is to model the relationship between X and θ using a latent variable model. If measurement invariance holds for X, the latent variable model should have the same form across groups defined by V (e.g., males and females). This prediction can be tested empirically. Matching is implicit in this latent variable approach through the chosen measurement model.

In this chapter, we adopt this second approach to examining measurement invariance using models in item response theory. The first approach, one conditioning on total scores, encounters potential problems when the number of items is small or when there is more than one latent variable underlying the scale (Meredith & Millsap, 1992; Millsap, 2011). Both of these are the case for the *SF-36*, and so the latent variable approach is preferred here. The next section provides a general description of this approach.

Research Methods

Item Response Theory and Measurement Invariance

Item response theory (IRT) consists of a collection of models for expressing the probability of a response to a test or questionnaire item as a function of the respondent's position on one or more latent variables. Item responses are usually discrete; examples include passing versus failing a cognitive test item, or selecting one's level of agreement from among five possible options on a questionnaire item. Scores on the latent variables are modeled as continuous measures in most cases. The number of latent variables that influence responses to a set of items is specified in the IRT model. Traditionally, only one such variable has been assumed (the *unidimensional* case), but more recently multiple latent variables have been incorporated in applications of IRT, especially in applications that do not involve cognitive tests (Reckase, 2009; see Chapter 2 in this volume for more detail). In a multidimensional situation, the IRT model can be related to the common factor model, which provides another representation for item-level data using multiple latent variables. The common factor model, in turn, can be viewed as a specific type of IRT model (Lord & Novick, 1968; Takane & de Leeuw, 1987).

The use of IRT for examining measurement invariance has a long history (Lord, 1980). The general idea is to begin with an IRT model that fits the data across all groups, and then examine invariance by either constraining model parameters through a nested sequence of models, or by directly testing group differences in model parameters. Historically, most applications of IRT to invariance questions have used unidimensional IRT models, and have focused on cognitive test items. In many cases the items under study were binary (i.e., scored dichotomously), as in multiple-choice cognitive test items. In contrast, many applications to noncognitive measures often encounter items with polytomous scoring (i.e., having more than two possible values) and possibly multiple latent variables. The use of polytomous items with multiple latent variables results in a greater number of model parameters in comparison to the simpler binary case, and they offer more opportunities for violations of the invariance principle.

A typical application of IRT to the examination of invariance occurs in a sequence of steps. The first step is *model selection*: we ask which IRT model is appropriate for the data at hand. Part of this selection step requires that the number of latent variables be specified. As used here, the latent variables of interest are those shared among multiple items; by analogy this is the common factors in factor analysis. How many latent variables influence the items in the set being analyzed? Furthermore, which latent variables relate to each item? Once the number of latent variables is specified, we must decide for each item whether more than one latent variable is relevant. It may be the case that while multiple variables are needed for the entire set of items, only one latent variable is important for any single item. Once the number of latent variables is specified, an appropriate IRT model is then chosen. This choice turns partly on the number of response options for each item. A number of possible models exist for polytomous response formats in the unidimensional case, for example. The choice may also be influenced by the type of item, along with any theory about how responses to the item are generated. Ultimately, the model choice will also use model fit information. Any model chosen at this step, therefore, must provide an adequate fit to the data so that the model can serve as a baseline for comparisons to further, more restricted models that incorporate invariance constraints. If a model that fits the data adequately in all groups cannot be found, further investigation of invariance is ill advised because the model fits will worsen typically as constraints are added.

A common explanation for poor model fit in the initial investigative stage is uncertainty about the number of latent variables underlying the items. Either this number varies across groups, and hence no model that stipulates the same number across groups will fit, or the number of latent variables is larger than first believed. If the number of latent variables does indeed vary across groups, this indicates a violation of measurement invariance and further modeling to compare parameter values across groups is not needed. If the number of latent variables is simply unclear, further exploratory analyses to assess the number of latent variables might be pursued, using a variety of statistical tools (see, for example, Brown, 2006).

Assuming that a model with adequate fit has been found to serve as a baseline, the next steps are to *examine invariance* in the parameter values for the chosen model. This phase of the analysis could pursue different options, but two broad approaches are (1) direct comparisons of parameters using Wald tests, or (2) likelihood-ratio (LR) tests that compare models with or without invariance constraints. The choice here depends in part on available statistical software. Some software programs can easily execute LR tests (e.g., Mplus (Muthén & Muthén, 1998–2012)), while other programs, IRTPRO, for example, can employ either method (Cai, du Toit, & Thissen, 2011). The type of measurement model will also affect the choice of method. Models for polytomous item responses are more easily handled using LR tests due, in part, to the large number of parameters to be estimated.

Regardless of which option is pursued, if the number of items is moderate or large, the number of tests of significance or model fit evaluations will grow quickly. When a large number of statistical tests are performed, Type I error inflation will result. In the measurement invariance context, a Type I error generally means we concluded that invariance is violated when no such violation is actually present in the data. To guard against this problem, procedures for controlling Type I error rate inflation are introduced. The key in doing so is to control the error rate without undermining the power to detect real violations of invariance. One flexible procedure that has been used with invariance applications in the past is the false discovery rate procedure (Benjamini & Hochberg, 1995). This procedure can be used in conjunction with any of the parameter comparison procedures described here.

The final step in the investigation of invariance, once items that appear to violate invariance have been identified, is to *decide what if anything should be done* about these items. The decision here will depend in part on the status of the scale under study. If the scale is under development, it may be relatively easy to drop biased items from consideration. If, however, it is an established, widely used scale, dropping items can mean that results using the scale will not be comparable across studies. One aspect of this process is to construct measures of "effect size" that evaluate the size of the group difference in model parameters. Effect size measures for unidimensional IRT models for binary items are available (Millsap, 2011). Measures for unidimensional models for polytomous items are less well developed, and extensions to the multidimensional models are rarer still. An additional issue to consider at this stage is the impact of the violations of invariance at the scale level. For example, when items scores are summed or averaged to create the scale score, what is the impact of the lack of invariance on the scale scores? In a scale consisting of many items, violations of invariance involving very few items may have little or no impact at the ale level. The degree of impact can be evaluated in several ways, as discussed later in this chapter. More detailed questions about the impact of violations of invariance with respect to the use of the test or questionnaire for diagnosis or prediction can also be addressed. Ultimately, a decision must be made about whether to retain or eliminate any item that violates invariance. If enough items are found to be violators, use of the scale itself in the groups being studied may be undermined.

Regardless of whether the items violating invariance are dropped or retained, explanations for the violations should be considered as well. Ideally, this line of investigation would be designed with some hypotheses about which items might violate invariance given the populations under study (Roussos & Stout, 1996). One framework for this approach is to regard violations of invariance as due to the presence of additional *nuisance latent variables* (Ackerman, 1992; Camilli, 1992; Mellenbergh, 1989; Shealy & Stout, 1993). In this scenario, the items are no longer measuring the same latent variables across groups presumably because the nuisance latent variables are functioning differently in the groups being compared. For example, suppose that two populations are being compared, one consisting of native English speakers, and another for whom English is a second language (ESL). Familiarity with the English language now becomes a potential nuisance variable that influences responses for items with substantial verbal content. Furthermore, this latent variable may have a stronger influence in the ESL group because the native English speakers are presumably more homogeneous on the nuisance latent variable. In this nuisance variable framework, seeking an explanation for violations of invariance entails considering what nuisance variables are likely to be operating in the context of the study, and then collecting data that would permit evaluations of the explanations.

In the next section we introduce data from the *SF-36* as the example we use to illustrate the process of examining measurement invariance in a health-related questionnaire. Each of the three steps just described is explored in more detail in the context of this example.

Application

The SF-36 Example

The *SF-36* (Ware, Snow, Kosinski, & Gandek, 1993) is a relatively brief, self-report health survey comprised of 36 questions, sorted into eight subscales, that yields a profile of patients' functional health and well-being. It is intended as a generic measure; it does not target a specific age, disease, or treatment group, and therefore is useful for general and specific patient populations. The *SF-36* is widely used in both clinical and research settings. The *SF-36* has a hierarchical structure that includes three levels: (1) 36 items; (2) eight subscales that aggregate 2–10 items each; and (3) two summary scales (Physical Health and Mental Health) that each aggregate four subscales. A series of factor analytic studies have been cited to confirm the invariance of the measurement structure of the scale across populations (Fukuhara, Ware, Kosinski, Wada, & Gandek, 1998; McHorney, Ware, & Raczek, 1993; Sullivan, Karlsson, & Ware, 1995; Ware et al., 1998). More complete detail of the history and development of the *SF-36*, including its psychometric properties (i.e., studies of reliability and validity, and normative data) is available in the *SF-36* user's manuals (Ware et al., 1993). In addition, a review of the development of the *SF-36* can be found in McDowell and Newell (1996).

The data example to be studied here consists of responses to the *SF-36* from 808 adult men and women who were participants in a five-year community-based study of resilience and healthy aging in the Phoenix, Arizona area. Ages of the participants ranged from 40 to 65 years old, with a mean age of 53.5. There were 355 women and 425 men in the original sample (unfortunately, a gender indicator was missing for 28 participants). For the analyses reported here, participants who were missing data on either gender or the *SF-36* items to be studied were dropped from the analyses, resulting in a total sample of 742, which included 339 females and 403 males. We used gender as the grouping variable for the invariance analyses.

As noted earlier, the complete 36-item *SF-36* scale yields eight subscale scores, divided into four physical health and four mental health subscales. The analyses reported here focus on two of the four mental health subscales: Role-Emotional (RE, three items) and Mental Health (MH, five items). The items are given in Table 17.1. These two subscales were selected for the present study because previous confirmatory factor analyses have shown them to be relatively pure measures of the general Mental Health factor in the *SF-36*, along with a third subscale (Keller et al., 1998). The third Social Functioning subscale, however, contains only two items, so we dropped this subscale when preliminary analyses including it led to numerical problems. It is worth noting that previous studies of invariance in the *SF-36* with respect to gender have either found no bias (Perkin, Stump, Monahan, & McHorney, 2006), or have found bias in very few items (Pollard, Johnson, & Dixon, 2013). Those studies, however, did not use latent variable modeling to test for invariance, and instead used variations of the first approach described earlier that employed a measured proxy matching strategy.

Table 17.1 SF-36 Items for the RE and MH Subscales

Role-Emotional (RE) Items:

During the past 4 weeks, have you had any of the following problems with your work or other regular daily activities as a result of any emotional problems (such as feeling depressed or anxious)?

RE1: Cut down the amount of time you spent on work or other activities (Yes or No)

RE2: Accomplished less than you would like (Yes or No)

RE3: Didn't do work or other activities as carefully as usual (Yes or No)

Mental Health (MH) Items:

These questions are about how you feel and how things have been with you during the past 4 weeks. For each question, please give the answer that comes closest to the way you have been feeling.

The response scale for all MH items is as follows:

1) All of the time

2) Most of the time

3) A good bit of the time

4) Some of the time

5) A little bit of the time

6) None of the time

MH1: Have you been a very nervous person?

MH2: Have you felt so down in the dumps that nothing could cheer you up?

MH3: Have you felt calm and peaceful?

MH4: Have you felt downhearted and blue?

MH5: Have you been a happy person?

Table 17.2 provides the response frequencies by gender across the eight items in the original response scale. Items MH3 and MH5 were reversed in scoring prior to analysis so that all items would correlate positively. The frequencies for these two items are displayed in their original form in Table 7.2. The low frequencies of response for some of the MH response categories compelled us to collapse some categories in both genders before beginning the analysis. For items MH3 and MH5, we combined categories 5 and 6. For items MH1, MH2, and MH4, we combined categories 1, 2, and 3. As a result, items MH3 and MH5 contained five response categories after recoding, and the remaining items each contained four categories.

Step One: Selecting the Baseline Model

The initial goal of an invariance analysis is to find an IRT model that provides an adequate fit to the data in all groups. Two important initial considerations in selecting a model are: (1) the nature of the item response scales, and (2) the expected number of latent variables underlying the items. The first issue is simple: Are the response scales binary (e.g., true/false) or polytomous (e.g., Likert-type scaling)? Mixtures of these two types of response scales across items are also common, and this is true for the *SF-36*: the RE subscale items are binary, while the MH subscale items are polytomous. As a result, different models will be needed for these different item types. This mixture of item types presents no problem for the software programs we used here.

Table 17.2 Item Response Percentages by Gender for RE and MH Items

	Males		*Females*	
	Yes	*No*	*Yes*	*No*
RE1	14.9	85.1	10.6	89.4
RE2	23.6	76.4	17.4	82.6
RE3	15.6	84.4	11.5	88.5

	Males					
	1	*2*	*3*	*4*	*5*	*6*
MH1	1.7	5.7	5.2	15.6	29.5	42.2
MH2	0.2	3.0	2.5	7.9	18.6	67.3
MH3	6.7	46.2	12.7	21.3	10.4	2.7
MH4	1.2	3.5	3.7	17.6	32.3	41.7
MH5	12.4	53.3	14.1	13.9	4.5	1.7
	Females					
	1	*2*	*3*	*4*	*5*	*6*
MH1	1.5	2.4	2.1	10.9	32.7	50.4
MH2	0.6	1.5	0.6	8.3	16.2	72.9
MH3	13.3	48.4	11.2	15.6	7.7	3.8
MH4	0.3	3.5	1.5	14.2	31.3	49.3
MH5	16.2	54.0	9.1	13.6	4.7	2.4

The second consideration noted earlier, that is, the number of latent variables, is usually more difficult to address. Prior research and theory involving the items under study can be a useful guide. Prior factor analytic evidence, however, may directly suggest a choice for the number of latent variables, especially when the items belong to a frequently used instrument. In the *SF-36*, the eight items have been shown previously to form two factors based on both confirmatory factor analyses and principal component analyses (Keller et al., 1998; Ware et al., 1998). These previous analyses have shown, too, that one general mental health factor may underlie the full set of eight items. If no previous analyses have addressed the number of latent variables underlying the items to be evaluated, either the latent variables must be investigated with the data at hand, or one must wait for independent studies to be conducted. If, on the other hand, one uses the data at hand to both explore dimensionality and examine invariance, there is a risk that the results of these numerous analyses may not cross-validate in future studies.

While factor analysis has been the traditional tool for exploring dimensionality in psychometrics, it is not always used optimally, and other statistical tools are now available. Standard exploratory factor analysis, it is well known, is designed for continuous measures, and can often lead to spurious results when applied to discrete item scores (Carroll, 1983; McDonald & Ahlawat, 1974). Also, researchers sometimes confuse principal component analysis and factor analysis. Principal component analysis is less optimal for exploring dimensionality in item-level data because it does not explicitly model measurement error, and it is less likely to match factor analytic results when the number of items in each scale is small (Widaman, 1993). In contrast, confirmatory factor analysis (CFA) is often a better option, if some theory about the likely number of factors is available and if the discrete version of the CFA model is used. CFA, moreover, provides a variety of fit information, along with detailed residuals for evaluating where the model does not fit. The CFA model can also be viewed as a special type of IRT model (Takane & de Leeuw, 1987). Thus, if a CFA model fits the data, an IRT model can be found that will also fit the data.

Other tools for exploring dimensionality exist that make fewer assumptions than factor analysis. The *DIMTEST* procedure (Nandakumar & Stout, 1993; Stout, 1987) is based on a general conception of "essential dimensionality" that seeks dominant latent dimensions, rather than attempting to model all of the latent variables. *DIMTEST* is designed for items with binary response scales; a version for polytomous items, *Poly-DIMTEST*, is also available (Li & Stout, 1995; Nandakumar, Yu, Li, & Stout, 1998). *DIMTEST* provides a test statistic that can be used to evaluate whether a single dominant latent dimension underlies the items. If, however, this hypothesis is rejected, the procedure does not suggest how many additional dimensions might exist. The *DETECT* index (Kim, 1994; Stout et al., 1996), alternatively, offers a procedure for assessing how many dominant latent variables underlie the items if more than one latent variable is present, and if each item is related to only one of the dominant dimensions. *DETECT* is based on the same conception of dimensionality as that of the *DIMTEST* procedures. In brief, *DETECT* evaluates whether a preliminary sorting of the items into different sets corresponding to hypothesized latent variables matches an ideal partitioning of items to dominant sets. The *DETECT* and *DIMTEST* procedures have the advantage of assessing dimensionality without the parametric assumptions that go along with factor analysis. For more information on the latest available tools for exploring dimensionality, see Svetina and Levy (2012).

Returning to our *SF-36* example, prior research would suggest that two common factors underlie the eight items, with one factor corresponding to the RE items and the other factor corresponding to the MH items. We used CFA to evaluate this hypothesis directly in *Mplus* (Muthén & Muthén, 1998–2012) under WLSMV estimation (Flora & Curran,

2004). The two gender groups were examined simultaneously in a multiple-group model. Also, CFA for ordered-categorical items was used here to account for the discrete response scales (Millsap & Tein, 2004). This CFA model required some special constraints for model identification purposes. The identification constraints were as follows:

1) The factor means were fixed to zero in the male group, and were left unconstrained in the female group.
2) The factor variances were fixed to one in the male group, and were left unconstrained in the female group.
3) The factor loadings for items RE1 and MH1 were constrained to invariance, but were not fixed to any value. The threshold parameter for RE1 was also constrained to invariance.
4) The unique factor variances of the three RE items were constrained to invariance.
5) The first threshold parameter of each of the MH items was constrained to invariance, and the second threshold of MH1 was constrained to invariance.

A full description of the identification constraints for the multiple-group CFA model for discrete measures can be found in Millsap and Tein (2004) or Millsap (2011).

We also evaluated a single-factor model, given that both scales are viewed as capturing aspects of a general mental health latent variable. Our results indicated that the single-factor model fit poorly, as shown in Table 17.3 in the row for the single-factor model. Results for the two-factor model are given in the row for Model CFA1. The chi-square statistic, a test of exact fit of the model to the data, led us to reject both models. The Root Mean Square Error of Approximation (RMSEA) is an index of approximate fit (Browne & Cudeck, 1993; Steiger & Lind, 1980). Values of the RMSEA less than 0.05 are generally considered to indicate good fit, with values between 0.05 and 0.08 indicating fair fit.

Table 17.3 Model Fit Statistics for CFA Models

Model		*Chisq*	*df*	*DIFF (df)* *RMSEA*	*CFI*	*WRMR*
Single-Factor	339.171	42	———	.138	.948	2.363
CFA1 (Baseline)	122.352	38	———	.077	.985	1.226
CFA2						
(Invar 16.644 (6) Loadings)	133.266	44	p = .0107	.074	.984	1.358
CFA3						
(Invar 10.425 (5) except RE3	128.806	43	p = .0641	.073	.985	1.297
CFA4						
(Invar 18.720 (12) Threshold)	142.915	55	p = .0955	.066	.985	1.393
CFA5						
(Invar 14.860 (5) Unique)	154.001	60	p = .0110	.065	.984	1.498
CFA6						
(Invar 8.013 (4) except MH3)	146.221	59	p = .0911	.063	.985	1.449

Note: Chisq = Chi-Square, df = degrees of freedom, DIFF = DIFFTEST from Mplus, RMSEA = Root Mean Square Error of Approximation, CFI = Comparative Fit Statistic, WRMR = Weighted Root Mean Square Residual

This index, too, would clearly reject the single-factor model, but would possibly retain the two-factor model. The Comparative Fit Index (CFI) offers a different conception of approximate fit, one that evaluates the fit of the proposed model against a "null model" that specifies no common factors. Values of the CFI above 0.95 are considered to indicate good fit (Hu & Bentler, 1995). This index would also retain the two-factor model. Finally, the WRMR is a relatively new index provided by the *Mplus* software. Values below 1.00 are considered optimal (Muthén & Muthén, 1998–2012). This index, however, did not support either model, although it was clearly worse for the single-factor model.

The evidence overall suggests that the two-factor model provides a better fit to the data; nevertheless, we also examined the model residuals for information about the sources of the lack of fit in this model. Again, *Mplus* provides local fit information in the form of residuals and modification indices, with the latter giving the expected improvement in the chi-square statistic if a model constraint were released while retaining all other constraints. The modification indices in the two-factor model did not provide a clear indication of why the model did not fit better. The most useful indices are those involving covariances among the unique factors, as these may indicate associations among the items that were not being modeled. None of these modification indices were especially large, with the exception of one index in each group that assessed the covariances between different MH items. Puzzlingly, a different pair of MH items was involved in each group, but we have no clear hypothesis for why these covariances should be nonzero. We therefore decided, for purposes of explication, to proceed with the hypothesis that two latent variables underlie the RE and MH items, with each item set loading on its own latent variable. Note that the estimated correlation between the two latent variables was nearly the same for males and females: 0.75 for males and 0.73 for females.

Once the number and configuration of the latent variables is decided, the next issue is the choice of the IRT model to be used. For binary items, common choices include the Rasch model (Rasch, 1960) and the two-parameter logistic (2PL) model (Lord & Novick, 1968). Models that would account for guessing behavior, such as the three-parameter logistic (3PL), would ordinarily be irrelevant outside of the context of cognitive ability testing. For polytomous items, the range of choices is wider still. Models in the Rasch family of models include the rating scale (Andrich, 1978a, 1978b) and partial credit models (Masters, 1982, 1985). The generalized partial credit model (Muraki, 1992) extends the partial credit model to permit greater flexibility, at the cost of the simpler interpretations afforded by the Rasch model structure. The graded response model (Samejima, 1969, 1972) is another choice that is outside of the Rasch family of models. This model is essentially a polytomous generalization of the 2PL binary model. Both the graded response model and the 2PL binary model can be shown to be equivalent to the common factor model in the discrete case (Kamata & Bauer, 2008; Takane & de Leeuw, 1987). For detailed discussions of the properties of all of these models, see Embretson and Reise (2000), De Ayala (2009), and Nering and Ostini (2010). As a rule, models in the Rasch family offer clearer measurement interpretations and statistical properties, but are more restrictive in their assumptions. Less restrictive models such as the 2PL, the generalized partial credit model, and the graded response model will fit the data more often, but may sometimes be difficult to interpret.

If the number of latent variables underlying the items exceeds one, a multidimensional IRT (MIRT) model is needed. The standard choice is the general compensatory MIRT model that permits each item to be influenced by each latent variable additively, apart from identification restrictions. To illustrate, let X_{ij} again represent the score for the ith person on the jth binary item. Let $\boldsymbol{\theta}_i = \boldsymbol{\theta}_{i1}, \boldsymbol{\theta}_{i2}, \ldots, \boldsymbol{\theta}_{ir}$, be a vector of scores on r latent variables for the ith person. Let $\mathbf{a}_j = (a_{1j}, a_{2j}, \ldots, a_{rj})$ be a vector of item discrimination parameters for the jth item, and let c_j be an intercept parameter for the jth item. Then the compensatory MIRT model for X_{ij} is:

$$P\left(X_{ij} = 1 \mid \theta_i, \mathbf{a}_j, c_j\right) = \Psi\left(c_j + \sum_{k=1}^{r} a_{jk}\theta_{ik}\right), \tag{17.2}$$

where Ψ is the logistic function:

$$\Psi(x) = \frac{exp(x)}{1 + exp(x)}. \tag{17.3}$$

In the special case of r = 1, the model is equivalent to the 2PL model. Note also that the MIRT binary model in (17.2) can be expressed using the cumulative standard normal or normal ogive function in place of the logistic. Psychometric software programs vary depending on whether the logistic or normal ogive (probit) form of the model is used.

The extension of the binary MIRT model to the polytomous case can again be done using either the logistic or the normal framework. From the viewpoint of model parameters, the change from the binary case only introduces multiple intercept parameters c_{jm}, with m = 1, 2, . . . , M – 1, and M being the number of response categories. A six-category item, for example, will require five intercept parameters, and each item has its own set of intercept parameters. The number of discrimination parameters is unchanged from the binary case. As noted earlier, the compensatory MIRT model and the discrete multiple-factor model are equivalent for discrete measures. This equivalence is most clear for the normal ogive form of the MIRT, which, itself, is an extension of the graded response model to the multidimensional case.

The compensatory MIRT model can, indeed, encompass many model structures as special cases. One such structure of particular interest in health outcomes research is the bifactor structure (Holzinger & Swineford, 1939; Reise, Morizot, & Hays, 2007; Chapters 2, 8, and 9 in this volume). In this model, all items are related to a single common latent variable (the general factor), and each item is also related to a second latent variable shared only among a subset of related items. These secondary latent variables that explain separate sets of items are denoted “group factors” in the factor analytic literature. The idea behind this particular model is that while all of the items share a common influence, a single latent variable is insufficient because the items also measure an additional set of latent variables. These additional latent variables are limited in their influence to mutually exclusive subsets of the items. For example, the *SF-36* contains four subscales that measure different aspects of mental health, but these subscale items are also thought to share a general mental health factor. This set of items therefore follows a bifactor structure in theory, with a general mental health factor and four potential group factors. Each item is influenced by two latent variables: the general factor and one group factor. All of the factors in the standard bifactor model are assumed to be mutually orthogonal, or uncorrelated.

In our *SF-36* example, it is clear that a MIRT model is needed, given the rejection of the single-factor model. We first attempted to work with a bifactor MIRT model with a general latent variable and two group latent variables using the IRTPRO software program (Cai, du Toit, & Thissen, 2011). Unfortunately, severe numerical and convergence problems were encountered with this model in multiple groups, leading us to abandon this model. We therefore chose to use a MIRT model with two latent variables, one for the RE items and one for the MH items.

To evaluate the fit of the MIRT baseline model, we again used IRTPRO with multiple-group estimation methods. The baseline model will fit the MIRT model in each gender group simultaneously, with no invariance constraints apart from those needed to identify the model. The two latent variables in the model were allowed to correlate within each group; the correlation was estimated conditionally given the identification constraints and the item allocations to the two latent variables. The identification constraints used were:

1) The variances of the latent variables were fixed to one in the male group, and were freely estimated in the female group.
2) The means of the latent variables were fixed to zero in the male group, and were freely estimated in the female group.
3) The discrimination parameter and the intercept for item RE1 were constrained to invariance across gender, but were not fixed in value.
4) The discrimination parameter and the first intercept parameter for item MH1 were constrained to invariance across gender, but were not fixed in value.

These choices were not the only possible ones for identification purposes. A thorough treatment of identification issues in MIRT models is beyond the scope of this chapter. Reckase (2009) is a good source for more information.

Table 17.4 provides some of the fit information given by IRTPRO for the baseline MIRT model in the Model IRT1 row of the table. The M_2 chi-square statistic (Maydeu-Olivares & Joe, 2005, 2006) would suggest rejection of the model, but the RMSEA value based on this statistic suggests a reasonably good approximate fit. The item-level chi-square statistics in each group (not shown in Table 17.4) yielded *p*-values that were all above 0.01, which also suggests a reasonably good fit at the item level. Local dependence statistics, which evaluate the presence of residual associations between pairs of items, also indicated no problems in either group with regard to fit. We concluded that the two-factor MIRT model could serve as a baseline model for further tests of invariance.

Table 17.4 Model Fit Statistics for IRT Models

Model	M_2	*df*	*LR Diff (df)*	*RMSEA*	*AIC*	*BIC*
IRT1						
(Baseline)	515.44	320	———	.03	9125.19	9392.54
IRT2						
(Invar 12.3 (6) Discrim)	537.78	326	p = .0556	.03	9125.46	9365.15
IRT3						
(Invar 6.2 (6) except RE3)	529.85	325	p = .2966	.03	9121.26	9365.55
IRT4						
(Invar 28.3 (17) intercept)	559.22	342	p = .0416	.03	9115.56	9281.49
IRT5						
(Invar 22.3 (14) except MH3)	548.92	338	p = .0719	.03	9117.60	9301.97

Note: M_2 = Limited information chi-square, df = degrees of freedom LR Diff = difference in the −2ln (likelihood), RMSEA = Root Mean Square Error of Approximation, AIC = Akaike Information Criterion, BIC = Bayesian Information Criterion

Step Two: Evaluating Measurement Invariance

The process of evaluating measurement invariance can follow a number of paths, depending on the nature of the baseline model and the goals of the investigation. Two broad approaches are commonly taken. The first conducts direct comparisons of item parameters across groups using test statistics known as Wald statistics (Wald, 1943). The Wald statistic compares the size of the difference in parameter values across groups to an appropriate standard error estimate, yielding a z-score. In sufficiently large samples, this z-score can be referenced to the standard normal distribution to test the null hypothesis of no group difference in the parameter values. The Wald statistic can be used in univariate form for tests involving a single parameter, or in multivariate form that tests a set of related parameters. In either the univariate or multivariate versions, a key requirement is that an accurate standard error measure be available. This Wald statistic approach is most useful when the item response scales are binary and only one latent variable is needed. When the model is multidimensional and the items are polytomous, the number of model parameters to be tested becomes substantial, and many Wald tests are needed to fully examine invariance.

The second commonly used approach to invariance testing in IRT uses the likelihood ratio (LR) statistic. In essence, this test evaluates the relative fit of two models: a model that constrains a set of model parameters to invariance, and a model that releases those constraints. To the extent that the latter model results in a likelihood value that is improved relative to the constrained model, the data suggest that invariance in the studied set of parameters is implausible. One advantage of the LR approach is its flexibility. Any number of parameters can be evaluated for invariance using the test, although rejection of invariance leaves open the question of which parameters are responsible. A disadvantage of the LR test is that it requires two separate model evaluations to obtain the required likelihood values. This fact may or may not be a limitation, depending on the availability of efficient software.

In the *SF-36* data, we opted for the LR approach because of the number of parameters involved. The IRTPRO software produces likelihood values for use in the required LR test. For purposes of comparison, we also pursued a model comparison approach using the Mplus program under a CFA model. Both sets of analyses included sequences of nested model comparisons. Both sequences proceeded from the initial baseline model described earlier: Model CFA1 in Table 17.3 for the CFA analyses, and Model IRT1 in Table 17.4 for the IRT analyses. In both cases, at least one item per latent variable was assumed to be partially or totally invariant for identification purposes. The two items used in both sets of models were RE1 and MH1. These items served as "anchor items" for purpose of the analyses. The use of anchor items in LR tests is needed for model identification purposes, but it can also create problems if the chosen anchors lack invariance (Glas & Verhelst, 1995; Rensvold & Cheung, 2001). Methods for choosing anchor items based on preliminary factor analyses have been found to be fairly successful (Woods, 2009).

Given that the CFA and MIRT models employed for the *SF-36* data are complementary in structure, our narrative considers, in parallel, the tests of invariance conducted using each method. As we will see, the two approaches lead to similar conclusions about invariance in the *SF-36* data.

We begin with tests of the first set of invariance constraints: invariance constraints on factor loadings in the CFA, and on the discrimination parameters in MIRT. For the models under consideration, these two sets of parameters are closely related in the population: higher loadings correspond to higher discrimination parameters. Model CFA2, in Table 17.3 imposes invariance on the factor loadings. The LR test for this model suggests that significant gender differences in factor loadings are present. Similarly, Model IRT2 in Table 17.4 imposes invariance constraints on the discrimination parameters. The LR test of that model is close to significance at p = 0.0556. Scrutiny of the residuals and modification indices for Model CFA2, and of the gender differences in estimates of the discrimination parameters from Model IRT1 in Table 17.4, suggests that the factor loading/discrimination parameter for item RE3 should be permitted to vary across groups. This change was introduced in both the CFA and IRT analyses, leading to Model CFA3 in Table 17.3 and Model IRT3 in Table 17.4. LR test results in both the CFA3 and IRT3 models suggest that no further relaxations of invariance constraints are needed in either case. One feature to note in Table 17.3 is that the RMSEA value has improved in Model CFA3 relative to the baseline Model CFA1, even though more constraints had been added. This effect is due to the "penalty" that the RMSEA imposes for including unnecessary parameters in the CFA1 model.

The next set of invariance tests concerns invariance in the threshold parameters in the CFA, and in the intercept parameters in MIRT. For item RE3, we did not constrain the MIRT intercept parameter to invariance because the discrimination parameter for that item had been found earlier to vary by gender; group differences in the "slope" (or discrimination) parameters almost surely imply differences in the location parameters. For all other items, invariance constraints were imposed on all intercept parameters in the MIRT analyses. Similarly, invariance constraints were imposed on all threshold parameters in the CFA model. These new sets of constraints led to Model CFA4 in Table 17.3 and Model IRT4 in Table 17.4. These constraints produced no significant lack of fit in the CFA, as shown by the LR test. In the test of Model IRT4 in Table 17.4, the results suggested statistically significant lack of fit in Model IRT4, with a p-value of 0.0416. This suggests that some intercept parameters differ by gender. To evaluate the source of this problem, we examined response frequencies in the different items and compared estimates of intercept parameters across gender from Model IRT3. We were also influenced by the CFA modeling results in the next step, which constrained the unique factor variances to invariance. On balance, it appeared that the intercept parameters for item MH3 might be the source of the problem. We therefore relaxed the invariance constraints on the MH3 intercepts, while retaining the other constraints from Model IRT4. This new model is Model IRT5 in Table 17.4. The results of the LR test for Model IRT5 in Table 17.4 suggest that no further releases of constraints on the intercept parameters are needed. Model IRT5 is the final MIRT model we tested.

In the CFA, some additional parameters remain to be evaluated for invariance, and these parameters have no direct counterpart in MIRT. These CFA parameters are the unique factor variances. In the population MIRT and CFA models, the unique factor variances are inversely related to the item discrimination parameters: higher unique factor variances correspond to smaller discrimination parameters. We tested a CFA model that imposed invariance on all unique factor variances: Model CFA5 in Table 17.4. The LR test for this model showed significant loss of fit in comparison to Model CFA4 in Table 17.4. Scrutiny of the residuals and modification indices for Model CFA5 suggested item MH3 as the source of the misfit. Model CFA6 was created in response. Model CFA6 retained the invariance constraints on the unique factor variances in Model CFA5, except for the constraint on MH3. The LR test for Model CFA6 indicated no further problems with the invariance constraints. Hence, Model CFA6 was the final CFA model we tested.

Table 17.5 gives the parameter estimates provided by Model IRT5. We transformed the intercept parameter estimates to difficulty parameter estimates in the case of the RE items, and to threshold parameter estimates in the case of the MH items. All item parameters are invariant except for the parameters for RE3 and the threshold parameters for MH3.

Table 17.5 Parameter Estimates From Model IRT5

RE Items		*Discrim*			*Difficulty*
RE1		4.21			–1.16
RE2		5.25			–.75
RE3		3.13 (1.48)*			–1.16 (–1.58)
MH Items	*Discrim*	d_1	d_2	d_3	d_4
MH1	1.36	–2.01	–1.01	.29	—
MH2	3.11	–1.93	–1.22	–.47	—
MH3	1.79	–1.58 (–1.46)	–.54 (–.62)	–.08 (–.19)	2.10 (1.74)
MH4	2.59	–1.71	–.76	.25	—
MH5	2.46	–1.78	–.91	–.45	1.40

* Estimates in parentheses for RE3 and MH3 are for females, with male estimates listed just before. Discrim = Discrimination parameter, d_m = mth threshold parameter.

The discrimination parameters for RE3 appear to be quite different, with the item being a more discriminating measure for males than for females. Males also have a somewhat higher difficulty parameter for RE3, suggesting that they will endorse the item less often. For MH3, the threshold parameters for males are more widely spaced than those for females. We would expect females to show more frequent endorsement of the higher categories for this item, and this is found in the data. It is also true, however, that the estimated means on the latent variables are higher for females than males. The means on the RE variable are 0 (i.e., fixed for identification purposes) and 0.57 for males and females respectively, and for the MH variable are 0 (fixed) and 0.21 for males and females respectively. Hence, females will tend to respond with higher item scores on all items if the items are indeed invariant.

Step Three: Effect Sizes and Decisions

Once the invariance analysis is completed and items that violate invariance have been identified, the practical question of what should be done about the violations will arise. One preliminary step that may help in the decision process is to create an "effect size" measure that assesses the size of the violation in some useful metric. For binary, unidimensional IRT models, a variety of these measures are available (see Millsap (2011) for a summary). One popular choice, particularly for the Rasch or 2PL models, is an area measure defined as the area separating the item response functions for each group. A simple unsigned area measure for two item response functions $P_{jk}(\theta) = P(X_{ij} = 1 | \theta_i)$ for the kth group, k = 1,2, is:

$$\int_{-\infty}^{\infty} | P_{j1}(\theta) - P_{j2}(\theta) | \, d\theta \tag{17.4}$$

where the brackets inside the integral denote absolute value. This statistic is denoted the "unsigned" area measure because it sums all discrepancies between the item response functions regardless of which function is greater at a given point. For the Rasch model, the area in (3) simplifies to the absolute value of the difference between the group-specific difficulty parameters. For the 2PL with discrimination parameters that vary across groups, the area in (3) simplifies to a function of the difficulty and discrimination parameters in the two groups, as illustrated later in this chapter.

For polytomous, unidimensional items, practical measures of effect size for violations of invariance are not yet in wide use. The item response functions in the polytomous case are not simple monotonic functions of the latent variable, unlike the binary item case. As a result, no simple area measures are available. One option is to plot the expected score function, which is the conditional expected score on the item given the latent variable. We can also describe this function as the nonlinear regression function for the item score regressed on the latent variable. It tells us what item response we would expect to see, on average, for people with a given latent variable score. If invariance is violated, the expected score functions will ordinarily also be different across groups. Plotting them permits visual comparisons between the group-specific score functions. Unfortunately, no summary measure that expresses the difference between the functions is yet available.

For the truly multidimensional case in which items are each influenced by multiple latent variables, no simple summary measures of effect size have been adopted for practical use. Plots of the item response functions are difficult to display if there are more than two latent variables, and even the two-dimensional case is difficult to visually process when plots from two groups are superimposed. The multidimensional case requires further research before usable effect size measures are available.

Effect size measures alone do not solve the decision problem concerning what to do about items that violate invariance. One strategy that has been used to address the problem is to evaluate the impact of the item-level violations on the scale-level score. The logic of this approach is that in a scale with a sufficient number of items, violations of invariance by a few items may have a negligible effect on the scale score. This could be due to the relatively small proportion of items that violate invariance, or to biases in the items that go in different directions, and are therefore countervailing at the scale level. To evaluate the impact of the violations of the invariance at the scale level, a simple approach is to compare the rank ordering of respondents over two versions of the scale, one with and one without the biased items. This comparison does not take into account the impact of the biased items on the mean of the scale, however. For situations in which actual latent score estimates are used, the impact of the biased items on the latent score estimates can be evaluated by generating score estimates from the full set of items, and from the subset of items that are invariant. Rank orderings of individuals on the resulting score estimates can then be compared.

A more systematic approach to evaluating the impact of item-level violations of invariance on the scale-level scores is provided by the DFIT system ("Differential Functioning of Items and Tests") (Raju, Van der Linden, & Fleer, 1995). This approach defines "differential test functioning" (DTF) by the expected difference in scale scores in the two groups, given the estimated item response functions in each group. This definition considers all scale items together, using whatever scoring function is to be used to calculate scale scores. It is also possible to test for the existence of nonzero DTF, using several possible test statistics. The DFIT method was originally designed for binary unidimensional items, but has been extended to the polytomous case (Flowers, Oshima, & Raju, 1999), and even to the multidimensional case (Oshima, Raju, & Flowers, 1997). Items showing substantial impact at the scale level would likely be removed from the instrument based on evidence provided by any of these methods, but as noted earlier, this action would depend heavily on the history of the scale.

Although all of these approaches are useful, it is sometimes valuable to ask whether the presence of biased items interferes with the actual use of the scale. Does the presence of biased items meaningfully impair the intended use of the scale? For example, if the scale is to be used for predictive purposes, do the biased items interfere with prediction? Or if the scale is used for diagnostic purposes, do the biased items render the diagnoses less accurate for one or more groups? At present, there is little research that explores how these questions might be answered. The impact of violations of measurement invariance on the use of scales for prediction has been studied (see Borsboom, Romeijn, & Wicherts (2008); Millsap (2011)). Less work is available on the impact of measurement bias on diagnosis. Millsap and Kwok (2004) demonstrated how measurement bias defined within the CFA model could be studied for its impact on sensitivity and specificity in diagnosis. In this particular application, the procedure assumes that invariance analyses have been completed using CFA, and then assesses the effects of the lack of invariance on sensitivity, specificity, and positive predictive value under a range of assumptions. Again, further research on the practical consequences of measurement bias is needed.

Returning to the *SF-36* example, Figure 17.1 displays the item response functions for males and females on item RE3. The value of the unsigned area measure in Equation (17.4) for this item is 0.10, a relatively small value (Raju, 1990). The item response functions for this item intersect, an example of nonuniform or bidirectional bias. The item does not favor one group or the other uniformly across the range of the latent variable. The effect size measure in this case suggests that the bias in this item is small. The situation for item MH3 is more complex because the item is polytomous, precluding use of the area measure in (3). As an alternative, Figure 17.2 displays the expected score functions for males and females. The horizontal scale is for the latent variable. The vertical axis gives possible scores on the item, starting at zero and going to a maximum of four. In practice, respondents can only receive integer scores (0, 1, 2, 3, 4), but the function is showing the average or expected value for individuals at any given latent score. For this reason, we can treat the vertical scale as continuous. The horizontal lines are for reference purposes. Figure 17.2 shows that the functions are closely matched for $\theta < 0$, but they diverge to

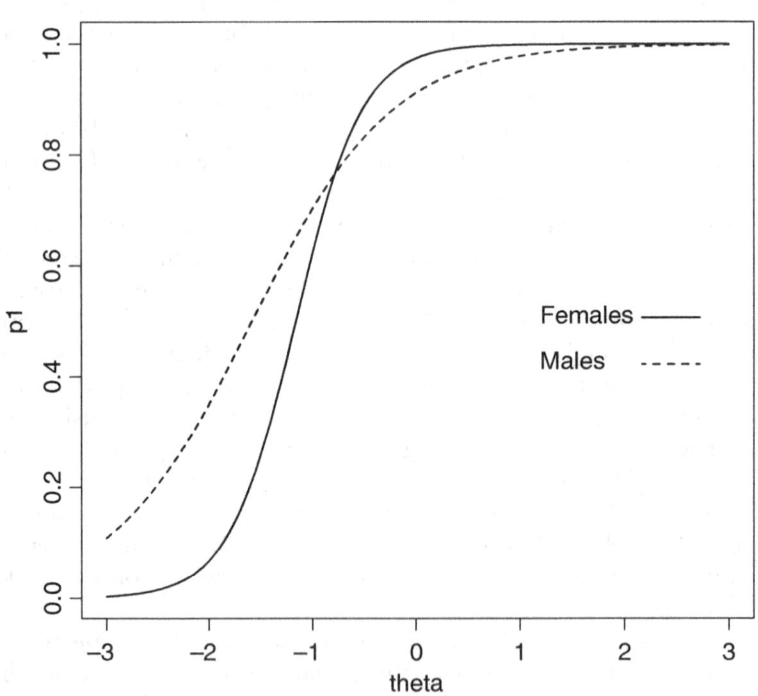

Figure 17.1 Item response functions for males and females for an item on the role emotional subscale of the SF-36.

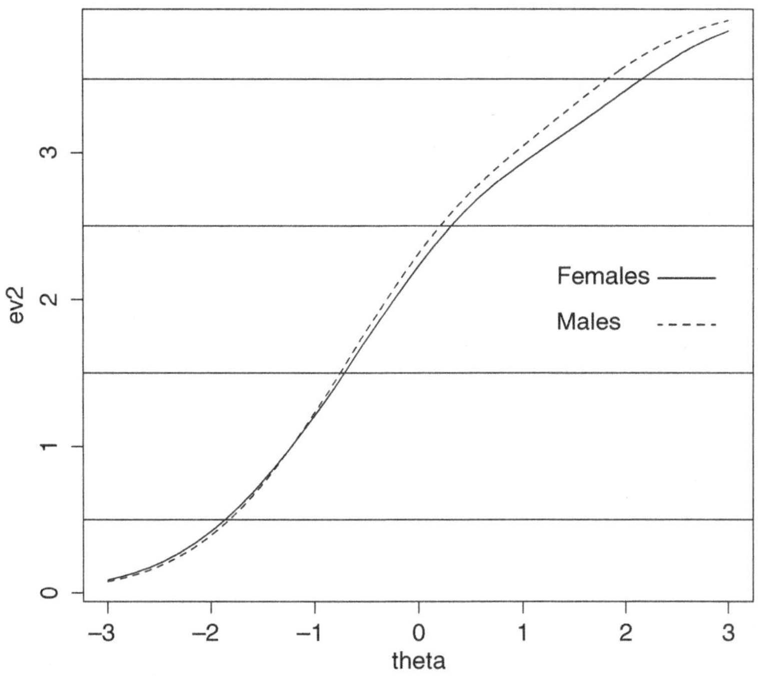

Figure 17.2 Expected score functions for males and females on an item on the mental health subscale of the SF-36.

some extent for $\theta > 1.0$. The size of the difference is not large however, even at its widest point. As measured by the discrepancy in expected score functions, the bias in this item is relatively small. The question of how the biases in the items RE3 and MH3 might affect the scale scores can probably be set aside here, given the small effect sizes at the item level. However, it may be more of a concern in subscale scores if the RE or MH subscales are used in practice because these are relatively short scales.

Summary

The investigation of measurement invariance is part of the general investigation of construct validity: Does the item or scale really measure what it is intended to measure? Health-related questionnaires and scales are now used widely across diverse populations defined by culture, language, geographical location, and health history. We would like to have confidence that when research is conducted or diagnoses are made across diverse populations, our health measures are not distorted by unanticipated influences. Unfortunately, the problem of empirically checking whether a survey item or scale is biased is not straightforward or simple, given that we generally have no "gold standard" measures for comparison. A number of statistical methods have been developed to address this difficult problem. This chapter has focused on model-based methods that evaluate measurement bias within a specific latent variable model for the items: item response theory.

Latent variable approaches for assessing measurement invariance have both advantages and disadvantages. One disadvantage is that the required models are based on assumptions that may not hold in the data. In some cases, a good baseline model may not be found, cutting short the entire investigation. The use of IRT requires the investigator to have some insight about the proper number of latent variables for the items being studied. This requirement is often not a major problem for measures that are already in wide use, as these measures typically have a history of research on the dimensionality of the measure. On the other hand, when new instruments are constructed, the dimensionality of the items is usually an open question. If little empirical information is available, it may simply be premature to investigate measurement invariance.

If an appropriate latent variable model can be found for the items, the advantages of the model-based approach become clear. First, model-based methods can handle situations in which multiple latent variables underlie the items. This multidimensional situation is likely to be the norm for many health-related measures. The *SF-36* was purposely designed to assess multiple dimensions of general health, for example. A second advantage of model-based methods is that scales based on relatively few items can still be effectively modeled and evaluated for invariance. Short scales pose difficulties for alternative methods that rely on measured proxy variables as substitutes for the latent variables. With a short scale, the total scale score is less reliable, and the unreliability tends to undercut the quality of the matching. This effect in turn leads to inaccuracy when testing for invariance (Meredith & Millsap, 1992). Many health-related scales are fairly short (e.g., less than 10 items), and so this matching problem may be significant.

Sample size demands for the use of item response theory or other latent variable methods can be substantial, depending on the model. Good results with the binary Rasch model can be achieved with several hundred cases. At the other extreme, MIRT models for large sets of polytomous items may require 1,000 cases or more to yield good results. The situations that require larger samples for latent variable methods are also the situations that are difficult to handle well using proxy variable methods. Proxy methods do perform better when the number of items is substantial, as long as the item set is roughly unidimensional. It is difficult, however, to construct a scale that is both unidimensional and that contains many items.

Finally, as we illustrated in this chapter, the use of models such as those in IRT to study measurement invariance requires some training and judgment on the part of the investigator. Critical thinking about the possible role of nuisance variables as explanations for violations of invariance is needed, both to interpret any results found, and to suggest additional data that might help evaluate such explanations. Furthermore, the analyses require the use of software that is unfamiliar to most health researchers, and the models themselves are still new to many. While descriptions of these models have traditionally been found only in technical journals or reports, this situation is changing, and there are now many more accessible accounts, as cited earlier, in the literature. We hope this chapter motivates readers to learn more about the use of IRT in studying measurement invariance.

Note: This work was supported in part by a grant from the National Institute on Aging (R01 AG 026006, Alex Zautra, PI).

References

Ackerman, T. A. (1992). A didactic explanation of item bias, item impact, and item validity from a multidimensional perspective. *Journal of Educational Measurement, 29*, 67–91.

Andrich, D. (1978a). A rating formulation for ordered response categories. *Psychometrika, 43*, 561–573.

Andrich, D. (1978b). Application of a psychometric rating model to ordered categories which are scored with successive integers. *Applied Psychological Measurement, 2*, 581–594.

Angoff, W. H. (1993). Perspectives on differential item functioning methodology. In P. W. Holland & H. Wainer (Eds.), *Differential item functioning* (pp. 3–23). Hillsdale, NJ: Lawrence Erlbaum Associates.

Benjamini, Y., & Hochberg, Y. (1995). Controlling the false discovery rate: A practical and powerful approach to multiple testing. *Journal of the Royal Statistical Society, Series B, 57*, 289–300.

Borsboom, D., Romeijn, J.W., & Wicherts, J.M. (2008). Measurement invariance versus selection invariance: Is fair selection possible? *Psychological Methods, 13*, 75–98.

Brown, T.A. (2006). *Confirmatory factor analysis for applied research*. New York: Guilford.

Browne, M.W., & Cudeck, R. (1993). Alternative ways of assessing model fit. In K.A. Bollen & J.S. Long (Eds.), *Testing structural equation models* (pp. 136–162). Newbury Park, CA: Sage.

Cai, L., du Toit, S.H.C., & Thissen, D. (2011). *IRTPRO: Flexible, multidimensional, multiple categorical IRT modeling*. Chicago, IL: SSI International.

Camilli, G. (1992). A conceptual analysis of differential item functioning in terms of a multidimensional item response model. *Applied Psychological Measurement, 16*, 129–147.

Carroll, J.B. (1983). The difficulty of a test and its factor composition revisited. In H. Wainer & S. Messick (Eds.), *Principles of modern psychological measurement*. Hillsdale, NJ: Lawrence Erlbaum Associates.

Cella, B., Yount, S., Rothrock, N., Gershon, R., Cook, K., Reeve, B., . . . Rose, M. (2007). The Patient-Reported Outcomes Measurement Information System (PROMIS): Progress of an NIH roadmap cooperative group during its first two years. *Medical Care, 45*(5 Suppl. 1), S3–S11.

De Ayala, R.J. (2009). *The theory and practice of item response theory*. New York: Guilford.

Dorans, N.J., & Holland, P.W. (1993). DIF detection and description: Mantel-Haenszel and standardization. In P.W. Holland & H. Wainer (Eds.), *Differential item functioning* (pp. 35–66). Hillsdale, NJ: Lawrence Erlbaum Associates.

Embretson, S.E., & Reise, S.P. (2000). *Item response theory for psychologists*. Mahwah, NJ: Lawrence Erlbaum Associates.

Flora, D. B., & Curran, P. J. (2004). An empirical evaluation of alternative methods of estimation for confirmatory factor analysis with ordinal data. *Psychological Methods, 9*(4), 466.

Flowers, C.P., Oshima, T.C., & Raju, N.S. (1999). A description and demonstration of the polytomous DFIT framework. *Applied Psychological Measurement, 23*, 309–326.

Fukuhara, S., Ware, J.E., Kosinski, M., Wada, S., & Gandek, B. (1998). Psychometric and clinical tests of validity of the Japanese SF-36 Health Survey, *Journal of Clinical Epidemiology, 51*(11), 1045–1053.

Glas, C.A.W., & Verhelst, N.D. (1995). Testing the Rasch model. In G.H. Fischer & I.W. Molenaar (Eds.), *Rasch models: Foundations, recent developments, and applications* (pp. 69–95). New York: Springer.

Holland, P.W., & Thayer, D.T. (1988). Differential item performance and the Mantel-Haenszel procedure. In H. Wainer & H. Braun (Eds.), *Test validity* (pp. 129–145). Hillsdale, NJ: Lawrence Erlbaum Associates.

Holzinger, K.J., & Swineford, F.A. (1939). A study in factor analysis: The stability of a bi-factor solution. *Supplementary Educational Monographs, 48*, University of Chicago, Chicago, IL.

Hu, L., & Bentler, P.M. (1995). Evaluating model fit. In R.H. Hoyle (Ed.), *Structural equation modeling: Concepts, issues, and applications* (pp. 76–99). Thousand Oaks, CA: Sage.

Kamata, A., & Bauer, D.J. (2008). A note on the relation between factor analytic and item response theory models. *Structural Equation Modeling, 15*, 136–153.

Keller, S.D., Ware, J.E., Bentler, P.M., Aronson, N.K., Alonso, J., Apolane, G., . . . Gandek, B. (1998). Use of structural equation modeling to test the construct validity of the SF-36 health survey in 10 countries: Results from the IQOLA project. *Journal of Clinical Epidemiology, 51*(11), 1179–1188.

Kim, H.R. (1994). *New techniques for the dimensionality assessment of standardized test data*. Unpublished doctoral dissertation, University of Illinois at Urbana-Champaign, Department of Statistics.

Li, H., & Stout, W. (1995). Assessment of unidimensionality for mixed polytomous and dichotomous item data: Refinements of Poly-DIMTEST. Paper presented at the annual meeting of the National Council on Measurement in Education, San Francisco.

Lord, F.M. (1980). *Applications of item response theory to practical testing problems*. Hillsdale, NJ: Lawrence Erlbaum Associates.

Lord, F.M., & Novick, M.E. (1968). *Statistical theories of mental test scores*. Reading, MA: Addison-Wesley.

Masters, G.N. (1982). A Rasch model for partial credit scoring. *Psychometrika, 47*, 149–174.
Masters, G.N. (1985). A comparison of latent-trait and latent-class analyses of Likert-type data. *Psychometrika, 50*, 69–82.
Maydeu-Olivares, A., & Joe, H. (2005). Limited and full information estimation and goodness-of-fit testing in 2^n contingency tables: A unified framework. *Journal of the American Statistical Association, 100*, 1009–1020.
Maydeu-Olivares, A., & Joe, H. (2006). Limited information goodness-of-fit testing in multidimensional contingency tables. *Psychometrika, 71*, 713–732.
McDonald, R.P., & Ahlawat, K.S. (1974). Difficulty factors in binary data. *British Journal of Mathematical and Statistical Psychology, 27*, 82–99.
McDowell, I., & Newell, C. (1996). *Measuring health: A guide to rating scales and questionnaires* (2nd ed.). New York: Oxford University Press.
McHorney, C.A., Ware, J.E., & Raczek, A.E. (1993). The MOS 36-Item Short-Form Health Survey (SF-36): II. Psychometric and clinical tests of validity in measuring physical and mental health constructs. *Medical Care, 31*(3), 247–263.
Mellenbergh, G.J. (1989). Item bias and item response theory. *International Journal of Educational Research, 13*, 127–143.
Meredith, W., & Millsap, R.E. (1992). On the misuse of manifest variables in the detection of measurement bias. *Psychometrika, 57*, 289–311.
Millsap, R.E. (2011). *Statistical approaches to measurement invariance*. New York: Routledge.
Millsap, R.E., & Kwok, O.M. (2004). Evaluating the impact of partial factorial invariance on selection in two populations. *Psychological Methods, 9*, 93–115.
Millsap, R.E., & Tein, J.Y. (2004). Assessing factorial invariance in ordered-categorical measures. *Multivariate Behavioral Research, 39*, 479–515.
Muraki, E. (1992). A generalized partial credit model: Application of an EM algorithm. *Applied Psychological Measurement, 16*, 159–176.
Muthén, L., & Muthén, B.O. (1998–2012). *Mplus user's guide* (7th ed.). Los Angeles, CA: Muthén & Muthén.
Nandakumar, R., & Stout, W. (1993). Refinements of Stout's procedure for assessing latent trait dimensionality. *Journal of Educational Statistics, 18*, 41–68.
Nandakumar, R., Yu, F., Li, H.H., & Stout, W. (1998). Assessing unidimensionality of polytomous data. *Applied Psychological Measurement, 22*, 99–115.
Nering, M.L., & Ostini, R. (2010). *Handbook of polytomous item response theory models*. New York: Routledge.
Oshima, T.C., Raju, N.S., & Flowers, C.P. (1997). Development and demonstration of multidimensional IRT-based internal measures of differential functioning of items and tests. *Journal of Educational Measurement, 34*, 253–272.
Osterlind, S.J., & Everson, H.T. (2009). *Differential item functioning* (2nd ed.). Los Angeles, CA: Sage.
Perkins, A.J., Stump, T.E., Monahan, P.O., & McHorney, C.A. (2006). Assessment of differential item functioning for demographic comparisons in the MOS SF-36 health survey. *Quality of Life Research, 15*(3), 331–348.
Pollard, B., Johnston, M., & Dixon, D. (2013). Exploring differential item functioning in the SF-36 by demographic, clinical, psychological and social factors in an osteoarthritis population. *BMC Musculoskeletal Disorders, 14*, 346.
Raju, N.S. (1990). Determining the significance of estimated signed and unsigned areas between two item response functions. *Applied Psychological Measurement, 14*, 197–207.
Raju, N.S., Van der Linden, W.J., & Fleer, P.F. (1995). IRT-based internal measures of differential functioning of items and tests. *Applied Psychological Measurement, 19*, 353–368.
Rasch, G. (1960). *Probabilistic models for some intelligence and attainment tests*. Copenhagen, Denmark: Danish Institute for Educational Research.
Reckase, M.D. (2009). *Multidimensional item response theory*. New York: Springer.
Reise, S.G., Morizot, J., & Hays, R.D. (2007). The role of the bifactor model in resolving dimensionality issues in health outcomes measures. *Quality of Life Research, 16*, 19–31.

Rensvold, R. B., & Cheung, G. W. (2001). Testing for metric invariance using structural equation models: Solving the standardization problem. In C. A. Schriesheim & L. L. Neider (Eds.), *Research in management* (vol. 1, pp. 25–50). Greenwich, CT: Information Age Publishing.

Roussos, L., & Stout, W. (1996). A multidimensionality-based DIF analysis paradigm. *Applied Psychological Measurement, 20*, 355–371.

Samejima, F. (1969). Estimation of ability using a response pattern of graded scores. *Psychometrika Monograph*, No. 17.

Samejima, F. (1972). A general model for free-response data. *Psychometrika Monograph*, No. 18.

Shealy, R., & Stout, W. (1993). A model-based standardization approach that separates true bias/DIF from group differences and detects test bias/DIF as well as item bias/DIF. *Psychometrika, 58*, 159–194.

Steiger, J. H., & Lind, J. M. (1980). *Statistically based tests for the number of common factors*. Paper presented at the annual meeting of the Psychometric Society, Iowa City, IA.

Stout, W. (1987). A nonparametric approach for assessing latent trait dimensionality. *Psychometrika, 52*, 589–617.

Stout, W., Habing, B., Kim, H. R., Roussos, L., Zhang, J., & Douglas, J. (1996). Conditional covariance-based nonparametric multidimensionality assessment. *Applied Psychological Measurement, 20*, 331–354.

Sullivan, M., Karlsson, J., & Ware, J. E. (1995). The Swedish SF-36 Health Survey: I. Evaluation of data quality, scaling assumption, reliability and construct validity across general populations in Sweden. *Social Science Medical, 41*(10), 1349–1358.

Svetina, D., & Levy, R. (2012). An overview of software for conducting dimensionality assessment in multidimensional models. *Applied Psychological Measurement, 35*, 659–669.

Takane, Y., & de Leeuw, J. (1987). On the relationship between item response theory and factor analysis of discretized variables. *Psychometrika, 52*, 393–408.

Wald, A. (1943). Tests of statistical hypotheses concerning several parameters when the number of observations is large. *Transactions of the American Mathematical Society, 54*, 426–482.

Ware, J. E., Kosinski, M., Gandek, B. G., Aaronson, N., Alonso, J., Apolone, G., . . . Sullivan, M. (1998). The factor structure of the SF-36® health survey in 10 countries: Results from the International Quality of Life Assessment (IQOLA) project. *Journal of Clinical Epidemiology, 51*(11), 1159–1165.

Ware, J. E., Snow, K. K., Kosinski, M., & Gandek, B. (1993). *SF-36® health survey manual and interpretation guide*. Boston, MA: New England Medical Center, The Health Institute.

Widaman, K. F. (1993). Common factor analysis versus principal component analysis: Differential bias in representing model parameters? *Multivariate Behavioral Research, 28*(3), 263–311.

Widaman, K. F., & Reise, S. P. (1997). Exploring the measurement invariance of psychological instruments: Applications in the substance abuse domain. In K. J. Bryant, *Alcohol and substance use research* (pp. 281–324). Washington, DC: American Psychological Association.

Woods, C. M. (2009). Empirical selection of anchors for tests of differential item functioning. *Applied Psychological Measurement, 33*, 42–57.

18 Detecting Faulty Within-Item Category Functioning With the Nominal Response Model

Kathleen S. J. Preston and Steven P. Reise

Introduction

For polytomous items with *m* ordered response categories, the nominal response model (NRM; Bock, 1972) allows researchers to estimate $m - 1$ category "boundary" discrimination (CBD) parameters. These CBD parameters provide important diagnostic information regarding item functioning. Specifically, in ordered polytomous data, a CBD parameter reflects the degree to which a particular response category distinction is useful in discriminating among individuals. Unfortunately, research applying the NRM model to ordered categorical responses is essentially nonexistent. Hence, we illustrate several potentially useful applications of the NRM including exploring whether: a) CBD parameters vary within an item, b) an item contains too many response options, and c) responses options are ordered. We also conducted Monte Carlo simulations to investigate the power of the likelihood-ratio and Wald tests to detect: a) different degrees of within-item variation in CBD parameters, and b) when a single within-item CBD parameter equals zero. Results support the utility of the likelihood-ratio and Wald tests for identifying items where response option choices are differentially discriminating, and for identifying items that contain poorly functioning response options.

The nominal response model (NRM; Bock, 1972, 1997; de Ayala, 2009, pp. 237–261; Ostini & Nering, 2006, pp. 16–24) is the most general divide-by-total (Thissen & Steinberg, 1986) item response theory (IRT) model. One attractive but underutilized feature of the NRM is that it allows researchers to estimate a slope parameter for each response category within a polytomous item with ordered categories. In turn, these category slope parameters can be transformed into category "boundary" discrimination (CBD) parameters. The size of a CBD indicates the amount of relative information provided by adjacent response categories (e.g., the degree to which a response in category 3 versus 2 differentiates among people on the latent trait). In reference to CBD parameters, "varied discriminating powers among categorical responses are essential features of the nominal response model" (du Toit, 2003, p. 559). The fact that CBD parameters in the NRM can vary within an item stands in stark contrast to the more commonly applied polytomous IRT models such as the graded response model (GRM; Samejima, 1969), or the generalized partial credit model (G-PCM; Muraki, 1992), wherein each item is characterized by a single overall item discrimination parameter (see Chapter 14).

Heretofore, the NRM has received relatively limited application to real-world measures (however, see Tokuda et al., 2009). Nevertheless, researchers have: a) described linking under the NRM (Baker, 1993), b) examined item parameter recovery (de Ayala & Sava-Bolesta, 1999; DeMars, 2003; Passos & Berger, 2004; Wollack, Bolt, Cohen, & Lee, 2002), c) developed indices to identify model violations (Glas, 1999), and d) explored the application of computerized adaptive testing (de Ayala, 1992). Researchers have also considered the use of the NRM to: a) test whether response categories on polytomous items are ordered (Samejima, 1996), and b) determine whether distractors on multiple-choice items provide additional information about examinee trait level (Thissen, 1976; Thissen, Steinberg, & Fitzpatrick, 1989).

Unfortunately, research on how to use the NRM as a basis for identifying the psychometric properties of specific response categories in ordered polytomous items has been lacking. Thus, in the following, we present real-data analyses of ordered categorical data to demonstrate the potential utility of the NRM in exploring whether: a) CBD parameters vary within an item, b) an item contains too many response options, and c) response options are ordered.

These example data analyses then serve to motivate a Monte Carlo investigation of the power of the likelihood-ratio and Wald tests to investigate two specific hypotheses regarding within-item CBD parameters. First, Monte Carlo data are generated where CBD parameters vary within items. The data are then fit to both the NRM and the G-PCM in order to estimate the power of the likelihood-ratio test to detect different degrees of within-item CBD variation. Second, Monte Carlo data will again be used to explore the power of the likelihood-ratio test to detect when a single CBD parameter within an item is zero (i.e., to detect when a response category distinction on a polytomous item is poorly functioning). Background information on polytomous IRT models is provided in the following section.

Research Methods

Polytomous IRT Models

It is important to distinguish between two types of polytomous IRT models that are referred to by Thissen and Steinberg (1986) as difference and divide-by-total models. The prototypical example of a difference model is Samejima's GRM (1969). In the GRM, the basic building block for item analysis is a threshold response curve that relates standing on a latent trait with the probability of responding above a between category threshold (e.g., on a four-point item, three threshold response curves are estimated that represent the probability of responding in category 0 versus 1, 2, 3; 0, 1 versus 2, 3; and, 0, 1, 2, versus 3). In the GRM, the threshold response curves within an item are constrained to have equal slope/discrimination parameters, and the probability of an individual scoring in any particular response category is found by subtracting adjacent threshold response curves.

Although the GRM (Samejima, 1969) is arguably more commonly applied, the present chapter focuses on the divide-by-total (Thissen & Steinberg, 1986) class of models, namely: a) the NRM (Bock, 1972, 1997), b) the partial credit model (PCM; Masters 1982), c) the rating scale model (RSM; Andrich, 1978a, 1978b), and d) the G-PCM (Muraki, 1992). In divide-by-total models, the basic unit for analysis is the distinction between each adjacent pair of response options considered independently (e.g., the probability of responding in category 2 versus 1, assuming the person has responded in either category 2 or 1). There are several critical differences between divide-by-total models and difference models (Thissen & Steinberg, 1986), such as the GRM, that are important to note (see also Andrich, 1995).

First, in divide-by-total models, a single equation can be written relating the latent trait with the probability of responding in a specific response category. Second, item location indices in divide-by-total models are not required to be ordered (except in the RSM), and are not interpreted as "threshold" parameters, but rather are "intersection" parameters that represent the point on the latent trait scale at which a response in category x is more likely than a response in category $x - 1$. Third, and most critical in terms of the present research, only divide-by-total models afford the possibility of varying CBD parameters within an item (see Ostini & Nering, 2006, p. 77, on why there is no heterogeneous case of the GRM). As a result, it must be recognized that the NRM is an appropriate baseline only for the more restricted divide-by-total models listed earlier, and thus the present findings are relevant only to this class of model.

The Nominal Response Model

The NRM (Bock, 1972, 1997) is considered the most general polytomous IRT model because all other divide-by-total IRT models are nested within or are constrained versions of the NRM (de Ayala, 2009; Ostini & Nering, 2006, p. 52; Thissen & Steinberg, 1986). In the NRM the conditional probability of an individual with trait level θ responding in category x ($x = 0 \ldots m_i$) on item i can be written:

$$P_{ix}(\theta) = \frac{\exp(a_{ix}\theta + c_{ix})}{\sum_{x=1}^{m} \exp(a_{ix}\theta + c_{ix})}, \tag{18.1}$$

where, for identification, $\Sigma\, a_{ix} = \Sigma\, c_{ix} = 0$.

In Equation (18.1), a set of slope and intercept parameters (a, c) are estimated for each response option within an item. These parameters represent the linear relation between the latent trait and the log-odds of responding in a given category. Thus, some authors have referred to the category slope a_{ix} parameters as "category discrimination" parameters (e.g., de Ayala, 2009)—the rate of change in log-odds of responding in a particular category. The category intercept parameters in Equation (18.1) are not intersection parameters (where on the latent trait scale two category response curves intersect), and cannot be interpreted thresholds (where on the latent trait scale the probability of a response in and above a given category is 50%), either. Rather, the category intercepts reflect the relative popularity of the response option; the larger the category intercept parameter, the greater relative frequency of responses in that category.

Thissen, Steinberg, and Fitzpatrick (1989) provide an alternative and more useful way of interpreting the parameters of the NRM. Assume the response categories are ordered and let x and $x' = x - 1$ represent two adjacent response options (e.g., category 3 and 2). Then the NRM for the choice between *two* options can be rewritten as shown in Equation (18.2).

$$P_{ix} \mid x = x \, or \, x' = \frac{1}{1 + \exp(-a_j^{*}\theta + d_j)}, \tag{18.2}$$

where $a_j^{*} = a_x - a_x'$ and $d_j = c_x' - c_x$.

In short, the probability of deciding between any two adjacent choices x and x' is a monotonically increasing 2-PL function when a^* is positive. Of course, a^* is only positive when the category slope a_x is larger than the category slope a_{x-1}. Thus, in an NRM response categories can be ordered by their slope parameters; higher slope for category x *vs.* x' means that the probability of responding to category x versus x' is a monotonically increasing function; as trait level goes up, the probability of selecting x over x' increases.

It is important to note that Equation (18.2) represents the probability of selecting response x versus x' assuming that the response is in either category x versus x'. If the categories are assumed to be ordered so that $x = x$ and $x' = x - 1$, then the $a^* = a_x - a_x'$ parameter provides the discrimination of the distinction between categories x and $x - 1$ considering only the dichotomous decision between category x and x'. For this reason, we subscript as a_j^* ($j = 1 \ldots m_i - 1$) and refer to these parameters as CBD parameters in order that they not be confused with category slope (a_x) parameters. For items with ordered response options, CBD parameters should never be negative. Large positive a_j^* indicate that the distinction between category x and x' is highly informative, while a_j^* near zero indicates that the distinction between category x and x' is meaningless; people (or raters) cannot differentiate between the response options.

Equation (18.2) introduces a second new term, namely, the intercept $d_j = c_x' - c_x$. The differences in c values from adjacent categories divided by the differences in a_x (i.e., a_j^*) produces an intersection parameter as shown in Equation (18.3).

$$c_j^* = \frac{c_{(x-1)} - c_x}{a_x - a_{(x-1)}}. \tag{18.3}$$

Intersection parameters represent the point on the latent trait scale where a response in adjacent categories is equally likely. Despite claims to the contrary in the literature, category intersection parameters have no other substantive interpretation—they are not relative difficulties of steps within a multistep problem and differences between category intersections are not "psychological" distances (Andrich, 1995, p. 116).

Now, given the formulation of the NRM in Equation (18.2), it is easy to show that other divide-by-total models are nested within the NRM (see de Ayala, 2009, p. 245; Ostini & Nering, 2006). For example, when all a_j^* parameters within and between items are constrained to equality (typically 1.0) this produces a partial credit model (Masters, 1982). If in addition, all c^* parameters are constrained to be equal between items, and it is assumed that intersections are ordered, this produces the rating scale model (Andrich, 1978a, 1978b). Finally, when a_j^* parameters are constrained to equality within items, but not between, this produces the G-PCM (Muraki, 1992). Thus, the restrictions imposed by the more constrained models such as the G-PCM can potentially be evaluated by comparing the decrement in fit relative to the NRM.

To better understand how various divide-by-total models are nested within the NRM, consider the G-PCM (Muraki, 1992). For $x = j$ the category response curves (CRCs) for the PCM are shown in Equation (18.4). Although this model is not a Rasch model, it is an unconstrained version of the Rasch PCM (Masters, 1982) where items are allowed to vary in discrimination.

$$P_{ix}(\theta) = \frac{\exp\sum_{j=0}^{x}\alpha_i(\theta - \delta_{ij})}{\sum_{r=0}^{m}[\exp\sum_{j=0}^{x}\alpha_i(\theta - \delta_{ij})]}, \tag{18.4}$$

where $\sum_{j=0}^{0}\alpha_i(\theta - \delta_{ij}) \equiv 0$.

In Equation (18.4), note that the δ terms are intersection parameters and equivalent to the intersections (c_j^*) in the NRM. The item discrimination a_i in the G-PCM parameter "indicates the degree to which category responses vary among items as θ level changes" (Muraki, 1992, p. 162). This single item discrimination parameter is in contrast with the NRM where a unique slope parameter is estimated for each category (with the constraint that they sum to zero), and where each response category distinction (i.e., 1 versus 2) has its own CBD parameter.

Finally, if we rewrite the G-PCM to include a_j^* parameters, then Equation (18.5) is simply an alternative way of writing the NRM. If a_j^* are equal within items, Equation (18.5) is the G-PCM and when a_j^* are fixed to 1.0 within and between items, Equation (18.5) is the PCM.

$$P_{ix}(\theta) = \frac{\exp \sum_{j=0}^{x} \alpha_{ij}^{*}(\theta - \delta_{ij})}{\sum_{r=0}^{m} [\exp \sum_{j=0}^{x} \alpha_{ij}^{*}(\theta - \delta_{ij})]}. \tag{18.5}$$

In short, for any set of category slope and intercepts modeled by Equation (18.1), if those values are transformed into category boundary discriminations and category intersection parameters, Equation (18.5) will produce the exact category response curves as Equation (18.1).

In closing, it is important to note that the item discrimination in the G-PCM is roughly equivalent to the (weighted) average of the CBD parameters in the NRM. However, there is a caveat to this claim. Specifically, different computer programs, such as MULTILOG (Thissen, 2003) and PARSCALE (Muraki & Bock, 1997), and IRTPRO (Cai, du Toit, & Thissen, 2012) operationalize divide-by-total models in slightly different ways. In practice, if a researcher estimates a G-PCM using MULTILOG by specifying all category discriminations to be equal within an item, the results will not exactly reproduce the parameters of the G-PCM when estimated on the same data set using PARSCALE. There are many reasons for the discrepancy (e.g., program defaults). However, Childs and Chen (1999) provide transformation equations to obtain comparable results for the G-PCM in PARSCALE and MULTILOG. More recently, IRTPRO utilizes a reparameterization of the divide-by-total models presented in Ostini and Nering (2006), allowing users to estimate any of the divide-by-total models by specifying constraints on a contrast matrix. In this chapter, we work with MULTILOG (Thissen, 2003) and IRTPRO (Cai, du Toit, & Thissen, 2012) exclusively.

Current Research Methods

Category Response Curves and Information in the Nominal Response Model

In this research, we simulate data where the CBD parameters have different properties; in some conditions they are constant within an item (producing the G-PCM), while in others they vary within items (producing the NRM), and in others one CBD is set to zero within an item. Because the NRM is rarely applied, in this section we provide a few visual demonstrations that we hope clarify how the parameters impact the category response curves and the amount of psychometric information an item provides. In all examples, and in the simulations to follow, we assume a four-point polytomous item with ordered response categories.

In Figures 18.1a and 18.1b the category response curves are contrasted for two items that differ in G-PCM item discrimination (i.e., CBD equal within an item), but have the same category intersection parameters of –1.5, 0, and 1.5. Specifically, in Figure 18.1a the item has a discrimination of 1.5 (a_x = –2.25, –0.75, 0.75, 2.25 in NRM) while in Figure 18.1b the item has a discrimination of 0.75 (a_x = –1.125, –0.375, 0.375, 1.125 in NRM). Clearly, the category characteristic curves are steeper in Figure 18.1a versus 18.1b. Accordingly, the category information curves for these two items shown in Figure 18.2a and 18.2b differ in height. Given Figure 18.2 it is tempting to conclude that the item discrimination is the determinant of the item information. However, we caution that items

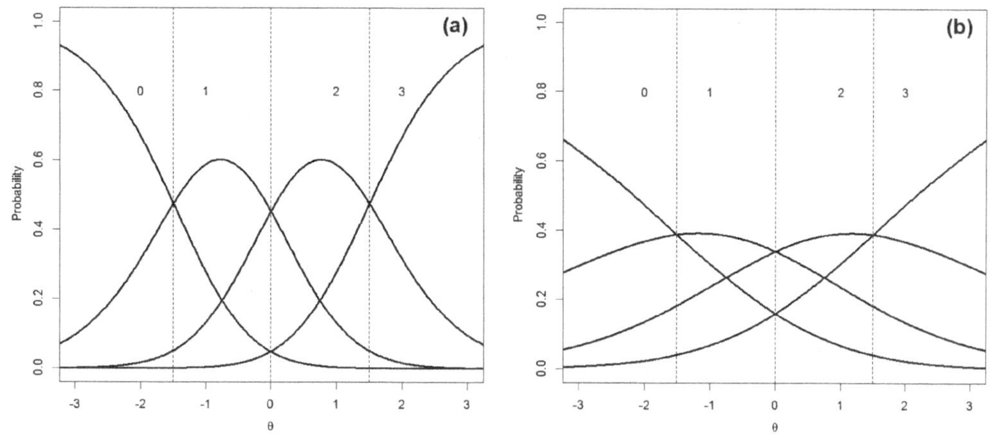

Figure 18.1 (a) Category response curves for an item modeled under the generalized partial credit model with high item discrimination of a* = 1.5. (b) Category response curves for an item modeled under the generalized partial credit model with low item discrimination of a* = 0.5.

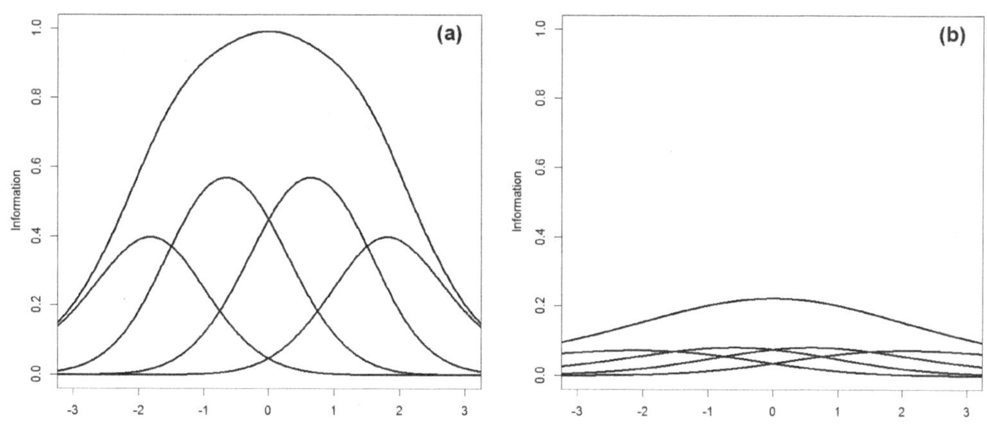

Figure 18.2 (a) Item and category information for an item modeled under the generalized partial credit model with high item discrimination of a* = 1.5. (b) Item and category information for an item modeled under the generalized partial credit model with low item discrimination of a* = 0.5.

with larger CBD parameters are not necessarily more informative than items with lower CBD parameters. The reason is that information in the NRM (as well as the G-PCM) is a function of both discrimination and the spread of intersection parameters (see Muraki, 1992, 1993).

In Figures 18.3a and 18.3b we display the category response curves and the information curves for an item with a^* = 1.5, 1.5, and 0.5 (a_x = –2.00, –0.50, 1.00, 1.50) and intersections –1.5, 0, and 1.5. The third CBD is lower than the first two. In Figure 18.3a we see that as the CBD goes toward zero the category response curves for the two adjacent options become flatter and more similar. If a^* equaled zero, the two category response curves would be identical and the intersection is undefined because the curves would be completely overlapping. Figure 18.3b demonstrates what happens to

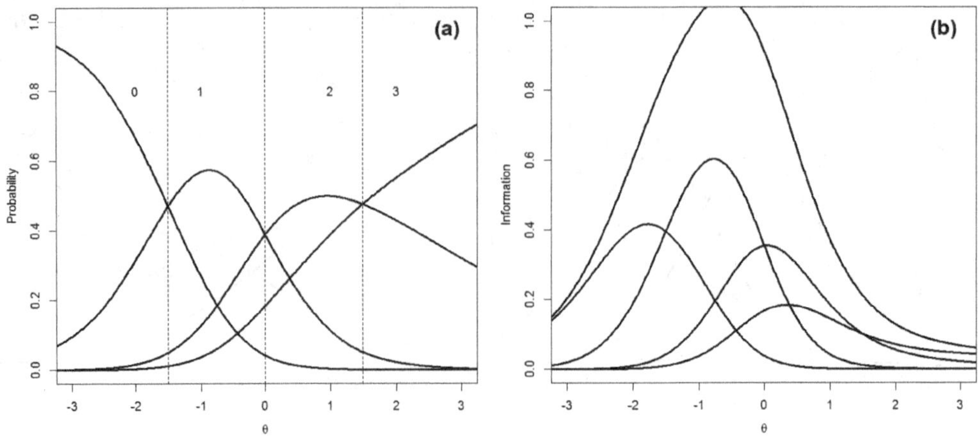

Figure 18.3 (a) Category response curves for an item modeled under the nominal response model with varying category boundary discrimination parameters of $a_1^* = 1.5$, $a_2^* = 1.5$, $a_3^* = 0.5$. (b) Item and category information for an item modeled under the nominal response model with varying category boundary discrimination parameters of $a_1^* = 1.5$, $a_2^* = 1.5$, $a_3^* = 0.5$.

the category and overall item information. Specifically, as a^* gets smaller, the relevant category distinction provides less information because the distinction between two categories is less meaningful.

In other words, in the present example a response in category 3 (as opposed to 2) is not as psychometrically informative as a response in category 1 (as opposed to 0). In such cases, a researcher may want to consider revising the item or rethinking the content used to anchor the response category. When a^* is zero, the response category distinction is completely nominal; that is, a response in category 3 does not indicate more of the trait than a response in category 2. In such cases, a researcher needs to consider the possibility that the item has too many response categories or poorly written anchors. For items that are scored by trained raters, a researcher may need to reconsider the training. At the very least, when category distinctions fail to discriminate, a researcher would not want to use a scoring strategy that aggregates raw integer item scores. Such a strategy is not justified unless all a^* are positive, at the least. We will return to this issue in the discussion.

Application

Because the research literature is so sparse, in order to motivate the Monte Carlo investigations to follow, in this section we use real data analyses to briefly illustrate potential applications of the NRM in diagnosing category functioning in ordered polytomous data.

1) Testing Whether CBD Parameters Vary Within an Item

As noted earlier, models such as the G-PCM model assume that CBDs are equivalent within an item, but not between. Specifying a single item discrimination (common CBD) within an item implies that response category distinctions are equally informative. As pointed out in Preston, Reise, Cai, and Hays (2011), there is essentially no research that investigates the equal within-item CBD hypotheses in personality, psychopathology, or

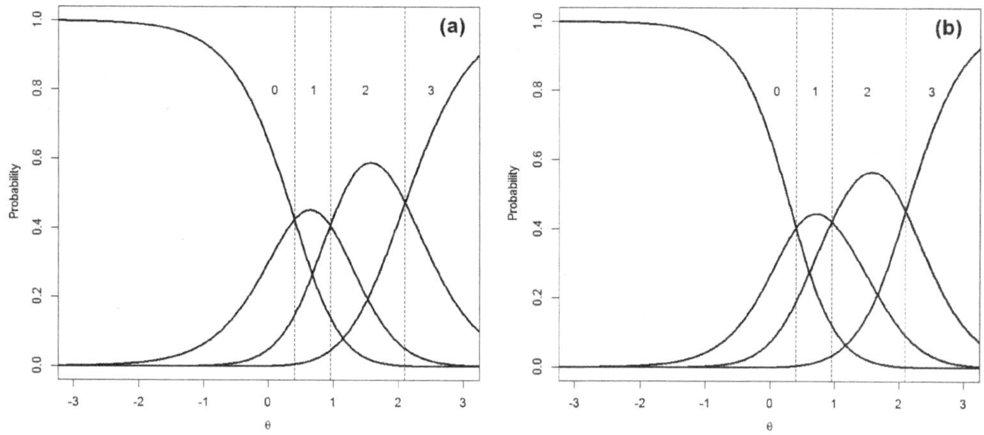

Figure 18.4 (a) Category response curves modeled under the generalized partial credit model for PROMIS® Depression Inventory item 24, "I felt that nothing was interesting," with an item discrimination of $a^* = 1.92$. (b) Category response curves modeled under the nominal response model for PROMIS® Depression Inventory item 24, "I felt that nothing was interesting," with with cateogry boundary discriminations of $a_1^* = 2.24$, $a_2^* = 1.37$, $a_3^* = 2.21$.

patient-reported outcomes measures. Thus, these authors used a Wald test comparing the NRM with the G-PCM to investigate the equal CBD hypothesis in the PROMIS® (Cella et al., 2007; Cella et al., 2010) emotional distress item pools. Specifically, multiplying the item parameters, standard errors, and item parameter covariances estimated in the NRM by specified linear orthogonal contrasts, they evaluated whether imposing within-item equality constraints on CBDs (i.e., the G-PCM) led to a significant change in χ^2 as determined via the Wald test. These authors argued that such tests are important because inappropriately forcing data into a restrictive model can seriously distort item properties (e.g., the information function) and subsequent item interpretation.

For example, in Preston, Reise, Cai, and Hays (2011), item #24 "I *felt that nothing was interesting*" taken from the PROMIS® Depression Inventory displayed a significant decrement in fit in going from the NRM to the G-PCM as judged by the Wald test. To better judge the consequences of this lack of fit, consider the following graphs. In Figures 18.4a and 18.4b the category response curves (CRCs) are presented for item #24 under the G-PCM and NRM, respectively. Under the NRM the item had CBDs of 2.24, 1.37, and 2.21, and a common slope parameter estimate under the G-PCM of 1.92. The dotted vertical lines in each figure mark the category intersection parameters. This is an item where the distinction between *never* (0) and *rarely* (1) as well as the distinction between *sometimes* (2) and *often/always* (3) are relatively more critical than the distinction between *rarely* (1) and *sometimes* (2). Inspection of the CRCs in Figures 18.4a and 18.4b reveals that the item does differ somewhat in functioning under the two models.

Another difference between the two models for item #24 is shown in Figures 18.5a and 18.5b, which show the item and category information functions under the G-PCM and NRM, respectively. Clearly, under the G-PCM the category information functions are relatively similar in height and range from approximately –1.0 to 3.0. In contrast, under the NRM, the category information is more widely spread over the entire trait range (from approximately –3.0 to 3.0). Accordingly, item information under the G-PCM appears unimodal and peaks near the mid-range of the trait scale, whereas information under the NRM is bimodal with peaks located nearly one standard deviation below the mean trait level and nearly two standard deviations above the mean trait level. In the present example, because of the bimodal nature of the item information curve the large first and third CBD increases information for the distinction between response categories 0 versus 1 as well as for the distinction between response categories 2 and 3, but creates a dip in the information for the distinction between response categories 1 and 2.[1] More interestingly, from a substantive perspective, significant CBD variation implies that the category distinctions are not equally informative in terms of scaling individual differences on the latent trait. For this reason, we believe it especially critical to use the NRM in order to test the equal CBD assumption prior to applying models such as the G-PCM, PCM, or RSM.

2) Evaluating Whether an Item Contains Too Many Response Options

As Reise argued (Reise, 2009; Reise & Waller, 2009), some traits may not be fully continuous and thus people cannot make distinctions at all levels of a continuum. In a related manner, some item content may simply not allow people to make fine level distinctions (e.g., between somewhat true of me and moderately true of me). Yet many researchers like to use five-, seven-, or nine-point rating scales to increase scale variance and hence internal consistency. If we are correct in our view that some items may contain too many categories, the NRM may be a useful tool in identifying such situations. Specifically, whenever a CBD is nearly zero, this suggests that adjacent categories are indistinguishable and that the distinction provides no useful information.

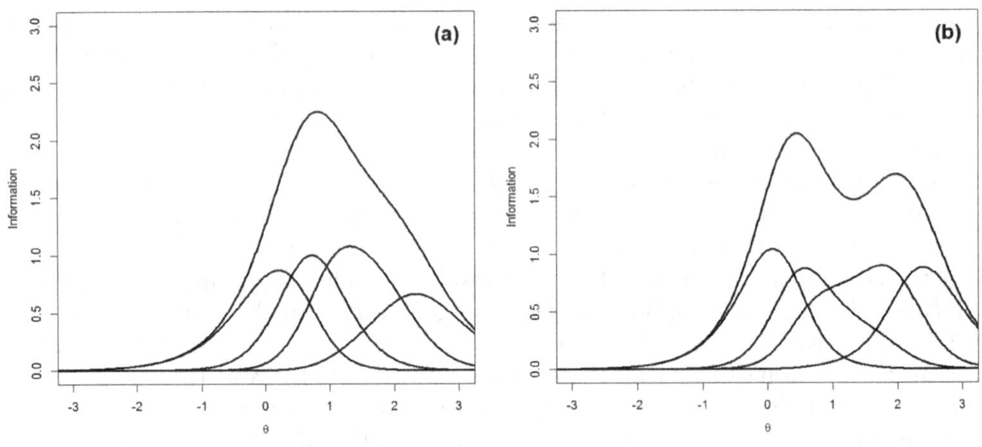

Figure 18.5 (a) Item and category information modeled under the generalized partial credit model for PROMIS® Depression Inventory item 24, "I felt that nothing was interesting," with an item discrimination of $a^* = 1.92$. (b) Item and category information modeled under the nominal response model for PROMIS® Depression Inventory item 24, "I felt that nothing was interesting," with cateogry boundary discriminations of $a_1^* = 2.24$, $a_2^* = 1.37$, $a_3^* = 2.21$.

1 However, note that the amount and location of category and item information is not solely determined by the CBD or slope parameters. Muraki (1992, 1993) has noted that information in a polytomous IRT model is a function of both the slopes and the relative spread of the category intersections.

To illustrate this phenomenon, we analyzed undergraduate student responses ($n = 1{,}059$) to an item questioning whether life would be interesting without emotions, a five-point response item taken from the Feelings facet of the Openness domain of the NEO-PI-R (Costa & McCrae, 1992) under the NRM and G-PCM. Under an NRM, the CBD parameters were $a^*_j = 0.04, 0.07, 1.09, 1.30$, whereas under the G-PCM the constrained slope parameter was 0.89. It appears that the only meaningful distinctions in this item are between categories 2 (neutral) versus 3 (agree), and 3 (agree) versus 4 (strongly agree). Distinctions between categories 0 (strongly disagree) versus 1 (disagree), and 1 (disagree) versus 2 (neutral), are essentially meaningless. This is exactly the type of finding where applying a G-PCM would seriously misrepresent the item.

3) Testing Whether Responses Options Are Ordered

In the application of most psychological scales, it is simply taken for granted that the response options (e.g., 1 . . . 5) are indeed ordered as intended—a response of 3 implies a higher trait standing than a response of 2. This practice is understandable; however, it is arguable that there are some contexts where it may be particularly interesting to study the ordering of categories. For example, on the NEO-PI-R (Costa & McCrae, 1992), a popular personality inventory, the middle response option is 3 (neutral). An interesting issue is whether neutral always falls between 3 (disagree) and 4 (agree).

Samejima (1996), among others, has shown that the NRM model can be used to evaluate category ordering. Specifically, categories are ordered if the a increase for each category (and thus a^* is positive). To illustrate such a situation, item #3 "I *generally try to be thoughtful and considerate*," taken from the Altruism facet of the Agreeableness domain of the NEO-PI-R (Costa & McCrae, 1992), was analyzed under the NRM and G-PCM. Under an NRM, CBD parameters were $a^*_j = -0.52, -0.21, 2.13$, and 1.98, indicating that those who responded in categories 1 (disagree) versus 0 (strongly disagree) or categories 2 (neutral) versus 1 (disagree) do not have higher trait levels of Altruism. However, the common slope parameter estimate under the G-PCM of 1.67 would not allow researchers to identify that the categories of the item are grossly out of order.

Power to Detect Within-Item CBD Variation

In what follows, we explore the power of the likelihood-ratio and Wald tests to: a) detect when CBDs vary within an item (indicating the constrained models such as the G-PCM are inappropriate), and b) to detect when a single within-item CBD equals zero (indicating that two categories are not differentiating and that there may be too many response options). Note that 25 years ago, Thissen and Steinberg (1986) suggested exactly such a test.

The detection of within-item variation in CBD is important for applied researchers for a variety of reasons. First, positive significant tests suggest that more constrained models, such as the G-PCM, may not be appropriate for modeling the item responses. The ability of a likelihood-ratio test to identify items where a CBD is zero is also important, for both technical and substantive reasons. Recall that when the category slopes for adjacent categories in an NRM are nearly equal, this results in a CBD parameter that is near zero. In turn, a CBD near zero implies that the probability of responding to category x versus $x - 1$ does not change as a function of the latent trait—either option is equally likely as a function of the latent trait. Thus, a CBD of zero indicates that a response distinction provides no unique information in terms of scaling individual differences.

Substantively, a finding of a near-zero CBD parameter indicates that: a) individuals cannot meaningfully distinguish between the response options and thus may rely on a response set in responding, b) the response options are not truly ordered, or c) in rated items, judges have not been properly trained to distinguish between certain rating options. Psychometrically, a finding of one or more near-zero CBD may imply that the item contains too many response options and the researcher may consider rewriting the item. Finally, if one or more CBD are zero, any scoring strategy (e.g., aggregating raw item scores or estimating scores under a G-PCM) will add nuisance variation into the estimate. In other words, if a model that assumes that higher item scores reflect more of the trait is incorrectly applied, distortion of the scaling of individual differences may occur (see also Preston, Reise, Cai, & Hays, 2011).

Given the above, in this chapter data analyses are divided into two parts. First, in Study 1a the power of the likelihood-ratio model differences test will be evaluated by simulating data under the NRM that varies in the average size of CBD and within-item CBD variation, and then forcing that data into the more constrained G-PCM. The degree to which the likelihood-ratio test is significant in comparing the G-PCM with the NRM conveys our ability to identify variation in within-item CBD. We also assessed the significance of the within-item CBD variation via the Wald test (Engle, 1984), which only requires estimation of the NRM and compares the within-item CBD parameters using orthogonal contrasts. In Study 1b, a similar procedure will be used to estimate the power of the likelihood-ratio and Wald tests to detect when a single within-item CBD equals zero. In other words, the power to detect that two response categories are indistinguishable.

Design

Several variables were either held constant or manipulated consistently across the following power studies. First, we fixed the test length to 25 items and the number of response categories to four, for all conditions. Many authors have shown that the number of items on a measure does not have a large impact on item parameter estimation using marginal maximum likelihood methods. Second, in both Studies 1a and 1b, we considered two sample size conditions: $N = 500$, and $N = 2{,}000$ because sample size is well known to affect item parameter estimation (De Ayala & Sava-Bolesta, 1999; DeMars, 2003). Third, in Studies 1a and 1b, within-item CBD parameters were simulated to vary within items (i.e., data were generated under a NRM). Fourth, in Study 1b, for each item one within-item CBD parameter was fixed to zero. Later in this chapter, we describe how CBDs and intersections were manipulated.

Study 1a

The average size of the within-item CBD parameters were: high = 1.50, medium 1.00, and low = 0.50. These values were chosen because when CBD parameters were set higher than 1.5 the resulting data sets have unrealistic precision (i.e., were nearly Guttman patterns) whereas data sets with CBD parameters below 0.50 had unrealistically poor properties. However, in order to create item sets that differed in the within-item spread of CBD parameters, values were generated using a uniform distribution that varied in the minimum and maximum values. Specifically, the minimum and maximum values originated at the average CBD values of either 1.50, 1.00, or 0.50. The minimum value of the uniform distribution was then decreased by increments of 0.25 and the maximum value was increased by increments of 0.25, creating a range that increased in increments of 0.5 across simulated conditions. The range increased in increments of 0.5 until the minimum CBD value was 0.25. Finally, we set the intersections in Study 1a to be –1.5, 0, and 1.5, respectively.

Study 1b

These conditions were slightly more complicated to generate. The specification of true CBDs followed Study 1a with the exception that for each item, the third CBD parameter was fixed to zero (actually 0.01). However, note that when a CBD is absolutely zero, this means that category response curves for the two response options are completely overlapping. One consequence is that the intersection parameter is no longer defined (see Equation (18.3)). To avoid this problem we set the third CBD to 0.01 so that a category intersection could be meaningfully defined.

Also, setting a CBD to near zero effects the response distribution in significant ways. For example, when we simulated 2,000 cases for a 25-item test with CBDs of 1.0 and intersections of –1.5, 0, and 1.5 (as in Study 1a), the response distribution was 13 percent in category 0, and 29 percent for categories 2, 3, and 4; this was judged unrealistic. Thus, to compensate for the near-zero CBD and create more realistic response distributions, we set the intersections in Study 1b to be –1.5, 0.5, and 1.5, respectively. For example, generating 2,000 cases for a 25-item test with CBD of 1.0 with intersections of –1.5, 0.5, and 1.5, the response distribution was 16 percent in category 0, 36 percent in category 1, 24 percent in category 2, and 24 percent in category 3.

For conditions evaluating the power of the likelihood-ratio test, a data set was generated using a simulation program written in *R* code (R Core Team, 2013). Item parameters were estimated under the NRM (CBD free) and then under the G-PCM using MULTILOG 7.03 (Thissen, 2003). In MULTILOG, mostly default conditions (e.g., assumed normal distribution) were used except that we set the estimation cycle limit to 100. Note that MULTILOG does not estimate or report NRM parameters or standard errors directly. Instead, model parameters and standard errors are estimated using linear contrasts. In turn, these contrasts need to be transformed into category slope and intercepts. In the present chapter, polynomial and triangle contrast matrices were specified for the estimation of category slopes and intercepts, respectively.

For a given set of likelihood-ratio test conditions, the simulation began by estimating the NRM for all items (i.e., where CBDs are all free) and then the G-PCM (where CBDs are equal within an item) was imposed on a single item by restricting the CBDs to equality within the item. The log-likelihood difference was calculated. Then the program cycled through and placed this constraint on item 2, and then on item 3, and so on. In each cycle only one item was free to have varying CBD parameters. Thus if the simulation condition had 25 items, then 25 distinct log-likelihood values were generated. This process of simulating data sets and computing log-likelihood differences continued until there were 1,000 replications per condition.

The test statistic was –2 times the difference between the log-likelihoods, which is χ^2 distributed with degrees of freedom (*df*) equal to the differences in the number of free parameters. The difference between estimated CBD parameters indicated two degrees of freedom because one common CBD parameter is estimated under the G-PCM and three CBD parameters are estimated for a four-category item under the NRM. Log-likelihood difference tests conducted for each item evaluated differences in G-PCM and NRM model fit. All tests were conducted using an alpha $\leq$ 0.05 rejection rate ($\chi^2 = 5.99$, $df = 2$, $\alpha < .05$).

For conditions evaluating the power of the Wald test, IRTPRO (Cai, du Toit, & Thissen, 2012) was used to estimate all item parameters for the NRM, using mostly default conditions. The maximization step cycle limit was set to 50, the estimation step cycle limit was set to 500, and the solution was evaluated at 49 evenly spaced quadrature points ranging from –6.0 to 6.0. IRTPRO output routinely includes CBD estimates as well as standard errors; the variance covariance matrix of the parameter estimates is also provided. Triangle contrasts were used to estimate all item parameters.

For each Wald test condition, the simulation began by estimating the NRM for all items, collecting the estimated CBD parameters, the standard errors, and the variance covariance matrix of the parameter estimates. For each item, we specified two orthogonal linear contrasts, specified by the following two by three matrix as contrast codes:

$$C_{2.3} = \begin{bmatrix} 1 & -1 & 0 \\ 1 & 1 & -2 \end{bmatrix}.$$

The first contrast compares CBD_1 versus CBD_2, and the second orthogonal contrast compares the average of CBD_1 and CBD_2 with CBD_3. When post-multiplied by a three by one matrix of CBD estimates (A), the result is a two by one matrix, $\lambda_{2.1} = C_{2.3}A_{3.1}$. Deriving the appropriate standard errors for these comparisons, we pre-and post-multiply the variance covariance matrix of the item parameter estimates ($\Sigma_{3.3}$) by the contrasts: $\Omega_{2.2} = C_{2.3}\Sigma_{3.3}C'_{3.2}$. Finally, the Wald test is: $W = \lambda'_{1.2}\Omega^{-1}_{2.2}\lambda_{2.1}$, which is evaluated using a chi-square distribution with two degrees of freedom ($\chi^2 = 5.99$, $df = 2$, $\alpha < .05$).

Results

Study 1a

The first three columns of Tables 18.1 and 18.2 list sample size condition (500, 2,000), average CBD, and range of CBD, respectively. The fourth column of Tables 18.1 and 18.2 presents the estimated power in terms of the proportion of significant likelihood-ratio difference and Wald tests, respectively. Consistent with the theory of the likelihood-ratio and Wald tests, when there is no variance in the CBD within items, the mean rejection rate is near the nominal alpha level of 0.05.[2] In the conditions where there was variation in CBD, as expected, power depended chiefly on the size of the within-item CBD spread—more variation leads to more power. Additionally, the Wald test is a bit more conservative than the likelihood-ratio test as evidenced by consistently lower rejection rates for all conditions. Finally, the power to detect variation in CBDs was also influenced by sample size; power was always greater when sample size was 2,000 rather than 500.

This latter effect can be understood by examination of the standard deviations of CBD parameter estimates that change markedly between 500 and 2,000. These values are shown in parentheses in the last four columns of Table 18.1 for the G-PCM and NRM, respectively. Clearly, the standard deviations are much larger in the $N = 500$ versus the $N = 2,000$ conditions, implying a large difference in parameter recovery accuracy. Additionally, the standard deviations for the parameter estimates are generally smaller and more consistent when estimated using IRTPRO than the standard deviations calculated from estimation using MULTILOG. However, note that because CBDs are randomly selected across items and replications within conditions, the standard deviations of the parameter estimates reflect both parameter estimation error and the range of variation specified within each condition. In short, these values are not empirical estimates of standard errors. Regardless

2 An additional study using 1,000 replications per condition was conducted where null conditions were studied across a wide range of conditions. However, the likelihood-ratio test always had the appropriate sampling distribution and thus the results are not reported. Results are available from the authors.

Table 18.1 Power of Likelihood-Ratio Difference Test Results for Zero Non-discriminating Parameters (1,000 Replications)

N	*Average a**	*a* Range*	*Power*	*G-PCM*	*NRM*		
				$\hat{a}^*$	$\hat{a}_1^*$	$\hat{a}_3^*$	$\hat{a}_3^*$
500	0.50	0.50 to 0.50	0.05[a]	0.50 (.07)	0.50 (.17)	0.50 (.14)	0.50 (.17)
500	0.50	0.25 to 0.75	0.19	0.51 (.11)	0.52 (.23)	0.52 (.21)	0.51 (.23)
500	1.00	1.00 to 1.00	0.04[a]	1.00 (.10)	1.01 (.21)	1.01 (.17)	1.01 (.22)
500	1.00	0.75 to 1.25	0.14	1.02 (.14)	1.03 (.26)	1.03 (.22)	1.02 (.26)
500	1.00	0.50 to 1.50	0.38	1.00 (.21)	1.03 (.38)	1.04 (.34)	1.02 (.37)
500	1.00	0.25 to 1.75	0.62	0.97 (.29)	1.03 (.52)	1.05 (.48)	1.03 (.51)
500	1.50	1.50 to 1.50	0.06[a]	1.50 (.13)	1.51 (.28)	1.51 (.20)	1.51 (.28)
500	1.50	1.25 to 1.75	0.11	1.51 (.16)	1.54 (.32)	1.53 (.25)	1.53 (.31)
500	1.50	1.00 to 2.00	0.32	1.50 (.23)	1.54 (.43)	1.54 (.35)	1.53 (.41)
500	1.50	0.75 to 2.25	0.54	1.47 (.30)	1.54 (.55)	1.55 (.50)	1.53 (.54)
500	1.50	0.50 to 2.50	0.67	1.44 (.39)	1.55 (.69)	1.57 (.64)	1.54 (.68)
500	1.50	0.25 to 2.75	0.77	1.39 (.48)	1.56 (.85)	1.58 (.79)	1.55 (.83)
2000	0.50	0.50 to 0.50	0.05[a]	0.50 (.03)	0.50 (.08)	0.51 (.07)	0.50 (.09)
2000	0.50	0.25 to 0.75	0.48	0.50 (.09)	0.51 (.17)	0.51 (.16)	0.50 (.17)
2000	1.00	1.00 to 1.00	0.05[a]	1.01 (.05)	1.01 (.09)	1.01 (.10)	1.01 (.08)
2000	1.00	0.75 to 1.25	0.38	1.00 (.10)	1.01 (.18)	1.01 (.17)	1.01 (.18)
2000	1.00	0.50 to 1.50	0.76	0.99 (.18)	1.02 (.31)	1.02 (.30)	1.01 (.32)
2000	1.00	0.25 to 1.75	0.89	0.96 (.26)	1.03 (.46)	1.03 (.44)	1.03 (.46)
2000	1.50	1.50 to 1.50	0.04[a]	1.50 (.07)	1.51 (.12)	1.50 (.10)	1.51 (.15)
2000	1.50	1.25 to 1.75	0.30	1.50 (.11)	1.51 (.19)	1.50 (.17)	1.51 (.20)
2000	1.50	1.00 to 2.00	0.67	1.47 (.19)	1.51 (.32)	1.50 (.31)	1.50 (.33)
2000	1.50	0.75 to 2.25	0.85	1.45 (.27)	1.52 (.46)	1.51 (.44)	1.49 (.46)
2000	1.50	0.50 to 2.50	0.91	1.41 (.35)	1.53 (.61)	1.52 (.58)	1.52 (.60)
2000	1.50	0.25 to 2.75	0.93	1.37 (.44)	1.54 (.75)	1.53 (.72)	1.48 (.74)

[a] These values should be 0.05 because the variance of $a^* = 0$.

of this confound, the results clearly demonstrate that the accuracy of item parameter estimates is critical in testing hypotheses about CBD variation.

Study 1b

Tables 18.3 and 18.4 display the results for the conditions where CBD vary within items, but one CBD is fixed to zero within each item for the likelihood ratio and Wald tests, respectively. These results are easy to summarize. When sample size is 2,000, the power to detect a nonfunctioning category is nearly perfect using both the likelihood-ratio and Wald tests. This remains true for the conditions where sample size is 500, except for the two conditions with the lowest average CBD (i.e., 0.50) and least range (0.50 to 0.50;

Table 18.2 Power of Wald Test Results for Zero Non-discriminating Parameters (1,000 Replications)

N	*Average a**	*a* Range*	*Power*	*NRM*		
				$\hat{a}_1^*$	$\hat{a}_2^*$	$\hat{a}_3^*$
500	0.50	0.50 to 0.50	0.04[a]	0.51 (.18)	0.51 (.15)	0.51 (.18)
500	0.50	0.25 to 0.75	0.14	0.51 (.18)	0.51 (.15)	0.51 (.18)
500	1.00	1.00 to 1.00	0.04[a]	1.02 (.22)	1.01 (.18)	1.02 (.23)
500	1.00	0.75 to 1.25	0.12	1.02 (.22)	1.01 (.18)	1.02 (.23)
500	1.00	0.50 to 1.50	0.36	1.03 (.22)	1.01 (.17)	1.01 (.23)
500	1.00	0.25 to 1.75	0.59	1.03 (.23)	1.01 (.18)	1.01 (.23)
500	1.50	1.50 to 1.50	0.05[a]	1.52 (.27)	1.51 (.21)	1.53 (.28)
500	1.50	1.25 to 1.75	0.10	1.53 (.27)	1.52 (.21)	1.53 (.28)
500	1.50	1.00 to 2.00	0.28	1.53 (.27)	1.52 (.21)	1.54 (.29)
500	1.50	0.75 to 2.25	0.49	1.53 (.28)	1.52 (.22)	1.54 (.30)
500	1.50	0.50 to 2.50	0.65	1.53 (.29)	1.52 (.23)	1.53 (.32)
500	1.50	0.25 to 2.75	0.74	1.55 (.31)	1.52 (.23)	1.53 (.32)
2000	0.50	0.50 to 0.50	0.03[a]	0.50 (.11)	0.50 (.08)	0.50 (.11)
2000	0.50	0.25 to 0.75	0.41	0.50 (.10)	0.50 (.07)	0.50 (.10)
2000	1.00	1.00 to 1.00	0.04[a]	1.00 (.12)	1.00 (.11)	1.00 (.14)
2000	1.00	0.75 to 1.25	0.37	1.00 (.11)	1.00 (.10)	1.00 (.12)
2000	1.00	0.50 to 1.50	0.75	1.01 (.11)	1.00 (.09)	1.00 (.11)
2000	1.00	0.25 to 1.75	0.88	1.01 (.11)	1.01 (.09)	1.00 (.11)
2000	1.50	1.50 to 1.50	0.05[a]	1.51 (.13)	1.50 (.10)	1.51 (.14)
2000	1.50	1.25 to 1.75	0.30	1.51 (.13)	1.51 (.10)	1.51 (.14)
2000	1.50	1.00 to 2.00	0.68	1.51. (.13)	1.51 (.10)	1.51 (.14)
2000	1.50	0.75 to 2.25	0.83	1.50 (.13)	1.50 (.10)	1.50 (.14)
2000	1.50	0.50 to 2.50	0.89	1.50 (.14)	1.51 (.11)	1.51 (.14)
2000	1.50	0.25 to 2.75	0.93	1.51 (.14)	1.51 (.11)	1.51 (.15)

[a] These values should be 0.05 because the variance of $a^* = 0$.

0.25 to 0.75). In those two conditions, power drops to 0.44 and 0.51, and 0.52 and 0.55 for the likelihood-ratio and Wald tests, respectively. These results are not too surprising. Overall, the Wald test was more sensitive to a single non-discriminating parameter as evidenced by the higher power-detection values for all the conditions using the Wald test.

In terms of its effects on the overall model likelihood, the difference between a CBD of 0.0 and 0.50 or 0.75 (max values in first two conditions) is perhaps not very large. In other words, the difference between the likelihood values for a model where the CBD are correctly estimated to be say, 0.75, 0.25, and 0.0 (i.e., the NRM), and a similar model that constrains CBD to equality, say 0.33, 0.33, and 0.33 (i.e., the G-PCM), is not great and thus it is difficult to detect that one CBD is zero. Contrast this example with the comparison of likelihoods between a model with true CBD parameters of 0.25, 2.75, and 0. When this data structure is forced into a G-PCM, parameter estimates should be around 1.0, 1.0,

Table 18.3 Power of Likelihood-Ratio Difference Test Results for One Non-discriminating Parameter (1,000 Replications)

N	*Average a**	*a* Range*	*Power*	*G-PCM*	*NRM*		
				$\hat{a}^*$	$\hat{a}_1^*$	$\hat{a}_2^*$	$\hat{a}_3^*$
500	0.50	0.50 to 0.50	0.439	0.34 (.06)	0.48 (.17)	0.50 (.16)	0.01 (.17)
500	0.50	0.25 to 0.75	0.512	0.35 (.09)	0.49 (.22)	0.52 (.22)	0.02 (.17)
500	1.00	1.00 to 1.00	0.914	0.66 (.08)	0.85 (.17)	1.04 (.18)	0.01 (.20)
500	1.00	0.75 to 1.25	0.906	0.67 (.11)	0.87 (.22)	1.06 (.25)	0.02 (.20)
500	1.00	0.50 to 1.50	0.908	0.67 (.16)	0.88 (.31)	1.07 (.37)	0.02 (.20)
500	1.00	0.25 to 1.75	0.910	0.66 (.22)	0.88 (.43)	1.08 (.51)	0.02 (.21)
500	1.50	1.50 to 1.50	0.986	0.99 (.10)	1.18 (.20)	1.61 (.24)	0.01 (.24)
500	1.50	1.25 to 1.75	0.987	1.00 (.13)	1.21 (.23)	1.63 (.30)	0.02 (.25)
500	1.50	1.00 to 2.00	0.983	1.00 (.18)	1.22 (.31)	1.64 (.42)	0.01 (.26)
500	1.50	0.75 to 2.25	0.981	0.98 (.24)	1.23 (.41)	1.65 (.57)	0.01 (.25)
500	1.50	0.50 to 2.50	0.975	0.96 (.30)	1.24 (.53)	1.64 (.70)	0.02 (.25)
500	1.50	0.25 to 2.75	0.962	0.94 (.37)	1.26 (.66)	1.65 (.84)	0.02 (.25)
2000	0.50	0.50 to 0.50	0.986	0.34 (.03)	0.48 (.08)	0.51 (.08)	0.00 (.08)
2000	0.50	0.25 to 0.75	0.970	0.34 (.08)	0.49 (.16)	0.51 (.17)	0.00 (.09)
2000	1.00	1.00 to 1.00	1.000	0.66 (.04)	0.85 (.08)	1.04 (.09)	0.00 (.10)
2000	1.00	0.75 to 1.25	1.000	0.66 (.08)	0.86 (.14)	1.04 (.18)	0.00 (.10)
2000	1.00	0.50 to 1.50	1.000	0.65 (.14)	0.87 (.26)	1.05 (.32)	0.00 (.10)
2000	1.00	0.25 to 1.75	0.999	0.64 (.21)	0.88 (.37)	1.06 (.47)	0.00 (.10)
2000	1.50	1.50 to 1.50	1.000	0.99 (.05)	1.18 (.10)	1.61 (.12)	0.00 (.12)
2000	1.50	1.25 to 1.75	1.000	0.98 (.09)	1.19 (.14)	1.60 (.20)	0.00 (.12)
2000	1.50	1.00 to 2.00	1.000	0.98 (.15)	1.20 (.24)	1.61 (.34)	0.00 (.12)
2000	1.50	0.75 to 2.25	1.000	0.97 (.22)	1.21 (.35)	1.61 (.49)	0.00 (.12)
2000	1.50	0.50 to 2.50	1.000	0.95 (.28)	1.23 (.46)	1.62 (.64)	0.00 (.12)
2000	1.50	0.25 to 2.75	0.999	0.93 (.35)	1.25 (.59)	1.61 (.78)	0.00 (.12)

and 1.0. In this case the likelihoods for the two models should differ greatly and power should be very high (0.99 in the last row of the fourth column of Table 18.3).

For the Wald test, the values in the λ matrix are directly influenced by the variation in the CBD parameters as determined by the orthogonal contrasts. Remember that the first orthogonal contrast compares CBD_1 to CBD_2, and the second orthogonal contrast compares the average of CBD_1 and CBD_2 to CBD_3. For instance, the λ matrix contains values of –0.18 and 0.64 when the true CBD parameters are 0.25, 0.75, and 0. However, when the true CBD parameters are 2.25, 2.75, and 0, then the λ matrix contains values of –0.57 and 4.07. In the first case, all of the CBD parameters are relatively small so the distance between the average of CBD_1 and CBD_2 to CBD_3 is not very large, producing a λ value of 0.64. In the latter case, however, the first two CBD parameters are very highly discriminating, so the distance between the average of CBD_1 and CBD_2 to CBD_3 is substantially more than in the first example, as evidenced by a much larger λ of 4.07. Therefore, it is not surprising that in conditions with widely varying CBD parameters, the Wald test is extremely powerful to detect the within-item CBD variation (1.00 in the last row of Table 18.4).

Discussion

The NRM (Bock, 1972) was originally designed to explore whether distracters in multiple-choice achievement tests provide additional information above and beyond that provided by the dichotomous correct and incorrect response distinction. Nevertheless, we argue that the model has a great deal of potential in the analysis of items that have ordered response categories such as are commonly used in education, health outcomes, and psychology. Specifically, the NRM may be useful for: a) testing the assumption of ordered response categories inherent in most psychological scales, b) evaluating the appropriateness of applying restricted models such as the G-PCM, and c) identifying items where CBD parameters are nearly zero. In addition, although not previously discussed, the NRM may also provide a tool: a) for conducting a fine-grained study of cross-cultural differences in category usage, c) studying the effects of collapsing or adding response categories to an item, and d) studying the effects of reverse wording.

In this chapter, we explored the power of the likelihood-ratio and Wald tests to detect variation in within-item CBDs (Study 1a) and the power to detect when a single CBD equals 0.0 (Study 1b). The results of Study 1a were generally supportive. However, when sample size was relatively small (i.e., $N = 500$), detection rates were modest (i.e., below the commonly cited standard of 0.80), unless the average CBD was high and the range of CBD was large. Although the detection rates appreciated substantially when sample size increased to 2,000, in many circumstances the ability to detect within-item variation in CBD was still below 0.80. For this reason, we recommend that researchers proceed cautiously with interpretation of this test in low sample size conditions, and recognize that in situations where there is modest variation in within-item CBDs, the G-PCM (where only a single item discrimination is estimated) may be statistically indistinguishable from a less restricted model.

In Study 1b we simulated data where CBD varies within items, but in addition one CBD was set to zero. When a CBD is zero, this indicates that the two adjacent response categories are not distinguishable, and should be collapsed prior to scoring, at the very least. We conjecture that such results can occur for a variety of reasons, including: a) the item is asking people to make a psychologically meaningless distinction (e.g., between being mostly happy and moderately happy), b) the item anchors are poor, or c) for items that are graded by trained raters, the training may be poor. The results of Study 1b demonstrated that under a variety of conditions, the power to detect a zero CBD parameter is very high, regardless of sample size.

Summary

NRM Versus G-PCM: Statistical and Practical Significance

In closing, we note that researchers have long been aware of the important difference between a statistically significant effect and a practically meaningful effect. In the present case, a researcher may conduct a likelihood-ratio test comparing the NRM with the G-PCM and discover that a number of items on a measure are better fit by the NRM. Such findings, as evidenced by results from the Wald test, imply that within-item CBD parameters are statistically significant from each other. Similarly, a researcher could use

Table 18.4 Power of Wald Test Results for One Non-discriminating Parameters (1,000 Replications)

N	*Average a**	*a* Range*	*Power*	*NRM*		
				$\hat{a}_1^*$	$\hat{a}_2^*$	$\hat{a}_3^*$
500	0.50	0.50 to 0.50	0.52	0.51 (.18)	0.51 (.16)	0.01 (.16)
500	0.50	0.25 to 0.75	0.55	0.51 (.18)	0.51 (.16)	0.01 (.16)
500	1.00	1.00 to 1.00	0.98	1.02 (.21)	1.02 (.17)	0.01 (.17)
500	1.00	0.75 to 1.25	0.97	1.02 (.21)	1.02 (.17)	0.01 (.17)
500	1.00	0.50 to 1.50	0.95	1.02 (.21)	1.01 (.18)	0.01 (.18)
500	1.00	0.25 to 1.75	0.91	1.03 (.23)	1.01 (.18)	0.01 (.19)
500	1.50	1.50 to 1.50	1.00	1.53 (.26)	1.52 (.20)	0.01 (.18)
500	1.50	1.25 to 1.75	1.00	1.53 (.26)	1.52 (.20)	0.01 (.18)
500	1.50	1.00 to 2.00	1.00	1.54 (.27)	1.52 (.21)	0.01 (.18)
500	1.50	0.75 to 2.25	1.00	1.54 (.27)	1.52 (.21)	0.01 (.18)
500	1.50	0.50 to 2.50	0.99	1.54 (.28)	1.53 (.22)	0.01 (.19)
500	1.50	0.25 to 2.75	0.98	1.53 (.29)	1.53 (.22)	0.01 (.19)
2000	0.50	0.50 to 0.50	0.99	0.50 (.09)	0.50 (.08)	0.01 (.08)
2000	0.50	0.25 to 0.75	0.97	0.50 (.09)	0.50 (.08)	0.01 (.08)
2000	1.00	1.00 to 1.00	1.00	1.00 (.10)	1.00 (.09)	0.01 (.08)
2000	1.00	0.75 to 1.25	1.00	1.01 (.10)	1.00 (.09)	0.01 (.08)
2000	1.00	0.50 to 1.50	1.00	1.00 (.10)	1.00 (.09)	0.01 (.08)
2000	1.00	0.25 to 1.75	1.00	1.01 (.10)	1.00 (.09)	0.01 (.08)
2000	1.50	1.50 to 1.50	1.00	1.50 (.11)	1.50 (.10)	0.01 (.07)
2000	1.50	1.25 to 1.75	1.00	1.51 (.11)	1.51 (.10)	0.01 (.08)
2000	1.50	1.00 to 2.00	1.00	1.51 (.10)	1.51 (.10)	0.01 (.08)
2000	1.50	0.75 to 2.25	1.00	1.50 (.11)	1.50 (.09)	0.01 (.08)
2000	1.50	0.50 to 2.50	1.00	1.50 (.11)	1.50 (.10)	0.01 (.10)
2000	1.50	0.25 to 2.75	1.00	1.50 (.11)	1.50 (.10)	0.01 (.09)

orthogonal contrasts to test significance of variation in the CBD parameters and discover that items have significantly varying CBD parameters. In turn, beyond indicating that the G-PCM may not be appropriate, such a finding potentially has two critical consequences. First, varying CBD parameters implies that the response category distinctions are differentially discriminating and this differential discrimination importantly affects the amount of psychometric information provided by different response options. Second, if CBD parameters vary within an item, any scoring function formulation (Andrich, 1978b; Muraki, 1997) that relies on consecutive integer weighting is incorrect and potentially misleading (du Toit, 2003, pp. 557–559; Preston, Reise, Cai, & Hays, 2011).

Unfortunately, fully demonstrating how the values of the CBD parameters affect item information and the scaling of individual differences is very complicated and would require a separate chapter. Nevertheless, even given the assumed accuracy advantages of the NRM, it is fair to ask, how important is it to correctly model items with varying CBD parameters, as opposed to simply treating these parameters as equal and applying the simpler G-PCM? In other words, is the increase in "fit" worth the sacrifice in parsimony, or does application of a restricted model lead to meaningful errors in terms of applications of IRT models such as: a) scaling individual differences, b) linking item parameters to different scales, c) studying differential item functioning, or d) computerized adaptive testing?

We have three observations regarding this issue. First, we believe the NRM is an incredibly useful tool for examining the psychometric properties of items, and should be routinely fit regardless of whether it is to be the final model used in applications. Second, we propose that the importance of capturing variation in CBD parameters depends on the size and configuration of that variation.

Third, we argue that ultimately the choice of model cannot solely be based on relative fit, but rather is a judgment call of the investigator. To make an informed judgment, a researcher should apply both the NRM and more restricted models such as the G-PCM. Category, item, and test information should then be calculated under each model and graphs carefully compared. It will sometimes be the case that even when CBD variation is significant, the graphs of item information for the two models will be highly similar. In addition, researchers may consider scoring individuals under both models and carefully comparing the order of individuals under each. In short, if a researcher decides to use a relatively poorer-fitting but more parsimonious model, he or she must be prepared to defend that decision based on empirical evidence that the applied consequences are minimal.

References

Andrich, D. (1978a) Application of a psychometric model to ordered categories which are scored with successive integers. *Applied Psychological Measurement, 2*, 581–594.

Andrich, D. (1978b). A rating formulation for ordered response categories. *Psychometrika, 43*, 561–573.

Andrich, D. (1995). Distinctive and incompatible properties of two common classes of IRT models for graded responses. *Applied Psychological Measurement, 19*, 101–119.

Baker, F. B. (1993). Equating tests under the nominal response model. *Applied Psychological Measurement, 17*, 147–162.

Bock, R. D. (1972). Estimating item parameters and latent ability when responses are scored in two or more nominal categories. *Psychometrika, 37*, 29–51.

Bock, R. D. (1997). The nominal categories model. In W. J. van der Linden & R. K. Hambleton (Eds.), *Handbook of modern item response theory* (pp. 33–49). New York: Springer.

Cai, L., du Toit, S. H. C., & Thissen, D. (2012). IRTPRO: Flexible, multidimensional, multiple categorical IRT modeling. Skokie, IL: Scientific Software International.

Cella, D., Riley, W., Stone, A., Rothrock, N., Reeve, B., Yount, S., et al. (2010). Initial item banks and first wave testing of the patient-reported outcomes measurement information system (PROMIS) network: 2005–2008. *Journal of Clinical Epidemiology, 63*, 1179–1194.

Cella, D., Yount, S., Rothrock, N., Gershon, R., Cook, K., Reeve, B., et al. (2007). The Patient-Reported Outcomes Measurement Information System (PROMIS): Progress of an NIH roadmap cooperative group during its first two years. *Medical Care, 45*(5 Suppl. 1), S3–S11.

Childs, R. A., & Chen, W. H. (1999). Software note obtaining comparable item parameter estimates in MULTILOG and PARSCALE for two polytomous IRT models. *Applied Psychological Measurement, 23*(4), 371–379.

Costa, P. T., & McCrae, R. R. (1992). Normal personality assessment in clinical practice: The NEO Personality Inventory. *Psychological Assessment, 4*, 5–13.

de Ayala, R. J. (1992). The nominal response model in computerized adaptive testing. *Applied Psychological Measurement, 16*, 327–343.

de Ayala, R. J. (2009). *The theory and practice of item response theory*. New York: Guilford.

de Ayala, R. J., & Sava-Bolesta, M. (1999). Item parameter recovery for the nominal response model. *Applied Psychological Measurement, 23*, 3–19.

DeMars, C.E. (2003). Sample size and the recovery of the nominal response model item parameters. *Applied Psychological Measurement, 27*, 275–288.

du Toit, M. (2003). *IRT from SSI: BILOG-MG, MULTILOG, PARSCALE, TESTFACT*. Chicago, IL: Scientific Software International.

Engle, R.F. (1984). Wald, likelihood ratio, and Lagrange multiplier tests in econometrics. In Z. Griliches & M.D. Intriligator (Eds.), *Handbook of economics* (vol. II, pp. 775–826). Elsevier.

Glas, C.A.W. (1999). Modification indices for the 2-PL and the nominal response model. *Psychometrika, 64*, 273–294.

Masters, G.N. (1982). A Rasch model for partial credit scoring. *Psychometrika, 47*, 149–174.

Muraki, E. (1992). A generalized partial credit model: Application of an EM algorithm. *Applied Psychological Measurement, 16*, 159–176.

Muraki, E. (1993). Information functions of the generalized partial credit model. *Applied Psychological Measurement, 17*, 351–363.

Muraki, E. (1997). A generalized partial credit model. In W.J. van der Linden & R.K. Hambleton (Eds.), *Handbook of modern item response theory* (pp. 153–164). New York: Springer.

Muraki, E., & Bock, R. D. (1997). *PARSCALE: IRT item analysis and test scoring for rating-scale data*. Chicago, IL: Scientific Software International.

Ostini, R., & Nering, M.L. (2006). *Polytomous item response theory models*, Thousand Oaks, CA: Sage.

Passos, V.L., & Berger, M.P.F. (2004). Maximum calibration designs for the nominal response model: An empirical evaluation. *Applied Psychological Measurement, 28*, 72–87.

Preston, K.S.J., Reise, S.P., Cai, L., & Hays, R.D. (2011). Using the nominal response model to evaluate response category discrimination in the PROMIS Emotional Distress item pools. *Educational and Psychological Measurement, 71*, 523–550.

R Core Team (2013). *R: A language and environment for statistical computing. R Foundation for Statistical Computing*, Vienna, Austria. ISBN 3–900051–07–0, URL www.R-project.org.

Reise, S.P. (2009). The emergence of item response theory models and the Patient Reported Outcomes Measurement Information Systems. *Austrian Journal of Statistics, 38*, 211–220.

Reise, S.P., & Waller, N.G. (2009). Item response theory and clinical measurement. *Annual Review of Clinical Psychology, 5*, 27–48.

Samejima, F. (1969). Estimation of latent ability using a response pattern of graded scores. *Psychometrika Monograph*, No. 17.

Samejima, F. (1996). Evaluation of mathematical models for ordered polychotomous responses. *Behaviormetrika, 23*, 17–35.

Thissen, D. (1976). Information in wrong responses to Raven's Progressive Matrices. *Journal of Educational Measurement, 13*, 201–214.

Thissen, D. (2003). *MULTILOG: Multiple, categorical item analysis and test scoring using item response theory* (Computer Software: version 7.03). Chicago, IL: Scientific Software International.

Thissen, D., & Steinberg, L. (1986). A taxonomy of item response models. *Psychometrika, 49*, 501–519.

Thissen, D., Steinberg, L., & Fitzpatrick, A.R. (1989). Multiple-choice models: The distractors are also part of the item. *Journal of Educational Measurement, 26*, 161–176.

Tokuda, Y., Okubo, T., Ohde, S., Jacobs, J., Takahashi, O., Omata, F., . . . Fukui, T. (2009). Assessing items on the SF-8 Japanese version for health-related quality of life: A psychometric analysis based on the nominal categories model of item response theory. *Value in Health, 12*, 568–573.

Wollack, J.A., Bolt, D.M., Cohen, A.S., & Lee, Y. (2002). Recovery of item parameters in the nominal response model: A comparison of marginal maximum likelihood estimation and Markov chain Monte Carlo estimation. *Applied Psychological Measurement, 26*, 339–352.

19 Multidimensional Test Linking

Jonathan P. Weeks

Introduction

In order to compare scores from two or more related tests it is necessary for them to be reported on a common scale. Various linking methods have been developed for this purpose, depending on the statistical properties of the tests and the data collection design (cf., Dorans, Pommerich, & Holland, 2007; Kolen & Brennan, 2004); however, most of these methods are premised on the assumption that a single construct is measured within and between tests. When a multidimensional model is applied to tests measuring more than one dimension it is important to consider the comparability of dimension-specific scores. The goal of this chapter is to provide a foundation for understanding multidimensional test score linking and various issues that should be considered in this process.

This chapter is organized into four main parts. The first part provides an overview of score linking within a unidimensional item response theory (IRT; Lord & Novick, 1968) framework and the correspondence to Procrustean transformations (Gower & Dijksterhuis, 2004; Mulaik, 1972) that serve as the basis for multidimensional test score linking. The second part presents the equations for score linking within a multidimensional item response theory (MIRT; Reckase, 2009) framework. This is followed by a section that lays out considerations for when it may or may not be appropriate to link scores multidimensionally. The final part provides a discussion of properties that should be evaluated as part of the linking process; these properties are addressed using empirical data from a large-scale mathematics assessment.

Research Methods

Methods for linking score scales have been around for more than a century (cf., Hull, 1922; Kelley, 1923). These methods include equipercentile equating (Braun & Holland, 1982; Kelley, 1923), linear raw-score methods (Angoff, 1971; Gulliksen, 1950; Kolen & Brennan, 2004; Levine, 1955), and IRT-based methods (Kim & Lee, 2006; Kolen & Brennan, 2004), among others. The focus of this chapter is primarily on linear transformations of score scales within an IRT framework when the item parameters for the tests of interest are estimated separately. Within this framework, the goal of the linking is to adjust the scores from different test forms so that the scores can be compared on a common scale and the forms can be used interchangeably. That is, the scores from all tests of interest must be transformed to the metric of a reference test (or a reference scale). The methods used to transform the scores are based principally on two characteristics: the equivalence (or lack thereof) of the examinee groups and the associated score distributions, and the statistical and construct-related properties of the test forms. The equivalence of the examinee groups is typically related to the data collection design while the properties of the tests are related to the various aspects of the test design (e.g., the construct of interest, difficulty, item format, etc.).

Data Collection Designs and Terminology

Three of the most common data collection designs (Kolen & Brennan, 2004) are the 1) randomly equivalent groups, 2) single-group with counterbalancing, and 3) nonequivalent groups common item design. In a randomly equivalent groups design each examinee group takes a different test form. The design assumes that the underlying distributions of true scores are equivalent for each group; hence, differences in observed performance can be attributed to differences in form difficulty. By adjusting the scores on each form to account for these differences, the scores across forms can be compared on a common scale. In a single-group design, the same examinees take each form. To minimize order effects in the linking, the administration of forms is typically counterbalanced (e.g., half of the examinees take Form X first and Form Y second while the other half takes Form Y first and Form X second). The transformation of scores then proceeds using the same methods employed for a randomly equivalent groups design.[1] When the groups are not equivalent—when the examinees come from different populations—differences between the tests and groups must be simultaneously considered (i.e., disentangling how much of the difference in scores is due to test difficulty versus group ability). In these instances, a nonequivalent groups common item design may be used to anchor the tests together. Under this design a given subset of items is administered on both tests and the relationship between performance on these common items across groups is used as the basis for linking the scores.

A variety of methods have been developed for linking test scores that are related in part to the associated data collection design; however, the terms used to differentiate between these methods are typically tied to the characteristics of the tests. Throughout this chapter I use three terms seemingly interchangeably (*linking, scaling*, and *equating*); however, these terms denote various assumptions with respect to the comparability of the constructs measured by each test as well as associated statistical specifications. My use of terms is generally consistent with those presented by Kolen (2004). *Linking* is a generic term for any approach used to make results comparable. *Scaling*[2] is a more restrictive term used to denote the linking of scores for tests that measure the same construct, yet differ with respect to test specifications (e.g., differences in content coverage or reliability). *Equating* is a restricted form of scaling where the test forms are constructed using the same test specifications and satisfy a set of specific criteria (addressed in the last part of this chapter).

Unidimensional Test Score Linking

Most of the methods developed for test score linking are premised on the assumption of unidimensionality (cf., Dorans, Pommerich, & Holland, 2007; Kolen & Brennan, 2004; Skaggs & Lissitz, 1986); that is, the assumption that the scores across test forms characterize examinee performance on a single construct. The primary focus of this chapter is

1 Because of practical considerations like test time and cost, the single-group design is rarely used.

2 In Kolen (2004), the term *calibration* is used instead of *scaling;* however, the term *calibration* is often used within an IRT context to distinguish between the simultaneous estimation of item parameters for multiple groups (concurrent calibration) and the estimation of item parameters for each test separately (separate calibration). To reduce confusion, the term *scaling* is used as the restricted form of linking.

on multidimensional score linking; however, the methods developed for unidimensional linking provide an important context for understanding linking within a multidimensional framework. The following section provides an overview of unidimensional IRT-based test score linking within a separate calibration framework. Readers familiar with these methods may wish to skip this section and jump to the discussion of Procrustean transformations that serve as the basis for multidimensional test score linking.

In item response theory, an examinee's response to a test item is modeled probabilistically as a function of the test taker's latent ability and the item's characteristics. Let the variable X_{ij} represent the response of examinee j to item i. Given a test consisting of dichotomously scored items, let $X_{ij} = 1$ for a correct item response and $X_{ij} = 0$ for an incorrect response. The item response curve for the two-parameter logistic model (2PL; Birnbaum, 1968) takes the following form:

$$P\left(X_{ij} = 1 \mid \theta_j, a_i, b_i\right) = \frac{exp\left(Da_i\left[\theta_j - b_i\right]\right)}{1 + exp\left(Da_i\left[\theta_j - b_i\right]\right)}, \tag{19.1}$$

where θ_j is an individual's latent ability on a single construct, a_i is the item discrimination (slope), b_i is the item difficulty, and D is a scaling constant. When items are polytomously scored (i.e., items with three or more score categories, as with constructed response items), the response X_{ij} can be coded using a set of responses $k = \{0, \ldots, K_i - 1\}$ where K_i is the total number of categories for the item. When the values of k correspond to successively ordered categories, the response probabilities can be modeled using a model like the generalized partial credit model (GPCM; Muraki, 1992), which takes the following form:

$$P\left(X_{ij} = k \mid \theta_j, a_i, b_{ik}\right) = \frac{exp\left[\sum_{v=1}^{k} Da_i\left(\theta_j - b_{iv}\right)\right]}{\sum_{h=1}^{K_i} exp\left[\sum_{v=1}^{h} Da_i\left(\theta_j - b_{iv}\right)\right]}. \tag{19.2}$$

where b_{ik} is a step-intersection parameter. The other parameters have the same interpretation as in the 2PL. Other models such as the three-parameter logistic model (3PL; Birnbaum, 1968), Rasch model (1960), and various polytomous models can be specified, but in many cases the linking equations are the same as those presented below for the 2PL/GPCM. For a more complete explication of unidimensional IRT-based linking methods for dichotomous and polytomous models, see Kolen and Brennan (2004) or Kim and Lee (2006).

The use of IRT in general, and for score linking, is premised on two strong, related, assumptions: local independence and unidimensionality. A set of items is considered locally independent if, for fixed values of the underlying construct, the item responses are statistically independent. In order for this to hold, the dimensional structure must be adequately specified within and across tests. More specifically, all of the items on the tests must measure a single construct. In the context of score linking, there is an added assumption that the item parameters are unbiased (e.g., that there is no differential item functioning between subpopulations). When these assumptions are met, and when the specified model fits the data, many IRT models share a property that makes IRT well suited for test linking: parameter invariance. That is, the parameters for a given item should be the same regardless of the subpopulation used to estimate them, and the ability for a given examinee should be the same regardless of the test administered.

Scaling and equating within an IRT framework is typically based on a common item design[3] that assumes invariance of the common item parameters across examinee groups and tests. When the item parameters for two or more tests are estimated concurrently using a multigroup approach (Bock & Zimowski, 1997; von Davier & von Davier, 2007), the common item parameters are usually constrained to be equal across groups while the latent ability distributions for each of the groups are allowed to vary (the mean and standard deviation of a reference group are typically fixed for identification purposes). This approach places all of the item parameter estimates and subsequent estimates of examinee abilities on a common scale. As an alternative to this approach, item parameters can be estimated separately for each test and then linked via a secondary process.

In the separate calibration approach the mean and standard deviation of the latent ability distributions are often constrained (e.g., to zero and one respectively) when estimating the item parameters. The linking then proceeds by using a linear scaling function to identify a set of coefficients that minimize the differences between common item parameter estimates. These linking coefficients are used to transform all of the item parameter and ability estimates for the focal tests and place them on the scale of the reference test. In cases where it is necessary to link scores from three or more forms, a chain-linking process (i.e., a series of linear transformations) can be used (Kolen & Brennan, 2004); however, additional error may be introduced via successive transformations. As an alternative to chain linking, a set of linking coefficients can be simultaneously estimated to transform the scores from each form directly to the reference scale (Haberman, 2009). Von Davier and von Davier (2007) show that when the various IRT assumptions are met, concurrent calibration is preferable to separate calibration insomuch that it reduces error in the linking; however, to provide a more explicit connection to various multidimensional linking methods, the separate calibration approach is described in more detail below.

With a separate calibration approach, the means and standard deviations of the scores on one or more tests are adjusted to resolve any differences between the test forms. A simple linear equation,

$$\theta_T = A\theta_F + B,$$

can be used to transform θ_F values to the θ_T scale (the subscripts F and T correspond to what I will refer to as the *from* scale and *to* scale respectively) where A and B are estimated coefficients that adjust the scale (variability) and location (mean) of the scores respectively. Because the item parameters are defined with respect to a θ scale, any transformation of the scale will necessarily require a change in the item parameters so that the expected response probabilities remain unchanged. It can be readily shown that a_i and b_{ik} for the 2PL and GPCM on the *from* scale can be transformed to the *to* scale by (Baker, 1992; Kim & Lee, 2006; Lord & Novick, 1968):

$$\begin{aligned} a_{iT} &= a_{iF} / A \\ b_{ikT} &= Ab_{ikF} + B . \end{aligned} \tag{19.3}$$

In practice, the parameters θ, a_i and b_{ik} for each test are unknown; hence, estimates of the parameters ($\hat{\theta}$, $\hat{a}_i$ and $\hat{b}_{ik}$ respectively) must be considered with respect to the linking.

3 Note that if a randomly equivalent group design is employed, the estimation can be run as a single group model or, in the case of separate calibration, the same identification constraints can be used for the latent ability distribution so that no subsequent linking is required (Kolen & Brennan, 2004).

Based on the assumption of parameter invariance, the goal is to find a set of coefficients that minimize the difference between the untransformed *to* scale and transformed *from* scale common item parameter estimates. Several approaches have been developed for this purpose. The mean/sigma (Marco, 1977) and mean/mean (Loyd & Hoover, 1980) methods, commonly known as moment methods, are the simplest approaches to estimating A and B because they only require the computation of means and standard deviations for various common item parameter estimates. For mean/sigma, only the difficulty parameters are used. That is,

$$A = \frac{\sigma\left(\hat{b}_T\right)}{\sigma\left(\hat{b}_F\right)}$$

$$B = \mu\left(\hat{b}_T\right) - A\left[\mu\left(\hat{b}_F\right)\right], \tag{19.4}$$

where $\mu()$ and $\sigma()$ are the means and standard deviations, taken over all $C \leq J$ common items and K_c response categories. One potential limitation of this approach is that it does not consider the slope parameters. The mean/mean, on the other hand, uses both the slope and difficulty parameters to estimate the linking coefficients where:

$$A = \frac{\sigma\left(\hat{a}_F\right)}{\sigma\left(\hat{a}_T\right)}$$

$$B = \mu\left(\hat{b}_T\right) - A\left[\mu\left(\hat{b}_F\right)\right]. \tag{19.5}$$

As an alternative to the moment methods, Haebara (1980) and Stocking and Lord (1983) developed characteristic curve methods that use an iterative approach to estimate the linking coefficients by minimizing the sum of squared differences between item characteristic curves (ICC) and test characteristic curves (TCC) for the common items for the two methods respectively. The Haebara method minimizes:

$$Q = \sum_{g=1}^{G}\sum_{c=1}^{C}\sum_{k=1}^{K_s}\left[P_{ck}\left(\theta_g\right) - P_{ck}^{*}\left(\theta_g\right)\right]^2, \tag{19.6}$$

while the Stocking-Lord method minimizes:

$$F = \sum_{g=1}^{G}\left[\sum_{c=1}^{C}\sum_{k=1}^{K_s}U_{ck}P_{ck}\left(\theta_g\right) - \sum_{c=1}^{C}\sum_{k=1}^{K_s}U_{ck}P_{ck}^{*}\left(\theta_g\right)\right]^2. \tag{19.7}$$

The θ_g are a set of G points on the *to* scale where differences in expected probabilities are evaluated, $P_{ck}\left(\theta_g\right)$ are expected probabilities based on the untransformed *to* scale common item parameter estimates, and $P_{ck}^{*}\left(\theta_g\right)$ are expected probabilities based on the transformed *from* scale common item parameter estimates.[4] To create the test characteristic curves

4 Extensions of the Haebara and Stocking-Lord method can be specified that consider a symmetric minimization of the criterion with or without quadrature weights (see Kim & Lee, 2006 for more information).

for the Stocking-Lord method, the scoring function U_{ck} must be included (particularly for polytomous items). These values are usually specified as $U_{ck} = \{0,\ldots,K_c - 1\}$ which assumes that the categories are ordered.

Procrustean Transformations

Multidimensional test score linking has its origins in Procrustean transformations (cf., Gower & Dijksterhuis, 2004; Mulaik, 1972). Simply put, the goal of Procrustean methods is to transform the values in a given matrix (e.g., a matrix of factor loadings or item slopes), $\boldsymbol{X}_F(N \times P_1)$, so that they align as closely as possible to values in a target matrix, $\boldsymbol{X}_T(N \times P_2)$. The simplest formulation of a Procrustean transformation is the minimization of:

$$H = \| \boldsymbol{X}_F \boldsymbol{T} - \boldsymbol{X}_T \|, \tag{19.8}$$

where $\boldsymbol{T}$ is a $P_1 \times P_2$ transformation matrix and the operator $\{\| \ \|\}$ is the matrix norm defined by the sums of squares.[5] Different variants of the transformation can be specified depending on the dimensions of $\boldsymbol{X}_F$ and $\boldsymbol{X}_T$ and any restrictions on the form of $\boldsymbol{T}$. The particular variations considered in this chapter are cases where $\boldsymbol{T}$ is an oblique transformation or an orthogonal rotation. In the latter case, the transformation will be denoted by $\boldsymbol{Q}$. The transformation matrices $\boldsymbol{T}$ and $\boldsymbol{Q}$ play one or two roles in the minimization of the difference between $\boldsymbol{X}_F$ and $\boldsymbol{X}_T$. Both matrices adjust for rotational indeterminacy in order to orient the values along the same axes within the multidimensional space, yet with the oblique transformation, $\boldsymbol{T}$, there is also an intrinsic scaling that adjusts the variability of each dimension in $\boldsymbol{X}_F$. With the orthogonal rotation, $\boldsymbol{Q}$, there are no adjustments made to the variability; hence, a separate scaling (dilation) matrix may be needed. In the latter case, the criterion to be minimized is:[6]

$$H = \| \boldsymbol{X}_F \boldsymbol{R} \boldsymbol{Q} - \boldsymbol{X}_T \| \text{ or } H = \| \boldsymbol{X}_F \boldsymbol{Q} \boldsymbol{S} - \boldsymbol{X}_T \|. \tag{19.9}$$

The matrices $\boldsymbol{R}$ and $\boldsymbol{S}$ correspond to pre-scaling and post-scaling transformations respectively. These are diagonal matrices of scaling coefficients. If the variability of each dimension is adjusted by a single constant, this is referred to as isotropic scaling; if the variability is adjusted differently for each dimension, this is referred to as anisotropic scaling. The final type of transformation that may be required is a translation of the values in $\boldsymbol{X}_F$. In this case, when no additional scaling matrix is specified, the criterion to be minimized is:

$$H = \| \boldsymbol{X}_F \boldsymbol{T} - 1\boldsymbol{a}' - \boldsymbol{X}_T \|, \tag{19.10}$$

where $\boldsymbol{a}' = \boldsymbol{a}'_F T - \boldsymbol{a}'_T$. The translation vector a essentially shifts the location of the means of each scale. There is no *a priori* defined sequence to multivariate transformations; that is,

5 Estimation of the various elements for rotation, scaling, and translation are presented in the following section in the discussion of test linking within a multidimensional item response theory framework.

6 It should be noted that a constrained oblique transformation for $\boldsymbol{T}$ can be specified with a pre-scaling and/or post-scaling transformation; however, for the purpose of this chapter only orthogonal transformations with an associated scaling matrix are considered. See Gower and Dijksterhuis (2004) for information on additional scaling transformations.

the sequence of rotation, scaling, and translation may occur in any order by restructuring the formulation of the minimization function accordingly. As such, a decision should be made regarding the sequence of transformations and applied consistently in any practical application of multidimensional linking.

The transformations presented above provide a simplified overview of the underpinnings of multidimensional test score linking, yet there are two other important considerations that can be addressed using Procrustean methods: the choice of a general reference scale and projection problems. The simplest formulation of the Procrustes problem seeks a solution to transform $\mathbf{X}_F$ onto the scale of $\mathbf{X}_T$ (a one-sided Procrustes problem); however, there may be instances where it is desirable to transform $\mathbf{X}_F$ and $\mathbf{X}_T$ to an "average" configuration. This is referred to as a two-sided Procrustes problem. The criterion to be minimized for two groups takes the following form:

$$H = \| \mathbf{X}_1 \mathbf{T}_1 - \mathbf{X}_2 \mathbf{T}_2 \|. \tag{19.11}$$

Because there is no longer a *to* scale and *from* scale, the subscripts are denoted by numbers. Notice also that instead of a single transformation matrix, each $\mathbf{X}$ has an associated $\mathbf{T}$. To illustrate the transformation to an "average" reference matrix, $\mathbf{G}$, the two-sided criterion can be reformulated as a generalized Procrustes problem (Gower & Dijksterhuis, 2004):

$$H = K \sum_{k=1}^{K} \| \mathbf{X}_k \mathbf{T}_k - \mathbf{G} \|, \tag{19.12}$$

where:

$$\mathrm{G} = K^{-1} \sum_{k=1}^{K} (\mathrm{X}_k \mathrm{T}_\mathrm{k}). \tag{19.13}$$

The two-sided approach is particularly relevant for multidimensional score linking in the implementation of oblique transformations. In order to obtain an oblique transformation that is symmetric, the two-sided criterion is minimized to estimate a single $\mathbf{T}$ (for a pair of tests) rather than $\mathbf{T}_k$.[7] On the other hand, it can be shown that the one-sided and two-sided approach in the estimation of $\mathbf{Q}$ both provide an orthogonal rotation. Hence, the simpler one-sided approach can be used to estimate $\mathbf{Q}$. As a further extension of the two-sided Procrustes problem, a generalized Procrustes approach could be used to link more than two test forms, although this approach has not been fully explored in the literature on multidimensional test score linking.

Another consideration in multidimensional test score linking is the number of dimensions underlying each test. The equations given earlier suggest that the dimensions of $\mathbf{X}_F$ and $\mathbf{X}_T$ are $(N \times P_1)$ and $(N \times P_2)$ respectively where $P_1 = P_2$. However, there may be instances where there are, say, four factors associated with $\mathbf{X}_F$ and three factors associated with $\mathbf{X}_T$ or, say, three factors associated with both $\mathbf{X}_F$ and $\mathbf{X}_T$ but with only two common factors. These scenarios may occur in K-12 assessments where tests are administered at different grade levels and it is possible that the measured constructs shift somewhat from grade to grade (this issue is discussed in more detail later). Some researchers may argue that

7 This is consistent with the notion of symmetric transformations in unidimensional linking presented by Haebara (1980).

linking scores on tests like these is not defensible while others may support the approach for the purpose of creating a single score scale for the common dimensions across tests.

When $P_1 \neq P_2$, $\boldsymbol{T}$ will not be a square transformation matrix. This is a projection Procrustes problem (Gower & Dijksterhuis, 2004). Different methods have been developed to handle cases where higher-dimensional matrices are projected onto lower-dimensional spaces and vice versa, but for the present discussion it can be shown that the correct solution for $\boldsymbol{T}$ and $\boldsymbol{Q}$ can be obtained by padding "missing" columns in $\boldsymbol{X}_F$ and/or $\boldsymbol{X}_T$ with zeros. For instance, with respect to the first example, $\boldsymbol{X}_F$ would be an $(N \times 4)$ matrix where all four columns include item slopes and $\boldsymbol{X}_T$ would be an $(N \times 4)$ matrix where the first three columns include item slopes and the fourth column includes all zeros.

There are number of additional constraints and/or extensions related to the transformations presented above that one might consider in order to address specific issues in multidimensional test linking, but it is beyond the scope of this chapter to delve into these constraints/extensions in more depth. The transformations discussed here represent key components that connect the linear transformations used in unidimensional test score linking to a multidimensional conceptualization of score linking. The reader interested in a more complete explication of Procrustes problems should consult Gower and Dijksterhuis (2004).

Multidimensional Test Score Linking

In the previous section, Procrustean methods were presented as the foundation upon which multidimensional test score linking is built (in a separate calibration context). In this section, extensions of the Procrustean transformations are provided for linking scores within a multidimensional item response theory framework. As in the unidimensional case, let the variable X_{ij} represent the response of examinee j to item i. Given a test consisting of dichotomously-scored items, let $X_{ij} = 1$ for a correct item response, and let $X_{ij} = 0$ for an incorrect response. The item response function for the multidimensional two-parameter logistic model (M2PL; Reckase, 1985) takes the following form:

$$P\left(X_{ij} = 1 \mid \theta_j, a_i, d_i\right) = \frac{exp\left(a_i' \theta_j + d_i\right)}{1 + exp\left(a_i' \theta_j + d_i\right)}, \tag{19.14}$$

where $\boldsymbol{\theta}_j$ is a vector of latent abilities in M dimensions, $\boldsymbol{a}_i$ is a vector of item slopes, and d_i is a scalar parameter related to item difficulty. When the item responses correspond to successively ordered categories, the response probabilities can be modeled using a model like the multidimensional generalized partial credit model (MGPCM; Yao & Schwarz, 2006), which takes the following form:

$$P\left(X_{ij} = k \mid \theta_j, a_i, d_{ik}\right) = \frac{exp\left[\sum_{v=1}^{k} a_i' \theta_j + d_{iv}\right]}{\sum_{h=1}^{K_i} exp\left[\sum_{v=1}^{h} a_i' \theta_j + d_{iv}\right]}, \tag{19.15}$$

where d_{ik} is a step-intersection parameter. The other parameters have the same interpretation as in the M2PL. As in the unidimensional case, other multidimensional models can be specified for dichotomous and polytomously scored responses; however, the M2PL/MGPCM will be used here because it aligns closely with the frequently used *common factor model* in factor analysis (Thurstone, 1931, 1935, 1947).

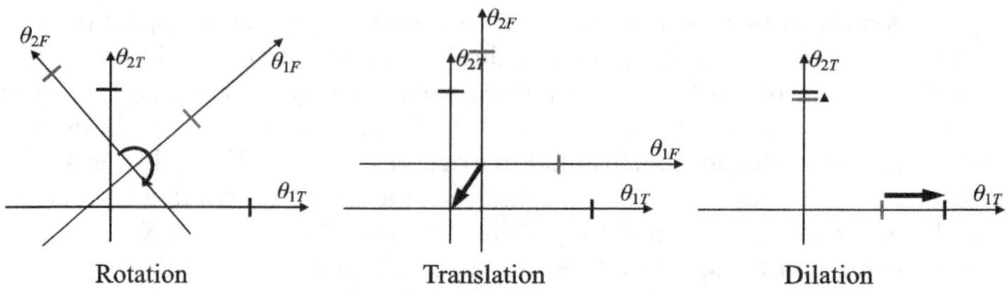

Figure 19.1 Transformations in multidimensional linking.

In order to establish a multidimensional scale across two or more forms, the item parameters can be estimated concurrently or separately. In the concurrent case, an extension of the multigroup method presented by Bock and Zimowski (1997) and von Davier and von Davier (2007) could be used where the common item parameters are constrained to be equal across groups. The latent ability distribution for a given group is usually specified as a reference group where the means and variances are fixed (typically with means equal to zero and variances equal to unity). Depending on the specified factor structure (e.g., an exploratory versus confirmatory structure), additional constraints may also be placed on the covariances for the reference group. The means, variances, and covariances for the remaining groups can be freely estimated. The end result of the concurrent calibration is that all of the item parameter and ability estimates will be on a common scale. As an alternative to the concurrent approach, the item parameters and examinee abilities can be estimated separately for each group. The linking then proceeds by finding linking coefficients that can be used to adjust for differences in the common item parameter estimates (or estimated latent ability distributions) for each group. In short, the goal is to implement a Procrustean transformation to place the results on a common scale. Building on the transformations described in the previous section, an explication of multidimensional separate calibration methods is presented below.

When conducting a separate calibration in the unidimensional case, a set of linking coefficients is estimated to adjust the location and scale of the ability distribution for the test being transformed. A corresponding transformation of the item parameters is made to maintain the expected probabilities of a given response. Similarly, in the multidimensional case, a set of coefficients can be estimated to adjust the scale and location for each of the modeled dimensions; however, a rotation may also be needed to align the dimensional axes. Figure 19.1 is a graphical representation of the various elements that must be resolved for linking tests in two dimensions;[8] the same premise holds for linking tests in more than two dimensions. In this figure, the axes with the labels θ_{1T} and θ_{2T} correspond to the *to* scales. The other set of axes correspond to the *from* scales. The goal of the linking process, conceptually, is to adjust the axes for the test being transformed so that they lie perfectly on top of the set of reference axes (i.e., adjusting for differences between the common item parameters). In general, this is a three-step process. The first step involves rotating the axes so that they are parallel. Once the axes are aligned, the *from* axes must be shifted so that the crosshairs lie on top of the *to* axes (translation). This is equivalent to adjusting the mean of the *from* distribution in a unidimensional context. The final step involves stretching or shrinking the scale associated with each axis so that

8 This illustration presumes an orthogonal transformation; however, the general premise of rotation, translation, and dilation holds for oblique transformations as well.

the perpendicular bars (representing the variability of each scale) lie on top of one another (scaling or dilation). This is equivalent to adjusting the standard deviation of the *from* scale in the unidimensional context.

MIRT Linking Equations

Several approaches have been developed to link tests on multiple dimensions with the key distinction being the rotation method (orthogonal vs. oblique) and dilation method (isotropic vs. anisotropic). In general, the parameters on the *from* scale can be transformed to the *to* scale via (Oshima, Davey, & Lee, 2000; Yao & Boughton, 2009):

$$\begin{aligned} a'_{iT} &= a'_{iF}T^{-1} \\ d_{ikT} &= d_{ikF} - a'_{iF}T^{-1}\mathbf{m} \\ \theta_{jT} &= \mathbf{T}\theta_{jT} + \mathbf{m}, \end{aligned} \tag{19.16}$$

where T is an oblique transformation matrix that adjusts for rotational indeterminacy and differences in variability, and $\mathbf{m}$ is a translation vector that adjusts for differences in difficulty on each dimension. Alternatively, the parameters can be transformed using an orthogonal rotation, Q, and an anisotropic scaling matrix, S (Min, 2007):

$$\begin{aligned} a'_{iT} &= a'_{iF}Q^{-1}S^{-1} \\ d_{ikT} &= d_{ikF} - a'_{iF}Q^{-1}\mathbf{m} \\ \theta_{jT} &= \mathrm{S}\left(\mathrm{Q}\theta_{jT} + \mathrm{m}\right). \end{aligned} \tag{19.17}$$

As an added constraint to this approach, S can be specified as a diagonal isotropic scaling matrix with a single dilation parameter (Li & Lissitz, 2000). This supposes that the variability of each dimension is adjusted by a constant value. It is useful to note that when the data are modeled using a between-item dimensional structure where each item only loads on a single dimension, Q will be an identity matrix and S will equal T.

As in the unidimensional case, the item parameters and linking coefficients are unknown and must be estimated. The simplest approach to estimating T is via unconstrained least squares:

$$\mathrm{T} = \left(\hat{a}'_F\hat{a}_F\right)^{-1}\hat{a}_F\hat{a}_T, \tag{19.18}$$

where $\hat{\mathbf{a}}$ is the matrix of common item parameter estimates for $\mathbf{a}$. In subsequent equations, $\hat{d}_{ik}$ is an estimate of d_{ik}. In general, the linking coefficients obtained via unconstrained least squares regression do not typically satisfy the symmetry property of equating (Lord, 1980); hence, additional constraints must be applied to the estimation of T to make it a symmetric transformation. In order to maintain the symmetry property, as well as the oblique transformation, T can be estimated using a two-sided Procrustes approach via alternating least squares (Gower & Dijksterhuis, 2004). On the other hand, T can be constrained to be orthogonal. In this case, a singular value decomposition of $\hat{a}'_F\hat{a}_T$:[9]

$$SVD\left(\hat{a}'_F\hat{a}_T\right) = U\Sigma V', \tag{19.19}$$

9 It is recommended that the values for X_F and X_T be mean centered prior to estimating the linking coefficients (Gower & Dijksterhuis, 2004; Schönemann & Carroll, 1970).

can be used to obtain the rotation matrix:

$$Q = VU' . \tag{19.20}$$

With orthogonal rotations it is possible for **Q** to produce a reflection rather than a pure rotation. This can be determined by examining [det(U) det(V)] where det is the determinant. If this value is negative, the sign in the final column of U or V can be changed to produce a rotation (Gower & Dijksterhuis, 2004). The diagonal matrix of anisotropic scaling coefficients can then be estimated as:

$$\mathrm{S} = \frac{diag\left(Q\,\hat{a}'_F \hat{a}_T\right)}{diag\left(Q\,\hat{a}'_F \hat{a}_F Q^{-1}\right)} . \tag{19.21}$$

If the dilation matrix is isotropic, the scaling coefficient, s, can be estimated as:

$$\mathrm{s} = \frac{trace\left(Qa'_F\ a_T\right)}{trace\left(a'_F\ a_F\right)} . \tag{19.22}$$

The translation vector **m** for both the oblique and orthogonal transformations can be estimated as:

$$\mathrm{m} = \left(\hat{a}'_F \hat{a}_F\right)^{-1} \hat{a}_F \left(\hat{d}_{ikF} - \hat{d}_{ikT}\right) . \tag{19.23}$$

In all of the equations used to estimate the multidimensional linking coefficients, only the item parameter estimates for the $C \leq J$ common items are used. These coefficients are then used to transform all of the item and ability parameter estimates to the reference scale.

In addition to the least squares methods presented earlier, researchers have developed multidimensional extensions of the unidimensional moment and characteristic curve methods (cf., Li & Lissitz, 2000; Min, 2007; Oshima, Davey, & Lee, 2000; Reckase & Martineau, 2004). Oshima and colleagues (2000) and Yao and Boughton (2009) compared multidimensional extensions of the moment and characteristic curve methods and found that the characteristic curve methods perform better than the moment methods in all cases. Li and Lissitz (2000) compared the performance of the multidimensional Stocking-Lord and a constrained least squares approach under four equating and vertical scaling conditions. They found that in all cases the least squares approach resulted in the smallest amount of linking error, particularly in the context of vertical scaling. Based on these findings, estimation of the multidimensional linking coefficients via constrained least squares is recommended.

When Is Multidimensional Score Linking Appropriate?

In practical applications of test linking, it is commonly assumed that all of the tests being linked measure a single construct; yet in many instances there are strong theoretical and empirical reasons to suspect that the construct of interest is multidimensional. Take, for example, subject areas like reading, mathematics, and science. A number of studies have been conducted to examine cognitive and content dimensions within these domains (cf., Abedi, 1994; Davis, 1972; Embretson & Wetzel, 1987; Geary, 2006; Gierl, Tan, & Wang, 2005; Kupermintz, Ennis, Hamilton, Talbert, & Snow, 1995; Kupermintz & Snow, 1997; Reckase & Martineau, 2004). In many cases, evidence of multidimensionality is present for both major and minor dimensions; however, almost all operational assessments of reading, mathematics, and science (e.g., K–12 state tests within the United States) treat the measured construct as unidimensional. There are a variety of explanations for this, but a key takeaway message is that evidence of underlying multidimensionality alone may be insufficient to justify the development of a multidimensional scale (or the subsequent linking of test scores on two or more dimensions). Other criteria such as reliability and interpretability must also be considered. The following section addresses subscore reliability, as it relates to the relative value of subscores versus total scores; score interpretability, as it pertains to construct shift; and common item requirements, as it relates to linking stability, in order to provide a context for when multidimensional test linking is appropriate.

Subscore Reliability

The Standards for Educational and Psychological Testing (American Educational Research Association, American Psychological Association, & National Council on Measurement in Education, 1999) state that "Scores should not be reported for individuals unless the validity, comparability, and reliability of such scores have been established." This standard applies to subscores as well as total scores. In the simplest case, raw subscores may be computed based on subsets of items within a given test. Alternatively, augmented subscores (Wainer et al., 2001) could be computed or factor scores/ability estimates from a multidimensional latent variable model could be estimated. An important consideration in all of these cases is whether the derived subscores are sufficiently reliable to be reported for individuals. In order to address this question, Haberman (2008) proposed a statistical method based on classical test theory (CTT) to evaluate whether subscores have added value relative to total scores.[10] The method is premised on the notion that subscores with added value are highly reliable and have correlations with the other subscores that are not very high. The approach relies on different regression-based estimates of true subscores and a comparison of the associated mean square error terms.

Consider an examinee, *j*, with a total raw score, S_j, and a raw subscore, S_{jk}, for skill *k*. The true score, T_j, associated with S_j is the average score for the examinee over repeated administrations of the same test or parallel forms of the test. Similarly, T_{jk} is the true subscore associated with S_{jk}. Haberman (2008) used three approaches to obtain estimates of the true subscores and the true subscore variance.

- $U_{jks} = \alpha_{ks} + \beta_{ks} S_{jk}$ is an estimate based on the raw subscore S_{jk}. This yields the following mean squared error: $\tau_{ks}^2 = E\left(\left[T_{jk} - U_{jks}\right]^2\right)$.
- $U_{jkx} = \alpha_{kx} + \beta_{kx} S_j$ is an estimate based on the raw total score S_j. This yields the following mean squared error: $\tau_{kx}^2 = E\left(\left[T_{jk} - U_{jkx}\right]^2\right)$.
- $U_{jkc} = \alpha_{kc} + \beta_{k1c} S_j + \beta_{k2c} S_{jk}$ is an estimate based on the raw total score S_j and the raw subscore S_{jk}. This yields the following mean squared error: $\tau_{kc}^2 = E\left(\left[T_{jk} - U_{jkc}\right]^2\right)$.

10 This method also holds in the consideration of augmented subscores (Wainer et al., 2001).

To compare the possible subscores, the proportional reduction in mean squared error (PRMSE) is considered relative to the variance of the true raw subscore $\tau_{k0}^2 = E\left(\left[T_{jk} - E\left(T_{jk}\right)\right]^2\right)$. The PRMSEs for each subscore are:

$$\begin{aligned} PRMSE_{ks} &= 1 - \tau_{ks}^2 / \tau_{k0}^2 \\ PRMSE_{kx} &= 1 - \tau_{kx}^2 / \tau_{k0}^2 \\ PRMSE_{kc} &= 1 - \tau_{kc}^2 / \tau_{k0}^2 . \end{aligned} \tag{19.24}$$

It is important to note that $PRMSE_{ks}$ is the reliability of S_{jk}. All of the PRMSE values range from zero to one, with values near one being more desirable. When $PRMSE_{ks}$ is less than $PRMSE_{kx}$, the subscore provides little added value relative to the total score. On the other hand, if $PRMSE_{ks}$ is greater than $PRMSE_{kx}$, the subscores provide more diagnostic information than the total score. Haberman suggests that $PRMSE_{kc}$ should only be used when it is substantively larger than the maximum of $PRMSE_{ks}$ and $PRMSE_{kx}$.

Haberman and Sinharay (2010) recast the CTT approach in a MIRT context and showed that the value:

$$PRMSE_{k\theta M} = 1 - \tau_{k\theta}^2 / \tau_{k0\theta}^2 , \tag{19.25}$$

is equal to the IRT marginal reliability (Adams, Wilson, & Wang, 1997) of the scores for dimension k where $\tau_{k\theta}^2$ is the dimension-specific error variance and $\tau_{k0\theta}^2$ is the dimension-specific total variance. When the items associated with a given subscore are modeled unidimensionally, the corresponding $PRMSE_{k\theta U}$ can be computed.[11] When $PRMSE_{k\theta M}$ is less than $PRMSE_{k\theta U}$, using the MIRT subscore provides little added value relative to the unidimensional subscore. On the other hand, if $PRMSE_{k\theta M}$ is greater than $PRMSE_{k\theta U}$, the MIRT subscore provides more diagnostic information than the corresponding unidimensional subscore. In addition to comparing PRMSE values within a CTT or MIRT framework, Haberman and Sinharay (2010) showed that these values can be compared across frameworks. For instance, $PRMSE_{ks}$ and $PRMSE_{k\theta M}$ could be compared to determine if there is added value to using MIRT subscores as opposed to raw subscores. They also showed that the results obtained using the CTT and MIRT approaches are generally comparable. As a point of clarification, within an IRT framework, the Haberman and Sinharay approach does not currently consider the added value of MIRT subscores relative to an overall unidimensional score.

With respect to the practicality of this method, Sinharay (2010) conducted an extensive review of operational programs that report subscores and employed a simulation to identify the characteristics that generally must be satisfied in order to have any hope of meeting the Haberman (2008) criterion. In short, he found that subscores should be comprised of a minimum of 20 items with disattenuated correlations between the subscores that are lower than 0.80. This assumes that the subscores are distinct, although the criterion may be satisfied for augmented subscores when there are fewer items and/or the disattenuated correlation between the subscores is less than 0.85. In either case, when the criterion is satisfied, modeling and linking parallel forms multidimensionally should be defensible. On

11 Haberman and Sinharay (2010) also established $PRMSE_{Vk\theta M}$, which is based on the test characteristic curves for each dimension.

the other hand, if the criterion is not satisfied, one may be better off treating the forms as essentially unidimensional and linking the scores as such.

Construct Shift

When multidimensional data are modeled unidimensionally using a latent variable model such as IRT, examinee abilities will be a linear weighted composite of abilities on the underlying dimensions (Reckase, 2009; Wang, 1986). This is akin to projecting scores from a multidimensional space onto a single linear composite within the space (Gower & Dijksterhuis, 2004). It can be shown that the weight of each dimension in the composite can be approximated by the eigenvector, $\boldsymbol{\omega}$, associated with the largest principal component of the matrix $\mathbf{a'a}$ where $\mathbf{a}$ is a matrix of factor loadings or item slopes. Based on this, the unidimensional item and ability parameters for the 2PL/GPCM can be approximated as a weighted composite of the M2PL/MGPCM parameters:

$$a_i = a_i' \omega$$
$$b_{ik} = \frac{-d_{ik}}{a_i' \omega}$$
$$\theta_j = \theta_j' \omega \,. \tag{19.26}$$

The vector $\theta_j' \omega$ is commonly referred to as a *reference composite*.

Conceptually, the contribution of a given factor in a composite score is based on the extent to which the items load on each dimension. A factor with higher loadings should weigh more heavily in the composite; hence, it should not come as a surprise that the weights for the reference composite are determined solely by the factor loadings/item slope parameters. To illustrate the idea of a composite visually, consider two hypothetical tests

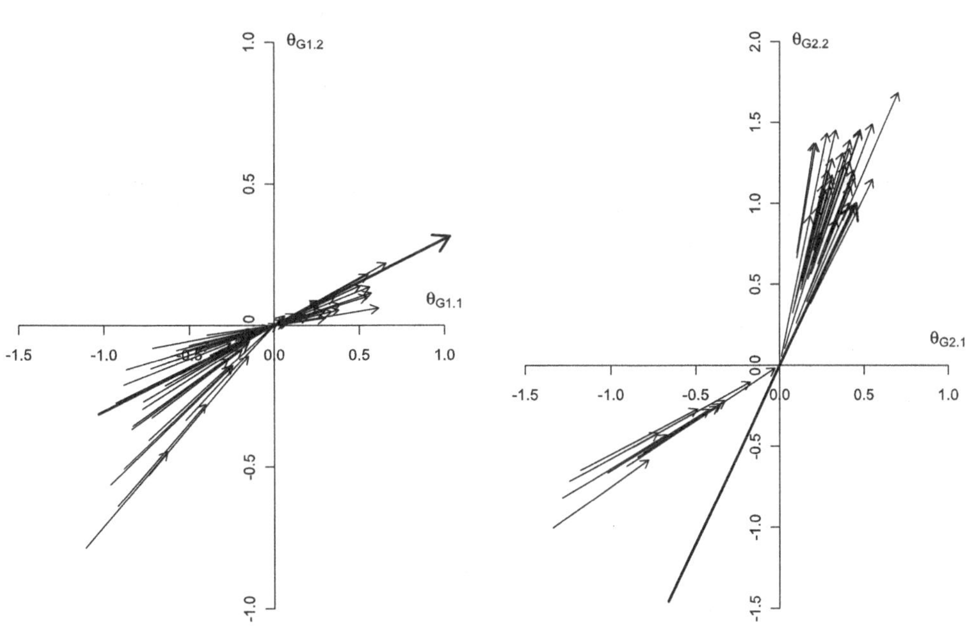

Figure 19.2 Vector representation of items and corresponding reference composites.

that each measure two dimensions (see Figure 19.2).[12] The short arrows correspond to a vector representation of items (Reckase, 2009). The base of the arrow for item i corresponds to the multidimensional item difficulty (MDIF):

$$MDIF_i = \frac{-d_i}{\sqrt{a_i' a_i}}, \tag{19.27}$$

which characterizes the signed deviation from the origin. The length of the arrow corresponds to the multidimensional discrimination (MDISC):

$$MDISC_i = \sqrt{a_i' a_i}\ . \tag{19.28}$$

Longer arrows represent more discriminating items (items with more weight in the composite score). The direction of the arrow corresponds to the relative weight of each dimension. The angle of the arrow, relative to a given axis, m, is:

$$\alpha_{im} = arccos\frac{a_{im}}{MDISC_i}, \tag{19.29}$$

where a_{im} is a specific element in a_i. Arrows that are more closely aligned with a given axis measure that dimension more predominantly. The items on the first test (the left panel) load primarily on θ_1, whereas the items on the second test load primarily on θ_2. The reference composite for each test is characterized by the long, dark arrows spanning from approximately (–1.0, 0.25) to (1.1, 0.4) in the left panel and (–1.5, 0.75) to (0.5, 1.0) in the right panel.

Given that there are no substantive differences in the magnitude of loadings on these two dimensions (i.e., the lengths of the individual arrows are about the same for items loading on the two factors respectively), θ_1 weighs more heavily in the composite for the first test simply because there are more items that measure that construct. Similarly, θ_2 weighs more heavily in the composite for the second test. If we assume that the axes are aligned, there is an obvious change in the direction of the reference composite between the tests. This coincides with Martineau's (2004) conception of construct shift, which he characterizes as a change in the proportional representation of dimensions at different points along the composite scale. More formally, construct shift can be characterized by the angle between the two reference composites. The angle between the composites for tests p and q can be computed as:[13]

$$\alpha_{pq} = cos^{-1}\left[\frac{\omega_p' \omega_q'}{\sqrt{\omega_p' \omega_p}\sqrt{\omega_q' \omega_q}}\right]. \tag{19.30}$$

When reporting scores on a common scale there is a strong assumption that the measured construct(s) can be interpreted in the same way at all points along the scale. As such, the

12 The subscripts G1 and G2 in the axis labels denote group (test) 1 and 2 respectively.

13 Note that cos(α_{pq}) = r_{pq} where r_{pq} can be interpreted as a correlation.

notion of a single construct (within and between tests) is sometimes interpreted as the presence of a single dominant factor with the possibility of several minor factors, for example, *essential unidimensionality* (Stout, 1987). This can be assessed by examining the extent to which the item covariances, conditional on examinee ability, are similar across scores. Conceptually, one can think about creating a reference composite for each ability level then comparing the direction of these composites. When the measurement direction of the composites differs substantively within and/or between tests—when there is construct shift—but the tests are modeled and linked unidimensionally, this raises questions about the comparability and interpretation of scores and any subsequent linking. One possible solution is to estimate the item parameters concurrently. Doing so will create a single reference composite that spans the multidimensional space for all of the tests being linked. This allows the scores to be compared on the same metric, but it does not resolve the problem of interpretation; what do scores on this composite scale mean substantively? If there is a clearer understanding of the underlying factors, it may be more valuable to model and link the tests multidimensionally.

Common Item Requirements

Based on a consideration of the Haberman (2008) criterion for the added value of subscores and/or an examination of potential construct shift a decision may be made to establish a multidimensional scale for two or more test forms. If the data for the forms were collected based on a randomly equivalent groups design, the scores across dimensions can be scaled by fitting a single-group multidimensional model; however, if a nonequivalent groups common item design is used, the number of common items available to establish the linking must be considered. There is no minimum criterion for the number of common items that should be used to link tests, either unidimensionally or multidimensionally. Many researchers use the rule of 20 percent or 20 items (whichever is greater) as a minimum, whereas some testing companies require a minimum of 15 common items (cf., Sykes, 1997).

In general, more common items should produce a more stable linkage between tests, but in an era of short tests, the number of available common items may be limited. Studies conducted by Vale (1986) and Kim and Cohen (1998) suggest that linking error, in the unidimensional case, can be relatively small with as few as five dichotomous common items while other studies suggest that 10 to 15 common items are required for the error to be considered "acceptable" (Hanson & Béguin, 2002; Kim, 2006; Kim & Cohen, 2002). That is, if the tests as a whole are not very long, it may be possible to link the tests with fewer than 20 common items; however, potential bias in estimates of ability may be non-ignorable (Weeks, von Davier, & Yamamoto, 2014).

To address the issue of common item requirements for multidimensional linking, Yao (2010) conducted a simulation study to link tests with a between-item dimensional structure and found that when the dimension-specific scores are highly reliable, the linking may be adequate with as few as 10 common items overall and two to four common items per dimension; however, given that simulation was used, these requirements seem optimistically small. Weeks (2013) conducted a resampling study using empirical data from an assessment spanning multiple years. He found that for a between-item dimensional structure with a more restrictive criterion for the magnitude of error, the linking may be adequate with as few as 15 to 20 items per dimension, although a minimum of around 20 to 30 common items per dimension is preferable. Li and Lissitz (2000) conducted a simulation that considered multidimensional linking for items with complex structure (i.e., within-item dimensionality). They found that 15 to 20 common items overall may be sufficient to conduct the linking.

Application

Dorans and Holland (2000) outlined a set of characteristics that are widely held as necessary for equating.[14] They include:

- Construct equivalence: The tests being equated should measure the same construct.
- Equal reliability: The test scores should have the same reliability.
- Score equity: Examinees' expected scores on the equated forms should be the same.[15]
- Symmetry of the equating function: The function used to transform scores from X to Y should be the inverse of the function used to transform scores from Y to X.
- Population invariance: The equating function used to transform scores from X to Y (or from Y to X) should be the same for all subpopulations.

In reality, none of these elements are likely to hold in the strictest sense (if they do, there is no need for equating), but they do provide a set of criteria by which to evaluate the comparability of equated scores. The goal of this section is to discuss these characteristics in the context of multidimensional test linking. To make the discussion more illustrative, empirical data from a large-scale mathematics assessment are presented.

Design

Six scales are created for each of four linking scenarios (a total of 24 scales) using two years of data from grades 5 and 6. The linking scenarios include two equating conditions and two vertical scaling conditions.

Equating Conditions:

- Grade 5—Year 1 and Year 2
- Grade 6—Year 1 and Year 2

Vertical Scaling Conditions:

- Grade 5 and Grade 6—Year 1
- Grade 5 and Grade 6—Year 1 and Year 2

For each condition three models are applied to the data: a unidimensional model, a multidimensional model based on an exploratory factor structure with two dimensions, and a multidimensional model based on a confirmatory factor structure tied to the content standards. The scales for each model in each condition are created using both separate and concurrent calibrations. The details regarding the models and estimation methods are described later.

Data

The data for the empirical illustration includes two years of item responses from a large-scale mathematics assessment in grades 5 and 6. There are around 58,000

14 These elements are based primarily on statements from Lord (1980).

15 Given the more practical test of equal reliability, for the present analysis, score equity is not evaluated.

examinees per grade, per year. Sixty-five percent of examinees are self-reported as white, 25 percent as Hispanic, 6 percent as black, and 3 percent as Asian/Pacific Islander. Thirty-four percent of examinees are on free or reduced lunch, and 9 percent are English language learners. The tests at each grade level include a combination of multiple-choice (MC) and constructed response (CR) items. Each year the grade 5 assessments include 54 MC items and 15 CR items. The grade 6 tests include 45 MC items and 15 CR items.

Each item on each of the grades 5 and 6 math assessments is associated with one of six content standards (based on the test blueprint): 1) Number Sense, 2) Algebra, Patterns, and Functions, 3) Statistics and Probability, 4) Geometry, 5) Measurement, and 6) Computational Techniques. In released reports, standards one and six and standards four and five are collapsed to produce four subscores: Std 1/6, Std 2, Std3, and Std 4/5. These standards are referred to here as "NUCO," "ALPF," "STPB", and "GEME" respectively (see Table 19.1).

The number of items associated with each of these standards does not change from year to year within a given grade; however, the proportional representation of each standard does change from grade to grade. In grade 5, nearly half of the items are NUCO items, but in grade 6 only 38 percent of the items measure this standard. ALPF and STPB are the least represented standards in grade 5 at 17 percent and 16 percent, respectively. In grade 6, there is a slight increase in the proportion of STPB items. There is also a notable increase in the proportion of grade 6 GEME items.

Table 19.2 shows the number of common items between tests for each dimension. In grade 5 there are a total of 33 common items (24%) between the Year 1 and Year 2 tests. In grade 6 there are 23 common items (19%) between the Year 1 and Year 2 tests, and between grades 5 and 6 there are 25 or 31 common items depending on whether the tests are linked using data from only Year 1 or if items are pooled across years within each grade prior to establishing the vertical scale. While the total number of common items in each case should be sufficient for unidimensional linking, the number of common items for most of the dimensions is quite small.

Table 19.1 Content Standard Identification and Proportional Representation by Grade

Standard	*Name*	*Description*	*Grade 5*	*Grade 6*
1/6	NUCO	Number Sense/Computational Techniques	47%	38%
2	ALPF	Algebra, Patterns, and Functions	17%	17%
3	STPB	Statistics and Probability	16%	18%
4/5	GEME	Geometry/Measurement	20%	27%

Table 19.2 Number of Common Items by Grade and Dimension

	NUCO	*ALPF*	*STPB*	*GEME*	*Total*
Grade 5 (Y1–Y2)	15	5	6	7	33
Grade 6 (Y1–Y2)	7	5	7	4	23
Grades 5–6 (Y1)	8	4	5	8	25
Grades 5–6 (Y1/Y2)	11	5	5	10	31

Dimensionality

Considerable work has been done over the years to identify the dimensions underlying mathematical ability. Geary (2006), for example, provides evidence from studies in psychometrics, cognitive psychology, and behavioral genetics to suggest that there are two primary cognitive dimensions. The first dimension is associated with numerical facility (i.e., arithmetic computation, number relations) and spans all ability levels from infancy to adulthood. The second dimension is associated with mathematical reasoning (i.e., evaluation of quantitative relationships and drawing conclusions based on quantitative information) and spans most ability levels for school-aged children and beyond. His cited studies also indicate that there is a set of factors related to complex skills like algebraic problem solving and estimation that are only present at higher ability levels. At the same time, there is evidence to suggest that these cognitive dimensions are intertwined with content domains. That is, answering a question correctly may require simple recall, problem solving, or abstract reasoning (Hegarty & Kozhevnikov, 1999).

On the other hand, Abedi (1994) examined the dimensionality of the 1990 and 1992 National Assessment of Educational Progress (NAEP) mathematics assessments using a confirmatory factor analysis where the five reported subscores (number and operations, measurement, algebra, geometry, and statistics) served as the basis for the number of dimensions. Although he did not compare this structure to one based on exploratory factors, he found that this model fit the data very well. In other words, this model provides some evidence in support of a content-based factor structure. However, other studies suggest that when content areas are used as the basis for the factor structure, the factor correlations can be quite high, suggesting that mathematics assessments may be better fit by a unidimensional model (cf., von Davier & Sinharay, 2007). The results from these various studies, among others, suggest that if an exploratory approach is used to identify the dimensional structure of a math test, one is likely to identify a combination of content and process dimensions; however, these dimensions may not be consistently identified across grades. In contrast, a content-based structure—across grades—may be defensibly identified using a confirmatory analysis.

For this illustration, the data were examined using both exploratory and confirmatory multidimensional factor structures (as well as a unidimensional structure). With respect to the exploratory structure, an analysis of the dimensional structure of the mathematics data was conducted using a combination of parallel analysis (Horn, 1965) and a vector approach developed by Reckase, Martineau, and Kim (2000). Parallel analysis is an extension of principal components analysis that compares the magnitude of principal components in the empirical data to randomly generated data with the same number of variables. The vector approach, on the other hand, considers changes in the angles between item vectors—characterized by factor loadings or MIRT slopes—as the number of modeled dimensions increases. Parallel analysis has been shown to perform well when the underlying factors in the data are orthogonal; however, the number of dimensions may be underidentified if the factors are correlated. In this case, the vector approach may more accurately identify the number of underlying factors. The results from the parallel analysis and vector approach were consistent and suggest the presence of three to four underlying factors in each grade-level test (two of which are major factors); however, a comparison of model fit suggests that the data are better characterized by two dimensions. The exploratory models were each applied using two factors.

Analyses

For all of the analyses, item parameters for the dichotomous items were estimated using the 2PL or M2PL; item parameters for the polytomous items were estimated using the GPCM or MGPCM. The data were modeled using three factor structures: 1) unidimensional, 2) two-factor within-item (exploratory), and 3) four-factor (confirmatory) simple structure based on the content standards. In each case the item parameters were estimated using IRTPRO (Cai, du Toit, & Thissen, 2012) via marginal maximum likelihood estimation.

For each factor structure, for each of the four linking scenarios described earlier, the item parameters for each test were first estimated separately for each test and then linked using a separate calibration approach (described later). The item parameters were then re-estimated concurrently such that the item parameters for the common items were constrained to be equal across groups. In linking scenario four where the items from Year 1 and Year 2 were pooled within each grade, the separate calibration approach proceeded by first estimating the item parameters within grade, across years concurrently and then estimating linking coefficients for the combined data. For the concurrent re-estimation, item parameters were estimated simultaneously using the data from both grades in both years. In all cases, the grade 5 and/or Year 1 test was treated as the reference scale and expected *a posteriori* (EAP) estimates of examinee ability were used.

With respect to the separate calibration approaches, in the unidimensional case, the Stocking-Lord method was implemented (with symmetry constraints) to maintain consistency with the linking of scales in operational use. In the multidimensional case, both for the exploratory and confirmatory factor structures, an oblique approach as well as orthogonal rotation with anisotropic scaling was used. For the oblique approach, symmetry constraints were applied. The estimation of linking coefficients for the separate calibrations were conducted using the plink package in R (Weeks, 2010).

Construct Equivalence

As described earlier, when a test measuring multiple dimensions is modeled unidimensionally, examinee ability can be treated as a weighted composite of the underlying dimensions. Simply put, the scores should coincide with the largest principal component in the data. When the dimensions are highly correlated, the resulting scores can be treated as essentially unidimensional; on the other hand, if the dimensions are uncorrelated or only moderately correlated, the interpretation of the reference composite is more ambiguous. Setting aside the interpretation of composite scores, given that the reference composite characterizes the relative weight of each dimension within a test, a comparison of the angle between the composites on the tests—after they have been scaled multidimensionally—can be used to assess construct equivalence within a multidimensional framework. The requirement of construct equivalence should be satisfied if this angle is sufficiently small, or when the correlation is close to unity (there is no research that provides a criterion for this difference).

Table 19.3 presents the angles between the reference composites, expressed as correlations (values near one indicate construct equivalence), for the parallel forms in grades 5 and 6 (in Year 1 and 2 respectively) as well as the nonparallel forms between grades 5 and 6 in Year 1. The angles between the reference composite based on the multidimensional concurrent calibrations and the reference composites for each of the separately calibrated, linked scales are also presented. In all cases the correlations are high and none substantively differs from unity. This is evidence of little to no construct shift between the forms.

Table 19.3 Angle Between Reference Composites (Expressed as Correlations)

Model	*Comparison*	*Grade 5*	*Grade 6*	*Grade 5–6*
EFA	Y1 Sep—Y2 Sep	0.999	0.996	0.994
	Y1 Sep—Y1/Y2 Con	0.950	0.951	0.951
	Y2 Sep—Y1/Y2 Con	0.951	0.955	0.957
CFA	Y1 Sep—Y2 Sep	0.995	0.998	0.946
	Y1 Sep—Y1/Y2 Con	0.998	0.999	0.998
	Y2 Sep—Y1/Y2 Con	0.995	0.999	0.946

Within grades one should expect this if the forms are designed to be parallel, whereas in the vertical scaling case where the test forms are not necessarily designed to be parallel, one might expect larger angles (lower correlations) between the composites. Regarding the differences between the reference composites from the separate calibration and the composites from the concurrent calibration, for the EFA comparisons, the composites based on the separate approach are more aligned than the separate and concurrent composites; however, the differences are still relatively small. In the CFA case, the composite for the concurrent calibration appears to be more closely aligned with the composite from the Year 1 separate calibration, as evidenced by the slightly lower correlation with the Year 1 separate calibration composite. Relative to the near perfect correlations for the within-grade conditions, particularly in the CFA case, there is some change—albeit small—in the angle for the between-grade linkage (e.g., 0.995 or 0.998 versus 0.946). This may be due in part to the change in representation of the NUCO and GEME standards from grades 5 to 6.

Equal Reliability

Table 19.4 presents marginal reliabilities (Adams, Wilson, & Wang, 1997) for each factor under each dimensional structure, for each grade-by-year. The table also includes columns (N Inc) that identify the additional number of items required in a given grade-year for each dimension to have the same reliability as the more reliable test dimension in the pair; this is based on a reformulation of the Spearman-Brown equation (Lord & Novick, 1968). These values are provided primarily to aid in the interpretation of differences between the marginal reliabilities. For example, the reliabilities of the scores for the STPB dimension in grade 5 are 0.77 and 0.76 in Years 1 and 2, respectively. An additional two items associated with this dimension would need to be added to the Year 2 test in order for both tests to have reliabilities of 0.77.

The unidimensional scores in both grades, across years, are quite reliable under both the separate and concurrent approach. Most of the dimension-specific scales are moderately reliable, while some scales (e.g., the first factor for the EFA model) are not very reliable. With respect to equal reliability, the unidimensional model arguably satisfies this condition. Under the separate approach, several of the scales across years appear to satisfy the condition, while others do not seem to meet the condition. Perhaps one of the most notable differences is between the separate and concurrent calibration results. The marginal reliabilities for the concurrently calibrated scales are virtually indistinguishable between forms within a given grade, across years. This is further evidence in favor of concurrent calibration. The between-grade differences in reliability

Table 19.4 Marginal Reliabilities

		Grade 5			Grade 6			Grade 5–6 (Year 1)
		Year 1	Year 2	N Inc	Year 1	Year 2	N Inc	N Inc
Separate Calibration	UD	0.93	0.93	5	0.93	0.94	6	6
	EFA D1	0.55	0.52	7	0.75	0.62	20	54
	EFA D2	0.82	0.81	4	0.83	0.80	7	7
	NUCO	0.89	0.88	2	0.85	0.86	1	20
	ALPF	0.77	0.81	14	0.72	0.76	10	19
	STPB	0.77	0.76	2	0.72	0.75	10	20
	GEME	0.74	0.78	13	0.78	0.81	10	0
Concurrent Calibration	UD	0.93	0.93	0	0.94	0.94	1	4
	EFA D1	0.62	0.61	0	0.54	0.55	1	20
	EFA D2	0.79	0.79	0	0.80	0.79	1	8
	NUCO	0.87	0.87	0	0.86	0.86	0	12
	ALPF	0.75	0.75	0	0.75	0.74	1	8
	STPB	0.71	0.71	1	0.75	0.75	1	1
	GEME	0.74	0.74	0	0.80	0.80	0	10

Table 19.5 Observed and Disattenuated Correlations by Grade

		UD	EFA D1	EFA D2	NUCO	ALPF	STPB	GEME
Grade 5	UD		**0.86**	**1.00**	**1.00**	**1.00**	**1.00**	**1.00**
	EFA D1	0.65		**0.36**	**0.82**	**0.80**	**0.87**	**0.95**
	EFA D2	0.90	0.25		**1.00**	**1.00**	**0.96**	**0.91**
	NUCO	0.93	0.60	0.83		**0.97**	**0.93**	**0.93**
	ALPF	0.86	0.54	0.78	0.78		**0.95**	**0.94**
	STPB	0.83	0.58	0.72	0.73	0.69		**0.96**
	GEME	0.83	0.64	0.69	0.74	0.69	0.70	
Grade 6	UD		**0.76**	**1.00**	**1.00**	**1.00**	**1.00**	**1.00**
	EFA D1	0.54		**0.22**	**0.90**	**0.66**	**0.78**	**0.56**
	EFA D2	0.91	0.14		**0.93**	**1.00**	**0.97**	**1.00**
	NUCO	0.91	0.61	0.77		**0.94**	**0.93**	**0.92**
	ALPF	0.85	0.42	0.80	0.75		**0.94**	**0.95**
	STPB	0.85	0.50	0.75	0.74	0.70		**0.94**
	GEME	0.88	0.37	0.85	0.77	0.73	0.73	

Note: Disattenuated correlations are located in the upper triangle.

are likely due, at least in part, to differences in the overall number of items in grades 5 and 6, 54 and 45 respectively. As such, it is not surprising that the number of items on the grade 6 test would need to be increased appreciably for the grade 6 scores to be as reliable as the grade 5 scores.

To further illustrate the impact of score reliability on the interpretation of dimension-specific scales, Table 19.5 presents the observed and disattenuated correlation between the ability estimates. The score reliabilities based on the concurrent calibration of items within each grade, across years, were used to disattenuate the correlations. The observed correlations between the CFA factors are positive and moderately high (0.69 to 0.78) while the correlations between the dimension-specific scores and the unidimensional scores are high (0.83 to 0.93). There is a low correlation between the factors for the EFA model, but moderate to high correlations with the unidimensional scores (0.54 to 0.91). However, after correcting for attenuation, most of the scales are indistinguishable from the unidimensional scale. Based on these results, there is strong evidence in favor of a unidimensional factor structure or, at best, a two-factor exploratory structure.

Symmetry of the Equating Function

The notion of symmetry of the equating function in the context of IRT is premised on the idea that true scores are equivalent across tests. This is consistent with the assumption of parameter invariance. If this assumption holds, the regression of $\hat{\theta}_{from}$ on $\hat{\theta}_{to}$ should produce linking coefficients that are a near inverse to the regression of $\hat{\theta}_{to}$ on $\hat{\theta}_{from}$. In practice, the symmetry requirement is likely to be violated except in cases where the scores on each test are highly reliable. Given the expectation of symmetry, scaling functions are commonly specified in a manner that imposes this constraint. For instance, if the correlation is constrained to be unity in the regression of scores between the *to* and *from* tests, the same coefficients will be estimated regardless of the choice of the reference scale. Differences between coefficients estimated with and without this constraint could be used as evidence for the satisfaction of the symmetry requirement. Stated differently, if the linking coefficients obtained via unconstrained least squares are not appreciably different from the coefficients obtained using a method that imposes the symmetry constraint, this is strong evidence in favor of a symmetric relationship between the score scales.

Table 19.6 presents the diagonal of $\boldsymbol{T}$ when estimated using an unconstrained oblique Procrustes approach or the diagonal of $\boldsymbol{QS}$ in the orthogonal Procrustes approach. These values are reported as T1, T2, T3, T4. The values for the translation vector $\mathbf{m}$ (m1, m2, m3, m4) are also included. Note that the translation vector is not dependent on the rotation/dilation; thus, it is the same for both the oblique and orthogonal approaches. The unidimensional linking coefficients and estimates of the group means and standard deviations from the concurrent calibration are also reported. Although the reported diag($\boldsymbol{T}$) coefficients are not strictly dilation parameters, they do provide some evidence for the comparability of the transformations. In almost all cases, the dilation coefficients estimated under the oblique transformation are lower than the corresponding coefficients estimated under the orthogonal approach. This indicates that as more restrictive constraints are placed on the linking coefficients to obtain symmetry, adjustments to the variability of dimension-specific scores are likely to be higher. The differences in the dilation coefficients between the oblique and orthogonal approach are small to moderate (< 0.01 to 0.08) with a mean difference of 0.027 across all EFA transformations. This suggests that even without the symmetry constraint, the transformations are fairly symmetric. It is not possible to explicitly evaluate the symmetry of the transformations for the CFA cases because the linking coefficients for both transformations are identical (as expected). While not an evaluation of symmetry, the linking coefficients can be compared to the estimated group means and standard deviations from the concurrent calibration to assess the extent to which the concurrent and separate approaches provide the same adjustments to the

Table 19.6 Dilation and Translation Coefficients and Concurrent Calibration Moments

				T1	*T2*	*T3*	*T4*	*m1*	*m2*	*m3*	*m4*
Grade 5	Separate Calibration	UD		1.06				0.01			
		EFA	Oblique	0.94	1.08			–0.02	0.04		
			Orthogonal	1.02	1.04						
		CFA	Oblique	1.03	1.45	1.04	1.02	0.19	–0.12	–0.21	0.10
			Orthogonal	1.03	1.45	1.04	1.02				
	Concurrent Calibration	UD		1.07				0.09			
		EFA		1.17	1.01			0.90	–0.44		
		CFA		1.78	1.63	1.50	1.63	0.34	0.01	0.01	0.16
Grade 6	Separate Calibration	UD		0.95				–0.09			
		EFA	Oblique	0.99	1.11			0.24	–0.16		
			Orthogonal	1.01	1.12						
		CFA	Oblique	1.04	0.99	1.00	1.01	0.10	0.01	0.30	–0.10
			Orthogonal	1.04	0.99	1.00	1.01				
	Concurrent Calibration	UD		1.01				0.09			
		EFA		1.37	1.12			0.30	–0.05		
		CFA		1.75	1.47	1.46	1.71	0.22	0.00	0.30	0.07
Grades 5–6	Separate Calibration (Year 1)	UD		0.99				0.14			
		EFA	Oblique	1.29	1.11			0.16	0.39		
			Orthogonal	1.30	1.11						
		CFA	Oblique	1.37	1.34	1.39	1.20	0.65	0.58	0.40	0.30
			Orthogonal	1.37	1.34	1.39	1.20				
	Concurrent Calibration	UD G5 Y2		1.08				0.12			
		UD G6 Y1		1.10				0.34			
		UD G6 Y2		1.13				0.42			
		EFA G5 Y2		1.03	1.15			–0.45	1.02		
		EFA G6 Y1		1.05	1.35			0.33	0.18		
		EFA G6 Y2		1.28	1.42			0.58	–0.02		
		CFA G5 Y2		1.77	1.65	1.52	1.66	0.28	0.14	0.00	0.17
		CFA G6 Y1		1.80	1.53	1.62	1.66	0.64	0.44	0.43	0.41
		CFA G6 Y2		1.83	1.62	1.61	1.76	0.82	0.36	0.68	0.38

underlying score distributions. In almost all cases, the concurrent calibration results in the largest adjustment to the variability of the scores; however, adjustments to the means are more ambiguous. There are no clear patterns in the magnitudes of translation coefficients and estimates of group means. This is likely due to the small numbers of common items for each dimension; the findings from Weeks (2013) suggest that a larger number of common items is needed to provide stable estimates of the translation coefficients, relative to the dilation coefficients.

Population Invariance

For equated scores to be considered comparable, the function used to transform the scores should be the same for all subpopulations. This implicitly assumes that the item parameters for each test are population independent. In the multidimensional case this corresponds, in part, to the notion of measurement invariance. Meredith (1993) outlined four types of measurement invariance.

- Configural invariance: The pattern and relative magnitude of zero and nonzero loadings is maintained across groups.
- Weak invariance: The loadings for each item are equal across groups.
- Strong invariance: The loadings and intercepts for each item are equal across groups.
- Strict invariance: The loadings, intercepts, and residual variances for each item are equal across groups.

Multidimensional linking within an MIRT context assumes strong invariance (the notion of strict invariance is really only applicable in cases where an error term is included in the model; this is not the case with MIRT). Measurement invariance is commonly examined for different subpopulations on a single test, but in the case of multidimensional score linking, invariance must be evaluated across test forms. Under the concurrent approach where there is no secondary linking, the item parameters across subpopulations can be examined via a comparison of model fit based on imposed versus relaxed constraints on various item parameters across groups. With separate calibration, differences between transformed score estimates based on linking coefficients obtained from the overall sample versus subpopulation samples can be used to test the invariance assumption. Dorans and Holland (2000) introduced a root expected mean squared difference (REMSD) statistic to quantify subpopulation differences. Adapted for the multidimensional context, the formulation is:

$$REMSD_m = \frac{\sqrt{\sum_{h=1}^{H} w_h E\{[e_{Th}(\theta_{Fm}) - e_T(\theta_{Fm})]^2\}}}{\sigma(\theta_{Tm})}, \tag{19.31}$$

where $e_T(\theta_{Fm})$ corresponds to the transformed *from* scale ability estimates for dimension m on the *to* scale based on the linking coefficients obtained using the overall sample, $e_{Th}(\theta_{Fm})$ corresponds to the transformed scores for subgroup h based on the linking coefficients obtained using data for the subgroup only, $w_h = N_h / N$ where N is the number of examinees overall and N_h is the number of examinees in the subgroup, $\sigma(\theta_{Tm})$ is the standard deviation of the *to* scale ability estimates, and E{ } is the expected value.

Using the math data, item parameters were estimated separately and concurrently for each of the grade-level tests for each of the three-dimensional structures using the complete data and the full subset of data for males and females, respectively (in practice, the invariance assumption should be evaluated for other relevant subpopulations). In a given grade, in a given year there are approximately 29,000 males and 28,000 females. In the separate case, linking coefficients for each of these groups were estimated using the orthogonal Procrustes approach. To provide a reference for the magnitude of REMSDs under the separate approach, REMSDs were also computed using ability estimates from the concurrent calibration.

Table 19.7 presents the REMSDs for the various linkages for each dimensional structure. In general, the differences between the overall transformation and the subpopulation

Table 19.7 Root Expected Mean Squared Deviations

		UD	*EFA D1*	*EFA D2*	*NUCO*	*ALPF*	*STPB*	*GEME*
Grade 5	Separate	0.016	0.111	0.171	0.007	0.019	0.041	0.009
	Concurrent	0.060	0.072	0.059	0.046	0.086	0.058	0.074
Grade 6	Separate	0.003	0.310	0.337	0.005	0.003	0.011	0.018
	Concurrent	0.028	0.045	0.071	0.041	0.005	0.028	0.081
Grades 5–6	Separate	0.013	0.159	0.312	0.040	0.039	0.050	0.013
	Concurrent	0.020	0.054	0.048	0.066	0.028	0.022	0.011

transformations are quite small, with the exception of the transformations for the EFA scales in the separate calibration case. This suggests that the exploratory factors may not have a consistent interpretation across subpopulations. In some instances the REMSDs for the separate case are slightly lower than the corresponding values in the concurrent case; however, the magnitude of the REMSDs are fairly comparable. In short, the transformations appear to be invariant for both the unidimensional and CFA models for both the separate and concurrent calibrations.

Summary

As the use of multidimensional models becomes more prevalent, it is useful to consider the extent to which the requirements for test equating are satisfied in the multidimensional case. I considered four of the requirements outlined by Dorans and Holland (2000). In order to ensure that the substantive interpretation of equated scores is comparable, it is necessary for the tests to measure the same constructs, to the same degree. To test the requirement of construct equivalence, a comparison of the angle between the reference composites for the two tests can be used to determine if there is a notable change in the measurement emphasis between tests. In order to satisfy the requirement of construct equivalence, the representation of each dimension should be the same across tests; hence, the angle between the composites should be small.

The requirement of symmetry of the equating function is premised on the idea that true scores are equivalent across tests. Unless the scores are highly reliable, this requirement is unlikely to be satisfied; however, linking equations can be constrained to impose symmetry, or in the case of concurrent calibration, symmetry is imposed directly. The issue of symmetric transformations for multidimensional test score linking in the separate calibration case has been adequately addressed in the literature on multidimensional linking, but it is possible to obtain symmetric transformations by estimating an oblique transformation matrix via a two-sided Procrustes approach or through the use of an orthogonal rotation. Finally, the requirement of population invariance can be checked by examining the stability of estimated linking transformation for subpopulations of examinees using an REMSD statistic. Comparable transformations (low REMSDs) are suggestive of construct equivalence across subpopulations.

Future Directions

The models and methods that form the basis for multidimensional test linking within an MIRT context have been in place for some time; however, the application of these methods in practice has been fairly limited. Much of the work up to this point has centered on extending unidimensional linking methods (within a separate calibration framework), but more research is needed to address the adequacy of the methods for linking tests empirically on multiple dimensions. Any work related to multidimensional linking in a separate calibration framework should also be compared against corresponding concurrent calibrations. In addition, more work is needed to establish criteria for when it is defensible to establish a multidimensional scale relative to modeling the data unidimensionally as well as to refine the evaluation of the equating requirements in the multidimensional case.

References

Abedi, J. (1994). *NAEP TRP Task 3e: Achievement dimensionality, section A*. Los Angeles, CA: National Center for Research on Evaluation, Standards, and Student Testing.

Adams, R. J., Wilson, M., & Wang, W. (1997). The multidimensional random coefficients multinomial logit model. *Applied Psychological Measurement, 21*(1), 1–23.

American Educational Research Association, American Psychological Association, & National Council on Measurement in Education. (1999). *Standards for educational and psychological testing*. Washington, DC: American Educational Research Association.

Angoff, W.H. (1971). Scales, norms, and equivalent scores. In R.L. Thorndike (Ed.), *Educational measurement* (2nd ed., pp. 508–600). Washington, DC: American Council on Education.

Baker, F.B. (1992). Equating tests under the graded response model. *Applied Psychological Measurement, 16*(1), 87–96.

Birnbaum, A. (1968). Some latent trait models and their use in inferring an examinee's ability. In F.M. Lord & M.R. Novick (Eds.), *Statistical theories of mental test scores* (pp. 397–479). Reading, MA: Addison-Wesley.

Bock, R.D., & Zimowski, M.F. (1997). Multiple group IRT. In W.J. van der Linden & R.K. Hambleton (Eds.), *Handbook of modern item response theory* (pp. 433–448). New York: Springer-Verlag.

Braun, H.I., & Holland, P.W. (1982). Observed-score test equating: A mathematical analysis of some ETS equating procedures. In P.W. Holland & D.B. Rubin (Eds.), *Test equating* (pp. 9–49). New York: Academic.

Cai, L., du Toit, S., & Thissen, D. (2012). *IRTPRO: Flexible professional item response theory modeling for patient reported outcomes* [Computer Program].

Davis, F. B. (1972). Psychometric research on comprehension in reading. *Reading Research Quarterly, 7*(4), 628–678.

Dorans, N.J., & Holland, P.W. (2000). Population invariance and the equatability of tests: Basic theory and the linear case. *Journal of Educational Measurement, 37*(4), 281–306.

Dorans, N.J., Pommerich, M., & Holland, P.W. (Eds.). (2007). *Linking and aligning scores and scales*. New York: Springer-Verlag.

Embretson, S.E., & Wetzel, C.D. (1987). Component latent trait models for paragraph comprehension tests. *Applied Psychological Measurement, 11*(2), 175–193.

Geary, D.C. (2006). Development of mathematical understanding. In W. Damon (Ed.), *Handbook of child psychology* (6th ed., pp. 777–810). New York: John Wiley & Sons.

Gierl, M.J., Tan, X., & Wang, C. (2005). *Identifying content and cognitive dimensions on the SAT* (Research Report No. 2005–11). New York: College Board.

Gower, J.C., & Dijksterhuis, G.B. (2004). *Procrustes problems*. New York: Oxford University Press.

Gulliksen, H. (1950). *Theory of mental tests*. New York: John Wiley and Sons.

Haberman, S.J. (2008). When can subscores have value? *Journal of Educational and Behavioral Statistics, 33*, 204–229.

Haberman, S.J. (2009). *Linking parameter estimates derived from an item response model through separate calibrations* (ETS Research Rep. No. RR-09–39). Princeton, NJ: Educational Testing Services.

Haberman, S.J., & Sinharay, S. (2010). Reporting of subscores using multidimensional item response theory. *Psychometrika, (75)*2, 209–227.

Haebara, T. (1980). Equating logistic ability scales by a weighted least squares method. Japanese *Psychological Research, 22*(3), 144–149.

Hanson, B. A., & Béguin, A. A. (2002). Obtaining a common scale for item response theory item parameters using separate versus concurrent estimation in the common item equating design. *Applied Psychological Measurement, 61*(1), 3–24.

Hegarty, M., & Kozhevnikov, M. (1999). Types of visual-spatial representations and mathematical problem solving. *Journal of Educational Psychology, 91*(4), 684–689.

Horn, J. L. (1965). A rationale and test for the number of factors in factor analysis. *Psychometrika, 30*(2), 179–185.

Hull, C. L. (1922). The conversion of test scores into series which shall have any assigned mean and degree of dispersion. *Journal of Applied Psychology, 6*(4), 298–300.

Kelley, T. L. (1923). *Statistical method.* New York: Macmillan.

Kim, J. (2006). Using the distractor categories of multiple-choice items to improve IRT linking. *Journal of Educational Measurement, 43*(3), 193–213.

Kim, S., & Cohen, A. S. (1998). A comparison of linking and concurrent calibration under item response theory. *Applied Psychological Measurement, 22*(2), 131–143.

Kim, S., & Cohen, A. S. (2002). A comparison of linking and concurrent calibration under the graded response model. *Applied Psychological Measurement, 26*(1), 25–41.

Kim, S., & Lee, W. (2006). An extension of four IRT linking methods for mixed-format tests. *Journal of Educational Measurement, 43*(1), 53–76.

Kolen, M. J. (2004). Linking assessments: Concept and history. *Applied Psychological Measurement, 28*(4), 219–226.

Kolen, M. J., & Brennan, R. L. (2004). *Test equating, scaling, and linking: Methods and practices* (2nd ed.). New York: Springer-Verlag.

Kupermintz, H., Ennis, M. M., Hamilton, L. S., Talbert, J. E., & Snow, R. E. (1995). Enhancing the validity and usefulness of large-scale educational assessments: I. NELS:88 mathematics achievement. *American Educational Research Journal, 32*(3), 525–554.

Kupermintz, H., & Snow, R. E. (1997). Enhancing the validity and usefulness of largescale educational assessments: III. NELS:88 mathematics achievement to 12th grade. *American Educational Research Journal, 34*(1), 124–150.

Levine, R. E. (1955). *Equating the score scales of alternative forms administered to samples of different ability* (Research Bulletin 55–23). Princeton, NJ: Educational Testing Services.

Li, Y. H., & Lissitz, R. W. (2000). An evaluation of the accuracy of multidimensional IRT linking. *Applied Psychological Measurement, 24*(2), 115–138.

Lord, F. M. (1980). *Applications of item response theory to practical testing problems.* Hillsdale, NJ: Lawrence Erlbaum Associates.

Lord, F. M., & Novick, M. R. (1968). *Statistical theories of mental test scores.* Reading, MA: Addison-Wesley.

Loyd, B. H., & Hoover, H. D. (1980). Vertical equating using the Rasch model. *Journal of Educational Measurement, 17*(3), 179–193.

Marco, G. L. (1977). Item characteristic curve solutions to three intractable testing problems. *Journal of Educational Measurement, 14*(2), 139–160.

Martineau, J. A. (2004). *The effects of construct shift on growth and accountability models.* Unpublished doctoral dissertation, Michigan State University, East Lansing, MI.

Meredith, W. (1993). Measurement invariance, factor analysis and factorial invariance. *Psychometrika, 58*(4), 525–543.

Min, K. (2007). Evaluation of linking methods for multidimensional IRT calibrations. *Asia Pacific Education Review, 8*(1), 41–55.

Mulaik, S. A. (1972). *Foundations of factor analysis.* New York: McGraw-Hill.

Muraki, E. (1992). A generalized partial credit model: Application of an EM algorithm. *Applied Psychological Measurement, 16*(2), 159–176.

Oshima, T. C., Davey, T., & Lee, K. (2000). Multidimensional linking: Four practical approaches. *Journal of Educational Measurement, 37*(4), 357–373.

Rasch, G. (1960). *Probabilistic models for some intelligence and attainment tests.* Copenhagen, Denmark: Danish Institute for Educational Research.

Reckase, M.D. (1985). The difficulty of items that measure more than one ability. *Applied Psychological Measurement, 9*(4), 401–412.

Reckase, M.D. (2009). *Multidimensional item response theory*. New York: Springer.

Reckase, M.D., & Martineau, J.A. (2004). *The vertical scaling of science achievement tests* (Research report for the Center for Education and National Research Council).

Reckase, M.D., Martineau, J.A., & Kim, J.-P. (2000). *A vector approach to determining the number of dimensions needed to represent a set of variables*. Paper presented at the annual meeting of the Psychometric Society. Vancouver, Canada.

Schönemann, P.H., & Carroll, R.M. (1970). Fitting one matrix to another under choice of a central dilation and a rigid motion. *Psychometrika, 35*(2), 245–255.

Sinharay, S. (2010). *When can subscores be expected to have added value? Results from operational and simulated data.* (ETS Research Rep. No. RR-10–16). Princeton, NJ: Educational Testing Services.

Skaggs, G., & Lissitz, R.W. (1986). IRT test equating: Relevant issues and a review of recent research. *Review of Educational Research, 56*(4), 495–529.

Stocking, M.L., & Lord, F.M. (1983). Developing a common metric in item response theory. *Applied Psychological Measurement, 7*(2), 201–210.

Stout, W.F. (1987). A nonparametric approach for assessing latent trait unidimensionality. *Psychometrika, 52*(4), 589–617.

Sykes, R.C. (1997). *Guidelines for the selection of anchor items for mixed (or single) item format tests.* Monterey, CA: CTB/McGraw-Hill.

Thurstone, L.L. (1931). Multiple factor analysis. *Psychological Review, 38*(5), 406–427.

Thurstone, L.L. (1935). *The vectors of mind.* Chicago, IL: University of Chicago Press.

Thurstone, L.L. (1947). *Multiple-factor analysis.* Chicago, IL: University of Chicago Press.

Vale, D. C. (1986). Linking item parameters onto a common scale. *Applied Psychological Measurement, 10*(4), 333–344.

von Davier, M., & Sinharay, S. (2007). An importance sampling EM algorithm for latent regression models. *Journal of Educational and Behavioral Statistics, 32*(3), 233–251.

von Davier, M. & von Davier, A.A. (2007). A unified approach to IRT scale linking and scale transformations. *Methodology: European Journal of Research Methods for the Behavioral and Social Sciences, 3*(3), 115–124.

Wainer, H., Vevea, J.L., Camacho, F., Reeve, B.B., Rosa, K., & Nelson, L. (2001). Augmented scores—"borrowing strength" to compute scores based on small numbers of items. In D. Thissen & H. Wainer (Eds.), *Test scoring* (pp. 343–387). Hillsdale, NJ: Lawrence Erlbaum Associates.

Wang, M.M. (1986). *Fitting a unidimensional model to multidimensional item response data: The effects of latent space misspecification on the application of IRT.* Paper presented at the Office of Naval Research Contractors Meeting.

Weeks, J.P. (2010). plink: An R package for linking mixed-format tests using IRT-based methods. *Journal of Statistical Software, 35*(12), 1–33.

Weeks, J.P. (2013). *Linking error in multidimensional vertical scaling.* Paper presented at the annual meeting of the National Council on Measurement in Education: San Francisco, CA.

Weeks, J. P., von Davier, M., & Yamamoto, K. (2014). Design considerations for the programme for international student assessment. In L. Rutkowski, M. von Davier, D. Rutkowski (Eds.), *A handbook of international large-scale assessment: Background, technical issues, and methods of data analysis* (pp. 259–275). Boca Raton, FL: Chapman Hall/CRC Press.

Yao, L. (2010). Multidimensional linking for domain scores and overall scores for nonequivalent groups. *Applied Psychological Measurement, 35*(1), 48–66.

Yao, L., & Boughton, K. (2009). Multidimensional linking for tests with mixed item types. *Journal of Educational Measurement, 46*(2), 177–197.

Yao, L., & Schwarz, R.D. (2006). A multidimensional partial credit model with associated item and test statistics: An application to mixed-format tests. *Applied Psychological Measurement, 30*(6), 469–492.

20 IRT for Growth and Change

John J. McArdle, Kevin T. Petway, and Earl S. Hishinuma

Introduction

The two terms used in the title, "IRT for Growth and Change," seem counterintuitive. After all, who studies growth or change using IRT? Perhaps it would be better to call this "A change analysis with repeated measures." In fact, there are several prior studies that set the stage for this use. And after all, we will do this, and we are going to suggest that you do too.

If, as we assume, you are doing longitudinal research, then you will know that the same construct needs to be measured at all occasions (from McArdle, 2008; McArdle & Nesselroade, 2014). This is primarily so we can look at changes in the individuals measured on this construct. It is not hard to correlate constructs over time; in fact, this is fairly easy. However, it is very hard to say that the construct is the same, but the score has also changed across time (see McArdle & Nesselroade, 1994, 2014). But we need to allow this feature so we can attribute change to the individuals and not the scale of measurement. This, of course, becomes very difficult to do if the same items have not been used at all occasions, although we have found a limited set where it is still possible to test out some ideas (see McArdle, Grimm, Hamagami, Bowles, & Meredith, 2009). Although we have tried other kinds of problems, we will take on a far easier problem here—where depression is measured in the same way over the high school years. The broad question we ask is, "How can we define growth and change?" (and see Lord, 1963; McArdle & Nesselroade, 1994, 2014)

The Longitudinal Item Response Theory (LIRT) Model

First, we need to have the same set of multiple items at each time (t = 1 to T) and we need a model where some aspect of the construct is allowed to change over time. This item score model can be written as Equation (20.1) with the addition of a change model of the common factor scores written here as Equation (20.2). Following this simple logic, the model of "Scalar Invariance" for multiple time point repeated measures data can be written as:

$$ln\{(Prob[\mathrm{i,t}]_n/1{=}Prob[\mathrm{i,t}]_n)\} = \lambda(\mathrm{i})\ F[\mathrm{t}]_n - \delta(\mathrm{i}), \tag{20.1}$$

where the probability of a correct response to every item (i) over time (t) is defined as the distance between the person's ability (λ(i) F[t]) and the item's difficulty (δ(i)). These, of course, are the characteristics we want to estimate. In noncognitive work such as this, the terms "correct and incorrect" should be generalized to words like "less or more" of an attribute and the scale should be expended to include all four choices (see Embretson & Reise, 2000; Reise & Henson, 2003).

To this specific item basis we can then examine changes over time in the common factor scores. For example, we just add a latent curve (Meredith & Tisak, 1990; Muthén & Khoo, 1998) approach. In this approach we write a score model for all the data and test it using a mean and covariance structure. The key difference now is we will apply this statistical model to the factor scores from the IRT. That is, we will write a model where the common factor scores of the items can change over time:

$$F[\mathrm{t}]_{\mathrm{n}} = G\{0\} + \{\Sigma_{(\mathrm{j}=1 \text{ to } \mathrm{t})}\ \Delta[\mathrm{j}]\} + u[\mathrm{t}]_{\mathrm{n}}, \tag{20.2}$$

so here each person has a constant latent score ($G\{0\}$) and an uncorrelated latent score over time (a unique score at each time, $u[\mathrm{t}]$), and where the only latent changes are organized by the accumulation of $\Delta[\mathrm{i,j}]$ for each common latent factor.

The first model of a single factor score over time we examine here is a baseline model with No-Change Scores (NCS) over time. Because the observations are repeated we only estimate one mean (μ_0), one common variance (ϕ^2), and one unique variance (ψ^2; as in McArdle, 2001). While we do not expect this model to fit, the NCS can be accomplished with various types of models of factorial invariance.

The second model for the same data is a *Linear Change Score* (LCS) model where a linear slope is added. This allows concepts of growth or decline, or just changes, and the level of the individual. To do this, we allow the slope to have a mean (μ_1) and variance of growth ($\phi_1{}^2$), and we usually allow a correlation with the initial level score ($\rho_{0,1}$). This growth is defined by a set of basis coefficients that demand an equal ($\omega[\mathrm{t}] = 1$) weighting of all the changes. Of course, equality of the changes is not necessary because changes can be different at different times. This is a latent growth component because the growth is independent of the uniqueness. This is also called constant change because mean slope represents the average amount of change per unit of time. In the present study, the constant change would identify the average increase or decline in depression per grade. We basically test the linear model as a simple hypothesis.

The next type of model is different again. It allows an *Auto-regressive Change Score* (ACS) component that relates a person's score to the amount of change they experience in a direct linear function of where they were at the prior time (by $t - 1$, where t = the time point of interest). In standard continuous time models, the strength of this relationship is assumed to be the same over time, so here the proportional parameter (β) is held equal from one time point to the next. It is sometimes referred to as proportional change because the amount of change a person experiences from one time point to the next is proportional to their score without any residual (e.g., innovation). Depending on the direction and size of this proportional change (β) as well as a person's score at the previous time point, one can have positive or negative change, and more or less change. In prior work we have shown how this model can create exponential growth (see McArdle & Hamagami, 1996, 2001).

In this same work we realized that we did not know the actual shape of changes on an a priori basis, so we explored two additional models here. First we tried a *Dual Change Score* (DCS) model where both additive and proportional influences are allowed to impact the latent accumulation of changes. This is a form of "partial adjustment" (as in McArdle & Hamagami, 1996), and we know that it allows for a combination of linear and exponential changes (in McArdle & Hamagami, 2001).

Next, we can try a *Triple Change Score* (TCS) model where the DCS is used but the basis of the changes ($\omega[\mathrm{t}]$) are allowed to be estimated—this will create an "optimal shape of changes" (i.e., a latent basis from Meredith & Tisak, 1990). We can fit and evaluate the TCS model (as done by McArdle & Nesselroade, 2014), and this can also be done if we simultaneously require that the basic measurement items are invariant over time, as we will do. These last two models are both exploratory forms of SEM that can be used to determine the type and amount of changes we have and the timing of these observations. More will be talked about in later discussions after we get some results for this TCS model.

These are all subsets of a model where we allow any changes to occur, and this can be fitted as a *Free Change Score* (FCS) model without any constraints on the factor scores. This is probably the most exploratory we can be. Clearly, the benefit of having an invariant item measurement structure (see Horn & McArdle, 1992; McArdle & Cattell, 1994) is that it allows a lot of patterns of change in the resulting common factor scores. This is intended to be a very general model of changes over time and, unless we have specific hypotheses, we can use it.

We can estimate these item and factor change parameters with standard *Maximum Likelihood Estimates* (MLE) following the lead of Meredith & Tisak (1990). Because all the models listed earlier are proper subsets of one another, we can examine these models for relative goodness of fit using standard likelihood expressions. Of course, we recognize that there are many more complex models for the factor score change (e.g., Grimm, An, McArdle, Zonderman, & Resnick, 2012; Grimm, McArdle, & Hamagami, 2007).

Prior Studies

The LIRT model is a direct descendant of several others used in the field now. The topic of repeated measures and change has been raised before by Lissitz (2006), and the specific work of Roberts & Ma (2006) is important here. They certainly suggest that a mixture of IRT and growth is an important topic, and they report that Andersen (1985) has presented a model for growth in repeated measures. We did not see this earlier, but we can assume that this model requires factorial invariance at the item level and then allows any kind of changes in the factor scores. This is similar to a model we have seen by Embretson (1991) where all types of changes are allowed in the factor scores. This work is summarized by McArdle and colleagues (2009), who assumed that a form of factorial invariance existed among, say, vocabulary items, even though not everything was measured at each time. Several models of age changes were considered afterward (in a second step).

Of course, the structural growth model presented by Muthén and Khoo (1998) where the items are fitted within a latent curve (Meredith & Tisak, 1990) structure is similar to what we are proposing. The main difference here is we will use an alternative representation of change in the factor scores—rather than fit model of latent curves, we will fit models of latent changes directly (as in Ferrer & McArdle, 2010; McArdle, 2001, 2008). The further work of Kaplan and Sweetman (2006) is of great interest here too. But we focus on the alternative definitions of the change model here. There is no doubt that this concept of "IRT and Growth" has been in use for a long time and we are simply adding some change model possibilities here.

Application

What we will do here is reexamine some longitudinal data on high school students' measure in 9th, 10th, 11th, and 12th grade levels on the *Center for Epidemiological Studies—Depression* Scale (CESD: from Radloff, 1977). Following the modeling work of McArdle, Johnson, Hishinuma, Miyamoto, & Andrade (2001), we will use only the 13 items of that scale that we had found to be a good measure of the negative affect component of depression. The data we will use is only a subset of the data collected as part of the *Hawaiian High School Health Survey* (HHSHS; see Andrade et al., 2006; Hishinuma,

Chang, McArdle, & Hamagami, 2012), and we will try to make this far easier to deal with than other models of IRT for Growth and Change.

RESEARCH METHODS

Participants

Data on N = 7,317 adolescents were collected over a five-year period from 1992 to 1996 in Hawai'i as part of the longitudinal survey study. The study organizers (the first author included) intentionally oversampled Native Hawaiian adolescents (see Andrade et al., 2006; Edman et al., 1999; Hishinuma, Andrade, Johnson, & McArdle, 2000; Johnson, Danko, Andrade, & Markoff, 1997; Prescott et al., 1998), and the data in general represent a sizeable sample of high school students in Hawai'i. For this study, sex and Native Hawaiian ancestry were of particular interest. There were 3,551 boys and 3,749 girls, and 4,848 students (67%) were of Native Hawaiian ancestry. A large sample size was necessary for greater precision with parameter estimates. Table 20.1 is a breakdown of the sample by year, sex, ethnicity, and grade level for a student's *first* assessment. Table 20.2 is a summary of the overall participation by describing how many students completed the CES-D one to four times.

The data used here were obtained as part of the National Center on Indigenous Hawaiian Behavioral Health (NCIHBH; formerly the *Native Hawaiian Mental Health Research Development Program*). Prior to the administration date of the *Hawaiian High Schools Health Survey* (HHSHS) (available upon request), students' parents were provided with written information regarding the study and the opportunity to decline participation (via postcard). Students who participated provided their active assent. This passive consent procedure on the part of parents was approved at the time of the study by the Institutional Review Board of the University of Hawai'i at Mānoa. Students were informed that their responses would be strictly confidential and that only group or aggregated data would be subsequently reported. Homeroom teachers (who had received training in the survey protocol a few weeks prior) assisted in reading aloud the consent information and survey instructions and handed out and collected the survey instruments upon completion. The majority of students required 30 to 45 minutes to complete the entire survey.

The design of our research was to oversample adolescents of Native Hawaiian ancestry, usually underrepresented in research in Hawai'i, and undersample members of other groups. Our participants were obtained from five different high schools on three of the islands of the archipelago, with the majority of the schools deliberately chosen to have high proportions of adolescents of Native Hawaiian ancestry. The schools included participants from rural and urban areas and permitted a reasonably representative sample of the Native Hawaiian adolescent population.

The non-Hawaiian comparison group was less representative, at least in terms of demographics. For example, persons of European-American and Japanese-American ancestry make up approximately 50 percent of the population of Hawai'i, yet they intentionally made up approximately 10 percent of the present sample. Although non-Hawaiians are often the majority groups in high schools in Hawaii, these students were very much in the minority in the schools assessed. In addition, the majority of the students of Native Hawaiian ancestry are also of other ancestral groups. In Hawai'i, those who have any Native Hawaiian ancestry are typically classified as Native Hawaiian. The non-Hawaiian participants most frequently were persons of European-American, Filipino-American, Japanese-American, and mixed non-Hawaiian ancestry. Most of our school-related data entailed too small a number of respondents for separate analyses of

Table 20.1 Sample Size by Year, Grade, Ethnicity, and Sex for Students' *First* Testing Session Only

		Boys		*Girls*	
		Hawaiian	*Non-Hawaiian*	*Hawaiian*	*Non-Hawaiian*
1992	**9th Grade**	241	27	241	23
	10th Grade	205	23	234	20
	11th Grade	168	27	228	20
	12th Grade	192	17	273	31
1993	**9th Grade**	368	202	418	220
	10th Grade	203	171	180	188
	11th Grade	153	191	172	181
	12th Grade	109	118	140	134
1994	**9th Grade**	365	193	408	197
	10th Grade	113	68	84	59
	11th Grade	76	52	61	41
	12th Grade	57	43	45	30
1995	**9th Grade**	0	0	0	0
	10th Grade	0	0	0	0
	11th Grade	17	20	19	20
	12th Grade	29	23	29	20
1996	**9th Grade**	0	0	0	0
	10th Grade	0	0	0	0
	11th Grade	0	0	0	0
	12th Grade	11	17	6	9
Total		2,307	1,192	2,538	1,193

Table 20.2 Sample Size by Number of Times Assessed, Sex, and Ethnicity

# Times	*Boys*		*Girls*		*Total*[a]
	Hawaiian	*Non-Hawaiian*	*Hawaiian*	*Non-Hawaiian*	
1 Year	1,327	663	1,349	648	4,054
2 Years	593	301	711	327	3,876
3 Years	290	167	338	152	2,841
4 Years	97	61	140	66	1,456

Notes: [a]Total = sum of sample sizes in row * # of times assessed. For example, 1,938 students were assessed two times, so the value in the "Total" column is 1,938 * 2 = 3,876. There were 12,227 total data points.

the different non-Hawaiian groups. Participants were assessed across successive years in a cross-sequential longitudinal design, with a new cohort of 9th graders introduced for the first three years as the 12th-grade cohort graduated. These individuals were assessed through the administration of the survey.

Measures

Depressive symptoms were assessed using the 20-item *Center for Epidemiological Studies-Depression* (CES-D) inventory (Radloff, 1977). "The CES-D scale is a short self-report scale designed to measure depressive symptomatology in the general population. The items of the scale are symptoms associated with depression which have been used in previously validated longer scales. The new scale was tested in household interview surveys and in psychiatric settings. It was found to have very high internal consistency and adequate test-retest repeatability. Validity was established by patterns of correlations with other self-report measures, by correlations with clinical ratings of depression, and by relationships with other variables which support its construct validity. Reliability, validity, and factor structure were similar across a wide variety of demographic characteristics in the general population samples tested. The scale should be a useful tool for epidemiologic studies of depression" (from Radloff, 1977, p. 385). Participants responded on a four-point scale to indicate how many days in a week the particular item applied to them. For all 20 items the standard response categories are: (1) "Rarely or none of the time (0–1 days)," (2) "Some or a little of the time (1–2 days)," (3) "A moderate amount of time (3–4 days)," and (4) "Most or all of the time (5–7 days)." For more details on the CES-D, see the substantive studies of Zimmerman and Coryell (1994), or the technical studies of Santor and Coyne (1997).

The unidimensionality of the four responses in the 20-item version has been extensively studied in the past (see Beals, Manson, Keane, & Dick, 1991; Bryant, 1999), and the literature has generally supported a multidimensional structure to the CES-D. It is common to see a four-common-factor model of the CES-D items, as initially resolved by Radloff (1977; also see Beals et al., 1991), and this includes the basic concepts of a "negative affect" factor, a "positive affect" factor, an "interpersonal" factor, plus a "somatic" factor. This study focuses on a 13-item subscale identified by Prescott and colleagues (1998) and subsequently checked by McArdle and colleagues (2001) and utilized by Hishinuma and colleagues (2012). Both Prescott and colleagues (1998) and McArdle and colleagues (2001) seem to believe these 13 negatively worded items captured the *negative affect* component of depression, arguably the most critical part of the construct. We ask the reader to refer to Table 20.3 for a list of the retained CES-D items to be restudied here.

The majority of this HHSHS sample (55.5%) completed the CES-D only once and this could be important for further analyses. But the remaining students (44.5%) took the measure two (26.5%), three (13.0%), or all four (5.0%) times, and we were able to link up their records in a longitudinal fashion. To retain the large sample size we will examine the models for everyone here, but we will retain when (at what grade level) they took the CES-D scale. That is, about 40.7 percent of the sample completed their first round of the CES-D in 9th grade, while about 17.8 percent had their first (and only) assessment in 12th grade. Not surprisingly, starting in the earlier years of the study meant a student was more likely to complete the CES-D multiple times. In order to complete all testings, the majority of 10th–12th graders had their first testing in either 1992 or 1993, while the majority of 9th graders began this testing in either 1993 or 1994.

Models

The Formal Basis of the Item Response Theory (IRT) Model

The basic item score model we will use is commonly attributed to Rasch (1960), but could alternatively be attributed to Lord (1953), or to Lord and Novick (1968). Recent

Table 20.3 Selected and Analyzed CES-D Items ("Negative Affect")

CES-D Original Item #	*Item used with the standard response categories are: (1) "Rarely or none of the time (0–1 days)," (2) "Some or a little of the time (1–2 days)," (3) "A moderate amount of time (3–4 days)," and (4) "Most or all of the time (5–7 days)."*
1	Felt bothered
2	Poor appetite
3	Felt blue
5	Trouble concentrating
6	Felt depressed
9	Life a failure
10	Felt fearful
11	Sleep restless
13	Talked less
14	Felt lonely
17	Crying spells
18	Felt sad
20	Lethargic

description and definitions of IRT can be found in Hambleton, Swaminathan, & Rogers (1991), McDonald (1999), Embretson and Reise (2000), or Bond and Fox (2001). Practical examples can be found in Reise and Henson (2003), Fraley, Waller, and Brennan (2000), and McArdle and colleagues (2007).

This starts with a model for the item-level scores measured at one time (and scored as incorrect = 0 or correct = 1) that can be written as:

$$ln\{(Prob(\mathrm{i})_n/1{=}Prob(\mathrm{i})_n)\} = \lambda(\mathrm{i})\ F_n - \delta(\mathrm{i}), \tag{20.3}$$

where we try to take care of the binary nature of the item scored (as incorrect = 0 or correct = 1), *ln* is the natural logarithm, the *Prob*(i) = the probability of a correct response by any person *n* (= 1 to *N*), the λ(i) is the factor loading or weight for all persons on that construct, the F_n is the person's individual score on the construct, and the δ(i) is the difficulty level of the item. This is often termed the "2PL model" because it requires two parameters for each item, the factor loading or weight (λ(i)]) and the difficulty level (δ(i)). To uniquely identify the common factor score we need to add a few constraints. First, we assume the mean of the factor at time 1 is nonexistent (ν[1] = 0). To identify (scale) the unobserved component we need to fix one of the loadings (λ(i) = 1, yes any one, or even the factor variance) to get a unique estimate of the factor variance (ϕ^2) and the rest of the loadings (λ(i)).

If we further assume all items are related to the factor in the same way (a practical assumption), we often fix all the loadings to be equal (as λ(i) = 1) and just estimate the factor variance (ϕ^2). This is a "1PL model" and it is usually written in exponential form to avoid the logarithm (see Rasch, 1960). The 1PL versus the 2PL model can be directly compared for fit in existing data sets, because the 1PL is simpler. In this un-exponetiated format of Equation (20.3) the 1PL model is intentionally simple—it basically means the probability of a correct response by a person is dependent only on their true score (F_n) on the construct (because all loadings are set to a value of $\lambda(i) = 1$) minus the difficulty level of the item ($\delta(i)$). This means (a) if the person has a much higher score than this item's difficulty level it turns out to be an easy item, (b) if this difference is close the item has a smaller probability of being answered correctly, but (c) if their true score is much lower than the difficulty level there is only a small chance they will get it right. As suggested earlier, in noncognitive work such as this, the terms "correct and incorrect" should be generalized to words like "less or more" of an attribute and multiple points on the scale should include all four choices (see Embretson & Reise, 2000; Reise & Henson, 2003).

What we want to do is estimate the true score for each person (F_n) and the difficulty level of the items ($\delta(i)$) at that time from a limited set of responses (0 or 1, or here 0, 1, 2, and 3) by the person to specific items and then see if this estimation fits the data at hand. We do make a lot of simplifying assumptions to carry this out. But when there are multiple items for the scale the idea of a singular construct can be tested. To examine this as a testable hypothesis we assume that all pairs of correlations among variables can be recreated by a single factor with equal loadings (see McDonald, 1999). This may not be true because people may use more than one resource to answer any particular question. In this case we assume there would be more than one factor present. In any case if we do assume that we have only one unobserved function, once the logarithms have been taken care of, we can show the same expectation for all items:

$$\sigma(i,j) = \lambda(i)\ \phi^2\ \lambda(j), \tag{20.4}$$

where the ϕ^2 is the expected variance of the common factor. This can be obtained as an estimate by assuming that all factor loadings are $\lambda(i) = 1$. In this way we can say the reason the model fails is that this expectation about the reason we can have these correlations is too simple (see McArdle, 2012). In any case, this model is considered testable because it can fail to fit the data at hand.

In an unrestricted case we estimate the difficulty levels using the means for all items as the sum of the thresholds. Here we introduce the inverse probability or probit function = $Prob^{-1}$ (the logistic function and the probit function can be translated by a constant 1.7; see McDonald, 1999), and $\tau(k)$ are item *thresholds* (see Muthén & Muthén, 2012). In the normal theory metric the thresholds are simply z-scores indicating how difficult it is for the group to shift from one response to the next. If there are only two valid responses (0 or 1), there is only one threshold, typically between –3 and +3, and the item difficulty is the proportion of ones (or the mean of the ones and zeros). The item threshold in this, or any other kind of model, indicates the expected point on the latent variable's scale at which an individual would be more likely to select the higher of two response options. In factor models with categorical indicators, there are $k - 1$ ordered thresholds, where k is the number of response categories associated with a particular item. The scale used here (CES-D) is a four-point Likert-type ordered scale, so all items have three thresholds representing the following shifts defined by thresholds: (1) category 0 to category 1, (2) category 1 to category 2, and (3) category 2 to category 3. When free to vary over time, the expected value of the latent variable needed to endorse a higher category is allowed to differ from one time point to the next.

The Formal Basis of a Longitudinal IRT (LIRT) Model

When we have multiple items at each time (t = 1 to T), we need a model where some aspect of the construct is allowed to change over time. This score model can be written as Equation (20.1) with the addition of a configuration of a trait where we have one trait ($F[t]_n$) at each time point that it is not related in exactly the same way. In such a case we might have a model of "Configural Invariance" written as:

$$ln\{(Prob[i,t]_n/1 = Prob[i,t]_n)\} = \lambda[i,t]\ F_n - \delta[i,t], \tag{20.5}$$

where many items have been measured over time (t = 1 to T). One way to understand this is to think of a construct as having a number of possible synonyms. They are very similar to the construct of interest, but may have subtle differences that make them context or time-specific (so they have different $\lambda[i,t]$ and $\delta[i,t]$). The items indicating a latent variable ($F[t]_n$) can exhibit different factor loadings ($\lambda[i,t]$), and these loadings can also differ over time such that a particular item can be more or less related to the construct of interest as time changes. As the strength of the relationship changes, so does the meaning of the latent variable that is being tested. Depending on the nature of these changes, certain items can become more (or less) important to the construct's definition, which affects interpretation of the results. Invariance at this stage would suggest the item-construct relationships do not change notably from one time point to the next, minimizing shifts in the definition of the construct.

Of course, the same construct may be present at each time. By a restriction that the factor loadings remain the same at each time point (so $\lambda[i,t] = \lambda[i]$), we have a model with "Metric Invariance" or invariance of the loadings as:

$$ln\{(Prob[i,t]_n/1 = Prob[i,t]_n)\} = \lambda[i]\ F[t]_n - \delta[i,t]. \tag{20.6}$$

Following this simple logic, the model of "Scalar Invariance" for multiple time point repeated measures data can be written as:

$$ln\{(Prob[i,t]_n/1 = Prob[i,t]_n)\} = \lambda(i)\ F[t]_n - \delta(i). \tag{20.7}$$

The way this is fit, every difficulty level ($\delta(i)$) is first transformed into an set of estimated item thresholds ($\tau(\kappa)$; see Muthén (1988) for convenience). Significant differences in the thresholds could indicate time-related "differential item functioning" (see McArdle, 1998). For example, an item threshold that changes from one time point to the next would suggest a different expected score is needed to select the higher response category, despite a constant construct score. A person could select a different response over time but end up with the same score at any time.

The assumption of the equality of the thresholds ($\tau[k,t] = \tau(k)$) or difficulty levels ($\delta[i,t] = \delta(i)$) over time) thus assuming the unique mean and variance are the same over time, and these are restrictions that could be imposed sooner. Of course, these could reflect another set of assumptions that may not be correct. The current software (e.g., Mplus and others) makes this an easy hypothesis to test, and it could be important. If in fact the items all can be said to have this property we would call this "Scalar Invariance." With continuous measurements we would call this "Strong Invariance"(from Meredith, 1993) but here the unique mean and its variance provide the same information.

To this invariant measurement basis we can then examine changes over time in the common factor scores. For example, we add a latent curve (Meredith & Tisak, 1990) approach, as done by Muthén and Khoo (1998). That is, the key difference now is we will apply all change models to the common factor scores from the IRT (as in McArdle et al., 2009). In the approach used here, we will write a latent change score model and test it using a mean and covariance structure. That is, we will write a model where the common factor scores for the items can change over time:

$$F[t]_n = G\{0\} + \{\Sigma_{(j=1 \text{ to } t)} \Delta[j]\} + u[t]_n, \tag{20.8}$$

so here each person has a constant score ($G\{0\}$) and an uncorrelated score over time (a unique score at each time, $u[t]$), and where the only changes are latent, and are organized by the accumulation of $\Delta[i,j]$ for each common factor (from McArdle, 2001, 2008, 2011; Ferrer & McArdle, 2010; as repeated from Equation (20.2)). This is the model for latent changes we will use because it is direct in the expected structure latent changes, and it takes into account the uncorrelated residuals ($u[t]$) that can easily confound ordinary observed changes (see Lord, 1963; McArdle & Nesselroade, 2014).

If we assume a rigid form of invariance exists (such as Scalar Invariance), then we can fit a few additional change models. We can think of this as a choice between: (*M0*) if $\Delta[j] = 0$, then we have a *no change score* (NCS) model; (*M1*) if $\Delta[j] = G\{1\}$, a single latent slope, then we have a *linear change score* (LCS) model; (*M2*) if $\Delta[j] = \beta\, F[t-1]$, so the future score is predictable from the immediate past score, then we have an *auto-regressive change score* (ACS) model of the first order; (*M3*) if $\Delta[j] = \beta\, F[t-1] + G\{1\}$, where both kind of changes are used, then we have a *dual change score* (DCS) model; and (*M4*) if $\Delta[j] = \beta\, F[t-1] + \Omega[t]\, G\{1\}$, where a DCS model is used but we estimate weights ($\Omega[t]$) to examine the contribution of the latent slopes to the latent changes, then we have a *triple change score* (TCS) model. In model fitting we can compare the fit and estimation of theoretical alternatives about both measurement invariance and changes in the latent scores (as in McArdle, 1997, 2011).

A Note on Model Misfit

When we have continuous scales of measurement, we could use *maximum likelihood estimation* (MLE) and the change models listed earlier are typically nested within one another so final likelihoods can be compared in the usual way (see McArdle, 1997, 2011). That is, all models are alternatives to the NCS, because they all include an intercept mean (μ_0) and variance (ϕ_0^2) and a common factor uniqueness (ψ^2), so they can be compared using standard likelihood ratio tests (as in Meredith & Tisak, 1990). Similarly, the LCS and ACS are nested versions of the DCS because this contains both kinds of parameters, and these models can be compared on a statistical basis to the DCS. A point has been made in prior work (McArdle, 2001, 2008) that the LCS and the ACS should not be compared to one another because they do not have the same parameters. But nesting is true of the DCS model, and the additional weights added in the TCS model compared to the DCS representations. And all structural models are restrictions on a generic FCS model that allows any means, variance, and correlations over time.

When a *weighted least squares mean and variance* (WLSMV) estimator is used the situation is slightly different (following Muthén & Muthén, 2012). When we make a comparison between nested models, the "observed" difference between the chi-square values is not correct and it needs to be rescaled. In computer programs like Mplus, the necessary adjustments are output, and the DIFFTEST argument can be used to make appropriate statistical comparisons between two nested models.

Multiple Group Models

When using any *structural equation model* (SEM) we can introduce differences in the mean levels of other variables by simply adding these variables to the model. If the regression parameters are zero we do not have any group mean differences. When using a *multiple group model*

(MGM) we can test hypotheses about differences in the same way, but here we first (a) split the groups up into independent data sources (usually independent categories), (b) force the parameters of the means of key variables to be equal (or invariant) to examine their equality over groups, and (c) we can add tests of the equality of variances as well. If we want we can test (d) whether regressions coefficients are equal over group, and this can be done in MGM with latent variables in an interaction model (as in McArdle & Prescott, 1992). We can use any number of groups desired as long as each individual goes in only one group.

Data Analyses

The negative affect subscale of the CES-D has not been evaluated very much in the literature. Prescott and colleagues (1998) found the dimension using an exploratory factor analysis but never tested the structure using a more hypothesis-driven approach like confirmatory factor analysis. McArdle and colleagues (2001) found this same combination using such an approach, a latent path model, and suggested that we use only 15 or 13 of the items (see pp. 122–126) instead of all 20 items. As a result, our first step was to investigate the stability of the structure of these 13 items across grade levels. For all models fitted here, the students' grade level is necessarily considered a proxy for both their varying age-at-measurement and their time-of-measurement.

The computer program Mplus (version 7.11) will be used for all analyses, but we know several other computer programs would give us the same estimates (e.g., see the Computer Appendix; Muthén & Muthén, 2012; cf., Rosseel, 2012). In general, we assumed all variables to be fitted were categorical indicators and used the WLSMV adjusted estimator with what the program authors (e.g., Muthén & Muthén, 2012) term a "delta" parameterization (see Prescott, 2004). We can say that, although WLSMV tends to be less efficient than MLE, particularly when there is incomplete data, it is much faster for models with multiple latent variables that are indicated by ordered categorical items (as we have here). Differences in model fit were determined using *scaled chi-square difference testing* (e.g., DIFFTEST). For the composite score models (see Table 20.8), we used what is termed a *robust maximum likelihood* (MLR) estimator because all modeled variables were considered continuous and ordered, but certainly skewed.

Grade-Level Invariance of CES-D-13

A student could have up to four time points if they participated every year from grades 9 through 12, though as previously noted, most students had only one time point. This meant our test of grade invariance was both longitudinal (for those 44.5% with more than one time point) and cross-sectional (55.5%). To overcome these issues we are estimating the model parameters in the typical way—by assuming "Missing at Random" assumptions (see Hishinuma et al., 2012; Little & Rubin, 1987).

Four models of invariance were evaluated allowing all types of changes in the factor scores (FCS). The first substantive model allowed both factor loadings and item thresholds to be free across grade levels (as in Equation (20.3))—a "Configural Invariance" model (after Meredith, 1993; and see Horn & McArdle, 1992). This approach was the most relaxed of the four substantive models tested because it only required a one common factor pattern at each of the four grades. The four models had the same hypothesized one-factor structure (13 items indicating one presumed dimension of negative affect), but the relationship between the construct and the items (i.e., the factor loadings) was not required to be equal over time. Similarly, the thresholds were not held equal, so we did not assume that the expected latent score needed to endorse a particular response was consistent from one grade level to the next. Neither of these constraints is required in real data, but these prove useful in interpretation. All latent means ($\nu[t] = 0$) were fixed to zero both for identification and because we cannot reliably make mean comparisons otherwise (because we may not be working with exactly the same construct). Good fit to the Configural Invariance model would indicate the construct's singular definition was consistent from one grade to the next, but it was not necessarily the same construct. That is, the selected CES-D items identify a construct we assumed was negative affect in all grades, but the optimal solution may be weighted differently.

The second model, often called the "Metric Invariance" model (from Meredith, 1993; see Horn & McArdle, 1992), tests the stability of the factor loadings by constraining them to be equal over time. This is much like saying the construct is the same at all occasions because we would measure it using the same weighted scores. That is, if the individual reaches a specific threshold we would say that behavior has the same psychological meaning at one time or another. Good fit to this Metric Invariance model extends the interpretation of the Configural Invariance model by narrowing the construct's definition (as stated earlier; see Equation (20.6)). This model allows for some changes in the factor means and variances too.

The third model fitted here was designed to evaluate the invariance of item thresholds (i.e., Scalar or Strict Invariance). Because of its categorical scaling, the unique variable has a mean ($\iota(i)$) that is not separated from its own unique variance ($\psi(i)^2$). This is typically the loss of information in binary or other categorical items, but not continuous items, and we lose a test of the independence of the mean and variance (e.g., perhaps the simplest case is a dichotomous item where the mean is a proportion correct, and the square of this is its variance). But this overall model allows a more complete invariance of the measurement model over all items and allows all changes, even in the latent means over time or over groups, to be done at the common factor level. In this model, the means of the latent variables ($\nu[t]$) were not constrained to zero (with the exception of the first group, or reference group, for identification).

Last, the fourth model fitted here was based on the one-parameter logistic model commonly used in IRT by constraining factor loadings to be equal within a grade level. This was the most restrictive model because it required every item to exhibit equal relationships with latent construct both across and within grade levels, and this is pretty hard to expect from existing scale data.

Change Score Models

Change in depression over time was the key question we were trying to answer, and it can be evaluated using several different change score models (Hishinuma et al., 2012; McArdle, 2001; McArdle & Hamagami, 2001). The basic idea here is primarily to show that we can use this approach to address multiple types of change. We examined a series of models: (1) a No Change Score (NCS) model; (2) a Linear Change Score (LCS) model; (3) an Auto-regressive Change Score (ACS) model; (4) a Dual Change Score (DCS) model; (5) a Triple Change Score (TCS) model; and, implicitly, (6) a Free Change Score (FCS) model (because it was fitted in the Strict Invariance models first). The DCS model can be used to represent most of the others, so it is depicted in the path diagram of Figure 20.1.

The NCS model builds off of the earlier grade-level Scalar Invariance model by specifying no latent changes to capture the differences between time points. That is, the model does not suggest there is a constant or proportional change component at play—changes occur from one time point to the next but are considered unrelated to each other and to previous time points.

The LCS, in contrast to the NCS, assumes there is a constant change at each time point by adding a slope mean and variance parameter on the change scores. This is exactly

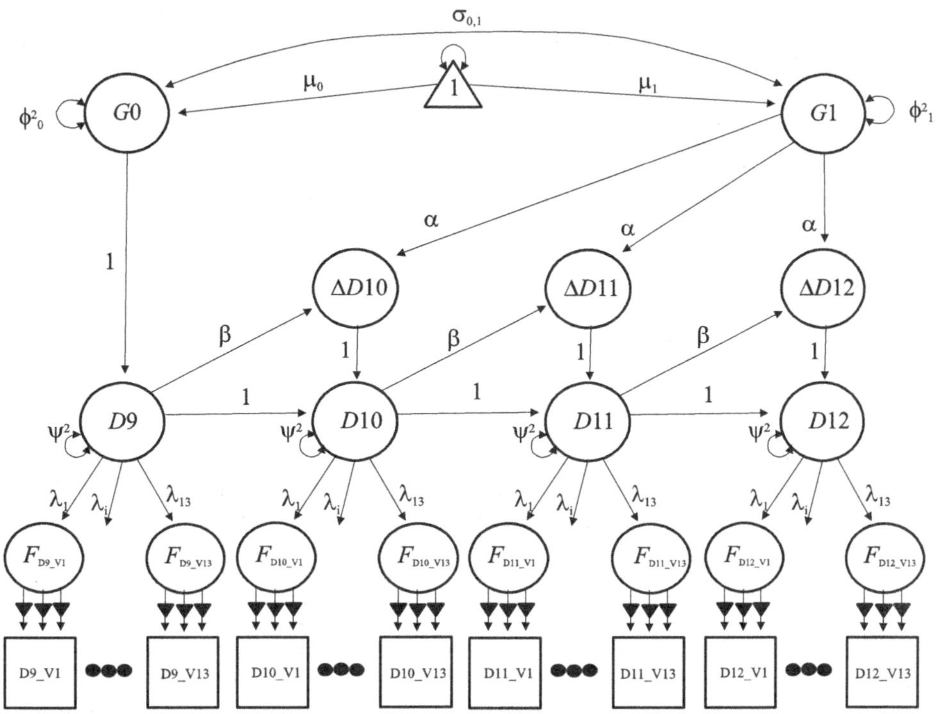

Figure 20.1 A Dual Change Model for the CES-D.

Notes: Only 13 items are used here and these are assume to be the result of one factor (D) held invariant over all four grades, Each of these items has three thresholds (denoted by the resister symbols) also held and these are also held invariant over all four grades.

what we would obtain with any linear change model (see Bryk & Raudenbush, 1987; Meredith & Tisak, 1990) but here it was fit as a sequential changes model (as in McArdle, 2001, 2008). The slope mean (μ_1), which describes the average amount of change observed from t – 1 to t, is freely estimated in this model. The slope variance ($\phi_1{}^2$) allows individual differences in changes, and this is estimated together with a covariance of level and slopes ($\phi_{0,1}$) so it does not matter how the basis is defined (i.e., where the starting point is assumed; but see Grimm et al., 2012).

The next ACS model focuses on proportional change, and allows the proportional (β) parameters to be estimated as predictors of the changes while constraining the slope mean and covariance to be nonexistent (0). For this reason, the ACS model is not nested with the LCS framework. In fact, this simple model is difficult to merge within the latent curve basis.

The DCS model combines the LCS and ACS models and this summation of additive and proportional impacts on the changes could be a better-fitting combination. For this reason both the LCS and the ACS are nested within this DCS model. This kind of model is depicted in Figure 20.1, and it allows changes of all kinds in the common factor scores even though the common factors are defined as being the same (i.e., invariant) over time. The question that can be asked is does the combination of both slopes and predictions from a prior time point outperform (in terms of fit to the data) the individual components.

Finally, the TCS model incorporates a relatively straightforward addition to the DCS. The weight for the first time point is set to $\omega[9] = 0$ while the weight for the change score from Time 1 (grade 9) to Time 2 (grade 10) is set at ω[10] = 1 (as in the LCS). The weights for the changes from Time 2 to Time 3 (at grade 11; ω[11]) and Time 3 to Time 4 (at grade 12; ω[12]) are freely estimated (at the values determined by ω[11] and ω[12]), so we can approximate a latent basis for the curve. If these weights are estimated from the data at unity then the optimal curve is linear. If not it can help tell us when (at what timing) it would be linear. So these weights could be estimated at any value based on the nature of the data. This allows for several grade-level based (or time-based) growth interpretations.

Sex and Ethnicity Models

As previously mentioned, sex and Native Hawaiian ancestry were the two demographic characteristics of most interest. Unfortunately, little has been done to understand how the intersection of sex and ethnicity relates to changes in depression for this population. We combined sex and Native Hawaiian ancestry to form a single grouping variable with four categories: (1) Native Hawaiian Males (HM), (2) Non-Native Hawaiian Males (NHM), (3) Native Hawaiian Females (HF), and (4) Non-Native Hawaiian Females (NHF). This new grouping variable was then included in the most constrained versions of the earlier DCS models to produce multiple-group DCS models. Group differences in the parameters of additive changes (μ_1), and proportional changes (β), as well as the unique variance (ψ^2), are of key interest now, and we set it up so the invariance of all these parameters can be examined.

For this set of comparisons, we examined both a model where CES-D scores were modeled as latent variables with categorical indicators (consistent with the other analyses discussed within) and a model where CES-D scores were represented as continuous composite scores. One allure in using composite scores is their simplicity and straightforwardness. They generally make complex models easier to handle by minimizing the number of parameters to manipulate, and for models with many dimensions, this is much more compatible with efficient MLE than models with categorical indicators. However, the composite scores themselves may not be as reliable or accurate as those implied by factor models. This is particularly true when there is a lot of noise or the items are not equally indicative of the construct. We evaluated both sets of multiple group DCS models to highlight differences between using latent variables and using composite scores to represent the subscale.

Results

Grade-Level Invariance Models

Table 20.4 presents the results of the measurement invariance analyses, including some of the parameters estimated using one group and then four groups (MGM). In order, we fit a Configural Invariance model (L^2 = 3899 with *df* = 1309) and a Metric Invariance model (L^2 = 3670 with *df* = 1345). Using the scaled χ^2 (e.g., the DIFFTEST) we found the measurement models to be close in fit (χ^2 = 65 on *df* = 36), so the concept of having one factor of depression that is invariant over time seems to fit these data well. This is not so surprising because we fit only the 13 previously selected items at each occasion.

The difference testing suggested the more constrained model, where all the thresholds were held constant too, particularly the Scalar Invariance model, did not fit the data as well as the more relaxed models (L^2 = 3899 with *df* = 1418). However, the other fit indices provided strong support for all models of invariance, and did not identify a model with notably different fit (ε_a = 0.015, TLI = 0.976). In fact, these indices leaned more in favor of the simpler, more constrained models (see Browne & Cudeck, 1993; Tanaka, 1993). Factor loadings and thresholds from the Scalar Invariance model are provided in Table 20.5.

Table 20.4 Model Fit and Means From Grade-Level Invariance Models

Parameter[a]	*Configural*	*Metric*	*Scalar*	*1PL*
N[9]	= 0	= 0	= 0	= 0
N[10]	= 0	= 0	−0.032 (−1.825)	−0.034 (−2.039)
N[11]	= 0	= 0	−0.035 (−1.962)	−0.038 (−2.165)
N[12]	= 0	= 0	−0.064 (−3.667)	−0.066 (−3.911)
Model Fit				
$L^2(df)$	3889(1309)	3678(1345)	3899(1418)	11721(1429)
Scaled χ^2 Diff. (df/p)	N/A	64.7(36 / .002)	275(73 / <.001)	2431(11 / <.001)
CFI / TLI	.974 / .973	.976 / .977	.975 / .976	.895 / .903
ε_α (90% CI)	.017 (.016–.017)	.016 (.015–.016)	.015 (.015–.016)	.032 (.032–.033)

Notes: [a]For fixed (mean) parameters, values in parentheses are the associated z-statistics; ε_α = root-mean-square error of approximation (RMSEA).

Table 20.5 Factor Loadings and Item Threshold Estimates From Scalar Invariance Model

Item	*Loading*	*Threshold*$_{0-1}$	*Threshold*$_{1-2}$	*Threshold*$_{2-3}$
Felt bothered	= 1	0.116	0.997	1.622
Poor appetite	0.891	0.243	1.052	1.750
Felt blue	1.298	0.280	0.920	1.512
Trouble concentrating	1.018	−0.512	0.369	1.116
Felt depressed	1.374	−0.029	0.718	1.298
Life a failure	1.224	0.620	1.224	1.742
Felt fearful	1.115	0.478	1.244	1.834
Sleep restless	0.981	0.045	0.748	1.365
Talked less	0.858	0.006	0.905	1.599
Felt lonely	1.259	0.195	0.858	1.397
Crying spells	1.256	0.687	1.212	1.698
Felt sad	1.381	0.074	0.886	1.463
Lethargic	1.140	0.146	0.923	1.545

Notes: Values are unstandardized coefficients from a model with factor variances fixed at one; scalar model constrained factor loadings and thresholds to be equal across time points, so these values represent all grades.

In a final model we tested whether these factor loadings were all equal. This model has only one parameter per item (the difficulty level $\delta(i)$), and was fitted as a probit (or logistic) model under the assumption that we constrained all loadings to be equal both across and within grade levels. This exceedingly simple 1PL model was found to be a significant departure (L^2 = 11721 with df = 1429) from all prior models, including the Scalar Invariance model, and the alternative indices of fit were not nearly as supportive of these stringent constraints.

Use of the Scalar Invariance model allowed us to evaluate both mean and variance differences in the factor of depression by grade levels (also their correlations over time).

Because we are talking about the same factor here, the means of this common factor seem to go down over time ($\nu[9] = 0$, $\nu[10] = -0.032$, $\nu[11] = -0.035$; $\nu[12] = -0.064$). That is, using grade level 9 as a reference, we find that there were lower depression scores on the same factor in later grades (especially 11th and 12th grade levels).

Because these are all essentially the fit of any changes at all (the FCS model), the latent variable variances estimated over the four grade levels can be different ($\sigma[9]^2 = 0.383$; $\sigma[10]^2 = 0.398$; $\sigma[11]^2 = 0.385$; and $\sigma[12]^2 = 0.386$). In addition, the latent variable correlations over the four grades are allowed (e.g., $\rho[9,10] = 0.605$; $\rho[9,11] = 0.505$; $\rho[9,12] = 0.541$; $\rho[10,11] = 0.584$; $\rho[10,12] = 0.545$; $\rho[11, 12] = 0.639$). Of course, in this part we are mainly concerned with the differences in the invariance of the measurement models.

Change Score Models

In Table 20.6 we present five alternative restrictive change models. The NCS is very poor fit ($L^2 = 9877$ with $df = 1429$), but it can be useful as a baseline model. In comparison,

Table 20.6 Model Fit and Parameter Estimates for Scalar Invariance Measurement With Alternative Latent Change Score Models of the Common Factor Scores

Parameter[a]	*NCS*[b]	*LCS*	*ACS*	*DCS*	*TCS*
μ_0	= 0	= 0	= 0	= 0	= 0
μ_1	= 0	−0.020 (−3.5)	= 0	−0.041 (−3.1)	−0.039 (−3.1)
Constant α	=1	=1	=1	=1	
LCS Weights $\Omega[\tau]$	= 0, =1, =1, =1	= 0, =1, =1, =1	= 0, =1, =1, =1	= 0, =1, =1, =1	= 0, =1, 0.958[c], 0.981[c]
Proportional β	= 0	= 0	−0.307 (−19.)	−0.806 (−13.)	−0.767 (−10.)
ϕ_0^2	0.253 (21.)	0.252 (21.)	0.182 (14.)	0.203 (14.)	0.208 (13.)
ϕ_1^2	= 0	= .0001*	= 0	0.132 (4.3)	0.124 (4.6)
$\phi_{0,1}$	= 0	−0.089 (−19)	= 0	0.161 (7.)	0.163 (7.)
Unique ψ^2	0.024 (9.)	0.177 (19.)	0.199 (22.)	0.179 (16.)	0.178 (15.)
Model Fit					
$L^2(df)$	9877 (1429)	4485 (1426)	3752 (1428)	3301 (1425)	3530 (1423)
Scaled χ^2 Diff (*df*/*p*)	636 (3 / < .001)	141 (2 / < .001)	73.6 (3 / < .001)	2.62 (2 / .270)	N/A
CFI / TLI	.914/.920	.969/.971	.976/.978	.981/.982	.979/.980
ε_α (90% CI)	.029 (.029–.030)	.018 (.017–.018)	.015 (.015–.016)	.014 (.013–.014)	.015 (.014–.015)

Notes: [a]Values in parentheses are the associated *z*-statistics; [b]Compared to the linear LCS; [c]The *z*-indices are typically based on changes from zero but here we want changes from one; *Though nested within the DCM, this model had a lower-fitting function and could not be compared using the Mplus DIFFTEST feature. The comparison model for the scaled chi-square difference test is the model to the right (e.g., TCS for DCS) of the model fitted.

both the LCS and the ACS seem to be reasonable change models (L^2 = 4485 with df = 1426 and L^2 = 3752 with df = 1428), especially the inclusion of the proportion ($\beta = -0.31$) in the ACS. But, as we expected, the DCS and TCS provided the best fit to the data (L^2 = 3301 with df = 1425 and L^2 = 3530 with df = 1423). The DCS suggests a small linear increment of slopes ($\mu_1 = -0.04$) with a larger exponential parameter (of $\beta = -0.81$) for the optimal combination. The TCS fit suggested the best timings for this model were when the loadings on the change scores were very close to unity ($\omega[9] = 0$; $\omega[10] = 1$; $\omega[11] = 0.958$; $\omega[12] = 0.981$). Because the last two models were not statistically distinct from each other (given results of the DIFFTEST), thus for parsimony, the DCS was considered the better model, and the best model for these data. With the exception of the NCS, all other models did actually fit the data pretty well, but they were statistically significant departures from the DCS. Suppressing the proportional coefficient ($\beta = 0$) seemed to have a larger impact on model fit than removing the constant slope parameter ($\mu_1 = 0$).

Sex and Ethnicity Models

The DCS model was fit as an MGM defined by sex and Native Hawaiian ancestry: (1) Native Hawaiian Males (HM), (2) Non-Native Hawaiian Males (NHM), (3) Native Hawaiian Females (HF), and (4) Non-Native Hawaiian Females (NHF). In these MGMs the proportional constraint (β) and the mean of the slope (μ_1), along with other parameters, were allowed to vary over groups. The results of some differences among groups are presented in Table 20.7.

At the initial time point we find the two Females groups (HF and NHF) are highest in their common factor score of depression (μ_0 = 0.23 and 0.21) and they get higher at each

Table 20.7 Multiple Group Parameter Estimates From a DCS Model With Categorical Indicators (all free μ, β, ϕ^2 and ψ^2)

Parameter[a]	*HM*	*NHM*	*HF*	*NHF*
μ_0	= 0	−0.384 (−7)	0.233 (7)	0.207 (5.)
μ_1	−0.058 (−2.8)	−0.114 (−3.2)	0.170 (6.)	0.080 (2.6)
Constant α	= 1	= 1	= 1	= 1
Proportional β	−0.668 (−5.)	−0.894 (−10.)	−0.817 (−9.)	−0.681 (−5.)
ϕ_0^2	0.126 (5.)	0.322 (4.5)	0.228 (7.)	0.277 (4.9)
ϕ_1^2	0.053 (1.2)	0.183 (3.4)	0.120 (2.9)	0.092 (1.6)
$\phi_{0,1}$	0.088 (2.4)	0.117 (3.0)	0.156 (4.7)	0.142 (2.7)
Unique ψ^2	0.203 (9.)	0.163 (7.)	0.179 (10.)	0.171 (7.)

Notes: [a]Values in parentheses are the associated z-statistics; Group model parameters are from the most constrained model (with free β); Model fit: χ^2 = 8407 (5694), $p < 0.001$; CFI = 0.968; TLI = 0.970; ε_α (90% CI) = 0.017 (.016–.017).); We combined sex and Native Hawaiian ancestry to form a single grouping variable with four categories: (1) Native Hawaiian Males (HM), (2) Non-Native Hawaiian Males (NHM), (3) Native Hawaiian Females (HF), and (4) Non-Native Hawaiian Females (NHF).

Table 20.8 Parameter Estimates From DCS with Composite Scores. Group Model Parameters Are From the Least Constrained Model (all free μ, β, ϕ^2 and ψ^2).

Parameter[a]	*HM*	*NHM*	*HF*	*NHF*
μ_0	0.590 (35.)	0.434 (16.)	0.820 (42.)	0.793 (24.)
μ_1	0.417 (7.)	0.528 (9.)	0.713 (13.)	0.563 (3.9)
Constant α	= 1	= 1	= 1	= 1
Proportional β	−0.783 (−7.)	−1.033 (−9.)	−0.920 (−14.)	−0.792 (−4.3)
ϕ_0^2	0.102 (4.6)	0.097 (2.4)	0.216 (9.)	0.235 (6.)
ϕ_1^2	0.048 (1.7)	0.134 (3.0)	0.152 (4.2)	0.111 (1.3)
$\phi_{0,1}$	0.066 (3.1)	0.111 (2.7)	0.162 (6.)	0.135 (2.7)
Unique ψ^2	0.163 (10.)	0.136 (8.)	0.209 (13.)	0.197 (6.)

Note: [a]Values in parentheses are the associated *z*-statistics. Model fit: χ^2 (*df*) = 44.5 (28), *p* = 0.025; CFI = 0.977; TLI = 0.981; ε_α (90% CI) = 0.019 (.007–.028).

grade (μ_1 = 0.17 and 0.08). The part of the change that is the prediction from one grade to another is strong (β = −0.82, −0.68) and this brings them down at each time quite a bit. The resulting change over grades is higher for the Females in both groups, especially for the Hawaiian Females, but is fairly low in general. In these cases the Males are have smaller mean parameters as a group, even though they have similar regressions. The individual differences at the beginning of 9th grade are highest for the NHM (ϕ_0^2 = 0.32) and they change a significant amount (ϕ_1^2 = 0.18 and $\phi_{0,1}$ = 0.12). The unique variance is highest for those in the HM group (ψ^2 = 0.23). Although only the Scalar Invariant measurement model is now invariant over time and groups, a variety of other models can be tested for invariance over groups in this framework.

In Table 20.8 we present the results from fitting the same kind of DCS model to a composite score of the same 13 items. We would basically make the same inferences from this starting point, but here the Females seem much more variable. For example, in this metric, the HF have the highest starting variance (ϕ_0^2 = 0.21), highest slope variance and covariance (ϕ_0^2 = 0.15, and $\phi_{0,1}$ = 0.16), and highest unique variance ψ^2 = 0.20). Other differences can also be found, and these could be tested for equality over groups.

Summary

We tried to make this analysis intentionally easier than other uses of these data (see Hishinuma et al., 2012), so it may not be complex enough to capture all the changes possible.

In this analysis we can see that the Depression items (at least these 13; see Table 20.3) seem to hold the Scalar Invariance over time, and this is all that is required to examine the changes in the same common factor scores. This is helpful because we can consider the changes at the latent variable level. The model results do show that the TCS change model is not needed, and this means the grades were probably equally spaced. But the results also show a DCS model is needed (more than the simpler LCS and ACS models) primarily because the previous time point incidence of Depression seemed to have a larger impact that the constant impacts of Depression.

And this occurs over and over again over grades. It seems as if prior lack of Depression sets the stage for later lack of Depression. Any model we use seems to have decline in Depression over grade levels. But this decline is an individual characteristic, and it is just the same kind of change as the group growth, but it naturally goes the other way. This broadly supports the idea of a decline in Depression over grades 9–12, with the exception of the Females, especially the Hawaiian Females.

Figure 20.2 is a display of the observed linear changes for each of the four groups. The groups exhibited very low levels of depression on average, never even reaching an average score of one (equivalent to response option 2, or "some or a little of the time"). Female students reported higher depression scores than Male students, but the only group to experience any increase over time was Non-Native Hawaiian Males, who eventually converged with Hawaiian Males. For both Males and Females, Native Hawaiians had higher scores overall and experienced minimal change, while Non-Native Hawaiians either started lower (Males) or ended up lower (Females) and seemed to have more meaningful change.

Keep in mind that Figure 20.2 simply shows the means of each group at each grade level, all of which had a significant amount of single-time participants. It is helpful to return to the equation for the DCS ($\Delta F[t] = \beta\, F[t-1] + G\{1\}$), to get a better sense of how a student's level of self-reported depression changed based on the model parameter estimates. If we apply the equation to the results of the multiple-group composite models, we find that the modal student at the beginning, in the 9th grade here (i.e., $F[t-1] = \mu_0$) experiences changes (over 10th–12th grade) that are relatively consistent with those implied by Figure 20.2.

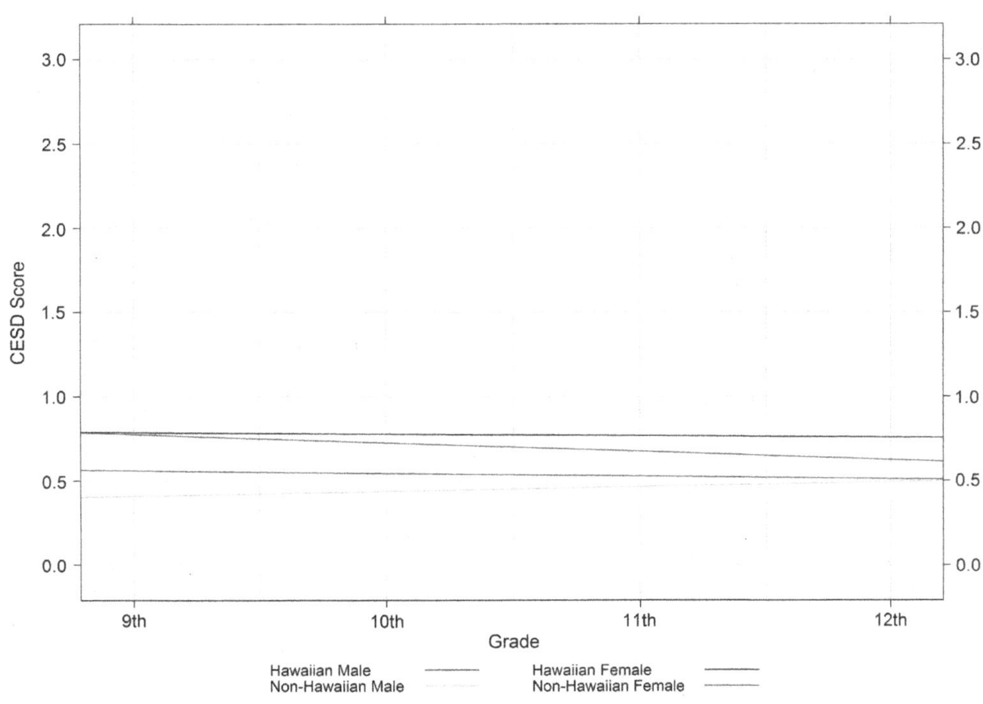

Figure 20.2 Observed linear relationship between CES-D scores and grades.

But it is important to note these results are as much a plausible summary of cross-sectional differences as they are a summary of longitudinal differences. It is possible the students in 10th through 12th grade levels would have reported less depression when they were in 9th grade than current 9th graders, and this would affect the overall means we observed and fitted in this model. So if the people who were higher (or lower) on Depression dropped out of the study in an consistent fashion, we would still have the correct parameters because Depression is a variable in this model (see Little & Rubin, 1987). Of course, the relation of Depression scores and other variables (e.g., Academic Performance) could be impacted by this selection of people as well (see Hishinuma et al., 2012). This basically requires further study of the selection of people to grade levels, and for those people who are present to take our survey.[1]

References

Andersen, E.B. (1985). Estimating latent correlations between repeated testings. *Psychometrika, 50*, 3–16.

Andrade, N.N., Hishinuma, E.S., McDermott, J.F., Johnson, R.C., Goebert, D.A., Makini, G.K., . . . Waldron, J.A. (2006). The National Center on Indigenous Hawaiian Behavioral Health Study of Prevalence of Psychiatric Disorders in Native Hawaiian Adolescents. *Journal of the American Academy of Child and Adolescent Psychiatry, 45*(1), 26–36.

Beals, J., Manson, S.M., Keane, E.M., & Dick, R.W. (1991). Factorial structure of the Center for Epidemiologic Studies–Depression scale among American Indian college students. *Psychological Assessment, 3*, 623–627.

Bond, T.G., & Fox, C.M. (2001). *Applying the Rasch model: Fundamental measurement in the human sciences*. Mahwah, NJ: Lawrence Erlbaum Associates.

Bryant, F.B. (1999). Measurement modeling: Identifying the constructs underlying the Center for Epidemiologic Studies Depression scale. *Behavioral Measurement Letter, 6*, 6–8.

Bryk, A.S., & Raudenbush, S.W. (1987). Application of hierarchical linear models to assessing change. *Psychological Bulletin, 101*(1), 147.

Browne, M., & Cudeck, R. (1993). Alternative ways of assessing model fit. In K. Bollen & S. Long (Eds.), *Testing structural equation models* (pp. 136–162). Newbury Park, CA: Sage.

Edman, J.L., Danko, G.P., Andrade, N., McArdle, J.J., Foster, J., & Glipa, J. (1999). Factor structure of the CES-D (Center for Epidemiologic Studies Depression scale) among Filipino-American adolescents. *Social Psychiatry and Psychiatric Epidemiology, 34*, 211–215.

Embretson, S. (1991). A multidimensional latent trait model for measuring learning and change. *Psychometrika, 56*, 495–515.

Embretson, S.E., & Reise, S. (2000). *Item response theory for psychologists*. Mahwah, NJ: Lawrence Erlbaum Associates.

Ferrer, E., & McArdle, J.J. (2010). Longitudinal modeling of developmental changes in psychological research. *Current Directions in Psychological Science, 19*(3) 149–154.

Fraley, R.C., Waller, N.G., & Brennan, K.A. (2000). An item-response theory analysis of self-report measures of adult attachment. *Journal of Personality and Social Psychology, 78*, 350–365.

Grimm, K.J., An, Y., McArdle, J.J., Zonderman, A.B., & Resnick, S.M. (2012). Recent changes leading to subsequent changes: Extensions of multivariate latent difference score models. *Structural Equation Modeling, 19*(2), 268–292.

1 Acknowledgments: The first author thanks the Department of Psychiatry, University of Hawaii, for the free public use of the longitudinal HHS data. This research is partly funded by an NIH-MERIT grant #AG07137-23 from the NIH-National Institute on Aging to the first author. All authors thank the Department of Psychiatry, University of Hawai'i at Mānoa. The HHSHS was supported by the National Institute of Mental Health (NIMH; R24 MH5015-01, R24 MH57079-A1). The contents of this chapter are solely the responsibility of the authors and do not necessarily represent the official views of the funding agencies.

Grimm, K.J., McArdle, J.J., & Hamagami, F. (2007). Nonlinear growth mixture models in research on cognitive aging. In K. van Montfort, H. Oud, & A. Satorra (Eds.), *Longitudinal models in the behavioral and related sciences* (pp. 267–294). Mahwah, NJ: Lawrence Erlbaum Associates.

Hambleton, R.K., Swaminathan, H., & Rogers, H.J. (1991). *Fundamentals of item response theory*. Newbury Park, CA: Sage.

Hishinuma, E.S., Andrade, N.N., Johnson, R.C., & McArdle, J.J. (2000). Psychometric properties of the Hawaiian culture scale—Adolescent version. *Psychological Assessment, 12*(2), 140–157.

Hishinuma, E., Chang, J., McArdle, J.J., & Hamagami, A. (2012). Potential causal relationship between depressive symptoms and academic achievement in the Hawaiian High Schools Health Survey using contemporary longitudinal latent variable change models. *Developmental Psychology, 48*(5), 1327–1342.

Horn, J.L., & McArdle, J.J. (1992). A practical and theoretical guide to measurement invariance in aging research. *Experimental Aging Research, 18*, 117–144.

Johnson, R.C., Danko, G.P., Andrade, N.N., & Markoff, R.A. (1997). Intergroup similarities in judgments of psychiatric symptom severity. *Cultural Diversity and Mental Health, 3*, 61–68.

Kaplan, D., & Sweetman, H.M. (2006). Finite mixture modeling approaches to the study of growth in academic achievement. In R.W. Lissitz (Ed.), *Longitudinal and value added models of student performance* (pp. 139–169). Maple Grove, MN: JAM Press.

Little, R., & Rubin, D. (1987). *Statistical analyses with missing data*. New York: John Wiley.

Lissitz, R.W. (Ed.) (2006). *Longitudinal and value added models of student performance*. Maple Grove, MN: JAM Press.

Lord, F.M. (1953). The relation of test score to the trait underlying the test. *Educational and Psychological Measurement, 13*, 517–548.

Lord, F.M. (1963). Elementary models for measuring change. In C.W. Harris (Ed.), *Problems in measuring change* (pp. 21–28). Madison: University of Wisconsin Press.

Lord, F.N., & Novick, M.P. (1968). *Statistical theories of mental test scores*. Reading MA: Addison-Wesley.

McArdle, J.J. (1997). Modeling longitudinal data by latent growth curve methods. In G. Marcoulides (Ed.), *Modern methods for business research* (pp. 359–406). Mahwah, NJ: Lawrence Erlbaum Associates.

McArdle, J.J. (1998). Contemporary statistical models for examining test bias. In J.J. McArdle & R.W. Woodcock (Eds.), *Human cognitive abilities in theory and practice*. Hillsdale, NJ: Lawrence Erlbaum Associates.

McArdle, J.J. (2001). A latent difference score approach to longitudinal dynamic structural analysis. In R. Cudeck, S. du Toit, & D. Sorbom (Eds.), *Structural equation modeling: Present and future* (pp. 342–380). Lincolnwood, IL: Scientific Software International.

McArdle, J.J. (2008). Latent variable modeling of differences and changes with longitudinal data. *Annual Review of Psychology, 60*, 577–605.

McArdle, J.J. (2011). Latent curve modeling. In R. Hoyle (Ed.), *Handbook of structural equation modeling*. New York: Oxford University Press.

McArdle, J.J. (2012). Testing the idea of general intelligence. *F&M Scientist, 1*, 27–66.

McArdle, J.J., & Cattell, R.B. (1994). Structural equation models of factorial invariance in parallel proportional profiles and oblique confactor problems. *Multivariate Behavioral Research, 29*, 61–101.

McArdle, J.J., Fisher, G.G., & Kadlec, K.M. (2007). Latent variable analysis of age trends in tests of cognitive ability in the health and retirement survey, 1992–2004. *Psychology and Aging, 22*(3), 525–545.

McArdle, J.J., Grimm, K., Hamagami, F., Bowles, R., & Meredith, W. (2009). Modeling life-span growth curves of cognition using longitudinal data with multiple samples and changing scales of measurement. *Psychological Methods, 14*(2), 126–149.

McArdle, J.J., & Hamagami, F. (1996). Multilevel models from a multiple group structural equation perspective. In G. Marcoulides & R. Schumacker (Eds.), *Advanced structural equation modeling techniques* (pp. 89–124). Hillsdale, NJ: Lawrence Erlbaum Associates.

McArdle, J.J., & Hamagami, F. (2001). Linear dynamic analyses of incomplete longitudinal data. In L. Collins & A. Sayer (Eds.), *Methods for the analysis of change* (pp. 137–176). Washington, DC: APA Press.

McArdle, J.J., Johnson, R.C., Hishinuma, E.S., Miyamoto, R.H., & Andrade, N.N. (2001). Structural equation modeling of group differences in CES-D ratings of native Hawaiian and non-Hawaiian high school students. *Journal of Adolescent Research, 16*(2), 108–149.

McArdle, J.J., & Nesselroade, J.R. (1994). Structuring data to study development and change. In S.H. Cohen & H.W. Reese (Eds.), *Life-span developmental psychology: Methodological innovations* (pp. 223–267). Hillsdale, NJ: Lawrence Erlbaum Associates.

McArdle, J.J., & Nesselroade, J.R. (2014). *Longitudinal data analysis using structural equation models*. Washington, DC: APA Books.

McArdle, J.J., & Prescott, C.A. (1992). Age-based construct validation using structural equation modeling. *Experimental Aging Research, 18*(3), 87–115.

McDonald, R.P. (1999). *Test theory: A unified approach*. Mahwah, NJ: Lawrence Erlbaum Associates.

Meredith, W. (1993). Factorial invariance from a measurement perspective. *Psychometrika, 58*, 525–543.

Meredith, W., & Tisak, J. (1990). Latent curve analysis. *Psychometrika, 55*(1), 107–122.

Muthén, B.O. (1988). Some uses of structural equation modeling in validity studies: Extending IRT to external variables. In H. Wainer & H.I. Braun (Eds.), *Test validity* (pp. 213–238). Hillsdale, NJ: Lawrence Erlbaum Associates.

Muthén, B.O., & Khoo, S.T. (1998). Longitudinal studies of achievement growth using latent variable modeling. *Learning and Individual Differences, 10*(2), 73–101.

Muthén, L., & Muthén, B.O. (2012). *Mplus 7.11: Computer Program File*. Santa Monica, CA.

Prescott, C.A. (2004). Using the Mplus computer program to estimate models for continuous and categorical data from twins. *Behavior Genetics, 34*(1), 17–40.

Prescott, C.A., McArdle, J.J., Hishinuma, E.S., Johnson, R.C., Miyamoto, R.H., Andrade, N.N., . . . & Carlton, B.S. (1998). Prediction of major depression and dysthymia from CES-D scores among ethnic minority adolescents. *Journal of the American Academy of Child & Adolescent Psychiatry, 37*(5), 495–503.

Radloff, L.S. (1977). The CES-D scale: A self-report depression scale for research in the general population. *Applied Psychological Measurement, 1*, 385–401.

Rasch, G. (1960). *Probabilistic models for some intelligence and achievement tests*. Copenhagen, Denmark: Danish Institute for Educational Research.

Reise, S.P., & Henson, J.M. (2003). A discussion of modern versus traditional psychometrics as applied to personality assessment scales. *Journal of Personality Assessment, 81*, 93–103.

Roberts, J.S., & Ma, Q. (2006). IRT models for the assessment of change across repeated measurements. In R.W. Lissitz (Ed.), *Longitudinal and value added models of student performance* (pp. 100–129). Maple Grove, MN: JAM Press.

Rosseel, Y. (2012). lavaan: An R package for structural equation modeling. *Journal of Statistical Software, 48*, 2, 1–36.

Santor, D.A., & Coyne, J.C. (1997). Shortening the CES-D to improve its ability to detect cases of depression. *Psychological Assessment, 9*, 233–243.

Tanaka, J. (1993). Multifaceted conceptions of fit in structural equation models. In K. Bollen & S. Long (Eds.), *Testing structural equation models* (pp. 181–204). Newbury Park, CA: Sage.

Zimmerman, M., & Coryell, W. (1994). Screening for major depressive disorders in the community: A comparison of measures. *Psychological Assessment, 6*, 71–74.

21 Summary

New IRT Problems and Future Directions

Dennis A. Revicki and Steven P. Reise

Introduction

The application of item response theory (IRT) models and analysis in health-related and other noneducational outcomes is progressing rapidly, and with these applications new problems are emerging. As applications to new health domains and diverse populations increase, we anticipate that new challenges will continue to be identified. The large-scale application of IRT models across a variety of health constructs as part of the National Institutes of Health–sponsored Patient Reported Outcomes and Measurement Information System (PROMIS®) project has identified a number of such challenges (Cella et al., 2007; Cella et al., 2010). For example, as we raised in Chapter 1, problems with multidimensionality, narrowly defined constructs, unipolar constructs, and non-normal data are becoming well recognized as real challenges for IRT analyses in the patient-reported outcomes (PRO) domain.

The chapters in the present volume demonstrate that there is a wealth of research on new IRT-based methods that will ultimately improve the quality of health outcomes measurement, including improved estimation methods (see Chapters 3 and 4), approaches for evaluating and handling multidimensional data (see Chapters 8 through 11), application of nominal (see Chapter 18) and nonparametric IRT models (see Chapter 5), and new approaches to modeling item response data relevant to noneducational measurement (see Chapters 12 and 13). In what follows, we briefly add commentary on some of the major issues in IRT applications in noneducational measurement.

Multidimensional Data

In the introductory chapter we noted that many PRO constructs are conceptually narrow. Nevertheless, they are not so narrow that they can be measured with a single test item. Indeed, for any construct, several items of differing content are required. If those items happen to share any common variance beyond the one targeted common dimension, the data will be multidimensional to some degree. Thus, multidimensionality in health-related domains is unavoidable. However, the question of how much multidimensionality is allowable to enable analysts to fit reasonable unidimensional IRT models remains in debate (see Chapter 2). At this point, many health-related measures may yield multidimensional data (e.g., emotional distress, fatigue, physical functioning), but they are considered "unidimensional enough" (i.e., a strong general dimension) to allow fitting of unidimensional IRT models. For these domains, it will be interesting to see whether future researchers are willing to trade off the simplicity of unidimensional models for the added complexity, but increased accuracy and validity of multidimensional models.

With that said, the chapters in the present volume demonstrate that advanced methods are being developed that enable researchers to explore the dimensionality of their ordinal item response data more effectively, and that provide for the fitting of more complicated multidimensional IRT models. Given these advances, we argue that such models should no longer be treated as "curiosities" relevant only to the more psychometrically inclined, but rather should be routinely estimated by applied researchers to determine whether they improve our understanding of the latent structure of health-related constructs, and the validity of clinical decisions based on resulting test or change scores.

For example, upper extremity and mobility subdomains have been identified as part of the PROMIS® physical function item bank (Hays et al., 2013) despite evidence that all the items are highly intercorrelated (i.e., there is a strong general factor). Bifactor and other multidimensional IRT models could be fit to these data to determine whether there are useful dimensional representations that better fit these data and that are interpretable and useful in some applied sense. This latter criterion is critical. We can rest assured that more complicated models will inevitably "fit better," and thus the key question is how much that improved fit provides gains in practical utility.

At this point, there is insufficient application of these types of advanced IRT models for health-related data, and it is largely unknown whether these modeling approaches can be used to advance our understanding of the measurement of health-related outcomes. We note, however, that just like unidimensional models, multidimensional models also assume that the data are locally independent, a property that may be difficult to achieve if the items do not conform to an independent cluster solution. Clearly, more work is needed on this and related issues.

Finally, we believe that multidimensional explanatory IRT models (see Chapter 12) may also be used to evaluate the meaning of item parameters and test scores in health-related data. In this approach the latent variables are viewed as based on the varying effects of item covariates and the items derive their meaning from the item and person covariates. One of the virtues of the explanatory IRT approach is that it forces researchers to think carefully and critically about item content, and which psychological and demographic covariates may be influencing the responses. Stated differently, these types of models encourage critical thinking about the response process. It will be very interesting to see where these explanatory types of models take us in the next 10 years. We know that they are being increasingly applied in educational measurement, and we expect to see an increase in health-related measurement as well.

Non-Normal Distributions and Unipolar Constructs

Many health-related constructs are not normally distributed in the general population, and often score distributions are highly skewed, with a substantial percentage of individuals endorsing no items. For example, as we previously noted, the PROMIS® pain behavior item bank is not normally distributed in the general population, and actually represents two distributions, one describing no pain versus pain and the other describing a relatively normal distribution of item responses in those respondents who have at least some pain. Also as noted, a hybrid nominal partial credit IRT model fit these data well (Revicki et al., 2009). Given recent advances in software and estimation, it may be possible to begin exploring various hybrid IRT models, although caution must be exercised as these types of models may be extremely complex to implement and interpret.

We also believe that the development of estimation techniques that do not assume normality (see Chapter 4) and nonparametric IRT models (see Chapter 5) may also advance our understanding of non-normally distributed health-related data, and provide alternative model fitting solutions. Currently, both these methodologies are underutilized in health outcomes measurement. Finally, the nominal response model may also contribute to our understanding of item functioning within various types of health outcomes data (see Chapter 18). Although the nominal response model is not new, we believe it can assist the analyst in further understanding the ordering of the within-item response categories, and the degree to which each category distinction provides useful information toward differentiating individual differences.

Related to the non-normality issue is the fact that many health-related constructs, such as pain interference and depression, can be considered as unipolar. In these cases, the latent construct does not span the entire continuum but the "best" end of the scale is when the trait is not present (no depression, no pain) and items can only be developed for the symptomatic end of the construct continuum. These types of constructs present a problem for fitting standard IRT models (e.g., graded response models, partial credit models, etc.), and may result in relatively large slope parameters and potentially biased threshold parameters. Indeed, it is easy to demonstrate that as the percentage of respondents scoring in the lowest category increases, the item slope parameter will increase as well, all else being equal and assuming that the item provides discrimination for individuals with some degree of ailment.

In our judgment, the application of unipolar item response models, as summarized by Lucke (see Chapter 13), represents a powerful approach for calibrating these type items. In the future, we expect that constructs such as pain interference may well be better represented by these types of models, where the latent trait scale begins at zero, and all zero responses are easily accommodated without impacting the overall metric for the latent trait scale. Although currently difficult to fit using standard, readily available IRT software, further examination of the unipolar item response models using PRO data is much needed. The resulting item parameters may increase our understanding of unipolar traits and may provide better-fitting and more interpretable parameter estimates. We foresee these models as being especially useful in terms of tracking change. Of course, as with all new proposed models, more work is needed.

Computerized Adaptive Testing

Although not included in this current book, computerized adaptive testing (CAT) represents a test administration method that capitalizes on the strengths of IRT analysis. In a CAT, participants are administered a small number of items from an item bank based on an algorithm that enables testing tailored to the individual. The first item may be selected from items located in the middle range of the latent construct (e.g., fatigue, physical function, etc.) or based on some other algorithm. For example, the first item may be selected to provide the maximum expected information over the prior distribution (normal distribution). Subsequent items are then selected targeting the posterior distributions, which converge to progressively narrow ranges as more items are administered. Additional items are selected until some set stopping rule is met, usually based on achieving a certain level of measurement precision. The implementation of CAT requires, ideally, large item banks, and some health constructs have narrow breadth that will make CATs challenging.

Research has demonstrated that multiple items are needed for very precise measurement across specific latent trait ranges, and that CAT scores outperform static short form scales (Choi et al., 2010; Lai et al., 2011). For example, a seven-item fatigue CAT demonstrated consistently better precision when compared with three seven-item static short-form scales, including a content-oriented short form (Lai et al., 2011). Continued improvement in item selection algorithms, conjoined with multidimensional models, may enable CATs to be briefer and as precise as longer static forms.

Clearly, there are advantages to implementing CAT for health outcomes assessment. The ability of CAT to provide precise and efficient assessment decreases burden on study participants without compromising measurement reliability. In practice, these brief tailored assessments can enable the relative efficient collection of multiple health domains and allow for a more comprehensive assessment battery for clinical research and practice. Further improvements in multidimensional CAT administration and item selection methods will make the tailored testing approach to health assessment even more feasible. Item banks and CAT based on item banks represent the future of health outcomes assessment.

Future Directions

These are exciting times for the development and psychometric evaluation of noneducational, typical performance measures. The widespread application of IRT methods is now becoming fairly standard as part of the patient-reported outcomes instrument development and evaluation process, and is well illustrated in the PROMIS® network project. While the IRT methods have helped improve the measurement of health outcomes, these methods have also uncovered a number of different challenges (see Chapter 1). For the future, we anticipate greater application of the IRT methods presented in the current book as possible solutions to those identified problems.

Although the present volume contains four chapters dedicated to multidimensional IRT (see Chapters 8 through 11), additional future work is much needed on dimensionality assessment (e.g., "essentially multidimensional"), item and person fit indices, and nonparametric exploratory methods. Increased application of the nominal IRT model (see Chapter 18) and nonparametric IRT models (see Chapter 5) in understanding item responses and data quality is also needed.

Research also needs to be conducted on whether the more advanced IRT methods provide better solutions for the psychometric evaluation of health outcomes data. Does application of the unipolar item response models or the multidimensional IRT models improve on model fit and if so, what applied benefit does the statistical rigor bring? In other words, we need increased understanding as to the advantages and disadvantages of these more advanced methods in health outcomes assessment. We also need a greater understanding as to which of these more advanced IRT methods work best with different types of item distribution data. This information is necessary to provide recommendations as to model selection and perhaps sequencing of different IRT models to provide the best-fitting solutions.

Better and more efficient estimation methods for IRT models will make fitting more complex, advanced models such as the bifactor, two-tier, and multidimensional IRT models more feasible. The more efficient estimation methods may also allow the fitting of more hybrid, combination models when relevant. We strongly encourage the development of new item response models for health outcomes data, an area where there is currently a paucity of work. In conclusion, we know that the application of IRT analysis is definitely a constituent part of current instrument development and psychometric evaluation of new and existing patient-reported outcome measures, and we expect that to become even more true in the foreseeable future. We hope the chapters provided herein provide a blueprint for that exciting future.

References

Cella, D., Riley, W., Stone, A., Rothrock, N., Reeve, B. Yount, S., et al. (2010). The Patient-Reported Outcomes Measurement Information System (PROMIS) developed and tested its first wave of adult self-reported health outcome item banks: 2005–2008. *Journal of Clinical Epidemiology, 63*, 1179–1194.

Cella, D., Yount, S., Rothrock, N., Gershon, R., Cook, K., Reeve, B., et al. (2007). The patient reported outcomes measurement information system (PROMIS): Progress of an NIH roadmap cooperative group during its first two years. *Medical Care, 45*, S3–S11.

Choi, S. W., Reise, S. P., Pilkonis, P. A., Hays, R. D., & Cella, D. (2010). Efficiency of static and computer adaptive short forms compared to full length measures of depressive symptoms. *Quality of Life Research, 19*, 125–136.

Hays, R. D., Spritzer, K. L., Amtmann, D., Lai, J.-S., DeWitt, E. M., Rothrock, N., . . . Krishnan, E. (2013). Upper extremity and mobility subdomains from the Patient-Reported Outcomes Measurement Information System (PROMIS®) adult physical functioning item bank. *Archives of Physical Medicine and Rehabilitation*, E-pub.

Lai, J.-S., Cella, D., Choi, S., Junghaenel, D. U., Christodoulou, C., Gershon, R., & Stone, A. (2011). How item banks and their application can influence measurement practice in rehabilitation medicine: A PROMIS fatigue item bank example. *Archives of Physical Medicine and Rehabilitation, 92*, 10 Suppl 1): S20–27.

Revicki, D. A., Chen, W. H., Harnam, N., Cook, K. F., Amtmann, D., Callahan, L. F., . . . Keefe, F. J. (2009). Development and psychometric analysis of the PROMIS pain behavior item bank. *Pain, 146*, 158–169.

Index